Advances in Drug Delivery Systems for Healthcare

From concept to clinic

Online at: https://doi.org/10.1088/978-0-7503-5613-8

IPEM–IOP Series in Physics and Engineering in Medicine and Biology

About the Series

The series in Physics and Engineering in Medicine and Biology will allow the Institute of Physics and Engineering in Medicine (IPEM) to enhance its mission to 'advance physics and engineering applied to medicine and biology for the public good'.

It is focused on key areas including, but not limited to:

- clinical engineering
- diagnostic radiology
- informatics and computing
- magnetic resonance imaging
- nuclear medicine
- physiological measurement
- radiation protection
- radiotherapy
- rehabilitation engineering
- ultrasound and non-ionising radiation.

A number of IPEM–IOP titles are being published as part of the EUTEMPE Network Series for Medical Physics Experts.

A full list of titles published in this series can be found here: https://iopscience.iop.org/bookListInfo/physics-engineering-medicine-biology-series.

Advances in Drug Delivery Systems for Healthcare

From concept to clinic

Edited by
Piyush Pradeep Mehta
Cipla R&D (India), Mumbai, India

Arpana Parihar
CSIR-Advanced Materials and Processes Research Institute (AMPRI), Bhopal, India

IOP Publishing, Bristol, UK

ISBN 978-0-7503-5613-8 (ebook)
ISBN 978-0-7503-5611-4 (print)
ISBN 978-0-7503-5614-5 (myPrint)
ISBN 978-0-7503-5612-1 (mobi)

DOI 10.1088/978-0-7503-5613-8

Version: 20240101

IOP ebooks

British Library Cataloguing-in-Publication Data: A catalogue record for this book is available from the British Library.

Published by IOP Publishing, wholly owned by The Institute of Physics, London

IOP Publishing, No.2 The Distillery, Glassfields, Avon Street, Bristol, BS2 0GR, UK

US Office: IOP Publishing, Inc., 190 North Independence Mall West, Suite 601, Philadelphia, PA 19106, USA

Dedicated to all our close individuals who provide positive energy for embarking on new things in life.

Contents

Preface

In the healthcare domain, new drug delivery technologies, green chemistry, computational intelligence, simulation know-how, and the Internet of Things have experienced significant growth over the past two decades. This paradigm shift is widely accepted and supported by pharmaceutical organizations, research institutes, and regulatory bodies for the promotion of sustainable healthcare practices. The book *Advances in Drug Delivery Systems for Healthcare: From Concept to clinic* attempts to address these diverse and essential aspects in the field of health care.

This reference text offers a comprehensive overview of cutting-edge technologies such as green synthesis, biomimicry, ionic liquid, artificial intelligence, machine learning, and simulation modelling. All these topics are directed towards nurturing sustainable advancements in healthcare. The book aims to explore topics related to a patient-centric approach, encompassing areas such as medical electronics, smart inhalers, personalized healthcare, and additive manufacturing. The book also delves into thought-provoking topics, including human ergonomics.

This book will serve as an essential reference source for readers seeking to comprehend how current technologies and materials, along with their advancements, can contribute to more efficient healthcare solutions. Each book chapter is systematically structured to tackle the challenging and pressing issues posed by life-threatening diseases, presenting advanced technologies as viable alternatives. Additionally, each chapter includes a Strengths, Weaknesses, Opportunities, and Threats (SWOT) analysis, offering readers a comprehensive situational assessment. Overall, this book stands as an essential reference for individuals seeking insights into the upcoming developments within the healthcare sector.

Certainly, both experts and non-specialist readers will find this book valuable for their day-to-day research work as it presents a unique mix of key topics, spanning from green synthesis to artificial intelligence and from medical electronics to human ergonomics. Briefly, it is an essential reference for those who want to learn about the upcoming developments in the healthcare sector.

Foreword

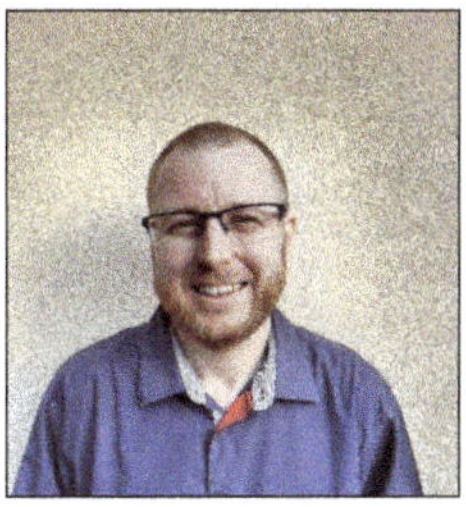

Innovation in drug delivery technologies stands at the forefront of modern healthcare, wielding profound implications for patients, practitioners, and the pharmaceutical industry as a whole. These advancements are pivotal in optimizing the effectiveness of pharmaceutical treatments while minimizing their potential side effects. The development of novel drug delivery methods, such as nanotechnology, targeted drug delivery systems, and biodegradable implants, not only enhances patient compliance but also expands the scope of therapeutic options available. Furthermore, these innovations facilitate the personalized medicine approach, tailoring treatments to individual patients' needs, leading to more precise and efficient healthcare outcomes. Beyond the clinical realm, drug delivery innovations have the potential to drive cost-efficiency in healthcare systems and contribute to the sustainable development of pharmaceutical manufacturing processes. In this era of rapid scientific progress, nurturing innovation in drug delivery technologies is indispensable in shaping a healthier, more patient-centric, and sustainable future for healthcare worldwide.

In the realm of healthcare, there exists an intricate web of innovation and discovery, connecting scientific ingenuity to the betterment of human lives. Within these pages, you are about to embark on a journey through this intricate web—a journey that traverses the multifaceted landscape of drug delivery systems. This book, *Advances in Drug Delivery Systems for Healthcare: From concept to clinic*, serves as your guide through a myriad of topics, each representing a distinct facet of advancement in the field of healthcare. As you turn the pages of this book, you will find a tapestry woven with the threads of innovation, from concept to realization, from laboratory research to commercialization, and from the fundamentals of chemistry to the sophisticated application of artificial intelligence. Together, these topics reflect the dynamic nature of drug delivery systems and their pivotal role in modern healthcare.

The book starts with the exploration of biomedical implants. These marvels of modern engineering bridge the gap between science and practical application, providing targeted drug delivery, enhanced diagnostics, and life-altering solutions. This chapter also represents the embodiment of scientific concepts transformed into commercialized reality. Delving into the realm of pharmaceuticals, you will uncover the transformative potential of green chemistry, where research not only revolutionizes the industry but also contributes to sustainable practices. From green chemistry, our journey takes us to the world of ionic liquid technology, where innovative substances hold the promise of enhancing drug solubility and stability, ultimately leading to more effective treatments. The future comes alive as we reach into the world of 3D and 4D bioprinting, where science fiction turns into reality. Witness how this groundbreaking technology has the potential to create functional tissues and organs, offering hope to those in need of life-saving transplants. Inspired by the elegance of Nature, biomimicry in drug delivery emerges as a theme, emphasizing the importance of understanding and mimicking natural processes to enhance drug delivery systems.

As our journey progresses, the spotlight shifts to personalized healthcare, where advances in genomics and individualized treatment plans pave the way for more effective and patient-centric therapies. The critical role of inhalation devices (dry powder inhalers and metered dose inhalers) in treating conditions like cystic fibrosis and chronic obstructive pulmonary disease is also explored. These devices have the power to significantly improve the lives of patients by delivering critical care directly to the lungs. The dedicated chapter of soft mist inhalers in delivering biologics presents yet another frontier in healthcare innovation. These devices offer a promising avenue for delivering complex therapeutic agents with precision and efficacy. Furthermore, artificial intelligence takes center stage as we investigate its current trends and future prospects in drug delivery. Witness how artificial intelligence is reshaping drug design, optimization, and delivery, ushering in an era of precision medicine. Machine learning further propels our exploration, as we delve into its current applications and future potential in the field of drug delivery. These systems continually adapt to the evolving demands of modern medicine.

The book also explores computational approaches employed in the field of drug delivery. The computational approaches for antibody-based targeted drug delivery strategies demonstrates how these models and simulations guide the design and optimization of precision medicine solutions. The book chapter of physiologically based pharmacokinetic modeling, with its diverse applications in institutes, industry, and regulatory agencies, provides a comprehensive view of how modeling techniques ensure drug safety, efficacy, and regulatory compliance. In the realm of medical electronics, the book explores future trends and market potential, offering a glimpse into how these technologies are poised to reshape healthcare and offer new possibilities for patient monitoring and treatment. Finally, book concludes with a focus on human ergonomics in the healthcare system. The human ergonomics chapter delve into the applications and challenges of optimizing healthcare environments and devices for the well-being of both patients and healthcare professionals.

As you embark on this journey through the pages of *Advances in Drug Delivery Systems for Healthcare: From concept to clinic*, may you gain not only knowledge but also instill innovative skills to design novel drug delivery platforms for healthcare management. The researchers, scientists, and experts who have contributed to this volume are the architects of a brighter, healthier future. Their work reminds us that the pursuit of knowledge and innovation is a never-ending journey, and the possibilities for improving human health are boundless. May this book serve as a beacon, guiding us toward a future where healthcare is not just a science but an art, where precision and compassion work hand in hand to heal, and where the boundaries of what is possible continue to expand.

Dr Tamás Sohajda
CEO – CarboHyde
www.cabohyde.com

Acknowledgements

The editors express their gratitude to all contributors for their dedicated and insightful work, as well as their unwavering support throughout the entire process.

Editor biographies

Piyush Pradeep Mehta

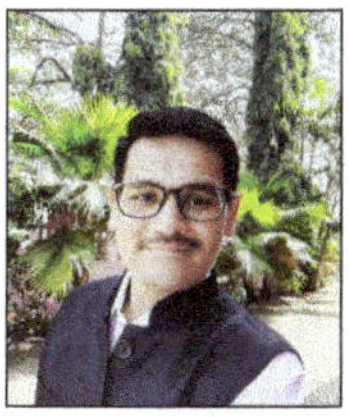

Dr Piyush Pradeep Mehta currently serves as a deputy manager in Cipla R&D, India. He earned his PhD from Bharati Vidyapeeth University, India, and an MBA from Sikkim Manipal University, India. With over nine years of experience in the pharmaceutical field, Dr Mehta actively contributes to pharmaceutical process and product development. His expertise spans formulation development, device design, and particle engineering, reflecting a solid understanding of fundamental concepts and principles. Recognized for his valuable contributions, Dr Mehta was elected as a Newton-Bhabha Fund, Royal Society of Chemistry (RSC) Researcher (2018—19). His work in pulmonary drug delivery earned him on-demand presentation opportunities from The Drug Delivery to the Lungs UK, specifically in the field of modified throat research. Dr Mehta holds credit for four device patents and has published over 50 articles, book chapters, and scientific communications in peer-reviewed journals. Additionally, he has successfully managed more than 20 international and national conferences, workshops, and scientific programs.

Arpana Parihar

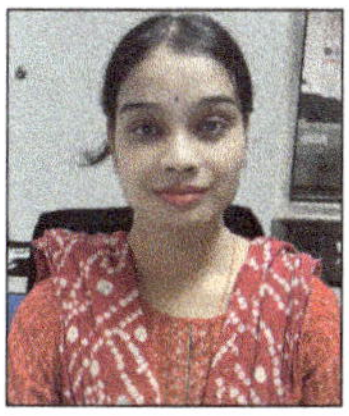

Dr Arpana Parihar is currently working as a Women Scientist B at CSIR-Advanced Materials and Processes Research Institute (AMPRI), Bhopal, MP, India, under the scheme of DST-WoS-B awarded by the Department of Science and Technology, Government of India. Dr Parihar has been awarded with prestigious GATE, CSIR-NET, and DST WoS B fellowships. Her research interests include synthesis and characterization of nanostructured materials, tissue engineering, targeted drug delivery systems, stem cell biology, fabrication of micro and nano sensors, point-of-care devices, and nanomedicine for healthcare applications. She has more than eight years of research and teaching experience at various prestigious institutes such as BARC, RRCAT, IITD, etc which fetched several peer-reviewed papers in national and international journals of repute. She has published over 50 articles and edited six books with renowned publishers.

List of contributors

Sara A Abouelmagd
Department of Pharmaceutics, Faculty of Pharmacy, Assiut University, Assiut, Egypt
and
Institute for Drug Development and Innovation Research, Assiut University, Assiut, Egypt

Punita Aggarwal
Department of Pharmacology and Toxicology, National Institute of Pharmaceutical Education and Research (NIPER)-Kolkata, Maniktala Main Road, Kolkata 700054, West Bengal, India

Ravikiran Allada
Novugen Pharma (Malaysia) Sdn Bhd, 3, Jalan Jururancang U1/21, Hicom-glenmarie Industrial Park, 40150 Shah Alam, Selangor, Malaysia

Hussain Ali
Christ University, Bangalore, Karnataka 560029, India

Ipek Arkca
Department of Bioengineering, İzmir Institute of Technology, İzmir 35430, Türkiye

Sangeeta Ballav
Cancer and Translational Research Centre, Dr D.Y. Patil Biotechnology and Bioinformatics Institute, Dr D Y Patil Vidyapeeth, Pune, Maharashtra, 411 033, India

Sumedh D Bahadure
National Institute of Pharmaceutical Education and Research, Guwahati, India

Sugato Banerjee
Department of Pharmacology and Toxicology, National Institute of Pharmaceutical Education and Research (NIPER)-Kolkata, Maniktala Main Road, Kolkata 700054, West Bengal, India

M Batıkan Kandemir
Departmant of Metallurgical and Materials Engineering, Muğla Sıtkı Koçman University, 48000 Muğla, Türkiye

Amitava Basu
Department of Commerce, Banwarilal Bhalotia College, G T Road, Ushagram, Asansol 713303, West Bengal, India

Soumya Basu
Cancer and Translational Research Centre, Dr D.Y. Patil Biotechnology and Bioinformatics Institute, Dr D Y Patil Vidyapeeth, Pune, Maharashtra 411 033, India

Seref Berk Atik
Department of Bioengineering, İzmir Institute of Technology, İzmir 35430, Türkiye

Kalpesh V Bhavsar
National Centre for Nanosciences and Nanotechnology, University of Mumbai, Kalina Campus. Kalina, Santacruz (E), Mumbai 400 098, India

Tamanna Bhuyan
Department of Applied Biology, School of Biological Sciences, University of Science and Technology Meghalaya, Meghalaya 793101, India

Sangeeta Deka
Indian Institute of Technology Guwahati, Guwahati 781039, India

Jayesh Dharwadkar
Cancer and Translational Research Centre, Dr D Y Patil Biotechnology and Bioinformatics Institute, Dr D Y Patil Vidyapeeth, Pune, Maharashtra, 411 033, India

Alperen Doğru
Department of Aircraft Technology, Aviation Higher Vocational School, Ege University, Izmir 35040, Turkey

Diana A Fernandes
Consultant and Founder, OnResp, Fruebjergvej 3, 2100 Copenhagen Ø, Denmark

Elisabeth Fink
Research Center Pharmaceutical Engineering GmbH (RCPE), Inffeldgasse 13, 8010, Graz, Austria

Ankit Gangarade
Terasaki Institute for Biomedical Innovation, Los Angeles, CA 90064, USA

Blassan P George
Laser Research Centre, Faculty of Health Sciences, University of Johannesburg, PO Box 17011, Johannesburg 2028, South Africa

Sude Gunes
Polymer Science and Engineering Master's Program, İzmir Institute of Technology, İzmir 35430, Türkiye

Sara A Hassan
Department of Pharmaceutics and Pharmaceutical Technology, Faculty of Pharmacy, Badr University in Assiut, Assiut, Egypt

Siddhanth Hejmady
Department of Pharmaceutical Sciences and Experimental Therapeutics, College of Pharmacy, University of Iowa, Iowa City, Iowa 52242, USA

Balaji Jayakrishnan
Business School, Vellore Institute of Technology (VIT), Chennai Campus, Kekottaiyur, Chennai, Tamilnadu 600127, India

Nani Kadrichu
Inspired—Pulmonary Solutions LLC

Ilango Kaliappan
SRM College of Pharmacy, SRM Institute of Science and Technology, Kattankulathur, India

Lakshmi Kanakaraj
Chettinad School of Pharmaceutical Sciences, Chettinad Academy of Research and Education, Chettinad Health City, Chennai 603103, Tamilnadu, India

Vivekanandan Kalaiselvan
Indian Pharmacopoeia, Commission, Ministry of Health and Family Welfare, Government of India, Sector 23, Rajnagar, Ghaziabad, UP 201002, India

Shahid Khan
Department of Biomedical Engineering, University of California, Davis, California 95616, USA

Darshana Khandge
Cancer and Translational Research Centre, Dr D Y Patil Biotechnology and Bioinformatics Institute, Dr D Y Patil Vidyapeeth, Pune, Maharashtra 411 033, India

Amanda Kirane
Department of Surgery, Stanford School of Medicine, Stanford University Medical Center, CA 94305, USA

Shital Kolhe
Department of Pharmaceutics, National Institute of Pharmaceutical Education and Research, Ahmedabad, Gujarat, India

Cansu İlke Kuru
Graduate School of Natural and Applied Sciences, Department of Biotechnology, Ege University, 35040 İzmir, Türkiye
and
Buca Municipality Buca Science and Art Center, 35390 Izmir, Türkiye

Deepak Kumar Sahel
Department of Pharmacy, Birla Institute of Technology and Science-Pilani, BITS-Pilani, Pilani 333031, Rajasthan, India

Ajay S Lale
Department of Biopharmaceutics and Clinical Development, Pharmaceutical Technology Center (PTC), Zydus Lifesciences Ltd, Ahmedabad, Gujarat 382 210, India

Surjendu Maity
Terasaki Institute for Biomedical Innovation, Los Angeles, CA 90064, USA

Shahid I Mir
Department of Pharmacy, BITS-Pilani, Hyderabad Campus, India

Prakash Muthudoss
A2Z4.0 Research and Analytics Private Limited, Chennai 600062, Tamilnadu, India

Subhamay Panda
Post Graduate Department of Zoology, Banwarilal Bhalotia College, G T Road, Ushagram, Asansol 713303, West Bengal, India

Amrit Paudel
Research Center Pharmaceutical Engineering GmbH (RCPE), Inffeldgasse 13, 8010, Graz, Austria
and
Graz University of Technology, Institute of Process and Particle Engineering, Inffeldgasse 13/3, 8010 Graz, Austria

Sudeep Pukale
Formulation Research and Development Division, Lupin Research Park, Lupin Pharmaceuticals, Inc., India

Manikandan Ramalingam
Chettinad School of Pharmaceutical Sciences, Chettinad Academy of Research and Education, Chettinad Health City, Chennai 603103, Tamilnadu, India

Gobi Ramasamy
Christ University, Bangalore, Karnataka 560029, India

Pintu K Rathod
Department of Pharmaceutical Sciences and Technology, Institute of Chemical Technology, Mumbai, Maharashtra, India

Ebrahim Saadat
Head of R&D, NovaGen Biopharmaceutical Co., Tehran, Iran

Anuj K Saini
Department of Biopharmaceutics and Clinical Development, Pharmaceutical Technology Center (PTC), Zydus Lifesciences Ltd, Ahmedabad, Gujarat 382 210, India

Amalendu Samanta
Department of Commerce, Banwarilal Bhalotia College, G T Road, Ushagram, Asansol 713303, West Bengal, India

Maitri S Sanghavi
Department of Biopharmaceutics and Clinical Development, Pharmaceutical Technology Center (PTC), Zydus Lifesciences Ltd, Ahmedabad, Gujarat 382 210, India
and
Research Scientist, Simcyp Ltd, Certara, Level 2, Acero, 1 Concourse Way, Sheffield City Centre, Sheffield S1 2BJ, United Kingdom

Paromita Sarbadhikary
Laser Research Centre, Faculty of Health Sciences, University of Johannesburg, PO Box 17011, Johannesburg 2028, South Africa

Mehmet Özgür Seydibeyoğlu
Department of Materials Science and Engineering, Izmir Kâtip Celebi University, 35620, İzmir, Türkiye
and
Thermoplastic Composites Application Center, Saxion University, The Netherlands

Saurabh Shahane
The Machine Learning Company, Maharashtra, India

Mahalaxmi Sharma
Bakson Homoeopathic Medical College and Hospital, Phase-I, Greater Noida, Uttar Pradesh 201310, India

Saurabh Sharma
Department of Surgery, Stanford School of Medicine, Stanford University Medical Center, CA 94305, USA

Angela Shony
National Centre for Nanosciences and Nanotechnology, University of Mumbai, Kalina Campus.Kalina, Santacruz (E), Mumbai 400 098, India

Manav Shirodkar
National Centre for Nanosciences and Nanotechnology, University of Mumbai, Kalina Campus. Kalina, Santacruz (E), Mumbai 400 098, India

Maargavi Singh
National Centre for Nanosciences and Nanotechnology, University of Mumbai, Kalina Campus. Kalina, Santacruz (E), Mumbai 400 098, India

Priya Singh
National Centre for Nanosciences and Nanotechnology, University of Mumbai, Kalina Campus.Kalina, Santacruz (E), Mumbai 400 098, India

M Sureshchandra
National Centre for Nanosciences and Nanotechnology, University of Mumbai, Kalina Campus.Kalina, Santacruz (E), Mumbai 400 098, India

Sachin S Surwase
Chemical and Biomolecular Engineering, Korea Advanced Institute of Science and Technology, Daejeon, South Korea
and
Department of Biomedical Engineering, Johns Hopkins University, Baltimore, USA

Humeyra Taskent Sezgin
Department of Bioengineering, İzmir Institute of Technology, İzmir 35430, Türkiye

Fulden Ulucan-Karnak
Department of Medical Biochemistry, Faculty of Medicine, Ege University, İzmir 35100, Türkiye
and
Institute of Health Sciences, Medical Biochemistry Department, Ege University, 35040, Bornova, Izmir, Türkiye

Arzu Uyar
Department of Bioengineering, İzmir Institute of Technology, İzmir 35430, Türkiye
and
Computational Science and Engineering Graduate Program, İzmir Institute of Technology, İzmir 35430, Türkiye

Mikhail Vora
National Centre for Nanosciences and Nanotechnology, University of Mumbai, Kalina Campus. Kalina, Santacruz (E), Mumbai 400 098, India

Chapter 1

Pharmaceutical implants: from concept to commercialization

Ebrahim Saadat, Pharm.D., Ph.D

The pharmaceutical implant is undoubtedly one of the big breakthroughs in novel drug delivery systems. Development of various implants in recent years confirms the important role of this special dosage form in the treatment of various chronic diseases. Many of the first line medicines and also newly developed therapeutic molecules have limited aqueous solubility and poor bioavailability, which limit oral administration. On the other hand, the chronic nature of many diseases needs long-term (and even lifelong) medication which decreases patient compliance and medication adherence. Apart from the bioavailability of the drug molecules, the pharmacokinetic profile is a vital issue in achieving satisfactory clinical outcomes. The big peak and valley in plasma concentration after administration of traditional dosage forms is a big challenge, especially in specific kinds of diseases like epilepsy, cardiac and those that require anticoagulant therapy. One of the big advantages of implantable drug delivery systems is a sustained release fashion of loaded drug molecules over a long period of time, which improves the pharmacokinetic profile of the medicines and also preserves the plasma concentration of drugs. This unique property of the implant system also decreases drug administration frequency and improves patient adherence to the medication. This chapter focuses on pharmaceutical implant drug delivery and explores various commercially available systems. Also, different polymers which have been used in the formulation of implant systems are introduced. Moreover, different industrial manufacturing methods for implants are explained.

1.1 Introduction

From ancient times, oral delivery has been the most common and widely used route of administration for various pharmaceuticals. In fact, oral drug delivery systems have been developed for the delivery of various therapeutics, especially in the past

doi:10.1088/978-0-7503-5613-8ch1

two decades. Lots of research has been conducted to deliver various peptides, proteins and small molecules via this route. Moreover, different sustained drug delivery systems have been developed for continuous delivery of drugs over time [1]. Despite all these developments, oral drug delivery systems face serious challenges, including lack of acceptable bioavailability for major peptides, proteins and hydrophobic molecules, the first pass metabolism which is responsible for extensive metabolism of many drugs, gastrointestinal disorders due to irritation effect of drug molecules (like Non-Steroidal Anti Inflammatory Drugs, NSAIDs) or their pharmacological side effects, higher does frequency, low medication adherence, high possibility of missed doses and also swallowing difficulties (dysphagia) in some patients especially in geriatric medicine [2–4]. Non adherence to medications is common in about 40%–50% of patients with chronic disease and causes 100 000 preventable deaths and 100 billion US dollars of health costs annually [5]. Also, it is reported that about 15%–20% of the geriatric population have some degree of swallowing difficulties [6]. Several drug delivery systems have been developed to overcome these limitations during the past couple of decades, including microparticulate delivery system, transdermal delivery systems, inhaler delivery, nanoparticulate drug delivery systems (like liposome, lipid nanoparticles, micelles) and implants. The main goals of all these delivery systems are sustained release of therapeutics and improved safety and efficacy of thc drug molecules.

Historically, the idea of implant drug delivery with its modern concept was introduced by Deansby and Parkes in 1938. They subcutaneously implanted estron compressed pellets into a castrated male chicken [1]. The concept of drug release from the polymeric membrane was introduced for the first time by Folkman and Long in 1960s [2]. They reported a novel method for systemic or local drug delivery by adding the therapeutic molecules in a silastic capsule which was implanted in the body. The main ideas behind the designing of the implant drug delivery are to reduce dose frequency by sustained drug release, reduce drug side effects, increase the medication adherence and patient compliance, increase the bioavailability of drugs, improve drug stability and reduce toxicity [3, 4]. In some medical fields, implant drug delivery has breakthrough achievements like interventional cardiology and contraception, while progress in the other areas is slower. Drug eluting stents (DES) are one of the most widely used implant delivery systems developed to date [5]. DES have revolutionized vascular disease treatment and especially coronary arteritis disease (CAD) by reducing restenosis risk of arthritis after angioplasty in comparison with non-eluting stents [6]. There are numerous implant delivery systems that have been developed in academia, research centers and industry, a number of which have been commercialized. Table 1.1 summarizes the implant delivery systems that have been commercialized since the 1970s.

Implant drug delivery is a successful system for delivery of drugs with poor water solubility and low bioavailability like most of the anticancers, contraceptives, antibiotics, analgesics, steroids, peptides and proteins [4, 7, 8]. Apart from the physicochemical properties and pharmacological class of the drug molecules, drug delivery to some parts of the body is a challenging issue. One of the good examples

Table 1.1. Implant delivery systems that have been commercialized since the 1970s.

Brand name	Loaded drug	Polymer	Indication	Manufacturer	Approval year
Ocusert®	Pilocarpine	PEVA	Glaucoma	Alza	1974
Zoladex®	Goserelin acetate	PLGA	Prostate cancer	AstraZeneca	1989
Norplant®	Levonorgestrel	Silicone	Contraception	Population council	1990
Vitrasert®	Ganciclovir	PEVA	Cytomegalovirus rhinitis	Bausch and Lomb	1996
Gliadel®	Carmustine	Silicone	Glioblastoma	Arbor Pharms	1996
Jadelle®	Levonorgestrel	Silicone	Contraception	Bayer AG	1996
Estring®	Estradiol	Silicone	Urogenital symptoms due to postmenopausal atrophy	Pfizer	2000
Viadur®	Leuprolide Acetate	PU	Prostate cancer	Bayer AG	2000
NuvaRing®	Etonogestrel and ethinylestradiol	PEVA	Contraception	Merck & Co.	2001
Cypher®	Sirolimus		Improving coronary luminal diameter	Cordis/Johnson & Johnson	2003
Taxus®	Paclitaxel		Tissue growth inhibitor	Boston Scientific Corporation	2004
Vantas®	Histrelin Acetate	Methacrylate	Prostate cancer	Endo Pharmaceuticals	2004
Nexplanon	Etonogestrel	PEVA	Contraception	Merck & Co.	2006
PROMUS element plus	Everolimus	Metal scaffold	Improving coronary luminal diameter	Boston Scientific Corporation	2015
Dextenza®	Dexamethasone	PEG	Ocular inflammation and pain	Ocular Therapeutix	2018
Durysta®	Bimatoprost	PDLLA/PLGA	Open-angle glaucoma	Allergan	2020

of such an organ is the ocular posterior chamber. Drug delivery to the eye is one of the tough issues due to its static and dynamic barriers [9].

Implants are typically presented in a cylindrical shape with a length of around 15–45 mm and a diameter of 2–10 mm. Apart from the other drug delivery systems, implants are administered via injection or insertion into the different parts of the body which release their payloads both locally or systemically. Implants are mostly injected into the muscles or subcutaneous tissues by means of an injection device or surgical implantation for systemic delivery, while other routes of administration are mostly intended for local delivery with negligible systemic absorption [10, 11]. There are also other implantation sites where implants are successfully administered, including intravaginal [12], intraocular [13], intrathecal [14], intravascular [15], intraperitoneal [16] and intracranial [17]. Intramuscular and subcutaneous implantation are the most trustful routes of application due to the high amount of adipose tissue which enhances slow drug absorption, lower localized inflammation and minimal innervation [18].

Implants are designed to deliver medicines in a sustainable fashion in a drug therapeutic window with the minimum fluctuation over a long period of time from one month to a year(s) [19]. In this regard, important items should be considered during the fabrication and design of such a system, including lack of toxicity, highest compatibility between excipient(s) and drug, patient compliance, stability, reproducibility, safety, efficacy and regulatory concerns. Implants like other delivery systems have some advantages and disadvantages. Tables 1.2 and 1.3 represent the advantages and disadvantages of an implant drug delivery system, respectively.

Introducing Zoladex® and Norplant® to the pharmaceutical market brought great progress in establishing implant drug delivery. Moreover, USFDA (United States Food and Drug Administration) approval of PROMUS Element, a DES, in 2015 was an impressive breakthrough in the treatment of CAD. Continuous research and development on this drug delivery system led to introducing two

Table 1.2. Advantages of an implant drug delivery system.

Patient compliance	Due to the low dosing frequency, patients get the benefit of sustained release of implant system.
Increasing the bioavailability	Implants bypass the hepatic first pass metabolism which may provide the possibility of lower loading dose per unit dose of implant.
Fewer side effects	Drugs follow zero-order kinetic release from implant systems which show sustained release over a long period of time without peaks and valleys in the plasma concentration. Moreover, implants release drug near the site of action which increases the efficacy and reduces side effects.
Higher drug stability	The stability of drugs in an implant in solid state would be higher than aqueous dosage forms.
Lower possibility of missed dose	Unlike the oral dosage form, the possibility of a missed dose is dramatically decreased with an implantable drug delivery system.

Table 1.3. Disadvantages of an implant drug delivery system.

Administration issues	Unlike the other dosage forms, implant drug delivery needs expert health care staff who are familiar with injection and implantation techniques. Moreover, in some cases the implantation may cause complications for patients.
Cost/benefit ratio	Developing implant systems is highly expensive. The benefits and costs of such systems should be carefully evaluated in advance.
Pain discomfort	Although the implantation is minimally invasive, pain and discomfort are a common side effect of almost all implant systems.
Toxicity	Implant systems follow zero-order release, but in the case of any accidental release a huge amount of drug may cause serious toxic effects.
Allergic reactions	Explantation due to allergic reactions to any components of the implant would be a challenging issue.

important ocular implants to the market, Dextenza® and Durysta® which were approved by the USFDA in December 2018 and March 2020, respectively [20]. Dextenza® (www.dextenza.com) which was introduced by Ocular Therapeutix is a polyethylene glycol-based implant which is conjugated with fluorescein and loaded with 0.4 mg dexamethasone. Dextenza® is a 3 mm cylindrical shaped resorbable implant which is administered through the intracanalicular route [21]. Pain and inflammation are common side effects of ocular surgery. In the US alone, more than 3.7 million cataract surgeries were performed in 2015 [22]. Control of inflammation and pain needs regular administration of corticosteroids like dexamethasone till 30 days after surgery. Dextenza® is indicated after ophthalmic surgery for the treatment of ocular pain and inflammation. Moreover, it is also used for allergic conjunctivitis [23].

Glaucoma, which is increasing intraocular pressure (IOP) is one of the most prevalent chronic ocular diseases. Glaucoma affected 2.9 million individuals, including 1.4 million women and 1.5 million men in the US population according to [24]. Treatment of glaucoma is based on surgery or long-life medication. Durysta® (www.durysta.com) is a poly (D,L-lactide), poly (D,L-lactide-co-glycolide), poly (D,L-lactide) acid end, and polyethylene glycol-based implant contains 10 µg bimatoprost for intracameral administration, which is used in patients with open-angle glaucoma (OAG) or ocular hypertension (OHT) to reduce IOP over a 4–6 months period [25]. This implant starts to release the content during the week of insertion.

Implants are classified into a wide range of applications. They are also classified by the materials used in their formulation. Basically, implants are classified as biomaterial-based systems which are mostly used as a drug carrier for long-term medication or which provide structural support or promote hemostasis, wound healing and supplement the function of localized tissues like dental and bone implants, orthopedic, cardiovascular, bare-metal or non-resorbable stents, artificial joints, ocular lenses and gastric implants. The latest examples are not used as a drug delivery platform but are widely used as therapeutic devices. Also, there is a class of implants which are used to deliver drugs for a long period of time by means of sensitive electromechanical pumps. The main focus of this chapter is biomaterial-based implants, which are used as a platform for the sustained delivery of different therapeutics.

1.2 Classification of implant drug delivery system

There are various classifications of pharmaceutical implants but the most important one is classification on the basis of release mechanism. The pharmaceutical implants are classified into two major groups of passive and active implants. Active implants release their cargo by means of energy like osmosis, pressure gradient as a driving force, but in contrast, passive implants release the payload by means of passive mechanisms like diffusion or matrix degradation. The passive implants are sub-categorized into degradable and non-degradable ones, depending on the nature of the materials which are used in their formulation.

1.2.1 Passive implants

There are various types of release mechanisms employed to release drugs from passive implants. These mechanisms are mainly diffusion mediated release, polymer degradation and erosion. There is no active driven force to release the drugs from such implants. The release rate is controlled by various parameters such as, polymer characteristics (molecular weight, crystallinity, etc) and the concentration, polymer/drug concentration, implant shape, dimension and surface morphology, various excipients, and drug specification. The passive implants are classified by the characterization of the polymer(s) which is used in their formulation as degradable and non-degradable.

1.2.1.1 Biodegradable implants

Biodegradable implants are one of the major groups of implant drug delivery systems. As the materials which are used in formulation and fabrication of implants degrade over time to safe metabolites, there is no need for any intervention (like surgery) to remove the system from the body. This is one of the most important characteristics of such systems whereby most of the pharmaceutical companies try to get benefit from kinds of delivery system. These kinds of polymers are degraded by enzymatic reaction or hydrolysis into the safe metabolites which are then exerted or absorbed by the body [26]. Various chemical bonds like amid, ester or anhydride on the backbone of these polymers make them susceptible to degradation. This unique characterization of such a system increases patient compliance and acceptability.

Various biodegradable polymers are introduced as an implant matrix in which thermoplastic aliphatic polyesters of lactide and glycolic acid are probably the most used polymers in the preclinical and clinical stages [27]. These polymers have been used since the 1970s as a suture and for drug delivery systems afterward [28]. Their unique features like biodegradability, biocompatibility, scalability, tunability of degradation kinetics, mechanical strength and ease of fabrication have made them an ideal candidate for developing various delivery systems. These polymers have

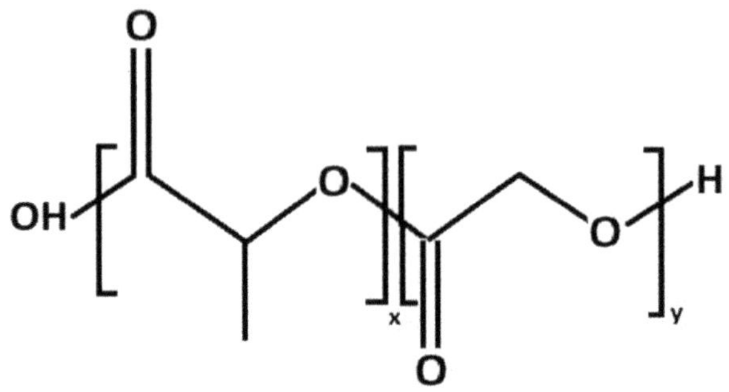

Figure 1.1. Chemical structure of PLGA.

been successfully used in various drug delivery systems including microsphere technology [29] and nanoparticulate drug delivery systems [30]. This range of polymers includes polylactic acid (PLA), polyglycolic acid (PGA) and ester of these two polymers, poly(lactic-co-glycolic acid) (PLGA); figure 1.1 represents the chemical structure of PLGA. These thermoplastic polymers degrade between one to over six months depending on their molecular weight, glass transition, co-polymer ratio and environmental conditions such as pH, temperature [31].

1.2.1.2 Polylactic acid (PLA)

PLA is a biocompatible and biodegradable polymer which was synthetized by Carothers for the first time with a low molecular weight in 1932 [32]. Higher molecular weight PLA was synthetized by Dupont in 1954 [33]. The main method of PLA manufacturing is fermentation of carbohydrate sources like corn starch. The FDA approved this polymer for use in medicinal and pharmaceutical products in 1997 [34]. Due to its thermal stability, it is used in different fabrication techniques including the spinning process, film casting, blow moulding and extrusion [35]. PLA is a white powder with a melting point of 55 °C and a glass transition temperature of 175 °C. Due to two stereoisomers of lactic acid (D and L), there are three types of PLA that can be synthetized by different isomers, D-lactic acid (PDLA) which is a crystalline polymer, hemi-crystalline poly L-lactic acid (PLLA) and a mixture of both isomers which led to amorphous D and L polylactic acid (PDLLA) [36]. PLA is soluble in a wide range of hydrophobic solvents including, chloroform, benzene, acetonitrile [35].

The degradation rate of various isomers is different as PDLA and PDLLA are degraded more rapidly than PLLA due to their crystalline structure [37]. Various rheological experiments showed that PLA exhibits Newtonian behaviors in low shear rates (less than 10 S^{-1}) and non-Newtonian behavior in higher shear rates (higher than 10 S^{-1}) [38, 39]. The rheological property of PLA is crucial for pre-formulation analysis, especially with the specific fabrication methods like extrusion and spinning processes. The effect of PLA isomers on the rheological specification was reported in 1990 [38]. It was reported that the shear viscosity of PDLLA increased with increasing the ratio of PLLA due to the crystalline nature of this isomer. Moreover, it was investigated that the viscosity of branched PLA was higher than the linear one in the Newtonian range, whereas in the non-Newtonian region the viscosity of branched PLA was lower due to the shear thinning behavior of this type of polymer [36].

PLA also exhibits acceptable mechanical properties like tensile and flexural strength in comparison with other popular polymers like polyethylene and polystyrene. Thermal and mechanical stability of polymers are two important factors during fabrication of implants with methods like extrusion. Several parameters are considered in extruders for successful implant manufacturing. For example, the ratio of the length to the diameter (L/D ratio) of the screw is one of the important items which impacts the thermal stability of the materials. Many materials need specific screws for processing, depending on their thermal stability. In the case of PLA, a screw with a low shear (L/D ratio between 24 and 40) was required to prevent the degradation induced by thermo-mechanical shearing during the extrusion process [40, 41]. PLA has several other medical applications, such as wound healing [42], tissue engineering [43], orthopedic devices [44], and developing drug delivery systems [45]. Due to the appreciated properties of PLA, perhaps it would be one of the most promising biomaterials for drug delivery and especially implants.

1.2.1.3 Polyglycolic acid (PGA)

PGA is a well-known, tough and low-cost polymer which has been developed since 1954 [46]. PGA was one of the first approved biocompatible and biodegradable polymers. Dexon® was the first absorbable suture, which was developed by American Cyanamide Co., using PGA [47]. PGA is the simplest aliphatic polyester that is synthetized by polymerization of glycolic acid. PGA has a glass transition between 35 °C and 40 °C and a melting point of 224 °C–227 °C [46]. PGA exhibits from amorphous to a highly crystalline polymer due to its simple structure. The crystallinity of PGA in Dexon® is in the range of 46%–52%, which decomposes rapidly within 2–4 weeks after implantation [48]. PGA shows a fast degradation profile and so it has not been used in sustained drug delivery systems alone. PGA is degraded to glycine, which is expelled by renal clearance via the citric acid cycle [49].

1.2.1.4 poly(lactic-co-glycolic acid) (PLGA)

PLGA is another interesting biodegradable and biocompatible polymer which is manufactured by ring opening co-polymerization of lactic acid and glycolic acid [49]. PLGA has various hydrophobic characteristics due to its molecular weight and also the ratio of lactic to glycolic acid monomers. At the higher ratio of the PGA/PLA, the hydrophobicity of the polymer decreases [31]. Moreover, the solubility and also degradation rate of the polymer is also tunable by the PLGA end group as well. Also, the crystallinity of this co-polymer is altered by its PGA/PLA ratio. At higher ratio of PGA content, PLGA exhibits lower crystallinity and polymer undergoes excessive hydrolyzation/degradation [50]. Randomly distributed PGA and PLA during the synthesis of PLGA leads to two different configurations of the polymer depending on the stereochemical configuration. If the configuration is regular, the polymer is called atactic but in the case of alternating stereochemical configuration the polymer is syndiotactic [51]. Sequencing is an important factor since it dramatically influences the degradation rate of the polymer, with random PLGA degrading much faster than sequenced one [52]. PLGA shows a higher degradation rate at the PLA/PGA of 50:50. PLGA has a glass temperature above 37 °C which makes it an ideal polymer for implantation [53]. PLGA is degraded from a couple of months to several years, depending on its molecular weight, PLA/PGA ratio, end terminal group and crystallinity [54]. PLGA is soluble in most solvents including, methylene chloride, acetone, tetrahydrofuran and ethyl acetate.

1.2.1.5 Polycaprolactone (PCL)

PCL was synthetized firstly by Carothers' group in the 1930s [55]. PCL is synthetized by polymerization of ε-caprolactone with cationic, anionic or coordination catalyst or via free radical ring opening polymerization of 2-methylene-1-3-dioxepane. PCL is a hydrophobic and semi-crystalline polymer with a melting point of 55 °C–60 °C [56]. PCL crystallinity decreases with increase in the molecular weight of the polymer. PCL has special characteristics which lead to an increase in its application either in industry or research centers. These unique specifications include, exceptional blend capacity with other polymers, low melting point and solubility in most solvents [57]. Other interesting specifications of PCL are tunable degradation kinetics, ease of fabrication and shaping [58]. PCL has quite a long degradation period from a couple of months to years, which is influenced by the molecular weight and environmental circumstances like pH, temperature or presence of specific enzymes [59]. The hydrophobicity of PCL leads to less water penetration and thus slow degradation rate. Apart from that, high-molecular-weight chains are composed of several ester bonds which require more time and water for cleavage.

The interesting blending capacity of PCL with other polymers along with its slow degradation profile, provide the possibility to synthesize various PCL co-polymers with tunable characteristics. One of the best examples of this co-polymerization is synthesis of PCL with polyethylene glycol (PEG). PEG exhibits appreciable hydrophilicity, compatibility and less toxicity. PEG–PCL shows lower degradation time due to the higher aqueous solubility and water permeability of the PEG derivative [60, 61]. Polymers with higher glass transition temperature and crystallinity exhibit limited motion and low free space, which all lead to low water penetration into the matrix of the polymer. Reducing the glass transition temperature and polymer crystallinity leads to higher water absorption and reduced the degradation time, accordingly [62]. Adding PEG to PCL leads to reducing the glass transition and also impacts on the crystallinity of PCL. PCL has been widely used in various fields like drug delivery and tissue engineering.

1.2.1.6 Other biocompatible polymers

Certainly PLA, PLGA and PCL are vastly used polymers in drug delivery due to their impressive physicochemical characterization, but there are also other biocompatible polymers which have been used in pharmaceutical and medical fields. These polymers include polyanhydrides, and polydioxanone [63, 64]. Polyanhydrides show rapid degradation time due to their high-water absorption. Thus, these series of polymers are suitable for fast releasing systems [65]. Polyphosphazenes are versatile polymers with a wide range of applications in tissue engineering, drug delivery and stimuli responsive materials. Thanks to its multifunctional chemical groups, it is possible to get more benefit from this group of polymers by various derivatizations [66].

1.2.1.7 Non-biodegradable implants

Apart from degradable implants which are degraded in the body over time, the non-biodegradable implants are composed of non-degraded materials which need further procedures for removal after implantation. Several types of implants introduced to the market, including Norplant® and Implanon® benefit from these series of polymers. Some of the mostly used polymers in the formulation of such implants are polysiloxane (silicones), poly(ethylene-vinyl acetate) (PEVA) and poly (urethanes).

1.2.1.8 Polysiloxane (silicones)

Polysiloxane is one of the important classes of organo-silicone synthetic material composed of silicone and oxygen. Figure 1.2 shows the typical structure of polysiloxane. Polysiloxane is widely used in pharmaceutical and medical fields due to its chemical stability, non-toxicity, biocompatibilities and elastomeric properties [67]. Polydimethylsiloxane (PDMS) is a commercially available polymer which is increasingly used in various drug delivery systems. PDMS has two methyl groups attached to a silicon atom. Polysiloxane is used in the various medical fields, including cardiac pacemaker leads, drainage implants in glaucoma, artificial skin, maxillofacial reconstruction, contact lenses, medical adhesives, and catheters [68]. Although polysiloxanes exhibit great potential for drug delivery, in the number of medical applications some limitations have occurred. For example, when siloxane implants are kept implanted for a long time in subcutaneous tissue, the implants are not immune to infection due to the empty space between the tissue and the device. This space between implant and tissue is removed by surface modification of the siloxane [69, 70]. For some medical applications, surface and bulk modification is necessary to make polysiloxane polymer more hydrophilic. Blending, co-polymerization and functionalization are some methods of polymer modification [71]. Several successful implant drug delivery systems have been launched by means of polysiloxane, for example, Femring® and Estring® are vaginal implants which are

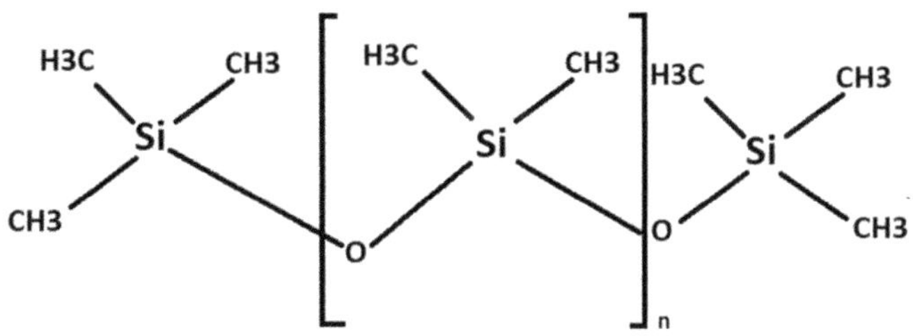

Figure 1.2. Chemical structure of polysiloxane.

loaded with estradiol acetate and estradiol, respectively. Both implants are indicated for hormone replacement therapy (HRT) in menopausal women. Another interesting implant which is fabricated by means of silicone rubber is Norplant® which delivers levonorgestrel via subcutaneous implantation [72, 73]. Norplant® is a cylindrical rod-shaped implant with dimensions of 2.4 × 34 mm.

1.2.1.9 Poly(ethylene-vinyl acetate) (PEVA)

PEVA is a biocompatible, transparent and thermoplastic co-polymer of polyethylene and vinyl acetate (VA) in which VA blocks are randomly distributed in a polyethylene backbone [74]. VA has a big impact on the physicochemical characterization of PEVA, including crystallinity, melting point, polarity and stiffness. Low-density polyethylene (LDPE) is a partially crystalline (50%–60%) polymer with a melting point around 110 °C. Co-polymerization of LDPE with VA residue leads to decrease in crystallinity and melting point of PEVA [75]. Increasing the VA content in PEVA (40%, W/W), decreases the melting point to a broad range between 45 °C and 55 °C and leads to an almost soft amorphous polymer [75–77]. The physicochemical characteristics of PEVA can be easily fixed by adjusting the VA content. VA softens the PEVA polymer and reduces the crystallinity by steric hindrance of acetate groups. This is one of the unique properties of PEVA in which, by adding the appropriate amount of VA, the crystallinity of the final polymer is adjusted without adding the migratory plasticizers. PEVA exhibits the glass transition between −35 °C and −25 °C [78]. PEVA is approved by the FDA as a safe non-drug product [79]. Its cytotoxicity, genotoxicity, irritation, sensitization, acute systemic toxicity and also cutaneous toxicity have also been well studied [80, 81].

Thanks to the flexible characteristics of PEVA, it has been processed by various techniques in the pharmaceutical industry including, hot melt extrusion (HME), spray coating, and injection molding [78, 82, 83]. This polymer is sterilized by gamma irradiation and ethylene oxide [84]. The low melting temperature, tunable plasticization and low hydroscopic characterization make PEVA a good candidate to manufacture implants with HME technique in the pharmaceutical industry. Unlike polyesters and polyurethanes which have hydroscopic characteristics, PEVA does not need a further drying process after the HME process, which leads to increased drug stability in the final dosage form. Because of all these versatile properties, several drugs have been formulated by means of PEVA during the last decade, and some of them are listed in table 1.4.

Several implantable delivery systems have been developed using PEVA polymer and introduced to the pharmaceutical market. Implanon® is a long-acting contraceptive PEVA-based implant containing 68 mg etonogerstrel, which delivers over three years. This 4 × 2 mm rod-shaped device is implanted subcutaneously 8 cm above the elbow [85]. Since 2010, the new equivalent of Implanon® was introduced to the market, called Nexplanon® which has two main differences. Nexplanon® is preloaded in the specific applicator which reduces the risk of insertion errors and also it is loaded with a radio-opaque material (barium sulfate) which detects by computed tomography (CT) scan or x-ray [86]. Probuphine® is another PEVA-based implant, approved by the FDA in 2016, which contains buprenorphine and is

Table 1.4. Drug molecules formulated with PEVA.

Brand name	Molecule(s)	Manufacturer	Indication
Progestesert®	Progesterone	Alza	Contraception
Implanon®	Etonogestrel	Merck & Co	Contraception
NuvaRing®	Etonogestrel/Ethinylestradiol	Merck & Co.	Contraception
Nexplanon®	Etonogestrel	Merck & Co.	Contraception
Probuphine®	Buprenorphine	Braeburn	Opioid addiction
Ocusert®	Pilocarpine	Alza	Glaucoma
Vitrasert®	Ganciclovir	pSividia/Bausch & Lomb	CMV retinitis
Iluvien®	Fluocinolone Acetonide	pSividia/Alimera Science	Chronic DME
Taxus®	Sirolimus	Cordis/Johnson & Johnson	Vascular restenosis
Actisite®	Tetracycline	Alza/Johnson & Johnson	Periodontitis

indicated for treatment of opioid addiction [87]. Probuphine® is composed of 25% wt.% PEVA and 75% wt.% buprenorphine. There are also several implants developed by means of PEVA in the field of ophthalmology. Ocusert® is one of the early developed ocular implants which contains 20 or 40 μg pilocarpine. The active ingredient in Ocusert® is embedded in an alginate gel and two rate controlling PEVA layers [88]. Ocusert® is a flat, flexible elliptical device with dimensions of 13.4 × 5.7 mm. Vitrasert® is another ocular implant that contains ganciclovir which is indicated for cytomegalovirus (CMV) retinitis. It is a tablet-shaped implant with a diameter of 2.5 mm and 1 mm thickness which was approved in 1996 by the FDA [89]. Iluvien® is another FDA-approved posterior ocular implant that contains 0.2 μg fluocinolone acetonide. Iluvien® is indicated for treatment of chronic diabetic macular edema (DME) based on PEVA polymer [90]. Apart from subdermal implants, there are also other inserts which were formulated by means of PEVA polymer. Nuvaring® (www.nuvaring.com) is a vaginal ring containing etonogestrel and estradiol for contraception [91]. Progestasert® is another example of a PEVA-based T-shaped intrauterine ring that contains progesterone which is used for long-term contraception [92].

PEVA is a well-established polymer for developing sustained release drug delivery systems and mainly implants. Its compatibility with a wide range of active ingredients, including small molecules, peptides and proteins make it an ideal carrier for major delivery platforms. Investigations showed that it is highly compatible with various fabrication methods with the highest stability profile.

1.2.1.10 Polyurethanes (PUs)

PUs are a wide range of polymers which are obtained by the co-polymerization of diisocyanate and diols/polyols in the presence of a suitable catalyst, as shown in figure 1.3 [93]. PUs were discovered by Otto Bayer in 1947 [94]. A wide range of PUs can be synthetized by the various substitutes. The physicochemical properties of PUs are tunable by selecting appropriate diisocyanate and polyols. PUs are the unique

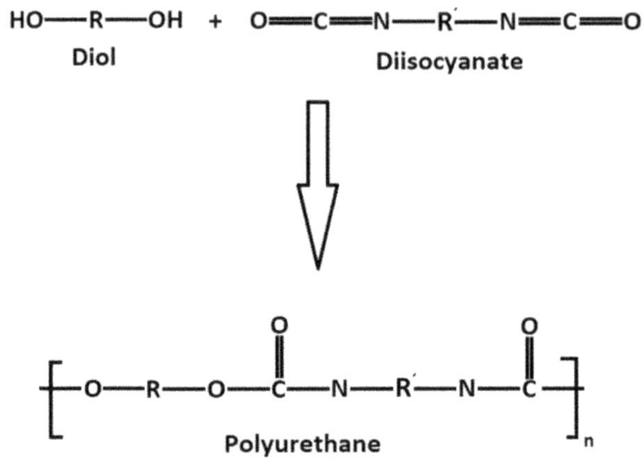

Figure 1.3. Copolymerization of diisocyanate and diols.

group of polymers which exhibit as a thermoplastic, elastomeric or thermosetting depending on the selected co-polymers. Polymerization of difunctional isocyanates and diols leads to linear PU, whereas crosslinked PU is synthetized by coupling tri or higher functional monomers.

In practice, PUs are composed of three segments; diisocyanates (aromatic or aliphatic), polyols (diols or triols) and chain extenders (diols or diamines). Aromatic diisocyantes are more reactive than aliphatic ones [93]. PUs made from aromatic diisocyantes are more sensitive to photodegradation, whereas aliphatic made PUs are more resistant to ultraviolate rays [95]. The structure of diisocyanates, polyols and chain extenders plays a significant role in the final characterization of PUs [96]. The polyol segment plays a major role in the physicochemical properties of PUs. For instance, polyester-based PUs are more susceptible to hydrolysis than polyether-based ones but introduction of alkyl side groups into a hydroxyl terminated polyester yields PUs that are more stable to hydrolysis [97].

The mechanical strength of PUs synthetized through simple polymerization of isocyanate and polyols is weak. Chain extenders play a significant role in modifying the mechanical characteristics of PUs, providing two thermodynamically incompatible blocks. The first part is a tough block which is composed of –NH-COO– and a chain extender and the second part which is the soft bock, is the polyol part [98, 99]. The hard blocks are responsible for mechanical strength, whereas the soft blocks give material flexibility. The chain extenders are low molecular weight bisamines or diols like 1,4-butandiol (BDO), 1,3-propanediol (PDO), ethylene diamine and putrescine [100]. So, the mechanical and physical characteristics of PUs are tunable by adjusting the appropriate type and number of chain extenders and diols used for polymerization. For instance, PUs with tough blocks content of 15–40 (wt%) are rather soft and rubbery elastomers, whereas PUs with tough blocks content of 45–60 (wt%) are hard elastomeric materials [100].

Because of flexible and tunable blocks in the architecture, PUs are extensively used as drug delivery vehicles. The chemistry of PUs can be modified to prepare pH-sensitive or thermosensitive polymers. For instance, adding groups such as amino and carboxyl (as pH-sensitive groups) provides pH sensitivity to the polymer. PUs based primarily on diisocyanate will provide temperature sensitivity [93]. Drug release from PU-based delivery systems is mainly based on the diffusion mechanism which is controlled by the permeability and thickness of the polymer matrix and also the solubility of the drug molecules in the polymeric matrix. Also, a release kinetic from the PU matrices will be dependent on various factors, including polymer composition, swelling ratio, drug loading and degradation rate [100–102].

1.2.1.11 Natural polymers

In addition to the synthetic polymers, there are also other natural polymers (biopolymers) which have been used in different drug delivery systems such as implants. These polymers include, chitosan, cellulose and hyaluronic acid. These biopolymers have many benefits, like biocompatibility, biodegradability and lack of toxicity, which make them an important choice for drug delivery application.

1.2.1.12 Chitosan

Chitosan is a natural polymer composed of randomly distributed N-acetyl-D-glucosamine and β-(1-4)-linked D-glucosamine block with one amine (NH_2) group and two hydroxyl groups (–OH) in each repeating glycosidic unit [103]. Figure 1.4 shows the chemical structure of chitosan. Chitosan is the second most abundant polysaccharide found in Nature after cellulose. Chitosan is extracted from deacetylation of chitin [104]. The main source of chitosan in Nature is the shells of crabs, prawns, lobsters and also the skeletons of various insects and mycelium of various fungi [105].

Chitosan is soluble in the dilute acids like formic acid, acetic acid and succinic acid. The physical characteristics of chitosan are highly dependent on the molecular weight and deacetylation degree. It is a hydrophilic polymer with appreciated hydration properties which has several medical and pharmaceutical applications. Chitosan has been used in different biomedical fields, such as tissue engineering and wound healing [106]. Chitosan has poor solubility in water; therefore, several modifications and derivatizations are suggested in the various functional groups to enhance the physicochemical properties of this biopolymer. Modifications to amino, hydroxyl or both amino and hydroxyl groups form N-modified, O-modified or N, O-modified chitosan derivatives. Incorporation of the carboxymethyl group at

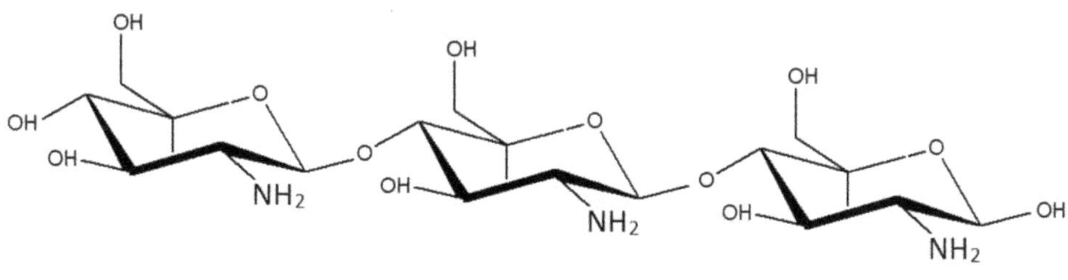

Figure 1.4. Chemical structure of chitosan.

the C6-hydroxyl group or at the NH2 functional group is an important modification for improving the solubility of chitosan [107].

A chitosan-modified implant has been extensively explored against osteomyelitis. Implant related infection is one of the serious challenges in orthopedic surgery [108]. Bacterial colonization and biofilm formation on an implant's surface cause serious tissue inflammation and disrupt the osseointegration process, which accelerates metal corrosion and eventually causes implant failure. Surface modification and coating of implants are employed to minimize the risk of bacterial film forming and improve the affinity of osteogenic cells to facilitate osseointegration. Due to the special characterization of chitosan, several chitosan-based implants were developed for the treatment of osteomyelitis [109]. Chitosan also has a broad-spectrum antibacterial effect against bacteria. Due to this impressive feature, chitosan implants have been explored for periodontal application as well [110].

1.2.1.13 Cellulose

Cellulose is a suitable natural polymer in Nature. It is an important part of plants which gives them structural strength. Cellulose was discovered by Anselme Payen in 1838 [111]. Cellulose is a high-molecular-weight polymer which is composed of β-1,4-anhydro-D-glucopyranose units. It is linked to an acetal molecule by covalent bonds between the C4 of the hydroxyl group and C1 of carbon. The solubility of cellulose is limited in aqueous and organic solvents because of strong inter- and intramolecular bonds. Different derivatives of cellulose can be synthetized by modification of the hydroxyl group of D glucose in its structure [112]. It can be modified by various derivatizations like esterification and etherification which alter the various specifications of this natural polymer, including water solubility and swelling properties, viscosity, adhesiveness, emulsifying properties and film forming [113, 114]. These derivatives have acceptable water solubility, safety, chemical stability, moldability and porosity [115, 116]. Moreover, cellulose derivatives show biocompatibility and biodegradability. For example, carboxymethyl cellulose is degraded during a couple of days in the presence of enzymes like cellulase [117]. Bacteria are another important source of cellulose. Bacterial cellulose is different from plant-derived cellulose in physicochemical properties like higher water content, high crystallinity (up to 80%), higher degree of polymerization and higher mechanical stability [118].

There are numerous studies that have been done on the medical applications of cellulose and its derivatives especially during the last two decades. For instance, cellulose nano crystals and cellulose nanofibers are under evaluation in various fields of medical indications like wound healing, tissue engineering, antibacterial and drug delivery formulation [119].

1.2.1.14 Hyaluronic acid (HA)

Hyaluronic acid (HA), figure 1.5, is a linear anionic polysaccharide composed of repeating units of disaccharides d-glucuronic acid (GlcA) and N-acetyl-d-glucosamine (GlcNAc) linked together through alternating β-1,3 and β-1,4 glycosidic bonds [120]. HA is an important part of the extracellular matrix, synovial fluid and

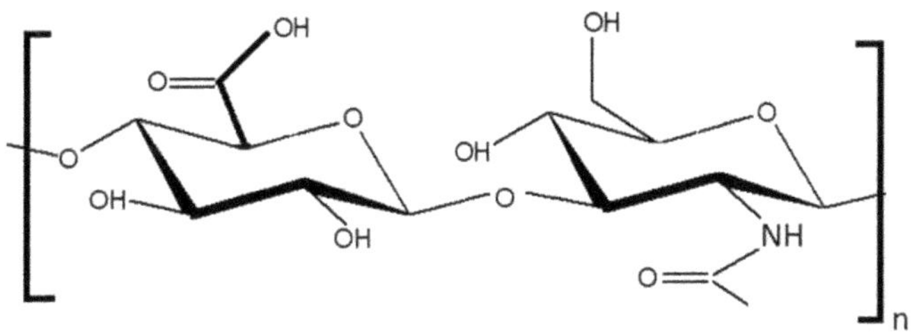

Figure 1.5. Chemical structure of hyaluronic acid.

vitreous humor. HA was first introduced in 1934 by Karl Meyer and John Palmer [121]. There are other sources of HA including rooster combs and shark fin. HA shows great biocompatibility, biodegradability and non-toxicity profile. HA solution exhibit shear thinning, non-Newtonian and viscoelastic behavior [122]. The shear thinning behavior of HA is due to the destruction of hydrogen bonds and numerous intramolecular interactions of the polymer by increasing the shear rate. Furthermore, HA solutions exhibit non thixotropic characterization while the polymer restores its shape and viscosity upon decreasing the shear rate [123]. HA swells up to a volume 1000-fold greater than its original solid volume, taking the full amounts of water [124]. Molecular weight and surrounding pH play an important role in water uptake of HA. Apart from these unique physicochemical characteristics, HA has several important biological roles. HA interacts with cells and tissues via specific ligands which trigger various biological pathways. These specific ligands include HA receptor for endocytosis (HARE), receptor for hyaluronate-mediated motility (RHAMM), lymphatic vessel endothelial hyaluronan receptor-1 (LYVE-1) and also cluster-determined 44 (CD-44) [125, 126]. Various studies confirm the critical role of HA in angiogenesis, cell migration and wound healing. Several studies showed that HA relieves corneal epithelial cell lesions by various mechanisms including, enhancing cell migration, upregulating repair response and inflammatory responses inhibition [127, 128].

HA is composed of several hydroxyl (–OH) and carboxylic acid (–COO) groups which make it an ideal polymer for derivatization and crosslinking [129]. Crosslinking of HA polymer alters the physicochemical characteristics. Crosslinked HA exhibits high viscosity, increases the average molecular weight, increases the viscoelasticity, decreases water solubility, increases mechanical strength, and prolongs the degradation time [130]. These unique properties of HA make it a great candidate to prepare a hydrogel system for implantation. Hydroxyl and carboxyl are two important functional groups in HA structure which enhance the crosslinking reactions. The most used crosslinkers for hydroxyl modifications are polyepoxides, aldehydes, and divinyl sulfones, while for carboxyl modification, are hydrazine, disulfide and 1-(3-Dimethylaminopropyl)-3-ethylcarbodiimide hydrochloride (EDC) [131–133].

Implantable HA based hydrogel is extensively investigated for ocular delivery [134, 135]. For example, in one study by Voss *et al* (2015) a hydrogel system was developed for subconjunctival glaucoma treatment using a biodegradable crosslinked hexamethylene diisocyanate-functionalized 1,2-ethylene glycol bis (dilactic acid). This hydrogel system released latanoprost over two months *in vitro*. The system enhanced the biocompatibility for human and rabbit Tenon's fibroblasts [136]. Crosslinked HA polymer has also been used extensively in aesthetic medicine as a soft tissue filler [137]. Due to the specific viscoelastic properties and excellent biocompatibility profile of crosslinked HA, this hydrogel system is implanted into the skin for augmentation and also for some dermal defects due to facial aging like wrinkles and rejuvenation. The durability of crosslinked HA in some formulations is reported to be several months [138].

1.2.2 Active implants

Unlike passive implants which release their cargo by mechanisms like diffusion, polymer erosion, matrix degradation and swelling, the active implants release the entrapped drug by continuous positive driving force. This force controls the drug release rate more precisely. The release kinetic from active implants is zero order or near zero order [139]. This release kinetic is an ideal pattern in sustained drug delivery systems. However, designing such an active implant is more costly and complex. The driving force in the active implants is divided into two categories: electromechanical devices and implant pumps [140]. The electromechanical devices benefit from microelectronic pumps which push drug at a constant rate. These devices are mainly based on microelectronics, which are not in the scope of this chapter. Implant pumps are those active systems which benefit from osmotic pumps or propellant infusion pumps which are discussed below.

1.2.2.1 Osmotic pumps

The concept of osmotic pumps is based on osmotic pressure. In these series of implants the drug is encapsulated in a reservoir which is surrounded by a semi-permeable membrane. This membrane controls the influx of fluid into the implant body through osmotic pressure. A constant hydrostatic pressure on the drug reservoir due to the steady efflux of fluid into the implant leads to the constant release of implant cargo [141]. The first osmotic pump was introduced by Rose and Nelson in 1955 [142]. Higuchi and Leeper introduced their osmotic pump in 1973 and made some modifications [143]. Alza corporation made several alterations to the osmotic pumps during the 1970s and 1980s [144]. Viadur® is a sterile, non-erodable, osmotically driven implant containing leuprolide acetate developed by Alza corporation on the basis of the Duros platform which was approved by the FDA in 2000 [145]. The Duros system was designed to deliver various drugs from several weeks to one year. While the Duros platform was designed to deliver a wide range of molecules, it has been mainly used for potent peptides and proteins for chronic diseases. In particular, Viadur® was used to deliver GnRH analog leuprolide to treat prostate cancer [146]. Duros is a cylindrical shaped implant with a typical diameter of 4–10 mm and a length of 45 mm. This system is composed of drug formulation, a piston and an osmotic engine. The drug formulation is separated from the osmotic engine by a piston. The piston part also seals the osmotic engine

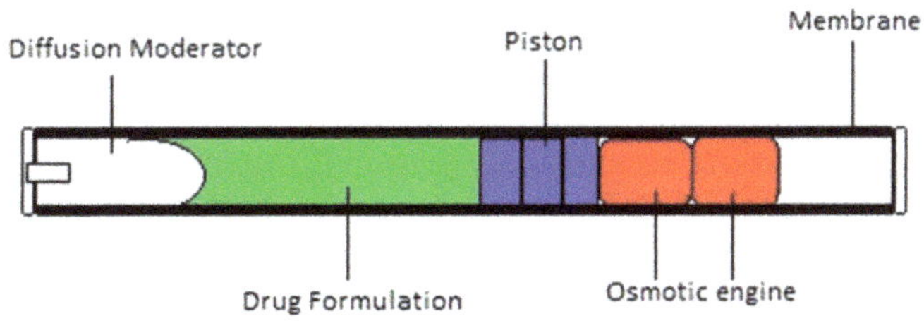

Figure 1.6. Typical scheme of a Duros implant.

from the drug reservoir. Body fluid is inhibited from entering into the drug reservoir by a diffusion moderator. Drug delivery rate is controlled by a specific polyurethan semi-permeable membrane which has antifouling properties during *in vivo* operation. The drug in the reservoir is loaded either in the form of dissolved or suspended formulation in an acceptable solvent. The role of solvents and also excipient is crucial for drug stability during the shelf life and also release period. Figure 1.6 shows the typical scheme of the Duros implant.

Another active implant on the basis of osmosis is Alzet® pump. This implant is designed to deliver its cargo between a day to six weeks. Alzet® pump contains a drug reservoir which is separated from a chamber by osmotic salt in a semi-permeable membrane. Water molecules enter the pump through a semi-permeable layer due to the high osmotic pressure. The volume of the chamber increases, which leads to compression of the flexible reservoir and drug release through the exit orifice, accordingly [147]. One of the big advantages of such a system is mitigation of 'burst release' which is a big obstacle especially in biodegradable matrices [4]. The minimum burst release and a precise release kinetic are crucial for drugs with a narrow therapeutic index. Various chemicals like antibodies, cytokines, growth factors, chemotherapeutics, hormones and peptides have been delivered by Alzet® pump [148].

1.2.2.2 Propellant infusion pump

One drawback of the osmotic pumps is a limited drug capacity due to the high amount of osmotic agent. In order to combat this challenge, a propellant infusion pump was designed. In this new design, a fluorocarbon gas provides a sustained driving force by a constant vapor pressure to release the drug. In this pump, a disk-shaped housing separates the chamber of fluorocarbon propellant from the drug formulation reservoir. The system contains a flow restrictor to ensure constant vapor pressure from the propellant at operating temperatures [3]. Infusaid is an example of such a design. Nine cancer patients in the terminal stage with chronic pain have been treated with continuous intrathecal infusion of morphine delivered by Infusaid pump, reported in one study at Howard University Hospital [149].

1.3 Implant manufacturing methods

There are a couple of fabrication methods developed for industrial scale manufacturing of implants. There are several factors which impact choosing the appropriate manufacturing methods including, physicochemical properties of active agent(s), physicochemical properties of polymer and excipient(s), costs, efficiency and properties of manufactured implants. Implants are fabricated through various methods, including hot melt extrusion (HME), solvent casting, compression, injection molding, and more recently, 3D printing. Implants manufactured through various fabrication methods exhibit different physical properties like surface morphology and porosity. So, the degradation rate and mechanism would be different and eventually the *in vitro* and *in vivo* release profiles of drugs would be different. Fialho *et al* (2005) compared two different manufacturing methods, HME and compression, to make intraocular implants. They found that the manufacturing method dramatically impacts on implant degradation and drug release [150].

1.3.1 Hot melt extrusion (HME)

Extrusion is a process of converting drug and excipients into a product by forcing it through the die under controlled conditions. This product is uniform in shape and density [151]. HME technology goes back to the 1930s. Extrusion is a well-known platform for processing materials which has been used in other industries as well. One of the excellent features of HME technique is the continuous manufacturing process. This kind of manufacturing technique affords a consistent product flow, ideally at relatively high throughput rates. HEM has been used in different pharmaceutical drug delivery systems and dosage forms, including granules, pellets, film, tablets, transdermal, transmucosal, and implants [152–156].

Extruders are typically composed of two parts. The first part is the conveying segment which transports materials and also performs some degree of mixing, and the second part is a dye system which is used to shape the extrudes. The HME technique has been used for both solid materials and semisolids. For the solid material, the heat is applied during the process to control the viscosity and flow of material through the extruder and also a dye which is called molten extruding. Semisolid materials are multiphase concentrated dispersions containing a high proportion of solid mixed with a liquid phase [157]. HME is an efficient method not only for fabrication of implants but also for improving the solubility and increasing the bioavailability of drugs with low aqueous solubility [158].

1.3.1.1 The HME process

The HME process is divided into four steps:

- Feeding the raw materials;
- Conveying of mass and entry to the die;
- Flow through the die;
- Exit from the die and downstream process.

There are various aspects in the four steps above, including powder flow, shear force, cooling rate, pressure, residence time, and shaping. During the HME, the temperature of the inside chamber increases due to the friction forces between materials. The additional heating energy is supplied through the electrical or liquid heating jacket mounted on the extruder's barrel. Thermal stability of drugs and other

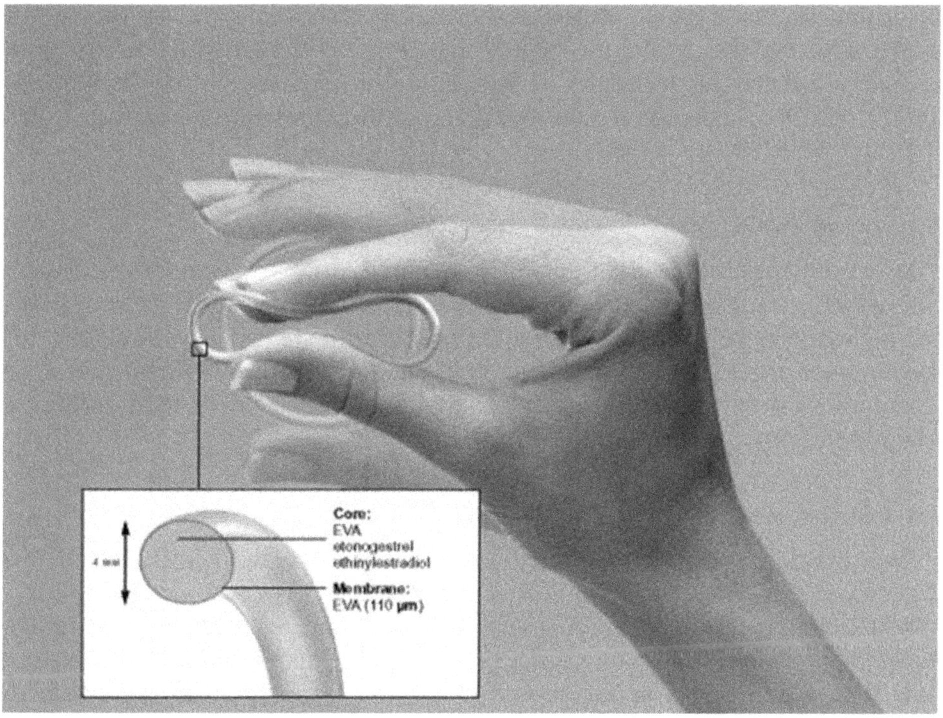

Figure 1.7. Typical scheme of Nuvaring® implant. From [219] with permission from Dove Medical Press Ltd.

materials is one of the main considerations during the HME process. Heating, pressure and also residence time are crucial factors that need to be precisely adjusted during the process. The HME process requires controlling different parameters like viscosity, elasticity, temperature, shear rate, extensional flow and slippage of the materials over the hot surface [159]. One of the main advantages of the HME process is that it is a well-known and mature engineering technology and most regulatory bodies including USFDA and European authorities have approved this technique [160]. Several implants have been fabricated and launched on the market using the HME technique. Implanon® and Nuvaring® (figure 1.7) have been developed by this technology using poly EVA co-polymer [161]. Moreover, Zoladex® and Depot-profact® are two LHRH (luteinizing hormone releasing hormone) agonists implant formulations which have been fabricated by HME technology [162].

1.3.2 Compression molding

Compression molding technique is simply compressing drug and excipient(s) under constant pressure within a mold until the materials flow and take the shape of the die. One of the important benefits of this method is ease of fabrication and also lack of requirement for use of various solvents during the process [163]. Moreover, normally there is no need for elevated temperatures, which makes this method suitable for sensitive substances like peptides and proteins [162]. One drawback of this method is the highly porous and irregular surface shape of the implants manufactured by this technique, which may lead to the irregular release profile and batch-to-batch inconsistency [150]. Also, the studies showed that implants manufactured by this method exhibited faster drug release in comparison with the other fabrication methods [53].

1.3.3 Solvent casting

In the solvent casting method, the polymer and drug (or other excipients) are dissolved in a suitable solvent, cast into a mold followed by solvent evaporation. Implants made by this method form a laminar or film-shaped structure. One of the disadvantages of this method is using a high amount of solvent, which causes a big concern about drug stability, toxicity and residual solvent in the final product and also environmental concerns [31].

1.3.4 Injection molding

Injection molding is another technique of implant fabrication. In this method, the polymer and drug molecules are heated and injected into the mold and solidify to form the implant. Injection molding has several advantages, including: (a) Implants with different shapes can be produced; (b) drug pellets can remain undissolved over a long time; (c) smoother surface morphology with lower porosity and cracks; and (d) dense drug pellets can be fabricated. Thermoplastic polymers such as PLGA and PLA are good candidates to use for this technique. Although this method is quite simple, studies showed that during the heating process the polymer molecular weight may decrease, with possible impacts on the drug release rate. In one study performed by Rothen-Weinhold *et al* it was shown that the PLA implants containing a somatostatin analog which were fabricated by injection molding exhibited lower molecular weight and polydispersity index in comparison with the extrusion method [164].

1.3.5 Three-dimensional printing (3D printing)

3D printers have been used to build up 3D objects by printing materials layer by layer [165]. The printers layer the materials hundreds of thousand times until the layers add up to design the objects. Till now, 3D printers have been used for fabrication of various dental and orthopedic implants and also protheses. 3D printing has become a more interesting technique in fabrication of various pharmaceutical dosage forms, especially after the first approval of levetiracetam porous tables 'Spritam' by the FDA in 2015 [166]. One of the big advantages of 3D printing is to customize medicine for specific groups of patients according to their situation and condition [167]. 3D printing enables pharmacists to manufacture customized formulations by adjusting formulations using computer-aided design (CAD) files. Therefore, 3D printers make it possible to personalize medicine in accordance with patients' age, weight, organ function and also underlying diseases [167].

3D printers can be used in fabrication of implants with biodegradable polymers which are filled with drug subsequently or coated with a rate controlling membrane [168]. In one study by Yang *et al* (2018) a hollow bullet-shaped implant was fabricated by 3D technique, loaded with a chemotherapeutic agent, cytoxan [169]. The fabricated implant showed rapid release due to its highly porous structure, which was solved by further coating the implant with PLA polymer. In another study, the PDLLA-based implant was fabricated and loaded with levofloxacin and tobramycin using ink jet 3D printers for treatment of chronic stage of osteomyelitis [168]. The drug release started from the surface, which continued to the inner core. 3D printing is a valuable method for quick manufacturing of implants in the research and development phase. The big challenge with the 3D printers is limited production capacity, which makes them an uncertain industrial manufacturing technique.

1.4 Drug release mechanisms from implantable delivery systems

Drug release from various bio-erodible and non-bio-erodible matrices occurs through different mechanisms. Understanding the underlaying release mechanism is crucial for optimizing the formulation and also the fabrication method. Different release mechanisms are introduced and well-studied by various drug delivery systems, including implant matrices. The drug release mechanism is highly depended on the drug molecule, physicochemical properties of the matrix and also implant surrounding conditions such as pH, ionic strength, presence of specific enzymes and temperature. The release mechanisms can be categorized into passive mechanism and active mechanism. Passive mechanisms include, diffusion, swelling and matrix degradation. Active mechanism examples are osmotic pressure and any other driving forces which induce drug release from the matrix.

There are various release kinetics explored depending on the different mechanism. These release kinetics are:

1. Fickian diffusion: $\delta\phi/\delta t = D\ (\delta^2\phi/\ \delta x^2)$

where, ϕ is drug concentration in a mole, t is time, D is diffusion coefficient and x, diffusion length.

2. Zero order: $Q_t = Q_0 + k_0 t$

where, Q_t is the amount of drug released in time t, Q_0 is the initial amount of drug in implant, k_0 is the release rate constant.

3. First order: $\ln Q_t = \ln Q_0 - K_1 t$

where K_1 is the release rate constant.

4. Higuchi: $Q_t = k_H t^{0.5}$

where k_H is the release rate constant.

5. Korsmeyer-Peppas: $M_t/M_\infty = kt^n$

where M_t/M_∞ is a fraction of the released drug at time t and n, is the diffusional exponent.

1.4.1 Release mechanisms from biodegradable matrices

The main release mechanisms from the biodegradable implants are diffusion, degradation or a mixture of both mechanisms [4]. Degradation mechanism is divided into surface erosion and bulk erosion [170]. During the surface erosion, the polymer starts to degrade from the outer layers by various physicochemical reactions like hydrolysis, enzymatic reactions and erosion. The ratio of surface to the volume of the implant is an important factor in erosion degradation intensity. Increasing the surface of the implants leads to a higher degree of surface erosion. Bulk erosion happens in the inner layer or core part of the implant by backbone degradation of the implant matrix. So apart from the physicochemical characteristics of the polymer matrix, drug and excipients, implant geometry and morphology are also important factors which impact the release mechanism and kinetics as well [171]. At the beginning phase of the release process, diffusion starts by dissolving the drug molecules in the surrounding solvent. Diffusion highly depends on the drug solubility in the implanted media solvent, diffusion coefficient, temperature, ionic strength and also pH of the medium [172]. The release rate is controlled by the degradation mechanism when the erosion is more prominent than diffusion. Water uptake or accessibility to the water is a key factor in degradation and drug release for matrices which are susceptible to hydrolysis. The degradation of semi-crystalline matrices occurs in two phases. In the first phase, the water molecules penetrate to the amorphous domains and hydrolyze the polymer. During the second phase, the entire domain of the polymer will be degraded along with amorphous regions [4]. During polymer hydrolysis the average molecular weight of the polymer decreases, which is an important index for drug release.

1.4.2 Release mechanisms from non-biodegradable matrices

Non-biodegradable implants are categorized into two groups depending on their design type. Matrix type and reservoir type. As explained earlier in the reservoir type implants, the drug molecules are entrapped in the semi-permeable membrane which controls drug release rate. In this type of implant, drug diffusion is the major release mechanism which is controlled by the important parameters including the membrane thickness, solubility and drug permeability across the membrane and diffusion coefficient of the drug [173]. In this type of implant, the release kinetic is zero order or near zero order. The release rate of such an implant is controlled by the semi-permeable membrane instead of drug concentration [174]. In fact, the driving release force is constant during the release period, assuming that the drug concentration in the reservoir is constantly in equilibrium with the core of the membrane. Matrix type implants follow diffusion-based release as the drug molecules are entrapped between the polymer chains and some portion of the drug may be entrapped on the surface of the implants, which leads to the initial 'burst release'. In this type of implant, water uptake, swelling and drug diffusion are the main release mechanisms which may deviate from the typical zero order release kinetic. In such a system the release rate is proportional to the drug concentration in the implant matrix [175].

1.5 Therapeutic applications of implantable drug delivery systems

The implant drug delivery system is an important platform for treatment of chronic diseases which need long-term medication. Some of the medical conditions and diseases even need long-life medication like glaucoma or some sort of cancer. Patients who suffer from these kinds of diseases should strictly adhere to their medication as relapsing from such a condition may deeply impact their health and prognosis. Some important therapeutic aspects of important implant drug delivery systems are discussed further.

1.5.1 Women's health

Implant drug delivery system in women's health is mostly focused on contraception and treating menopausal syndrome. Norplant® is the first developed implant in the field of women's health which was approved by the FDA in 1990 [176]. This implant delivers levonorgestrel as a contraceptive agent and the pregnancy rate was reported to be less than 1% [177]. Jadelle® is a newer version of Norplant which is a five-years non-biodegradable implant that was introduced by Bayer pharmaceuticals [178]. It is a rod-shaped implant, 2.5 mm in diameter and 43 mm in length. Estring® (www.estring.com) is an intravaginal ring (IVR) with an outer diameter of 55 mm which was introduced by Pfizer and approved by the FDA for treatment of menopause symptoms [179]. This ring is loaded with 2 mg estradiol and releases its cargo 90 days after implantation [180]. Nuvaring® is another IVR with an outer diameter of 54 mm which is developed by Merck that delivers 120 μg etonogestrel and 15 μg ethinylestradiol in three weeks [181]. Nexplanon® is a newer contraceptive implant which delivers 68 mg etonogestrel over three years [182]. Nexplanon® has two main differences from Implanon. First, it has a specific applicator for subcutaneous insertion and second, it contains a specific radio-opaque material (barium) which can be detected easily via x-ray or CT-Scan.

1.5.2 Ocular diseases

Several intraocular implants have been developed and introduced to the market for various ocular complications. These implants and insets are mainly indicated for ocular infection, controlling IOP and post-surgery inflammation. Table 1.5 summarizes the intraocular inserts and implants. Iluvine® is a sustained release fluocinolone acetonide implant which releases over three years to treat DME [90]. Iluvine® is a nonerodable intravitreal implant which is injected into the back of the eye [183]. Retisert® is a fluocinolone acetonide implant introduced by Bausch & Lomb which is indicated for treatment of uveitis that releases the drug during 30 months [184]. The fluocinolone acetonide tablet is entrapped in an elastomeric silicon cup containing the orifice for release of drug molecules. The tablet inside the reservoir is coated by polyvinyl alcohol (PVA) which creates a membrane between the tablet and the orifice that serves as a barrier for drug release from the cup [185]. Vitrasert® which was introduced by Bausch & Lomb, is a ganciclovir implant that is indicated for treatment of cytomegalovirus rhinitis [186]. Vitrasert® is made of PVA and EVA

Table 1.5. Intraocular inserts and implants.

Brand name	Active molecule	Polymer	Indication	Manufacturer
Ocusert®	Pilocarpine	PEVA	Glaucoma	Alza
Vitrasert®	Ganciclovir	PEVA	Cytomegalovirus rhinitis	Bausch & Lomb
Iluvien®	Fluocinolone acetonide	Silicone	Chronic DME	pSividia/Alimera Science
Retisert®	Fluocinolone acetonide	PVA	Uveitis	Bausch & Lomb
Ozurdex®	Dexamethasone	PLGA	DME	Allergan
Dextenza®	Dexamethasone	PEG	Ocular inflammation and pain	Ocular Therapeutix
Durysta®	Bimatoprost	PDLLA/ PLGA	Open-angle glaucoma	Allergan

polymers and implanted into the posterior segment of the eye. Ozurdex® contains 0.7 mg dexamethasone embedded in PLGA polymer and implanted into the vitreous cavity. Ozurdex® is indicated for the treatment of uveitis and macular edema following Branch Retinal Vein Occlusion (BRVO) and Central Retinal Vein Occlusion (CRVO) [187]. As stated earlier, Dextenza® is a polyethylene glycol implant loaded with 0.4 dexamethasone indicated for the treatment of ocular inflammation and pain following ophthalmic surgery. Durysta® which was introduce by Allergan, is a poly (D,L-lactide), poly (D,L-lactide-co-glycolide), poly (D,L-lactide) acid end, and polyethylene glycol-based implant contains 10 μg bimatoprost which is used for the treatment of IOP in patients with open-angle glaucoma [188]. Durysta® is a cylindrical shaped implant with a length of 1 mm.

1.5.3 Cancer therapy

Cancer therapy needs long-term treatment and in some cases the treatment is lifelong. Apart from the chronic nature of cancer diseases, most anticancer drugs are hydrophobic compounds with low bioavailability. Also, due to their poor solubility in an aqueous media the injectable formulation of such drugs is quite complicated. In order to prepare a suitable injectable dosage form, some excipients and co-solvents have been used in such formulations but further clinical studies have shown some level of toxicity reactions [189, 190]. The best example of such excipients is Cremophor® which is extensively used in some Taxane formulations. Serious side effects have been reported after administration of formulations containing Cremophor®, including anaphylactoid reactions, hepatotoxicity and renal toxicity [191]. Various drug delivery systems have been introduced for the delivery of anticancer drugs without such toxic excipients, including liposome [192], polymeric micelle [193], solid lipid nanoparticles [194] and also implants [195].

Table 1.6. Implantable anticancer drug.

Brand	Active molecule	Indication	Manufacturer
Zoladex®	Goserelin acetate	Prostate cancer	AstraZeneca
Gliadel®	Carmustine	Glioblastoma	Arbor pharms
Viadur®	Leuprolide acetate	Prostate cancer	Bayer AG
Vantas®	Histrelin acetate	Prostate cancer	Endo Pharmaceuticals
GemRIS®	Gemcitabine	Bladder cancer	Taris Biomedical

The implant has a unique platform in cancer drug delivery due to its flexible characteristic in which drugs with various physicochemical properties can be loaded into such a system. Lots of research has been done to deliver anticancer agents including chemicals, peptides and proteins to the cancerous cells via an implant drug delivery system [196–198]. The first anticancer implant, Zoladex® (www.zoladex.com), was introduced by AstraZeneca, which was approved in 1898 by the FDA [199]. Zoladex® is a cylindrical rods-shaped implant 10 mm in length that contains a potent synthetic decapeptide analogue of luteinizing hormone-releasing hormone (LHRH), goserelin acetate for the treatment of advanced prostate cancer and advanced breast cancer in premenopausal and perimenopausal women [200]. The matrix of Zoladex® is composed of D,L-lactic and glycolic acids co-polymer. This implant is presented in two doses of 3.6 and 10.8 mg of goserelin, which are released over 28 days and 12 weeks, respectively [201]. Another breakthrough in cancer therapy was achieved by introducing Gliadel® (www.gliadel.com) by Arbor pharms. Gliadel® is a wafer of carmustine, a nitrosourea alkylating agent, which is indicated for the treatment of patients with high-grade glioma [202]. The matrix of Gliadel® is composed of co-polymer of poly[bis (p-carboxyphenoxy)] propane and sebacic acid in a 20:80 molar ratio [203]. Gliadel® is a sterile, off-white-to-pale-yellow wafer 1.45 cm in diameter and 1 mm thick. Each wafer contains 7.7 mg of carmustine and 192.3 mg of a biodegradable matrix [204]. The next implant which was introduced in 2004 is Vantas®, which is a non-biodegradable implant of Histrelin acetate for the treatment of prostate cancer [205]. This implant is composed of a non-biodegradable diffusion-controlled reservoir consisting of 2-hydroxyethyl methacrylate, 2-hydroxypropyl methacrylate co-polymers [206]. The Vantas® implant is a small thin flexible tube which consists of a 50-mg Histrelin acetate drug core inside a 3.5 cm by 3 mm, cylindrical shaped reservoir [207]. Table 1.6 summarizes the implantable anticancer drugs for the treatment of various cancers.

1.5.4 Central nervous system (CNS) complications

Probuphine® is an EVA-based implant containing 74.2 mg buprenorphine which is indicated for the maintenance treatment of opioid dependence in patients who have achieved and sustained prolonged clinical stability at low-to-moderate doses of a transmucosal buprenorphine-containing product [208]. It is a rod-shaped implant with a dimension of 26 mm in length and 2.5 mm in diameter. It is implanted sub dermally and releases the drug for up to six months [209]. LiRIS® is another implant which was designed by scientists from Massachusetts Institute of Technology (MIT) introduced to relieve symptoms associated with interstitial cystitis, such as bladder pain and voiding dysfunctions [210]. This implant which is currently being evaluated in a phase two clinical trial, contains lidocaine hydrochloride, either 200 or 650 mg, which is designed to provide zero order release for the first 24 h following 14 days first-order release fashion [211].

1.5.5 Other chronic diseases

Supprelin®-LA is an implant which is used for the treatment of central precocious puberty (CPP) in children, once a year. This implant, which is designed on the basis of hydron technology, is inserted subcutaneously in the inner aspect of the upper arm and continuously releases approximately 65 mcg/day over 12 months of the gonadotropin releasing hormone (GnRH) analog, Histrelin [212].

1.6 Clinical trials

The implant drug delivery system is one of the robust and effective platforms for continuous drug therapy especially for chronic conditions. In this regard, many research centers and pharmaceutical companies have been developing several implant systems some of which have entered into the various stages of clinical trial. Table 1.7 summarizes some of the implant systems which are getting through the various phases of clinical trials for safety and efficacy.

1.7 Current obstacles and future prospective

The implant is one of the important drug delivery systems, especially among specific populations like geriatrics and patients who may need lifelong medication. As mentioned earlier, the implant drug delivery system has lots of advantages over many conventional dosage forms but design, formulation, industrial manufacturing, clinical trials and also regulatory issues are the main challenges in introducing drugs via this delivery system. One of the important challenges in developing an implant drug delivery system is the biodegradability and biocompatibility of the matrix polymer. Safety and non-toxicity of the polymer matrix and its degraded residuals are the main important issues in selecting such macromolecules. Since implants are maintained for a long time in the body, minimal or no adverse reaction should be seen from the polymer matrix. All implant components including drug cargo, implant matrix and other excipients should be non-toxic, non-carcinogenic, hypo-allergic, and chemically stable at the implantation site. Moreover, the implant material should not be modified or altered by the surrounding tissue or the implant should not cause any inflammatory reactions to the implantation site. In fact, the biocompatibility of implants is a two-way process that involves the time dependent of the host (patient) on the implant and also the effect of the implant on the host.

As per international guidelines and specifically per WHO and FDA, all implantable materials should comprehensively be tested for biocompatibility, bioreactivity and stability [213]. Even for biodegradable implants, excessive studies

Table 1.7. Implant systems in clinical trial.

Name	Drug	Polymer/carrier	Indication	Phase	Identifier	Company
PA5108	Latanoprost	Polymer-drug conjugate	Control of mild-moderate glaucoma	1	NCT04060758	PolyActiva Pty Ltd
PA5436	Levofloxacin	Polymer-drug conjugate	Delivers a bolus dose of levofloxacin after cataract surgery	1	NCT04682288	PolyActiva Pty Ltd
OTX-TIC	Travoprost	polyethylene glycol-based hydrogel	Control of open-angle glaucoma or ocular hypertension	2	NCT05335122	Ocular Therapeutix
DLP 160	Naltrexone	PLGA	prevention of relapse to opioid dependence	1	NCT05304364	Delpor
DLP 114	Risperidone	PLGA	Antipsychotic	2	NCT04418466	Delpor
iDose	Travoprost	Titanium	Control of open-angle glaucoma or ocular hypertension	3	NCT03519386	Glaukos Corporation

are required for the safety evaluation of degraded products. Several serious complications may happen in the case of non-biocompatibility of implant components including, infection, tissue sensitivity or damage, inflammation, platelet adhesion, thrombosis, fibrosis, allergic reaction and severe immune responses. Blood compatibility of implantable materials is one of the important and crucial issues. When a biomaterial is exposed to the blood, certain proteins are adsorbed and, on the basis of the adsorbed proteins, the platelet aggregates on the surface of the implanted biomaterial. This platelet aggregation may cause thrombosis in some cases, which may result in blockage of blood flow and embolism, which is a serious medical complication [214]. The surface modification of implants is an accepted idea to minimize the risk of blood complications, especially in implants which are in direct contact with blood like implants which are used in coronary artery stenosis. The role of various hydrophilic coating materials like polyethylene oxide, heparin, albumin or other hydrophilic polymers were studied [215, 216]. Such materials prevent cell or protein adhesion to the surface of implanted biomaterials by steric hindrance or electrostatic repulsion. Tissue biocompatibility is also an important factor which needs to be considered before implant design and formulation. The classical signs of tissue reaction to the implant are reddening, swelling, pain, inflammation, fever and infection. Other offensive reactions occur after the primary tissue reactions mediated by immune cells, including neutrophils, eosinophils and macrophages. The role of these cells is phagocytosis of the death tissue or implanted particulates [217]. Macrophages start to repair the damaged tissue by forming a scaffold which is called granulation tissue. The granulation tissue starts to surround the implant. If the phagocytosis system cannot eliminate the implant, then the body tends to completely isolate it by forming a fibrous membrane capsule around it [217]. The formation of a capsule around the implant (encapsulation) is mediated by fibroblasts originating in perivascular connective tissue [218].

Another important factor in implant design and formulation is patient compliance. Normally, implanting and explanting is done by a physician or surgeon during the noninvasive procedure. Although the process is noninvasive or minimally invasive, there are some possible complications for some patients. If the administered implant is non-biodegradable, then there would be an extra process of removal needed which may decrease patient compliance. Apart from patient compliance, health care training is a key factor which needs to be considered during the product launch to the market. Physicians need to be well trained for implanting and explanting and also be informed about the possible adverse effects of an administered implant system.

Cost effectiveness is also the crucial point which needs to be considered during the development phase of each drug delivery system. Formulation complexity, manufacturing cost, expensive clinical trials and also regulatory issues make the implant drug delivery system an expensive option for patients, especially in under-developed countries and uninsured markets. Introducing new therapies for chronic diseases, including monoclonal antibodies, gene, cell and immunotherapy and also other alternative drug delivery systems on one hand, and also cost effectiveness and patient compliance on the other hand cause most large international pharmaceutical

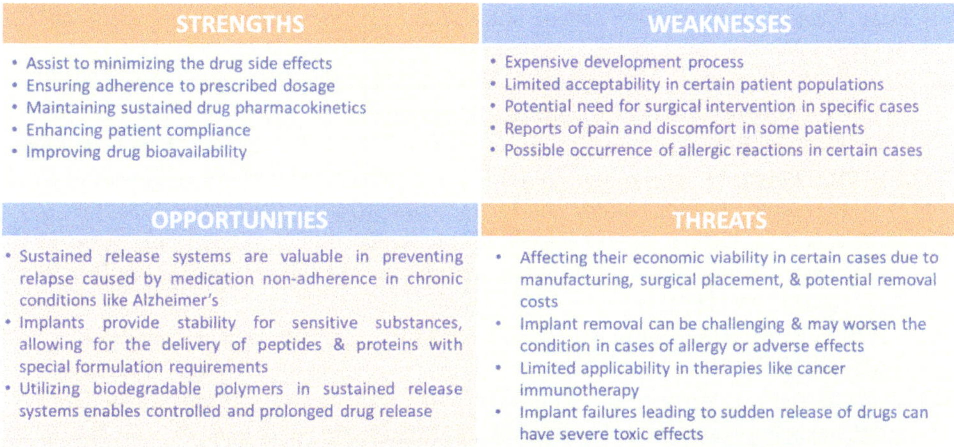

Figure 1.8. The SWOT analysis for pharmaceutical implants.

companies to focus less on developing complicated implantable drug delivery systems. The strengths, weaknesses, opportunities and threats (SWOT analysis) for a brief overview of pharmaceutical implants is represented in figure 1.8.

1.8 Conclusion

Developing new drug molecules is a challenging and costly process. Sustained delivery of old drug molecules which have a clear safety and efficacy profile seems to be feasible. The implant delivery system is one of the promising platforms for zero-order or near-zero-order release kinetic, *in vivo*. Moreover, during the past several decades, the implantable drug delivery system has shown reasonable clinical outcomes in various fields of therapy. However, patient compliance, cost effectiveness, regulatory issues, clinical trial challenges and also the safety and efficacy of this type of delivery system should be deeply considered.

References

[1] Kleiner L W, Wright J C and Wang Y 2014 Evolution of implantable and insertable drug delivery systems *J. Control. Release* **181** 1–10

[2] Peppas N A 2013 Historical perspective on advanced drug delivery: how engineering design and mathematical modeling helped the field mature *Adv. Drug Delivery Rev.* **65** 5–9

[3] Rajgor N, Patel M and Bhaskar V 2011 Implantable drug delivery systems: an overview *Syst. Rev. Pharm.* **2** 91–5

[4] Kumar A and Pillai J 2018 Implantable drug delivery systems: an overview *Nanostructures for the Engineering of Cells, Tissues and Organs* (Elsevier) 473–511

[5] Htay T and Liu M W 2005 Drug-eluting stent: a review and update *Vasc. Health Risk Manag.* **1** 263–76
[6] Bønaa K H, Mannsverk J, Wiseth R, Aaberge L, Myreng Y and Nygård O *et al* 2016 Drug-eluting or bare-metal stents for coronary artery disease *New Engl. J. Med.* **375** 1242–52
[7] Abdelkader H, Fathalla Z, Seyfoddin A, Farahani M, Thrimawithana T and Allahham A *et al* 2021 Polymeric long-acting drug delivery systems (LADDS) for treatment of chronic diseases: inserts, patches, wafers, and implants *Adv. Drug Delivery Rev.* **177** 113957
[8] Mohtashami Z, Esmaili Z, Vakilinezhad M A, Seyedjafari E, Akbari and Javar H 2020 Pharmaceutical implants: classification, limitations and therapeutic applications *Pharm. Dev. Technol.* **25** 116–32
[9] Gaudana R, Ananthula H K, Parenky A and Mitra A K 2010 Ocular drug delivery *AAPS J.* **12** 348–60
[10] Wong I, Teoh S, Yeoh A and Lingam G 2013 Sustained-release ganciclovir implant as prophylaxis for cytomegalovirus retinitis in a child undergoing bone marrow transplantation *Eye.* **27** 890–1
[11] De Oliveira L G, Figueiredo L A, Fernandes-Cunha G M, Machado L A and Dasilva G R 2015 Methotrexate locally released from poly (ε-caprolactone) implants: inhibition of the inflammatory angiogenesis response in a murine sponge model and the absence of systemic toxicity *J. Pharm. Sci.* **104** 3731–42
[12] Benagiano G, Gabelnick H and Farris M 2008 Contraceptive devices: intravaginal and intrauterine delivery systems *Exp. Rev. Med. Devices* **5** 639–54
[13] Bourges J, Bloquel C, Thomas A, Froussart F, Bochot A and Azan F *et al* 2006 Intraocular implants for extended drug delivery: therapeutic applications *Adv. Drug Delivery Rev.* **58** 1182–202
[14] Bottros M M and Christo P J 2014 Current perspectives on intrathecal drug delivery *J. Pain Res.* **6** 615–26
[15] Jang J-S, Song Y-J, Kang W, Jin H-Y, Seo J-S and Yang T-H *et al* 2014 Intravascular ultrasound-guided implantation of drug-eluting stents to improve outcome: a meta-analysis *JACC: Cardiovasc. Interv.* **7** 233–43
[16] Eriguchi N, Aoyagi S, Okuda K, Tamae T, Fukuda S and Kanazawa N *et al* 2000 Successful surgical treatment for implanted intraperitoneal metastases of hepatocellular carcinoma *J. Hepato-Biliary-Pancreat. Surg.* **7** 520–3
[17] Gernert M and Feja M 2020 Bypassing the blood–brain barrier: direct intracranial drug delivery in epilepsies *Pharmaceutics* **12** 1134
[18] Fumimoto Y, Matsuyama A, Komoda H, Okura H, Lee C M and Nagao A *et al* 2009 Creation of a rich subcutaneous vascular network with implanted adipose tissue–derived stromal cells and adipose tissue enhances subcutaneous grafting of islets in diabetic mice *Tissue Eng. Part C: Methods* **15** 437–44
[19] Pons-Faudoa F P, Ballerini A, Sakamoto J and Grattoni A 2019 Advanced implantable drug delivery technologies: transforming the clinical landscape of therapeutics for chronic diseases *Biomed. Microdev.* **21** 1–22
[20] Allyn M M, Luo R H, Hellwarth E B and Swindle-Reilly K E 2022 Considerations for polymers used in ocular drug delivery *Front. Med.* **8** 2963
[21] Ibach M J, Zimprich L, Wallin D D, Olevson C, Puls-Boever K and Thompson V 2022 In clinic optometrist insertion of dextenza (dexamethasone ophthalmic insert 0.4 mg) prior to cataract surgery: the PREPARE study *Clin. Ophthalmol.* **16** 2609–15

[22] Moshirfar M, Milner D and Patel B C 2020 *Cataract Surgery* (Treasure Island, FL: StatPearls Publishing)
[23] Lee A and Blair H A 2020 Dexamethasone intracanalicular insert: a review in treating post-surgical ocular pain and inflammation *Drugs* **80** 1101–8
[24] Gupta P, Zhao D, Guallar E, Ko F, Boland M V and Friedman D S 2016 Prevalence of glaucoma in the United States: the 2005–2008 national health and nutrition examination survey *Invest. Ophthalmol. Vis. Sci.* **57** 2905–13
[25] Sirinek P E and Lin M M (ed) 2022 Intracameral sustained release bimatoprost implants (Durysta) *Seminars in Ophthalmology* (Taylor and Francis)
[26] Claes L and Ignatius A 2002 Development of new, biodegradable implants *Der Chirurg* **73** 990–6
[27] Balakrishnan P, Geethamma V, Sreekala M S and Thomas S 2018 *Polymeric Biomaterials: State-of-the-Art and New Challenges. Fundamental Biomaterials: Polymers* (Amsterdam: Elsevier) pp 1–20
[28] Bîrcă A, Gherasim O, Grumezescu V and Grumezescu A M 2019 Introduction in thermoplastic and thermosetting polymers *Materials for Biomedical Engineering* (Amsterdam: Elsevier) pp 1–28
[29] Prajapati V D, Jani G K and Kapadia J R 2015 Current knowledge on biodegradable microspheres in drug delivery *Expert Opin. Drug Deliv.* **12** 1283–99
[30] Zhao K, Li D, Shi C, Ma X, Rong G and Kang H *et al* 2016 Biodegradable polymeric nanoparticles as the delivery carrier for drug *Curr. Drug Deliv.* **13** 494–9
[31] Makadia H K and Siegel S J 2011 Poly lactic-co-glycolic acid (PLGA) as biodegradable controlled drug delivery carrier *Polymers.* **3** 1377–97
[32] Lunt J 1998 Large-scale production, properties and commercial applications of polylactic acid polymers *Polym. Degrad. Stab.* **59** 145–52
[33] Lowe C E 1954 Preparation of high molecular weight polyhydroxyacetic ester *Google Patents* US277726A
[34] Farah S, Anderson D G and Langer R 2016 Physical and mechanical properties of PLA, and their functions in widespread applications—a comprehensive review *Adv. Drug Delivery Rev.* **107** 367–92
[35] Xiao L, Wang B, Yang G and Gauthier M 2012 Poly (lactic acid)-based biomaterials: synthesis, modification and applications *Biomed. Sci. Eng. Technol.* **11** 247–82
[36] Saeidlou S, Huneault M A, Li H and Park C B 2012 Poly (lactic acid) crystallization *Prog. Polym. Sci.* **37** 1657–77
[37] Fukushima K, Hirata M and Kimura Y 2007 Synthesis and characterization of stereoblock poly (lactic acid)s with nonequivalent D/L sequence ratios *Macromolecules* **40** 3049–55
[38] Fang Q and Hanna M A 1999 Rheological properties of amorphous and semicrystalline polylactic acid polymers *Ind. Crops Prod.* **10** 47–53
[39] Hamad K, Kaseem M and Deri F 2011 Rheological and mechanical characterization of poly (lactic acid)/polypropylene polymer blends *J. Polym. Res.* **18** 1799–806
[40] NatureWorks L 2005 *Sheet Extrusion Processing Guide* (NatureWorks LLC: Minnetonka, MN)
[41] Carrasco F, Cailloux J, Sánchez-Jiménez P and Maspoch M L 2014 Improvement of the thermal stability of branched poly (lactic acid) obtained by reactive extrusion *Polym. Degrad. Stab.* **104** 40–9

[42] Bi H, Feng T, Li B and Han Y 2020 In vitro and *in vivo* comparison study of electrospun PLA and PLA/PVA/SA fiber membranes for wound healing *Polymers* **12** 839
[43] Grémare A, Guduric V, Bareille R, Heroguez V, Latour S and L'heureux N *et al* 2018 Characterization of printed PLA scaffolds for bone tissue engineering *J. Biomed. Mater. Res.* A **106** 887–94
[44] Zhao C, Wu H, Ni J, Zhang S and Zhang X 2017 Development of PLA/Mg composite for orthopedic implant: tunable degradation and enhanced mineralization *Compos. Sci. Technol.* **147** 8–15
[45] Vlachopoulos A, Karlioti G, Balla E, Daniilidis V, Kalamas T and Stefanidou M *et al* 2022 Poly (lactic acid)-based microparticles for drug delivery applications: an overview of recent *Adv. Pharm.* **14** 359
[46] Singh V and Tiwari M 2010 Structure-processing-property relationship of poly (glycolic acid) for drug delivery systems 1: synthesis and catalysis *Int. J. Polym. Sci.* **2010**
[47] Schmitt E E and Polistina R 1969 Polyglycolic acid prosthetic devices *US Patent* 3463158 Frazza E J and Schmitt E E 1971 A new absorbable suture *J. Biomed. Mater. Res. Symp.* **5** 43–58
[48] Williams D 1982 Biodegradation of surgical polymers *J. Mater. Sci.* **17** 1233–46
[49] Maurus P B and Kaeding C C 2004 Bioabsorbable implant material review *Oper. Tech. Sports. Med.* **12** 158–60
[50] Muddineti O S and Omri A 2022 Current trends in PLGA based long-acting injectable products: the industry perspective *Expert Opin. Drug Deliv.* **19** 559–76
[51] Dechy-Cabaret O, Martin-Vaca B and Bourissou D 2004 Controlled ring-opening polymerization of lactide and glycolide *Chem. Rev.* **104** 6147–76
[52] Gentile P, Chiono V, Carmagnola I and Hatton P V 2014 An overview of poly (lactic-co-glycolic) acid (PLGA)-based biomaterials for bone tissue engineering *Int. J. Mol. Sci.* **15** 3640–59
[53] Stewart S A, Domínguez-Robles J, Donnelly R F and Larrañeta E 2018 Implantable polymeric drug delivery devices: classification, manufacture, materials, and clinical applications *Polymers* **10** 1379
[54] Danhier F, Ansorena E, Silva J M, Coco R, Le Breton A and Préat V 2012 PLGA-based nanoparticles: an overview of biomedical applications *J. Control. Release* **161** 505–22
[55] FJv N, Hill J W and Carothers W H 1934 Studies of polymerization and ring formation. XXIII. 1 ε-Caprolactone and its polymers . *J. Am. Chem. Soc.* **56** 455–7
[56] Okada M 2002 Chemical syntheses of biodegradable polymers *Prog. Polym. Sci.* **27** 87–133
[57] Nair L S and Laurencin C T 2007 Biodegradable polymers as biomaterials *Prog. Polym. Sci.* **32** 762–98
[58] Merkli A, Tabatabay C, Gurny R and Heller J 1998 Biodegradable polymers for the controlled release of ocular drugs *Prog. Polym. Sci.* **23** 563–80
[59] Woodruff M A and Hutmacher D W 2010 The return of a forgotten polymer—polycaprolactone in the 21st century *Prog. Polym. Sci.* **35** 1217–56
[60] Escobar Ivirico J L, Salmeron Sanchez M, Sabater i Serra R, Meseguer Duenas J M, Gomez Ribelles J L and Monleón Pradas M 2006 Structure and properties of poly (ε-caprolactone) networks with modulated water uptake *Macromol. Chem. Phys.* **207** 2195–205
[61] Sabater i Serra R, Escobar Ivirico J, Meseguer Dueñas J, Andrio Balado A, Gómez Ribelles J and Salmerón Sánchez M 2007 Dielectric relaxation spectrum of poly

(ε-caprolactone) networks hydrophilized by copolymerization with 2-hydroxyethyl acrylate *Eur. Phys. J.* E **22** 293–302

[62] Castilla-Cortázar I, Más-Estellés J, Meseguer-Dueñas J M, Ivirico J E, Marí B and Vidaurre A 2012 Hydrolytic and enzymatic degradation of a poly (ε-caprolactone) network *Polym. Degrad. Stab.* **97** 1241–8

[63] Uhrich K E, Cannizzaro S M, Langer R S and Shakesheff K M 1999 Polymeric systems for controlled drug release *Chem. Rev.* **99** 3181–98

[64] Lakshmi S, Katti D and Laurencin C 2003 Biodegradable polyphosphazenes for drug delivery applications *Adv. Drug Delivery Rev.* **55** 467–82

[65] Doppalapudi S, Jain A, Khan W and Domb A J 2014 Biodegradable polymers—an overview *Polym. Adv. Technol.* **25** 427–35

[66] Khalid Z, Ali S and Akram M 2018 Review on polyphosphazenes-based materials for bone and skeleton tissue engineering *Int. J. Polym. Mater. Poly. Biomater.* **67** 693–701

[67] Rahimi A and Mashak A 2013 Review on rubbers in medicine: matural, silicone and polyurethane rubbers *Plast. Rubber Compos.* **42** 223–30

[68] McMillin C R 1994 Elastomers for biomedical applications *Rubber Chem. Technol.* **67** 417–46

[69] Keshvari H, Ourang F, Mirzadeh H, Khorasani M and Mansouri P 2008 Collagen immobilization onto acrylic acid laser-grafted silicone for using as artificial skin: *in vitro* *Iran. Polymer J.* **17** 14965–115

[70] Okada T and Ikada Y 1991 Modification of silicone surface by graft polymerization of acrylamide with corona discharge *Makromol. Chem.: Macromol. Chem. Phys.* **192** 1705–13

[71] Abbasi F, Mirzadeh H and Katbab A A 2002 Bulk and surface modification of silicone rubber for biomedical applications *Polym. Int.* **51** 882–8

[72] Foye W O 2008 *Foye's Principles of Medicinal Chemistry* (Lippincott Williams & Wilkins)

[73] Touitou E and Barry B W 2006 *Enhancement in Drug Delivery* (Boca Raton, FL: CRC Press)

[74] Salyer I and Kenyon A 1971 Structure and property relationships in ethylene–vinyl acetate copolymers *J. Polym. Sci. Part A-1: Polym. Chem.* **9** 3083–103

[75] Zhang Q, Lin W, Yang G and Chen Q 2002 Studies on the phase structure of ethylene-vinyl acetate copolymers by solid-state 1H and 13C NMR *J. Polym. Sci., Part B: Polym. Phys.* **40** 2199–207

[76] Brogly M, Nardin M and Schultz J 1997 Effect of vinylacetate content on crystallinity and second-order transitions in ethylene–vinylacetate copolymers *J. Appl. Polym. Sci.* **64** 1903–12

[77] Arsac A, Carrot C and Guillet J 2000 Determination of primary relaxation temperatures and melting points of ethylene vinyl acetate copolymers *J. Therm. Anal. Calorim.* **61** 681–5

[78] Almeida A, Possemiers S, Boone M, De Beer T, Quinten T and Van Hoorebeke L *et al* 2011 Ethylene vinyl acetate as matrix for oral sustained release dosage forms produced via hot-melt extrusion *Eur. J. Pharm. Biopharm.* **77** 297–305

[79] Schneider C, Langer R, Loveday D and Hair D 2017 Applications of ethylene vinyl acetate copolymers (EVA) in drug delivery systems *J. Control. Release* **262** 284–95

[80] Persico A M, Calia E and Keller F 1997 Implants for sustained drug release over the somatosensory cortex of the newborn rat: a comparison of materials and surgical procedures *J. Neurosci. Methods* **76** 105–13

[81] Langer R, Brem H and Tapper D 1981 Biocompatibility of polymeric delivery systems for macromolecules *J. Biomed. Mater. Res.* **15** 267–77
[82] Gokhale A, McConnell J, Loxley A and Mitchnick M 2009 Combination devices to protect women from sexual transmission of HIV *Drug Deliv. Technol.* **9** 18–21
[83] Tambe S, Singh S, Patri M and Kumar D 2008 Ethylene vinyl acetate and ethylene vinyl alcohol copolymer for thermal spray coating application *Prog. Org. Coat.* **62** 382–6
[84] Massey L 2005 *The Effect of Sterilization Methods on Plastics and Elastomers* (New York: William Andrew)
[85] Fischer M A 2008 Implanon: a new contraceptive implant *J. Obst. Gynecol. Neonatal Nurs.* **37** 361–8
[86] Palomba S, Falbo A, Di Cello A, Materazzo C and Zullo F 2012 Nexplanon: the new implant for long-term contraception. A comprehensive descriptive review *Gynecol. Endocrinol.* **28** 710–21
[87] Itzoe M and Guarnieri M 2017 New developments in managing opioid addiction: impact of a subdermal buprenorphine implant *Drug Des. Devel. Ther.* **10** 1429–37
[88] Lavik E, Kuehn M and Kwon Y 2011 Novel drug delivery systems for glaucoma *Eye* **25** 578–86
[89] Anselmo A C and Mitragotri S 2014 An overview of clinical and commercial impact of drug delivery systems *J. Control. Release* **190** 15–28
[90] Syed Y Y 2017 Fluocinolone acetonide intravitreal implant 0.19 mg (ILUVIEN®): a review in diabetic macular edema *Drugs* **77** 575–83
[91] Roumen F J and Mishell D R 2012 The contraceptive vaginal ring, NuvaRing®, a decade after its introduction *Eur. J. Contracep. Reprod. Health Care* **17** 415–27
[92] Pharriss B B, Erickson R, Bashaw J, Hoff S, Place V A and Zaffaroni A 1974 Progestasert: a uterine therapeutic system for long-term contraception: I. Philosophy and clinical efficacy *Fertil. Steril.* **25** 915–21
[93] Basu A, Farah S, Kunduru K, Doppalapudi S, Khan W and Domb A 2016 Polyurethanes for controlled drug delivery *Advances in Polyurethane Biomaterials* (Cambridge: Woodhead) pp 217–46
[94] Bayer O 1947 Das di-isocyanat-polyadditionsverfahren (polyurethane) *Angew. Chem.* **59** 257–72
[95] Irusta L and Fernandez-Berridi M 2000 Aromatic poly (ester–urethanes): effect of the polyol molecular weight on the photochemical behaviour *Polymer* **41** 3297–302
[96] Ibarboure E, Baron A, Papon E and Rodriguez-Hernandez J 2009 Self-assembly of graft polyurethanes having both crystallizable poly (ε-caprolactone) blocks and soft poly (n-butyl acrylate) segments *Thin Solid Films* **517** 3281–6
[97] Kim B S and Kim B K 2005 Enhancement of hydrolytic stability and adhesion of waterborne polyurethanes *J. Appl. Polym. Sci.* **97** 1961–9
[98] Ping P, Wang W, Chen X and Jing X 2007 The influence of hard-segments on two-phase structure and shape memory properties of PCL-based segmented polyurethanes *J. Polym. Sci., Part B: Polym. Phys.* **45** 557–70
[99] Caracciolo P C, Buffa F and Abraham G A 2009 Effect of the hard segment chemistry and structure on the thermal and mechanical properties of novel biomedical segmented poly (esterurethanes) *J. Mater. Sci., Mater. Med.* **20** 145–55
[100] Cherng J Y, Hou T Y, Shih M F, Talsma H and Hennink W E 2013 Polyurethane-based drug delivery systems *Int. J. Pharm.* **450** 145–62

[101] Johnson T J, Gupta K M, Fabian J, Albright T H and Kiser P F 2010 Segmented polyurethane intravaginal rings for the sustained combined delivery of antiretroviral agents dapivirine and tenofovir *Eur. J. Pharm. Sci.* **39** 203–12

[102] Yu L, Zhou L, Ding M, Li J, Tan H and Fu Q *et al* 2011 Synthesis and characterization of novel biodegradable folate conjugated polyurethanes *J. Colloid Interface Sci.* **358** 376–83

[103] Aranaz I, Mengíbar M, Harris R, Paños I, Miralles B and Acosta N *et al* 2009 Functional characterization of chitin and chitosan *Curr. Chem. Biol.* **3** 203–30

[104] El Knidri H, Belaabed R, Addaou A, Laajeb A and Lahsini A 2018 Extraction, chemical modification and characterization of chitin and chitosan *Int. J. Biol. Macromol.* **120** 1181–9

[105] Iber B T, Kasan N A, Torsabo D and Omuwa J W 2022 A review of various sources of chitin and chitosan in nature *J. Renew. Mater.* **10** 1097

[106] Pandey A R, Singh U S, Momin M and Bhavsar C 2017 Chitosan: application in tissue engineering and skin grafting *J. Polym. Res.* **24** 1–22

[107] Chopin N, Guillory X, Weiss P, Bideau J L and Colliec-Jouault S 2014 Design polysaccharides of marine origin: chemical modifications to reach advanced versatile compounds *Curr. Org. Chem.* **18** 867–95

[108] Roderick M R, Sen E S and Ramanan A V 2018 Chronic recurrent multifocal osteomyelitis in children and adults: current understanding and areas for development *Rheumatology* **57** 41–8

[109] Tao F, Ma S, Tao H, Jin L, Luo Y and Zheng J *et al* 2021 Chitosan-based drug delivery systems: from synthesis strategy to osteomyelitis treatment—a review *Carbohydr. Polym.* **251** 117063

[110] Sah A K, Dewangan M and Suresh P K 2019 Potential of chitosan-based carrier for periodontal drug delivery *Colloids Surf.* B **178** 185–98

[111] Marchessault R and Sundararajan P 1983 *Cellulose. The Polysaccharides* (Amsterdam: Elsevier) pp 11–95

[112] Alavi M and Nokhodchi A 2020 Antimicrobial and wound treatment aspects of micro-and nanoformulations of carboxymethyl, dialdehyde, and TEMPO-oxidized derivatives of cellulose *Rec. Adv. Macromol. Biosci.* **20** 1900362

[113] Mischnick P and Momcilovic D 2010 Chemical structure analysis of starch and cellulose derivatives *Adv. Carbohydr. Chem. Biochem.* **64** 117–210

[114] Hopson C, Villar-Chavero M M, Domínguez J C, Alonso M V, Oliet M and Rodriguez F 2021 Cellulose ionogels, a perspective of the last decade: a review *Carbohydr. Polym.* **274** 118663

[115] Hu W, Chen S, Yang J, Li Z and Wang H 2014 Functionalized bacterial cellulose derivatives and nanocomposites *Carbohydr. Polym.* **101** 1043–60

[116] Dai L, Cheng T, Duan C, Zhao W, Zhang W and Zou X *et al* 2019 3D printing using plant-derived cellulose and its derivatives: a review *Carbohydr. Polym.* **203** 71–86

[117] Oprea M and Voicu S I 2020 Recent advances in composites based on cellulose derivatives for biomedical applications *Carbohydr. Polym.* **247** 116683

[118] Ogrizek L, Lamovšek J, Čuš F, Leskovšek M and Gorjanc M 2021 Properties of bacterial cellulose produced using white and red grape bagasse as a nutrient source *Processes* **9** 1088

[119] Ullah H, Santos H A and Khan T 2016 Applications of bacterial cellulose in food, cosmetics and drug delivery *Cellulose.* **23** 2291–314

[120] Laezza A, Pepe A and Bochicchio B 2022 Elastin-hyaluronan bioconjugate as bioactive component in electrospun scaffolds *Chem. Eur.* J **28** e202201959

[121] Salwowska N M, Bebenek K A, Żądło D A and Wcisło-Dziadecka D L 2016 Physiochemical properties and application of hyaluronic acid: a systematic review *J. Cosmet. Dermatol* **15** 520–6
[122] Safari A, Cervantes M J and Emami N 2016 Viscoelastic behaviour effect of hyaluronic acid on reciprocating flow inside mini-channel *Lubr. Sci.* **28** 521–44
[123] Rwei S-P, Chen S-W, Mao C-F and Fang H-W 2008 Viscoelasticity and wearability of hyaluronate solutions *Biochem. Eng. J.* **40** 211–7
[124] Guter M and Breunig M 2017 Hyaluronan as a promising excipient for ocular drug delivery *Eur. J. Pharm. Biopharm.* **113** 34–49
[125] Spadea A, Rios de la Rosa J M, Tirella A, Ashford M B, Williams K J and Stratford I J *et al* 2019 Evaluating the efficiency of hyaluronic acid for tumor targeting via CD44 *Mol. Pharm.* **16** 2481–93
[126] Mondalek F G, Fung K-M, Yang Q, Wu W, Lu W and Palmer B W *et al* 2015 Temporal expression of hyaluronic acid and hyaluronic acid receptors in a porcine small intestinal submucosa-augmented rat bladder regeneration model *World J. Urol.* **33** 1119–28
[127] Bhattacharya S, Ghosh A, Maiti S, Ahir M, Debnath G H and Gupta P *et al* 2020 Delivery of thymoquinone through hyaluronic acid-decorated mixed Pluronic® nanoparticles to attenuate angiogenesis and metastasis of triple-negative breast cancer *J. Control. Release* **322** 357–74
[128] Price R D, Myers S, Leigh I M and Navsaria H A 2005 The role of hyaluronic acid in wound healing: assessment of clinical evidence *Am. J. Clin. Dermatol* **6** 393–402
[129] Tiwari S and Bahadur P 2019 Modified hyaluronic acid based materials for biomedical applications *Int. J. Biol. Macromol.* **121** 556–71
[130] Vorvolakos K, Isayeva I S, Luu H-M D, Patwardhan D V and Pollack S K 2011 Ionically cross-linked hyaluronic acid: wetting, lubrication, and viscoelasticity of a modified adhesion barrier gel *Med. Devices: Evid. Res.* **4** 1–10
[131] Burdick J A and Prestwich G D 2011 Hyaluronic acid hydrogels for biomedical applications *Adv Mater.* **23** H41
[132] Highley C B, Prestwich G D and Burdick J A 2016 Recent advances in hyaluronic acid hydrogels for biomedical applications *Curr. Opin. Biotechnol.* **40** 35–40
[133] Bayer I S 2020 Hyaluronic acid and controlled release: a review *Molecules* **25** 2649
[134] Akbari E, Imani R, Shokrollahi P and Heidari keshel S 2022 Corneal sustained delivery of hyaluronic acid from nanofiber-containing ring-implanted contact lens *J. Biomater Appl.* **37** 992–1006
[135] Lai J-Y, Ma D H-K, Cheng H-Y, Sun C-C, Huang S-J and Li Y-T *et al* 2010 Ocular biocompatibility of carbodiimide cross-linked hyaluronic acid hydrogels for cell sheet delivery carriers *J. Biomater. Sci. Polym. Ed.* **21** 359–76
[136] Voss K, Falke K, Bernsdorf A, Grabow N, Kastner C and Sternberg K *et al* 2015 Development of a novel injectable drug delivery system for subconjunctival glaucoma treatment *J. Control. Release* **214** 1–11
[137] Gold M 2009 The science and art of hyaluronic acid dermal filler use in esthetic applications *J. Cosmet. Dermatol* **8** 301–7
[138] Romagnoli M and Belmontesi M 2008 Hyaluronic acid–based fillers: theory and practice *Clin. Dermatol* **26** 123–59

[139] Gong W, Liu Y, Mei D-Y, Yang M and Mei X-G 2015 Preparation, release and pharmacokinetics of a risperidone elementary osmotic pump system *Drug Dev. Ind. Pharm.* **41** 464–9

[140] Staples M, Daniel K, Cima M J and Langer R 2006 Application of micro-and nano-electromechanical devices to drug delivery *Pharm. Res.* **23** 847–63

[141] Lee M Y, Lee J H, Lee H S, Choi J-J, Jang J and Choi H *et al* 2015 Continuous topical drug delivery using osmotic pump in animal cochlear implant model: continuous steroid delivery is effective for hearing preservation *Acta Oto-Laryngologica* **135** 791–8

[142] Jerzewski R L and Chien Y W 2017 Osmotic drug delivery *Treatise on Controlled Drug Delivery* (Boca Raton, FL: CRC Press) pp 225–53

[143] Almoshari Y 2022 Osmotic pump drug delivery systems—a comprehensive review *Pharmaceuticals* **15** 1430

[144] Lee P I and Li J X 2010 *Evolution of Oral Controlled Release Dosage forms. Oral Controlled Release Formulation Design and Drug Delivery* (New York: Wiley) pp 21–31

[145] Stevenson C L, Santini J T and Langer R 2012 Reservoir-based drug delivery systems utilizing microtechnology *Adv. Drug Delivery Rev.* **64** 1590–602

[146] Fowler J E, Flanagan M, Gleason D M, Klimberg I W, Gottesman J E and Sharifi R 2000 Evaluation of an implant that delivers leuprolide for 1 year for the palliative treatment of prostate cancer *Urology* **55** 639–42

[147] Gullapalli R, Wong A, Brigham E, Kwong G, Wadsworth A and Willits C *et al* 2012 Development of ALZET® osmotic pump compatible solvent compositions to solubilize poorly soluble compounds for preclinical studies *Drug Deliv.* **19** 239–46

[148] Sharma A, Kumar D and Painuly N 2018 A review on osmotically controlled drug delivery systems *Asian J. Pharm. Res. Dev.* **6** 101–9

[149] D'Orsay D B, DeWitty R L and Dennis G C 1987 The Infusaid pump in the management of intractable cancer pain *J. Natl. Med. Assoc.* **79** 305

[150] Fialho S L and Silva Cunha A 2005 Manufacturing techniques of biodegradable implants intended for intraocular application *Drug Deliv.* **12** 109–16

[151] Simões M F, Pinto R M and Simões S 2019 Hot-melt extrusion in the pharmaceutical industry: toward filing a new drug application *Drug Discov. Today* **24** 1749–68

[152] Chaturvedi K, Gajera B Y, Xu T, Shah H and Dave R H 2018 Influence of processing methods on physico-mechanical properties of Ibuprofen/HPC-SSL formulation *Pharm. Dev. Technol.* **23** 1108–16

[153] Vo A Q, Feng X, Pimparade M, Ye X, Kim D W and Martin S T *et al* 2017 Dual-mechanism gastroretentive drug delivery system loaded with an amorphous solid dispersion prepared by hot-melt extrusion *Eur. J. Pharm. Sci.* **102** 71–84

[154] Pimparade M B, Vo A, Maurya A S, Bae J, Morott J T and Feng X *et al* 2017 Development and evaluation of an oral fast disintegrating anti-allergic film using hot-melt extrusion technology *Eur. J. Pharm. Biopharm.* **119** 81–90

[155] Crowley M M, Zhang F, Koleng J J and McGinity J W 2002 Stability of polyethylene oxide in matrix tablets prepared by hot-melt extrusion *Biomaterials* **23** 4241–8

[156] Cossé A, König C, Lamprecht A and Wagner K G 2017 Hot melt extrusion for sustained protein release: matrix erosion and *in vitro* release of PLGA-based implants *AAPS PharmSciTech.* **18** 15–26

[157] Tadmor Z and Klein I 1970 *Engineering Principles of Plasticating Extrusion* (New York: Van Nostrand Reinhold Company)

[158] Serajuddin A T 1999 Solid dispersion of poorly water-soluble drugs: early promises, subsequent problems, and recent breakthroughs *J. Pharm. Sci.* **88** 1058–66
[159] Shah R D, Kabadi M, Pope D G and Augsburger L L 1994 Physicomechanical characterization of the extrusion-spheronization process. I. Instrumentation of the extruder *Pharm. Res.* **11** 355–60
[160] Breitenbach J 2002 Melt extrusion: from process to drug delivery technology *Eur. J. Pharm. Biopharm.* **54** 107–17
[161] LAARHOVEN V A N and Vromans J H 2003 H. Influence of supersaturation on the release properties of a controlled release device based on EVA copolymers *J. Control. Release* **87** 210–3
[162] Ganesh K, Yang S, Schillace S, Vita V, Wang Y and Ehmann K F *et al* 2022 A review of manufacturing techniques for subcutaneous drug delivery implants *Procedia CIRP* **110** 329–34
[163] Jivraj M, Martini L G and Thomson C M 2000 An overview of the different excipients useful for the direct compression of tablets *Pharm. Sci. Technol. Today* **3** 58–63
[164] Rothen-Weinhold A, Besseghir K, Vuaridel E, Sublet E, Oudry N and Kubel F *et al* 1999 Injection-molding versus extrusion as manufacturing technique for the preparation of biodegradable implants *Eur. J. Pharm. Biopharm.* **48** 113–21
[165] Norman J, Madurawe R D, Moore C M, Khan M A and Khairuzzaman A 2017 A new chapter in pharmaceutical manufacturing: 3D-printed drug products *Adv. Drug Delivery Rev.* **108** 39–50
[166] Kotta S, Nair A and Alsabeelah N 2018 3D printing technology in drug delivery: recent progress and application *Curr. Pharm. Des.* **24** 5039–48
[167] Prasad L K and Smyth H 2016 3D Printing technologies for drug delivery: a review *Drug Dev. Ind. Pharm.* **42** 1019–31
[168] Wu W, Ye C, Zheng Q, Wu G and Cheng Z 2016 A therapeutic delivery system for chronic osteomyelitis via a multi-drug implant based on three-dimensional printing technology *J. Biomater. Appl.* **31** 250–60
[169] Yang N, Chen H, Han H, Shen Y, Gu S and He Y *et al* 2018 3D printing and coating to fabricate a hollow bullet-shaped implant with porous surface for controlled cytoxan release *Int. J. Pharm.* **552** 91–8
[170] Wu D-Q and Chu C-C 2008 Biodegradable hydrophobic–hydrophilic hybrid hydrogels: swelling behavior and controlled drug release *J. Biomater. Sci. Polym. Ed.* **19** 411–29
[171] Soo P L, Cho J, Grant J, Ho E, Piquette-Miller M and Allen C 2008 Drug release mechanism of paclitaxel from a chitosan–lipid implant system: effect of swelling, degradation and morphology *Eur. J. Pharm. Biopharm.* **69** 149–57
[172] Siepmann J and Siepmann F 2008 Mathematical modeling of drug delivery *Int. J. Pharm.* **364** 328–43
[173] Fu Y and Kao W J 2010 Drug release kinetics and transport mechanisms of non-degradable and degradable polymeric delivery systems *Exp. Opin. Drug Deliv.* **7** 429–44
[174] Tobias I S, Lee H, Engelmayr G C, Macaya D, Bettinger C J and Cima M J 2010 Zero-order controlled release of ciprofloxacin-HCl from a reservoir-based, bioresorbable and elastomeric device *J. Control. Release* **146** 356–62
[175] Huang X and Brazel C S 2001 On the importance and mechanisms of burst release in matrix-controlled drug delivery systems *J. Control. Release* **73** 121–36

[176] Watkins E S 2010 From breakthrough to bust: the brief life of Norplant, the contraceptive implant *J. Women's Hist.* **22** 88–111
[177] Mansour D, Inki P and Gemzell-Danielsson K 2010 Efficacy of contraceptive methods: a review of the literature *Eur. J. Contracept. Reprod. Health Care* **15** 4–16
[178] Sivin I, Wan L, Ranta S, Alvarez F, Brache V and Mishell D R *et al* 2001 Levonorgestrel concentrations during 7 years of continuous use of Jadelle contraceptive implants *Contraception* **64** 43–9
[179] Karp D R, Jean-Michel M, Johnston Y, Suciu G, Aguilar V C and Davila G W 2012 A randomized clinical trial of the impact of local estrogen on postoperative tissue quality after vaginal reconstructive surgery *Urogynecology* **18** 211–5
[180] Ibe C and Simon J A 2010 Continuing medical education: vulvovaginal atrophy: current and future therapies (CME) *J. Sex. Med.* **7** 1042–50
[181] Thurman A R, Clark M R, Hurlburt J A and Doncel G F 2013 Intravaginal rings as delivery systems for microbicides and multipurpose prevention technologies *Int. J. Women's Health* **5** 695–708
[182] Stabile G, Foti C, Mordeglia D, De Santo D, Mangino F P and Laganà A S *et al* 2022 Alternative insertion site of nexplanon: description of a case report and systematic review of the literature *J. Clin. Med.* **11** 3226
[183] El-Ghrably I, Steel D H, Habib M, Vaideanu-Collins D, Manvikar S and Hillier R J 2017 Diabetic macular edema outcomes in eyes treated with fluocinolone acetonide 0.2 μg/d intravitreal implant: real-world UK experience *Eur. J. Ophthalmol.* **27** 357–62
[184] Taban M, Lowder C Y and Kaiser P K 2008 Outcome of fluocinolone acetonide implant (Retisert™) reimplantation for chronic noninfectious posterior uveitis *Retina* **28** 1280–8
[185] Kang-Mieler J J, Rudeen K M, Liu W and Mieler W F 2020 Advances in ocular drug delivery systems *Eye* **34** 1371–9
[186] Barar J, Aghanejad A, Fathi M and Omidi Y 2016 Advanced drug delivery and targeting technologies for the ocular diseases *Bioimpacts* **6** 49–67
[187] Pielen A, Feltgen N, Isserstedt C, Callizo J, Junker B and Schmucker C 2013 Efficacy and safety of intravitreal therapy in macular edema due to branch and central retinal vein occlusion: a systematic review *PLoS One* **8** e78538
[188] Shirley M 2020 Bimatoprost implant: first approval *Drugs Aging* **37** 457–62
[189] Engels F K, Mathot R A and Verweij J 2007 Alternative drug formulations of docetaxel: a review *Anti-Cancer Drugs* **18** 95–103
[190] Merisko-Liversidge E, Sarpotdar P, Bruno J, Hajj S, Wei L and Peltier N *et al* 1996 Formulation and antitumor activity evaluation of nanocrystalline suspensions of poorly soluble anticancer drugs *Pharm. Res.* **13** 272–8
[191] Gelderblom H, Verweij J, Nooter K and Sparreboom A 2001 Cremophor EL: the drawbacks and advantages of vehicle selection for drug formulation *Eur. J. Cancer* **37** 1590–8
[192] Zhang J A, Anyarambhatla G, Ma L, Ugwu S, Xuan T and Sardone T *et al* 2005 Development and characterization of a novel Cremophor® EL free liposome-based paclitaxel (LEP-ETU) formulation *Eur. J. Pharm. Biopharm.* **59** 177–87
[193] Saadat E, Amini M, Khoshayand M R, Dinarvand R and Dorkoosh F A 2014 Synthesis and optimization of a novel polymeric micelle based on hyaluronic acid and phospholipids for delivery of paclitaxel, *in vitro* and *in-vivo* evaluation *Int. J. Pharm.* **475** 163–73

[194] Chen D-B, Yang T-Z, Lu W-L and ZHANG Q 2001 In vitro and *in vivo* study of two types of long-circulating solid lipid nanoparticles containing paclitaxel *Chem. Pharm. Bull.* **49** 1444–7

[195] Hiremath J G, Khamar N S, Palavalli S G, Rudani C G, Aitha R and Mura P 2013 Paclitaxel loaded carrier based biodegradable polymeric implants: preparation and *in vitro* characterization *Saudi Pharm.* J **21** 85–91

[196] Kannan S and Nallaiyan R 2020 Anticancer activity of Samarium-coated magnesium implants for immunocompromised patients *ACS Appl. Bio Mater.* **3** 4408–16

[197] Maher S, Kaur G, Lima-Marques L, Evdokiou A and Losic D 2017 Engineering of micro-to nanostructured 3D-printed drug-releasing titanium implants for enhanced osseointegration and localized delivery of anticancer drugs *ACS Appl. Mater. Interfaces* **9** 29562–70

[198] Wang Y, Sun L, Mei Z, Zhang F, He M and Fletcher C *et al* 2020 3D printed biodegradable implants as an individualized drug delivery system for local chemotherapy of osteosarcoma *Mater. Des.* **186** 108336

[199] Johnson A R, Forster S P, White D, Terife G, Lowinger M and Teller R S *et al* 2021 Drug eluting implants in pharmaceutical development and clinical practice *Exp. Opin. Drug Deliv.* **18** 577–93

[200] Weber G F 2015 Hormone therapy *Molecular Therapies of Cancer* (Springer) pp 303–32

[201] Noguchi S, Kim H J, Jesena A, Parmar V, Sato N and Wang H-C *et al* 2016 Phase 3, open-label, randomized study comparing 3-monthly with monthly goserelin in pre-menopausal women with estrogen receptor-positive advanced breast cancer *Breast Cancer* **23** 771–9

[202] Roux A, Caire F, Guyotat J, Menei P, Metellus P and Pallud J 2017 Carmustine wafer implantation for high-grade gliomas: evidence-based safety efficacy and practical recommendations from the Neuro-oncology Club of the French Society of Neurosurgery *Neurochirurgie* **63** 433–43

[203] Ghadi R, Muntimadugu E, Domb A, Khan W and Zhang X 2017 Synthetic biodegradable medical polymer: polyanhydrides *Science and Principles of Biodegradable and Bioresorbable Medical Polymers* (Amsterdam: Elsevier) pp 153–88

[204] Nkanga C I, Fisch A, Rad-Malekshahi M, Romic M D, Kittel B and Ullrich T *et al* 2020 Clinically established biodegradable long acting injectables: an industry perspective *Adv. Drug Delivery Rev.* **167** 19–46

[205] Chaudhary K, Patel M M and Mehta P J 2019 Long-acting injectables: current perspectives and future promise *Crit. Rev. Ther. Drug Carrier Syst.* **36** 137–81

[206] Rafael D, Melendres M M R, Andrade F, Montero S, Martinez-Trucharte F and Vilar-Hernandez M *et al* 2021 Thermo-responsive hydrogels for cancer local therapy: challenges and state-of-art *Int. J. Pharm.* **606** 120954

[207] Mane A, Maheshwari N, Ghode P, Sharma M C and Tekade R K 2019 Approaches to the Development of Implantable Therapeutic Systems *Biomaterials and Bionanotechnology* (Amsterdam: Elsevier) pp 191–224

[208] Shephard C J and Drovandi A D 2019 Sustained-release subdermal buprenorphine implants: the future of opioid use disorder management? *J. Pharm. Pract. Res.* **49** 41–9

[209] Barnwal P, Das S, Mondal S, Ramasamy A, Maiti T and Saha A 2017 Probuphine® (buprenorphine implant): a promising candidate in opioid dependence *Ther. Adv. Psychopharmacol* **7** 119–34

[210] Kim H, Lee S H, Wentworth A, Babaee S, Wong K and Collins J E *et al* 2022 Biodegradable ring-shaped implantable device for intravesical therapy of bladder disorders *Biomaterials* **288** 121703

[211] Watanabe T, Sadahira T, Watanabe M, Maruyama Y, Wada K and Sekito T *et al* 2022 Intravesical indwelling lidocaine-releasing devices for IC/BPS *World Acad. Sci.* J **4** 1–7

[212] Silverman L A, Neely E K, Kletter G B, Lewis K, Chitra S and Terleckyj O *et al* 2015 Long-term continuous suppression with once-yearly histrelin subcutaneous implants for the treatment of central precocious puberty: a final report of a phase 3 multicenter trial *J. Clin. Endocrinol. Metabol* **100** 2354–63

[213] Masaeli R, Zandsalimi K and Tayebi L 2019 Biomaterials evaluation: conceptual refinements and practical reforms *Ther. Innov. Regul. Sci.* **53** 120–7

[214] Nuss K M and von Rechenberg B 2008 Biocompatibility issues with modern implants in bone-a review for clinical orthopedics *The Open Orthop.* J **2** 66

[215] Amiji M and Park K 1993 Surface modification of polymeric biomaterials with poly (ethylene oxide), albumin, and heparin for reduced thrombogenicity *J. Biomater. Sci. Polym. Ed.* **4** 217–34

[216] Zhang M, Chan C H, Pauls J P, Semenzin C, Ainola C and Peng H *et al* 2022 Investigation of heparin-loaded poly (ethylene glycol)-based hydrogels as anti-thrombogenic surface coatings for extracorporeal membrane oxygenation *J. Mater. Chem.* B **10** 4974–83

[217] Park H and Park K 1996 Biocompatibility issues of implantable drug delivery systems *Pharm. Res.* **13** 1770–6

[218] Anderson J M and Jiang S 2017 Implications of the acute and chronic inflammatory response and the foreign body reaction to the immune response of implanted biomaterials *The Immune Response to Implanted Materials and Devices* ed B Corradetti (Springer) pp 15–36

[219] Roumen F J M E 2008 Review of the combined contraceptive vaginal ring, NuvaRing® *Therapeut. Clin. Risk Manage.* **4** 441–51

Chapter 2

Green chemistry-assisted pharmaceuticals—research, revolution, and revenue

Paromita Sarbadhikary and Blassan P George

The growing demand for medicine and healthcare systems on a global scale is increasingly burdening the pharmaceutical industry, which in turn highlights it as a major environmental pollution creator. Adoption of green chemistry as a preliminary idea by pharmaceutical companies in the 1990s has grown to be a major promising approach in improvement of environmental performance as well as industrial sustainability. This chapter provides a comprehensive overview and introduction to green chemistry and engineering principles, focused domains of research and strategies for the synthesis process of active pharmaceutical ingredients and drug candidates with reduced environmental risk, waste recycling, decreased solvent usage, and environmentally friendly manufacturing techniques. We also discuss certain notable examples of industrial scale production of pharmaceutical drugs utilizing green chemistry approaches. Additionally, we highlight the status, future opportunities, key promoters and challenges for improving and embracing the green chemistry perspective as a major future goal for sustainability of pharmaceutical industry.

2.1 Introduction

Although we are in the 21st century, an era of globalization, artificial intelligence and robotization, an outbreak of the COVID-19 pandemic, 100 years after the last pandemic, shows the vulnerability of humankind to invisible threats. Over the last few decades, the frequency of emergence of several viral diseases like Ebola virus, Zika virus, and COVID-19, antibiotic resistant bacterial infections, cancer and several aging-related disorders have been on the rise. This necessitates investment and addressing of the most important global healthcare challenges such as manufacture and access to better and more effective drugs with the aim to improve healthcare systems to efficiently tackle the present and emerging situations of

doi:10.1088/978-0-7503-5613-8ch2

healthcare problems. Thus, over the years, the pharmaceutical industry has been given a great deal of responsibility of human health as a fundamental need of every individual in society. In this regard, the pharmaceutical sector has played an important role over the years to ensure effective drug manufacturing that aids in prevention, therapy, treatment, and improvement of a patient's life [1–3].

The increasing burden of the global healthcare system is well reflected in the growth, revenues, and sales data, which makes the pharmaceutical sector one of the chemical industries with the highest profits [4–7]. As per several collections of marketing statistics, by 2017 the global pharmaceutical industry had revenues of $996 billion, which crossed a value of approximately $1.40 trillion in 2021 itself, with a predictable annual growth rate of 11.34%, representing a projected over $2.4 trillion from 2021 to 2028 [8–10]. Such tremendous growth in the pharmaceutical industry has also contributed to it being a major global polluter, generating ~1.9 million tonnes of carbon dioxide annually. Moreover, as per reports, in the pharmaceutical industry, the multiple steps-based organic synthetic routes result in ~25–100 kg of waste generation for every 1 kg of manufactured product, which is the highest as compared to any other chemical industry [5, 11]. Thus, due to the lack of information and realization of the toxic impact of chemicals, over many decades the pharmaceutical industry became the main hub for production of a high volume of hazardous waste by-products and air, water and land pollutants which is mainly contributed by high energy requiring conventional synthetic routes and intensive use of a variety of petrochemical precursors and organic solvents for separation and purification [5, 12].

Thus, the growing interest and public concern about environmental pollution and chemical toxicity in living forms led to the introduction of 'greener' methods in pharmaceutical industries, in an effort for waste minimization and sustainability [5, 12]. This article highlights the efforts of pharmaceutical companies and global drug regulatory agencies to adopt a green chemistry approach to practice environment-friendly production of pharmaceutical products in expanding the therapeutic opportunities along with the major purpose of waste reduction, as well as sustainable growth. The chapter extensively focuses on the current status and main approaches of green chemistry research in pharmaceutical industry and potential gaps and research areas that need to be examined in the future.

2.2 The rise of green chemistry: a revolution

In an effort to deal with the hazardous effects of pharmaceutical waste on the environment and living beings, green chemistry approaches have gained popularity since the 1990s. It is a branch of science that is primarily concerned with the development, design, and use of chemical products and processes to minimize or completely eliminate the use and production of harmful substances [13].

2.2.1 History and principle of green chemistry

It was in 1991, for the first time that the green chemistry concept was theorized by Paul Anastas and Roger Garrett as an idea of designing eco-friendly products and procedures to address the environmental problems imposed by chemicals and their synthesis processes. However, by that time the concept was known as 'benign by design', which was later termed 'green chemistry' by Joe Breen, which gained popularity in 1995 in the United States during Presidential Green Chemistry Challenge (PGCC) [14–16]. Thus, as per the United States Environmental Protection Agency (US EPA), green chemistry is said to be the design of chemical products and processes that reduce or eliminate the use or generation of hazardous substances. Green chemistry applies across the life cycle of a chemical product, including its design, manufacture, use, and ultimate disposal. Green chemistry is also known as sustainable chemistry [15]. Anastas and Warner (1998) introduced the twelve principles of green chemistry, which then became the effective guiding principles of green chemistry as represented in figure 2.1 [14, 15, 17].

Later, in 2003, at the first conference on 'Green Engineering: Defining the Principles' held in Florida, nine principles known as The Sandestin Declaration were developed and presented as green engineering principles to promote sustainability, human and environmental welfare [18]. The nine principles of green engineering proposed by The Sandestin Declaration are listed below. The pharmaceutical business became the first industry sector to embrace the field of green chemistry in the late 1990s due to Dr Berkeley Cue's endeavours, which helped launch the first corporate program ever to do so [19]. Later, in 2005, ACS Green Chemistry Institute and a handful of pharmaceutical companies established ACS Green Chemistry Institute Pharmaceutical Roundtable (ACS GCIPR) to promote hazardless and economically competitive chemical synthesis [20]. According to Tucker (2006), pharmaceutical green chemistry can be defined as the quest for benign synthetic

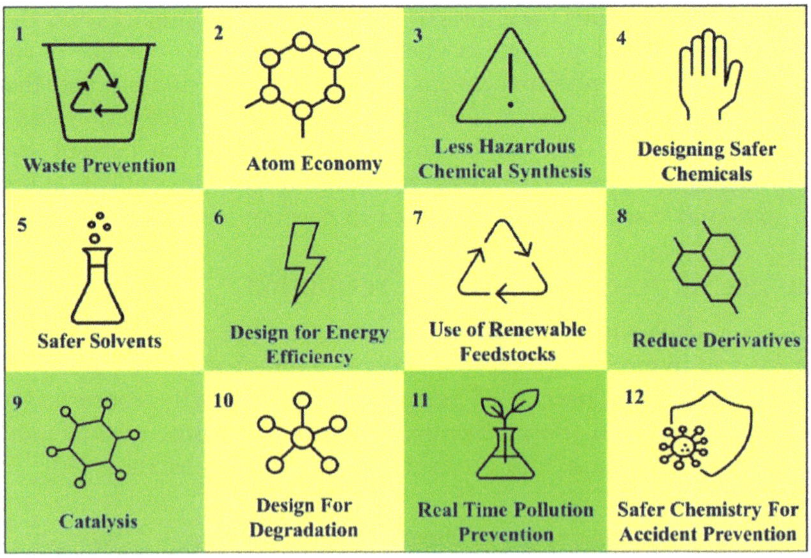

Figure 2.1. Twelve guiding principles of Green Chemistry as proposed by Anastas and Warner. Reproduced from [12] with permission from Elsevier, copyright (2021).

processes that reduce the environmental burden within the context of enabling the delivery of our current standard of living [21].

2.2.1.1 The nine principles of green engineering proposed by The Sandestin declaration

1. Engineer processes and products holistically, use systems analysis, and integrate environmental impact assessment tools.
2. Conserve and improve natural ecosystems while protecting human health and wellbeing.
3. Use life-cycle thinking in all engineering activities.
4. Ensure that all material and energy inputs and outputs are as inherently safe and benign as possible.
5. Minimize depletion of natural resources.
6. Strive to prevent waste.
7. Develop and apply engineering solutions, while being cognizant of local geography, aspirations, and cultures.
8. Create engineering solutions beyond current or dominant technologies; improve, innovate, and invent (technologies) to achieve sustainability.
9. Actively engage communities and stakeholders in development of engineering solutions.

2.2.2 Green chemistry metrics in the pharmaceutical industry

The accomplishments of green chemistry over time in managing pharmaceutical industry induced environmental toxicity directed the measurement of green chemistry to estimate manufacturing improvements as a corporate priority. This resulted in the introduction of vital metrics (table 2.1) to assess the environmental impact and compare various synthesis methods for a specific product. Two of the first, most popular, effective and relatively simple metrics are the environmental factor (E) and the atom economy (AE) [5, 15]. Based on the concept of modified E factors (cEF and sEF) and process complexity, Roschangar *et al* (2015) introduced the novel concept of Green Aspiration Level™ (GAL), as an unbiased metric to balance the performance of green chemistry processes across the pharmaceutical industry in terms of measurement (figure 2.2) [22]. In 2022, as directed by United Nations Sustainable Development Goal 12 (UN SDG 12), Roschangar *et al* (2022) proposed iGAL 2.0 as a better representation of the metric intended to overcome the barriers currently associated with iGAL. The major objective of UN SDG 12 is to substantially reduce the production of waste by 2030, dependent on a vision of catalysing the manufacturing of greener active pharmaceutical ingredients (APIs) across the globe. Hereby, authors introduced convergence (CV) and yield (YD), as new key sustainability indicators (KSI), in context to process efficiency and optimization. YD, which is a measure of overall process productivity, is defined as the overall yield of the longest linear step sequence from an iGAL rule-aligned starting material to the final APIs. CV is an indicator of how directly the starting materials are assembled into the APIs, thus signifying the API process design efficiency. They also presented

Table 2.1. List of green chemistry metrics applicable for the pharmaceutical industry.

Metrics	Equation	Reference
Environmental factor (E)	$E - \text{factor} = \frac{\sum \text{mass(Input materials)} - \text{mass (Product)}}{\text{mass (Product)}}$	[24]
Atom economy (AE)	$AE\ (\%) = \frac{\text{Molecular weight of final product}}{\sum \text{molecular weight (Raw materials)} + \sum \text{molecular weight (Reagents)}} \times 100$	[25]
Process mass intensity (PMI)	$PMI = \frac{\sum \text{mass (Input materials including process water)}}{\text{mass (Product)}}$	[26]
Complete E factor, (cEF),	$cEF = \frac{\sum \text{mass(Raw materials)} + \sum \text{mass (Reagents)} + \sum \text{mass(Solvents)} + \sum \text{mass(Water)} - \text{mass (Product)}}{\text{mass (Product)}}$	[22]
Simple E factor, (sEF)	$sEF = \frac{\sum \text{mass(Raw materials)} + \sum \text{mass (Reagents)} - \text{mass (Product)}}{\text{mass (Product)}}$	[22]
Percent ideality	$\%\text{ideality} = \frac{\text{no. of construction reactions + no. of strategic redox reactions}}{\text{total no. of reactions}}$	[27]
Process complexity	$\text{Complexicity} = \%\ \text{Ideality} \times \text{total no. of reactions}$ $= \text{no. of construction reactions} + \text{no. of strategic redox reactions}$	[22]
Transformation-GAL (tGAL)	$tGAL = \frac{xEF}{\text{Average Complexicity}}$ $GAL = tGAL \times \text{Complexicity}$ (Where, xEF = sEF or cEF)	[22]
Relative process greenness (RPG)	$RPG = \frac{GAL(xEF)}{xEF(\text{actual})}$ (Where, xEF = sEF or cEF)	[22]
Relative (green) process improvement (RPI)	$RPI = RPG\ (\text{Current process}) - RPG(\text{Earlier process})$	[22]
Relative (process) complexity improvement (RCI)	$RCI = I - \frac{\text{Complexicity (Current process)}}{\text{Complexicity (Earlier process)}}$	[22]
Overall green process improvement (PI)	$PI = \frac{RPI + RCI}{2}$	[22]
Pharmaceutical waste index (mGAL)	$mGAL = \frac{(\text{average cEF} \times 100)}{(\text{average FMW})}$	[22]
Innovation green aspiration level (iGAL)	$iGAL = \frac{(mGAL \times FMW)}{1000}$	[23, 28]
iGAL RPG	$RPG = \frac{(iGAL)}{(cEF)} \times 100\%$ (where, cEF = PMI – 1)	[23, 28]
Convergence (CV)	$CV_{iGAL} = \frac{1}{ss_{avg}} \times 100\% = \frac{SM}{SSS} \times 100\%$	[23]

FMW (free molecular weight); cEF (commercial waste); SS (subprocess steps) SM (starting materials) and SSS (sum of subprocess steps).

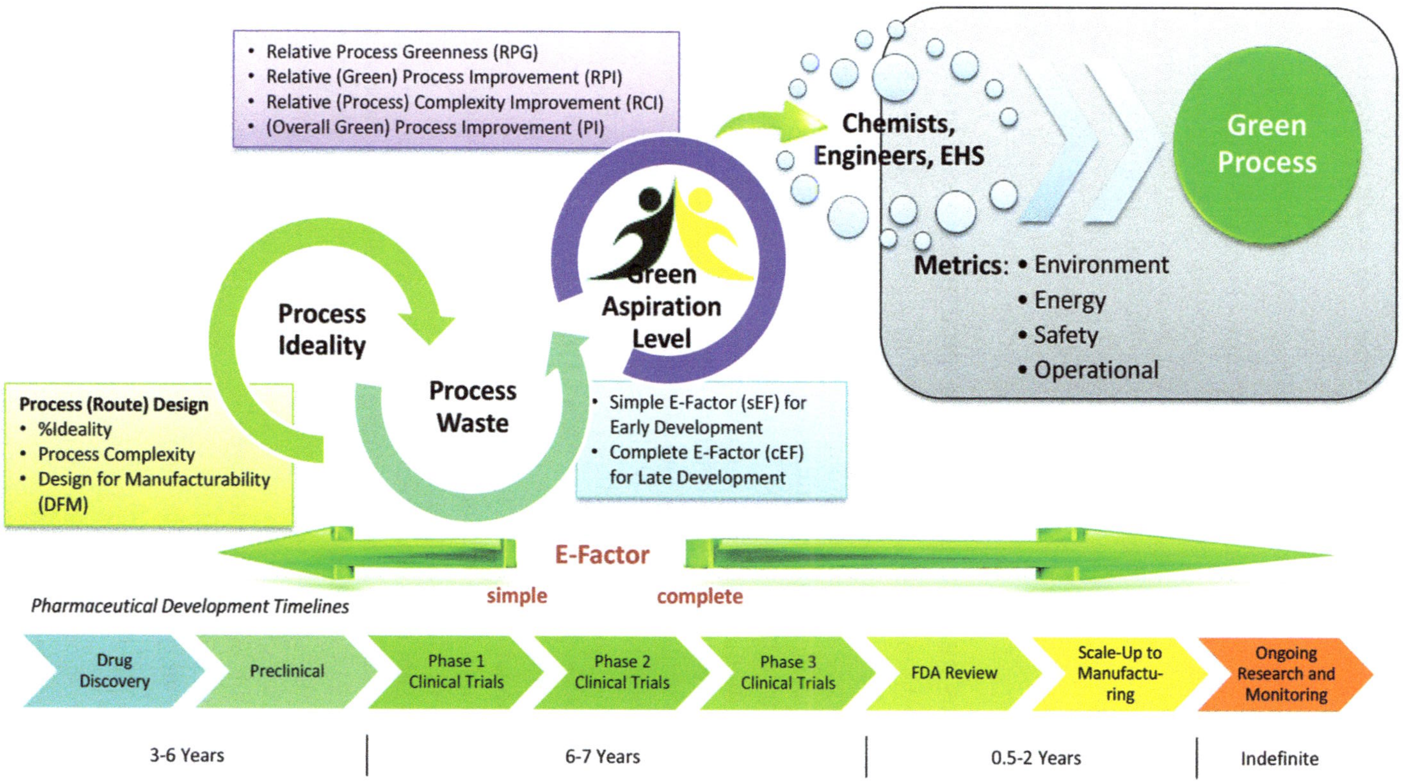

Figure 2.2. Development of green pharmaceutical processes utilizing the Green Aspiration Level concept. Reproduced from [22] with permission from The Royal Society of Chemistry, Copyright (2015).

an innovative convergence equation that can be applied to Computer-Aided Synthesis Planning (CASP) algorithms [15, 23]. The authors further proposed a new iGAL 2.0 statistical model, where the relationship of waste to the KSI is expressed via regression.

$$\ln(\mathrm{cEF}) = 6.913 - (3.130 \times \mathrm{CV}_{\mathrm{iGAL}}) - (1.987 \times \mathrm{YD})$$

The improved metric iGAL 2.0 provides significant improvement with respect to (a) environmental aspect by allowing one to identify possibly underachieving and environmentally concerning processes, as well as (b) economic value by reducing waste which correlates to lower API production costs. Thus, adoption of iGAL 2.0 by pharmaceutical companies worldwide as a uniform metric system will thereby influence comparing the synthesis process' sustainability performance with industry standards [23].

2.3 Green techniques and strategies in the pharmaceutical industry

Two main categories of pharmaceutical drugs include new chemical entities (NCEs) and APIs. In general, due to several factors like time restraints, NCE amount required for activity analysis, dubiety regarding the lead development and high cost during the discovery process, limits the utilization of green chemistry principles in the synthesis of NCEs. In comparison to NCE synthesis, more environmental waste is generated during API manufacturing as a result of complexity and huge amounts involved in the synthesis reactions [29]. Therefore, the application of several green chemistry approaches in synthesis of API and intermediates has gained impetus in the pharmaceutical industry [5, 15]. Much of the relevant literature has discussed in detail case studies of industrially manufactured bestselling United States Food and Drug Administration (FDA)-approved drugs by green synthesis methods [5, 12, 15, 19]. In this section, we have compiled figure 2.3, for highlighting the advantages of green approaches over conventional approaches for the synthesis of certain drugs [5, 15, 30].

In this section we mainly focus on the green approach-based technologies and chemistries for synthesis of pharmaceuticals, which include:

(1) **Selecting no solvents or green solvents (preferably water):** A survey across multiple pharmaceutical companies revealed that solvents comprise the principal component of all materials used in synthesis of APIs. Thus as per green chemistry approaches, certain criteria are considered for assessing the environmental impact of a solvent, such as carbon footprint, biodegradability, water solubility, ability to give rise to volatile organic compounds, easy recyclability, production from a renewable feedstock, reactivity and stability, flammability, life cycle, human and environmental toxicity and final cost [15, 31–33]. Based on all these factors several pharmaceutical companies, Pfizer, AstraZeneca, GlaxoSmithKline and Sanofi have reported solvent selection guides [34]. The evaluation of greenness of a solvent is based on factors of environmental and health safety, and energy demand depending on its utilization in the synthesis process as well as its recovery [34, 35]. Thus, the major challenge for applying green chemistry

S.No	Target Drug	Modification in the Mechanism	Outcome
1	Sertaline Hydrochloride	Use of Green chemistry technology in commercial process (combined process)	●Pollution prevention ●Reduced energy and water use ●Double overall product yield
2	Pregabalin	Replacing all the chemical solvents with water	●Reduction in the use of energy by 83% ●Elimination in usage of Mandelic acid ●Reduction in the usage of the starting material
3	Sitagliptin	Use of the enzymatic process in the mechanism of production of the drug	●Elimination of metal catalyst ●Reduction the generation of the waste ●Improved yield.
4	Doramectin	Replacement of biocatalysts in the synthesis process.	●40% Increase in efficiency of the reaction ●Reduced production of the by-products ●Reduced waste generation in purification
5	Ibuprofen	Reduction of process from 6 steps to 3 steps with the incorporation of atoms of reactants directly into the product.	●Increased atom utilization ●Small amounts of by-products ●Decreased need for waste disposal.
6	Gemifloxacin	Use of biocatalysis for the manufacturing of the drug	●Reduced generation of waste. ●Use of less energy ●Decreased processing time.
7	Atorvastatin	Manufacturing of the drug using enzymatic catalysis	●Increase in volumetric productivity ●Economical and envionment friendly ● Decreased generation of waste
8	Simvastatin	Optimization of both enzymatic and chemical process with use of engineered enzyme with low cost feedstock.	●Elimination of use of hazardous compounds ●Significant increase in the yield by 97% ●Biodegradable waste with biological treatment.

Figure 2.3. Advantageous outcomes of green synthetic approaches over conventional synthesis routes for listed pharmaceutical drugs. Reproduced from [12] with permission from Elsevier, copyright (2021).

principles is to eliminate solvents from the reaction mixture, if possible, otherwise choosing safer, greener and more efficient solvents. Practically, achieving solvent-less reactions at the industrial scale can be hazardous leading to serious accidents. The best known green solvent or cosolvent in industrial scale reactions is water, which, due to its relatively easier removal process, results in high atom economy and low waste generation and can be used in a range of processes such as in reaction examinations, biocatalysis, and in product isolation [15]. However, there are various commercial reactions that cannot adopt water as a solvent, thus green chemistry teams have researched and proposed alternative solvents and reaction media to replace several undesirable category solvents, which also offers the benefits of comprehensive catalyst recovery and recycling [15, 36, 37].

(2) **Green catalyst:** Other than the contribution of solvent in commercial manufacturing of APIs, the choice of catalytic process and the involved catalysts also critically influence the greenness of the synthesis reactions [15, 38–40]. The pharmaceutical industry is one of the primary consumers of precious metal catalyst globally, which are used to enhance and expedite chemical transformations that are normally impossible to gain in their absence. Precious metal catalysts like palladium, platinum, rhodium, and ruthenium etc are required in the synthesis of APIs as well as the recovery process. However, these noble metals are expensive, in limited abundance and reserves, potentially lethal and their extraction and isolation result in substantial environmental footprint. Thus, as a complementary and green

approach non-precious metal catalysts, particularly copper, cobalt, nickel, and iron catalysts, are of interest as commercial catalysts because of several reasons like: (a) low cost; (b) relatively less toxicity; (c) they permit new methods of catalysis for challenging heterocyclic and sterically-encumbered substrates; (d) are effective in allowing new reactivities such as unconventional electrophilic coupling partners; and (e) offer green chemistry opportunities with low carbon footprint in terms of CO_2 emission [40–42].

Specific catalyst-based reaction/transformation related to green synthesis of pharmaceuticals involves:

(a) **Catalytic C–H bond activation reactions:** Direct Green C–H activation and functionalization reactions have vast potential in the pharmaceutical industry and are involved in several reactions like coupling, dehydrogenation, eliminations and/or oxidation reactions. These reactions offer several advantages: (a) significant atom economy due to shorter synthesis steps and exclusion of the intermediate functional group insertion step; (b) reduction of the mass intensity and step-count of the synthesis processes by eradicating the requisites for pre-functionalization steps; and (c) reduced waste generation. The major areas which contribute to green C–H activation toward sustainability and in largescale synthesis involve: (i) catalytic methods such as metal catalysis, chemical catalysis, metal complexes-based homogeneous catalytic reactions, heterogeneous catalytic methods with solid counterpart, enzymatic catalysis and organo-catalysis; and (ii) averting and substituting the greener solvents, molecular oxygen, static directing groups and metal-based electro-catalysis [15, 43].

(b) **Asymmetric organocatalysis:** Organocatalysis is a well-established process for catalytic asymmetric synthesis of low-to medium-molecular-weight organic chiral molecules where an inorganic element is not part of the active reaction transition. Organocatalysis is an inherent green chemistry toolbox due to its environmentally benign synthetic methodology with facile reaction course, selectivity and environment-friendly chemistry of being nontoxic, ready availability, moisture and air tolerance, stability and easy handling, as well as biocompatibility of many organocatalysts. However, with the aim of augmenting the sustainability of making the asymmetric organocatalysis, several different approaches are being investigated and applied: (i) the first approach focuses on intensification and activation techniques, such as catalyst immobilization, flow setups, high pressure or light mechanical activation, microwave, or ultrasound, that can be used to increase yields, hasten reactions, make it easier to isolate products, or produce new reactivities; (ii) the second approach involves the use of either solvent-free conditions or greener reaction media such as water, ionic liquids, deep eutectic solvents, supercritical solvents and green solvent alternatives [44–47].

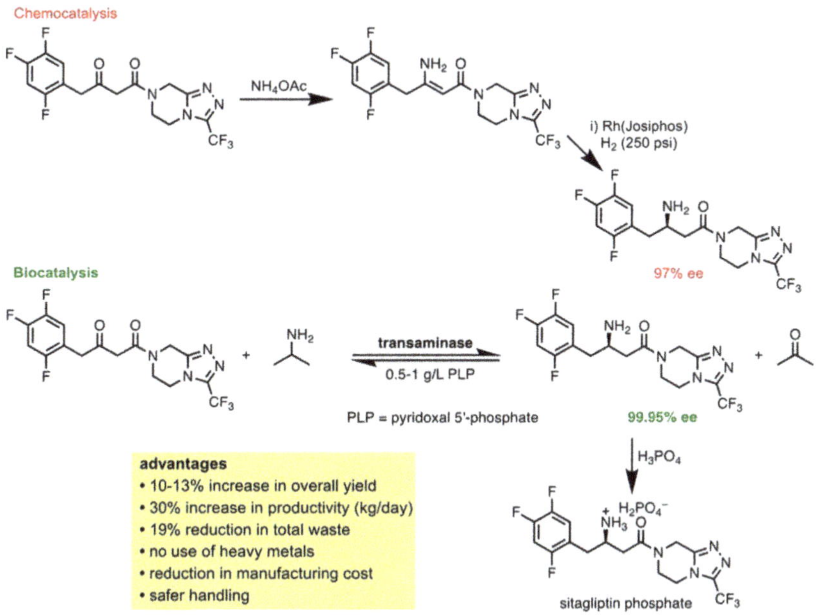

Figure 2.4. Comparison between chemical and biocatalytic synthesis of Sitagliptin. Reproduced from [29] John Wiley & Sons. Copyright 2020 Wiley-VCH Verlag GmbH & Co. KGaA, Weinheim.

(c) **Biocatalysis:** Biocatalysis is a powerful tool for green chemistry and cost-effective processes in the pharmaceutical industry for the syntheses of small chiral drugs molecules, which otherwise present challenges for being synthesised as single stereoisomers resulting in either introduction of additional steps to recycle the undesired enantiomers, and/or most cases ending up in generating more waste. Thus, enzymatic catalysis and biocatalysis are becoming more common in environmentally friendly and sustainable growth of pharma companies due to advantages of high chemo-, regio- and enantioselectivity, use of water as a green reaction medium, no trace metal-based product contamination, no requirement of any protection/deprotection steps, and are carried out under mild conditions of ambient temperature and pressure. Thus, chemoenzymatic catalysis has the potential to increase energy efficiency with reduction in hazardous waste generation. Based on the ability of enzymes to catalyse a wide range of transformations, several pharmaceutical drugs such as Atorvastatin, Cephalexin, Amoxicillin, Pregabalin, Sitagliptin, Dexamphetamine, Glasdegib, Simvastatin, Sulopenem, Montelukast Boceprevir, Telaprevir, Esomeprazole etc have been synthesised bio-catalytically at commercial scale (figures 2.4–2.6) [29, 48, 49].

(3) **One-pot cascade synthesis:** The concept of a one-pot synthesis comprises implementation of all reactions in a single reactor for continuous reactions,

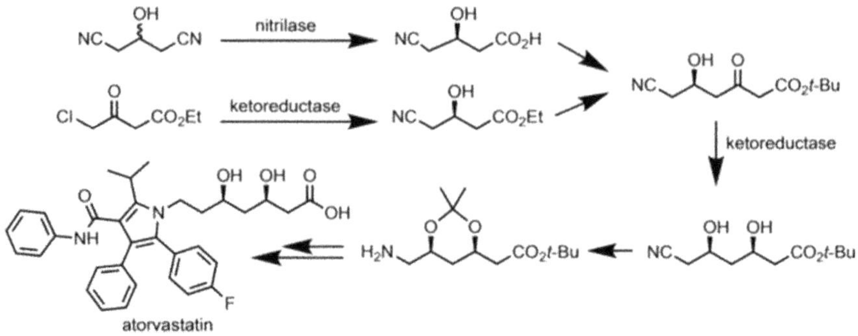

Figure 2.5. Biocatalytic synthesis of Atorvastatin. Reproduced from [29] John Wiley & Sons. Copyright 2020 Wiley-VCH Verlag GmbH & Co. KGaA, Weinheim.

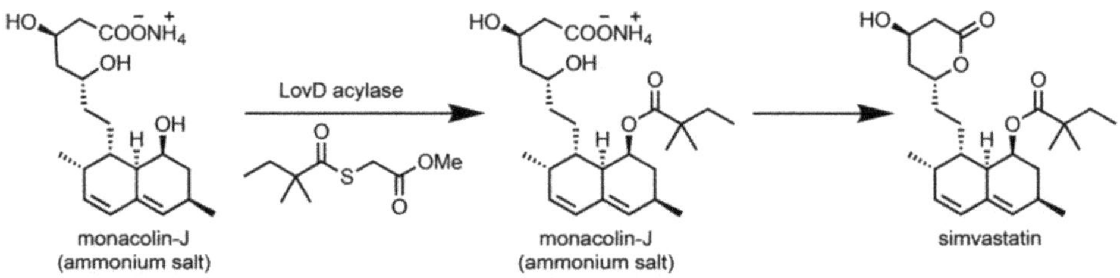

Figure 2.6. Whole-cell biocatalytic synthesis of Simvastatin. Reproduced from [29] John Wiley & Sons. Copyright 2020 Wiley-VCH Verlag GmbH & Co. KGaA, Weinheim.

which offers the advantages of [1] lowering the final waste generation along with the reaction time and effort and [2] reduces the need for a time-consuming intermediate separation and purification process, eventually increasing the chemical yield [15, 50].

(4) **Multicomponent reactions (MCRs):** MCRs are a subtype of one-pot cascade reaction where more than two starting materials are mixed to form a high regio- and stereoselective structurally complex single organic molecule, assimilating either all or a majority of the atoms of the starting reactants. Furthermore, MCR presents a direct method to create diversity as well as complexity in a particular procedure, with an irreversible flow of the reactions to provide a yield almost approaching 100%, along with water as a major by-product. Thus, compared to the traditional stepwise linear synthetic process, MCR strategy accomplishes several green chemistry and sustainability principles, largely due to the advantages of the AE, including savings in time and energy, waste minimization, eco-friendliness, shortened steps, efficient use of human efforts and others, simplified purification steps, mild conditions, high convergence, and high yield of the final product. Several popular and classical MCRs such as Biginelli, Bucherer–Bergs, Gewald reactions, Groebke–Blackburn–Bienayme, Hantzsch, Kabachnik–Fields, Mannich, Orru, Petasis, Passerini, Strecker, Ugi, Willgerodt–

Kindler, etc are used for green chemistry approach-based synthesis of many API and key intermediates [15, 51, 52].

(5) **Green drug delivery formulations:** The application of green chemistry principles is not only linked to early drug synthesis stages but applies to the manufacturing of commercial products to accomplish reduced drug doses needed to achieve the therapeutic goal. The majority of new drug candidates as well as old pharmaceuticals faces the challenges of low aqueous solubility and poor oral absorption, resulting in the generation of an enormous waste output per production unit. New drug delivery approaches and platforms like spray-dried dispersions (SDDs), make use of solid amorphous dispersions developed by spray-drying, comprising a molecular mixture of drugs with poor-solubility in a homogeneous and noncrystalline polymeric carrier. Thus, SDD technology has the potential for 10-fold enhancement of the bioavailability of oral drugs as well as offering substantial green chemistry advantages. Thus, such drug delivery platforms influence the whole drug-development process towards a greener and more sustainable approach by reducing the waste generation due to efficient screening, non-progression of drug candidates, lower dose requirements and during manufacturing as well as the after-dosing drug amount that is released into the environment. Thus, as predicted, implementation of SDD technology for all low-solubility drugs, can prevent hazardous pharmaceutical waste generation totalling in tons per year [53]. Following the adoption of green chemistry methodologies and technologies, several pharmaceutical industries have been awarded with Presidential Green Chemistry Challenge awards due to green synthesis of popular APIs, and development of other pharmaceutical relevant green process [54]. Other than pharma-based drug manufacturing processes, another major concern for environmental pollution is pressurized metered-dose inhalers (pMDIs) which are used in the management of lung diseases like asthma and chronic obstructive pulmonary disease (COPD). Hydrofluorocarbon propellants in pMDIs are a major source of greenhouse gas (GHG) emissions, accounting for almost 0.03% of global GHG annually [55, 56]. Thus, in an effort to maintain pMDIs as one of the viable and valuable therapeutics there is a need for alternatives with favourable environmental, physical, and toxicological properties, use of next generation low GWP propellants 1, 1-difluoroethane (HFA-152a) hydrofluoroolefin (HFO)-1234ze(E) is encouraged as replacement options to currently used hydrofluoroalkane (HFA)-134a and HFA-227ea [57].

2.4 Current status and future opportunities for green chemistry adoption in the global pharmaceutical market

Established in 2005, ACS GCIPR, which started with only three US based founding member companies (Pfizer, Merck, and Eli Lilly), have expended globally with about 25 members, 16 associate members and 4 affiliate members as of 2022 [58].

2.4.1 Green chemistry drivers

Along with the growth of green chemistry over the past 20 years, the idea of sustainable development has attracted significant attention on both an industrial and societal level. In the late 1980s, the term sustainability was first introduced by Brundtland, defined as meeting the needs of the present generation without compromising the ability of future generations to meet their own needs [14]. The majority of pharmaceutical firms have made green chemistry a key component of their business strategy for achieving their sustainability goals and targets [59, 60]. Sustainable chemistry is the subcategory within the field of sustainability, while green chemistry is a subset of sustainable chemistry and development [61]. Thus, sustainable development is the ultimate goal that can be achieved with the embracing of green chemistry [14]. As per the research findings, implementation of green chemistry in the pharmaceutical industry is driven by both internal (cost savings and management commitment) and external (regulatory requirements and stakeholder pressures) key factors, among which cost savings and regulation are the top two drivers, and these are summarized as [62, 63]:

(1) **Cost benefits:** Green pharmaceutical chemistry's ability to reduce costs is becoming more and more crucial due to the constant growing pressures on the pharmaceutical industry to reduce healthcare costs globally. Thus, several different factors such as lower costs of materials and energy, efficient production, waste removal costs, upgraded employee wellbeing and reduced insurance expenses, contribute to the cost savings of a pharma company [63].

(2) **Environmental impacts and regulations:** The international pharmaceutical industry is governed by a number of environmental laws, including those enacted by the FDA in accordance with the 1969 National Environmental Policy Act (NEPA), the European Medicines Agency (EMA) in accordance with Article 8 [3] of Directive 2001/83/EC, and incentive programs like the Swedish National Pharmaceutical Strategy (NPS). The main aim of such global drug regulatory agencies is to evaluate the potential environmental risks associated with medicinal products and to take appropriate measures to limit the potential impacts [64–66]. Chemical manufacturing regulations such as Evaluation and Authorization of Chemicals (REACH) and the US Toxics Substances Control Act (TSCA) and the EU Registration, address the manufacture, importation, use, and disposal of specific chemicals related to the production of APIs [67, 68]. Further, EPA's Toxics Release Inventory (TRI) also serves as a useful tool for assessing certain toxic chemicals released into the environment, annually or otherwise managed as waste by pharmaceutical manufacturing sectors in the US [69]. However, conversely, regulatory guidelines have also become hurdles for quick adoption of green chemistry processes, because of re-certification of FDA policies involved with changes made in the production process, which is both costly and time consuming [62].

Other more or less influential drivers of greem chemistry like (i) improving reputation among stakeholders, affected due to poor management of negative event news, lack of corporate integrity, pricing policies and transparency; (ii) increased demands to intensify the effectiveness of its manufacturing processes and the effects of its products' useful lives; (iii) increasing customer demands requesting more information on sustainable practices; (iv) sustainable, responsible and impact (SRI) investors pressure; and (v) attracting and retaining talents by enhancing worker wellbeing and minimizing adverse effects on the environment, also play important roles in driving the green pharmaceutical chemistry [70].

The pharmaceutical industry has been pressured by the COVID-19 pandemic to adopt and build strong, sustainable drug supply chains, whereby there has been a lot of interest in using flow chemistry techniques to attain continuous manufacturing to satisfy the growing demand for drugs [71]. According to a World Economic Forum (WEF) report published in November 2021, continuous manufacturing could 'revolutionize' the drug manufacturing process by enabling greater personalization of each medication made on-demand and eliminating the need for shipping across multiple locations [72]. Moreover, as an important aspect, implementation of continuous manufacturing in pharmaceutical industry has the potential for advancing both 'sustainability benefits' and 'green chemistry benefits' [71, 73–75]. From a sustainability perspective, continuous manufacturing can address various green chemistry principles, which include (a) waste minimization (recycling, improved yield, coupling unit operations, and upgraded process control), (b) energy efficiency (energy transfer between unit operations and steady-state operation), and (c) process safety (real-time monitoring and controlling techniques and reduction in reactor volume) [71, 73]. However, it is also noteworthy to mention that continuous manufacturing is not always associated with sustainability benefits, under certain circumstances, application of continuous manufacturing leads sustainability to be either neutral or decreased, thus it is the decision process by the manufacturers whether to implement continuous manufacturing as the production mode [71].

2.4.2 Green chemistry barriers

Research conducted by Matus *et al* (2012) and Green Chemistry & Commerce Council (GC3) engaged T Fennelly & Associates, Inc. (TFA) provided comprehensive analyses of key deterrents which affect the growth and readiness for adoption of green chemistry. This includes cultural, economic, incumbency, metrics, organizational, regulatory, supply chain complexity, technical, switching risk, lack of proficiency about available methods and techniques, supply and demand and transparency [63, 76–78]. In addition to the above-stated green chemistry-related barriers, pharmaceutical industries face certain specific challenges such as (i) regulatory requirements with applied changes at each phase of development and manufacturing of APIs of a drug, and (ii) time pressure to deliver drugs faster. Thus, due to time constraints and high financial investments pharmaceutical companies have a low tolerance for delays in bringing new drugs to market, and they also have to recover their costs from the sales of drugs that have already been released to the market [22, 63, 78].

Due to strict enforcement of environmental regulations, greater resources, and education in the U.S. and Europe, the adoption of green chemistry practices is strongly led by these countries resulting in a steady decline in TRI releases from the pharmaceutical industry. However, the increasing global pressures on manufacturing of medicines and outsourcing API manufacturing and R&D by many US- and Europe-based 'big pharma' due to cost advantages and workforce have led countries like India and China to become the major contributors to environmental pollution from drug manufacturing [63, 70, 78, 79]. According to reports, the main obstacles to green chemistry engineering and adoption in India are: (a) a lack of green technologies; (b) a lack of connections between green chemistry solution providers and industry; (c) scale-up and commercialization; (d) a lack of understanding of the fundamentals of green chemistry and engineering; (e) misconceptions that green chemistry is difficult and complex and therefore unsuitable for small- and medium-sized businesses; and (f) regulatory obstacles. However, over the past few years, generic drug pharma and API manufacturers in India have begun to invest interest and advances in using green chemistry principles, as shown by the data, which shows that 92% use green chemistry principles, 80% use metrics, over two thirds use green chemistry resources like the Solvent Selection Guide, 60% support green chemistry education and awareness, and 64% are involved in external green chemistry collaborations [4, 80, 81]. Similarly, China faces significant obstacles to the adoption of green pharmaceutical chemistry, including: (a) the conflicting goals of economic growth and environmental protection; (b) regulatory and bureaucratic hurdles; (c) a lack of funding for research; (d) technical hurdles; (e) a scarcity of necessary knowledge; (f) a lack of industrial engineering capacity; and (g) economic and financial obstacles [82]. However, government energy efficiency and environmental standard and economic policies, have positively driven the application of green chemistry in China as with the a variety of newly reported innovations in the fields of green flame retardants, biomass utilization, biopolymers, alternative solvents, and catalysis [82–84].

In a systematic literature review study, Milanesi *et al* (2020), identified five major challenges in the application of sustainability in the pharmaceutical industry which represent opportunities for future research: (a) social sustainability in terms of market access; (b) relationship between mature and emerging markets; (c) waste management and advanced resolutions; (d) relationship between innovation and sustainability of new disruptive drugs; and (e) economic sustainability of the health system [59].

2.5 Future perspective

With the implementation of regulations, policies, strategies, and innovations by the US EPA, REACH legislations of the European Union and ACS GCIPR, the last two decades have witnessed the practice of green chemistry by many pharmaceutical industries, wherever possible logistically [15, 63, 85, 86]. Over the years from 1996 to 2022, several pharmaceutical industries have received awards from the Presidential Green Chemistry Challenge program, due to their efforts to employ green chemistry resulting in reduction in solvent usage and waste disposal expenses along with energy efficiency benefits, green drug design and green synthesis of selective pharmaceuticals. According to estimates, each year green chemistry technologies collectively cut down on the release of 7.8 billion pounds of carbon dioxide into the atmosphere, 826 million pounds of hazardous chemicals and solvents, and over 21 billion gallons of water [54]. According to a recent report, the global market of green chemistry showed an exponential growth of 48.5% with a representation of about $98.5 billion by 2020 from $2.8 billion in 2011 [87, 88]. As a result of direct or indirect benefits of implementation of pharmaceutical green chemistry, US EPA's TRI reported a 7% decrease in environmental release of chemical waste over the years from 2004 to 2013, with an almost 60% reduction in the discharge of potentially harmful substances like methyl isobutyl ketone, trichloroethylene, and hydrochloric acid [15, 88].

In the pharmaceutical sector there is a myth that one must forgo performance and cost to perform green chemistry, which limits the appreciation of the full potential of green chemistry. However, in practicality, there are myriad examples whereby implementation of innovative as well as award-winning green chemistry research and technologies has resulted in the benefits of decreasing API manufacturing costs [38, 89–91]. For example, as per reports, with an estimated $14 million in annual savings, Merck has benefited by the adoption of an improved manufacturing process for Primaxin, [92]. Despite the successful cases of adoption of green pharmaceutical chemistry as both environmentally safer and sustainable alternatives, the overall adoption rates and progress remain sluggish, measured in decades. The research conducted by Veleva *et al* (2017 and 2018), reveals that mostly big pharma has adopted green chemistry to a certain extent, however, the key manufacturers of the bulk of today's global drugs i.e., manufacturers of APIs and generic drugs have not yet accepted green chemistry, which is well reflected from average green chemistry score of 11 for the big pharma versus 2 for generic drug companies [63, 70]. Thus, accelerated integration of green chemistry in pharma companies can be accomplished by some strong strategies like: (a) increasing financial, operational, and government investment into corporations to foster business, progress and global collaboration; (b) improving technical direction and education related to green chemistry and engineering; and (c) approving and supporting proactive and logical strategies and fast track approval in regulatory process [63, 78, 93]. The strengths, weaknesses, opportunities and threats (SWOT analysis) for a brief overview of green chemistry in the pharmaceutical industry are represented in figure 2.7.

In silico tools and/or computational approaches hold great promise as a future aspect in the promotion and success of green chemistry principles in pharmaceutical industries. With the consideration of various aspects of green chemistry, strategic applications of computer-assisted synthesis design (CASD) and critical assessment of protein structure prediction techniques could be effective methods to use in contemporary drug design and discovery. Such approaches could allow early prediction of toxicity profiles and metabolism by living beings, thus helping in avoiding the development of thousands of unnecessary drugs. In one study, the molecular editing concept discussed how computational tools can be used to change,

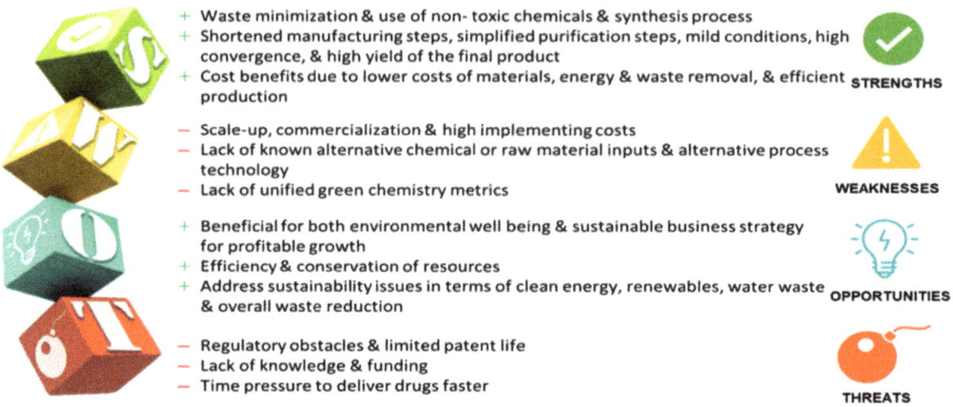

Figure 2.7. Strengths, weaknesses, opportunities and threats (SWOT analysis) for green chemistry in aspects of the pharmaceutical industry.

insert or remove atoms in highly functionalized chemicals, in addition to editing accomplished through site-specific C–H functionalization, heteroaromatic reduction, ring contraction or expansion, as well as avoiding a fictitiously time-consuming synthesis of analogues, and overcoming synthetic obstacles [94]. Computational approaches such as the public Comparative Toxicogenomic Database (CTD) (http://ctdbase.org/), Adverse outcome pathways (AOPs) and multi-criteria decision analysis (MCDA) algorithms are conceptual frameworks intended to assess hazards to human health and the environment by utilization pathway-based data. These computational tools in combination with machine learning and artificial intelligence could provide a great platform for regulatory decision-making process in chemical risk management with the company and the approving authorities during and after drug design phase [15, 94, 95]. Furthermore, along with saving time and money, reducing waste and adapting to such advanced computational approaches will also promote and prioritize the efforts of the US EPA to reduce animal testing [96]. The future of green synthesised pharmaceuticals will therefore involve integrated chemical databases with Web servers, followed by AI-guided green synthesis.

2.6 Conclusion

In this chapter, we have focused on the importance and practices of green synthesis of pharmaceuticals with emphasis on certain important green methods like choice of safer and greener raw starting materials, no solvents or greener solvents, greener and safer alternative synthetic routes, biocatalysis, advanced chemistries like one-pot synthesis, and multicomponent reactions, continuous processing as well as greener ways of drug delivery, for the sustainable growth and feasibility of pharmaceutical industries. Without a dedication to create a healthy environment, the pharmaceutical industry's mission of achieving longer, healthier, and more productive human lives and ecosystems cannot be achieved. Thus, as shown in figure 2.8 the imperative application of green chemistry holds potential in several aspects of the

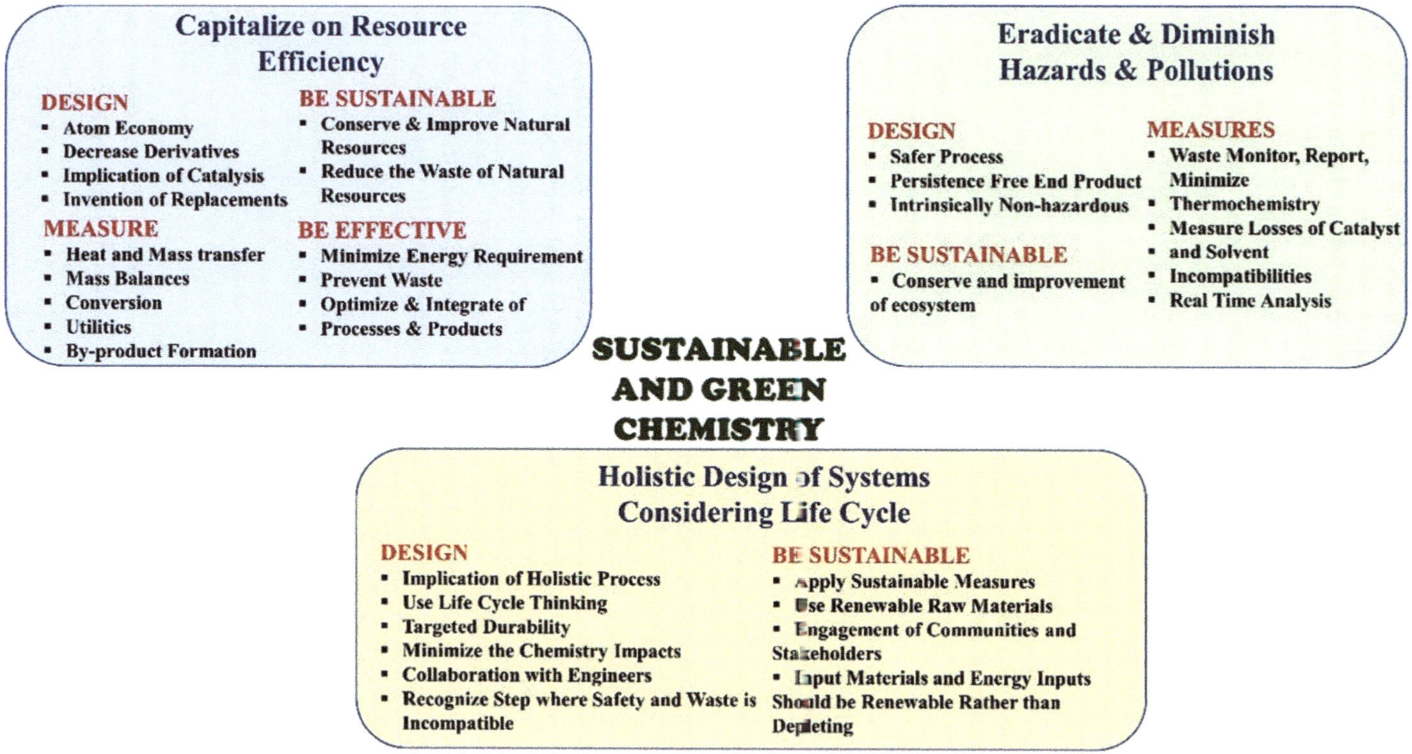

Figure 2.8. Fundamental idea of green chemistry in several aspects of the pharmaceutical industry. Reproduced from [15] with permission from American Chemical Society, copyright (2022).

pharmaceutical industry such as in the reduction of toxic substances and pollution lowest to the molecular level, resource efficiency benefits, and developing safe pharma-based drugs or chemicals. Although, among all chemical industries, the pharmaceutical industry is the first one to adopt and embrace green chemistry, green chemistry growth still seems to be naïve with respect to the extensive growing burden in healthcare sectors. Thus, more awareness and collaborative efforts are needed from government regulatory bodies, companies, financial investors, researchers, and consumers to overcome some of the barriers that have slackened the adoption and flow of green chemistry, especially in small pharmaceutical companies and significantly in countries like India and China.

Funding

This work is supported by the South African Research Chairs initiative of the Department of science and technology and National Research Foundation of South Africa (Grant No. 98337), South African Medical Research Council (Grant No. SAMRC EIP007/2021) as well as grants received from as well as grants received from the NRF Research Development Grants for Y-Rated Researchers (Grant No. 137788), the University Research Committee (URC), University of Johannesburg and the Council for Scientific and Industrial Research (CSIR)-National Laser Centre (NLC).

Acknowledgments

The authors sincerely thank the South African Research Chairs initiative of the Department of science and technology and National Research Foundation (NRF) of South Africa, South African Medical Research Council (SAMRC) and Laser Research Centre (LRC), University of Johannesburg. Research reported in this book chapter was supported by the South African Medical Research Council (SAMRC) through its Division of Research Capacity Development under the Research Capacity Development Initiative from funding received from the South African National Treasury. The content and findings reported/ illustrated are the sole deduction, view and responsibility of the researcher and do not reflect the official position and sentiments of the SAMRC.

Conflicts of interest

The authors declare no conflict of interest.

References

[1] Role of Pharmaceutical Products Manufacturing in Human Society. 2020. https://www.cironpharma.com/blog/role-of-pharmaceutical-products-manufacturing-in-human-society/

[2] Saxena K, Balani S and Srivastava P 2022 The role of pharmaceutical industry in building resilient health system *Front. Public Heal* **10** 964899

[3] Health and Pharmaceuticals. https://www.llorenteycuenca.com/en/sector/salud-e-industria-farmaceutica/

[4] Veleva V R, Cue B W, Todorova S, Thakor H, Mehta N H and Padia K B 2018 Benchmarking green chemistry adoption by the Indian pharmaceutical supply chain *Green Chem. Lett. Rev.* **11** 439–56

[5] Gupta P and Mahajan A 2015 Green chemistry approaches as sustainable alternatives to conventional strategies in the pharmaceutical industry *RSC Adv.* **5** 26686–705

[6] Analyzing the Global Pharmaceutical Industry 2022 https://www.researchandmarkets.com/reports/5680874/analyzing-the-global-pharmaceutical-industry-2022?utm_source=BW&utm_medium=PressRelease&utm_code=k2zh89&utm_campaign=1782294+-+Analyzing+the+%241.4+Trillion+Global+Pharmaceutical+Industry+2022&utm_exec=ch

[7] Pharmaceutical Manufacturing Market Size, Share & Trends Analysis Report By Molecule Type, By Drug Development Type, By Formulation, By Routes of Administration, By Sales Channel, By Age Group, And Segment Forecasts, 2021–2028 https://www.grandviewresearch.com/industry-analysis/pharmaceutical-manufacturing-market

[8] Elder D 2022 Green chemistry *Eur. Pharm. Rev.* https://www.europeanpharmaceuticalreview.com/article/168537/green-chemistry/

[9] Zhang C 2018 Hazardous reagent substitution: a pharmaceutical perspective *Green Process Synth* **7** 387–8

[10] Bandichhor R 2018 Introduction to hazardous reagent substitution in the pharmaceutical industry *Hazardous Reagent Substitution* (Cambridge: Royal Society of Chemistry) ch 1

[11] Fortunak J M 2009 Current and future impact of green chemistry on the pharmaceutical industry *Future Med. Chem.* **1** 571–769

[12] Mishra M, Sharma M, Dubey R, Kumari P, Ranjan V and Pandey J 2021 Green synthesis interventions of pharmaceutical industries for sustainable development *Curr Res Green Sustain Chem.* **4** 100174

[13] Green Chemistry in the Pharma Industry: Sustainable Pastures for Those Who Innovate CAS. https://www.cas.org/resources/cas-insights/sustainability/green-chemistry-pharma-industry (accessed 2 March 2023)

[14] Sheldon R 2010 Introduction to green chemistry, organic synthesis and pharmaceuticals *Green Chemistry in the Pharmaceutical Industry* (Wiley) ch 1

[15] Kar S, Sanderson H, Roy K, Benfenati E and Leszczynski J 2022 Green chemistry in the synthesis of pharmaceuticals *Chem. Rev.* **122** 3637–710

[16] Sauer N N 1999 *Green Chemistry: Frontiers in Benign Chemical Syntheses and Processes* ed P T Anastas and T C Williamson (New York: Oxford University Press) p 360

[17] Anastas P T and Warner J C 1998 *Green Chemistry: Theory and Practice* (New York: Oxford University Press)

[18] Abraham M A and Nguyen N 2003 Green engineering: defining the principles *Results from the Sandestin Conf.* vol 22 (Environmental Progress)

[19] Dunn P J, Wells A S and Williams M T 2010 *Green Chemistry in the Pharmaceutical Industry* (Wiley)

[20] Diorazio L J, Richardson P, Sneddon H F, Moores A, Briddell C and Martinez I 2021 Making sustainability assessment accessible: tools developed by the ACS green chemistry institute pharmaceutical roundtable *ACS Sustain. Chem. Eng* **9** 16862–4

[21] Tucker J L 2006 Green chemistry, a pharmaceutical perspective *Org. Process Res. Dev.* **10** 315–9

[22] Roschangar F, Sheldon R A and Senanayake C H 2015 Overcoming barriers to green chemistry in the pharmaceutical industry-the Green Aspiration Level™ concept *Green Chem.* **17** 752–68

[23] Roschangar F, Li J, Zhou Y, Aelterman W, Borovika A and Colberg J *et al* 2022 Improved iGAL 2.0 metric empowers pharmaceutical scientists to make meaningful contributions to united nations sustainable development goal 12 *ACS Sustain Chem. Eng.* **10** 5148–62
[24] Sheldon R A 2007 The E factor: fifteen years on *Green Chem.* **9** 1273–83
[25] Trost B M 1991 The atom economy—a search for synthetic efficiency *Science* **254** 1471–7
[26] Jimenez-Gonzalez C, Ponder C S, Broxterman Q B and Manley J B 2011 Using the right green yardstick: Why process mass intensity is used in the pharmaceutical industry to drive more sustainable processes *Org. Process Res. Dev.* **15** 912–7
[27] Gaich T and Baran P S 2010 Aiming for the ideal synthesis *J. Org. Chem.* **75** 4657–73
[28] Roschangar F, Zhou Y, Constable D J C, Colberg J, Dickson D P and Dunn P J *et al* 2018 Inspiring process innovation: via an improved green manufacturing metric: IGAL *Green Chem.* **20** 2206–11
[29] Sharma S, Das J, Braje W M, Dash A K and Handa S 2020 A glimpse into green chemistry practices in the pharmaceutical industry *Chem. Sus. Chem.* **13** 2859–75
[30] Mishra M, Sharma M, Dubey R, Kumari P, Ranjan V and Pandey J 2021 Green synthesis interventions of pharmaceutical industries for sustainable development *Curr. Res. Green Sus. Chem.* **4** 100174
[31] Sneddon H F 2016 Tools for facilitating more sustainable medicinal chemistry *RSC Green Chemistry* (Cambridge: Royal Society of Chemistry)
[32] Scott J L and Sneddon H F 2018 Green solvents *Green Techniques for Organic Synthesis and Medicinal Chemistry* (Wiley) 2nd edn
[33] Breeden S W, Clark J H, Macquarrie D J and Sherwood J 2012 Green solvents *Green Techniques for Organic Synthesis and Medicinal Chemistry* (Wiley)
[34] Byrne F P, Jin S, Paggiola G, Petchey T H M, Clark J H and Farmer T J *et al* 2016 Tools and techniques for solvent selection: green solvent selection guides *Sustain. Chem. Process.* **4** 7
[35] Capello C, Fischer U and Hungerbühler K 2007 What is a green solvent? A comprehensive framework for the environmental assessment of solvents *Green Chem.* **9** 927–34
[36] Alfonsi K, Colberg J, Dunn P J, Fevig T, Jennings S and Johnson T A *et al* 2008 Green chemistry tools to influence a medicinal chemistry and research chemistry based organisation *Green Chem.* **10** 31–6
[37] Lipshutz B H and Ghorai S 2014 Transitioning organic synthesis from organic solvents to water. What's your e Factor? *Green Chem.* **16** 3660–79
[38] Cue B W 2012 Green chemistry strategies for medicinal chemists *Green Techniques for Organic Synthesis and Medicinal Chemistry* (Wiley)
[39] Watson W J W 2012 How do the fine chemical, pharmaceutical, and related industries approach green chemistry and sustainability? *Green Chem.* **14** 251–9
[40] Bryan M C, Dunn P J, Entwistle D, Gallou F, Koenig S G and Hayler J D *et al* 2018 Key Green Chemistry research areas from a pharmaceutical manufacturers' perspective revisited *Green Chem.* **20** 5082–103
[41] 2022 Global Precious Metal Catalyst Market Outlook to 2028 *Market Research Reports* BQ0400 https://www.bluequarkresearch.com/reports/global-precious-metal-catalyst-market (accessed 2 April 2023)
[42] Maes J, Mitchell E A and Maes B U W 2016 Base metals in catalysis: from zero to hero *RSC Green Chemistry* (Cambridge: Royal Society of Chemistry)
[43] Tomin A, Bag S and Török B 2012 Catalytic C–H bond activation reactions *Green Techniques for Organic Synthesis and Medicinal Chemistry* (Wiley)

[44] Krištofíková D, Modrocká V, Mečiarová M and Šebesta R 2020 Green asymmetric organocatalysis *Chem. Sus. Chem.* **13** 2828–58
[45] Zhang W-Z, Nanda S and Luo S 2018 Practical asymmetric organocatalysis *Green Techniques for Organic Synthesis and Medicinal Chemistry* (Wiley)
[46] Bhowmick K C and Chanda T 2018 Asymmetric organocatalysis in aqueous media *Green Techniques for Organic Synthesis and Medicinal Chemistry* (Wiley)
[47] Zhang L, Cui L, Luo S and Cheng J P 2012 Supported asymmetric organocatalysis *Green Techniques for Organic Synthesis and Medicinal Chemistry* (Wiley)
[48] Lalonde J 2018 Biocatalysis ed W Zhang and B W Cue *Green Techniques for Organic Synthesis and Medicinal Chemistry* (New York: Wiley) pp 161–84
[49] Wu Q and Tao J 2012 Biocatalysis *Green Techniques for Organic Synthesis and Medicinal Chemistry* ed W Zhang and B W Cue (Wiley)
[50] Hayashi Y 2016 ChemInform abstract: pot economy and one-pot synthesis *Chem. Inform.* **47** 12258
[51] Wang Z and Domling A 2022 Multicomponent reactions in medicinal chemistry *Multicomponent Reactions towards Heterocycles* (Wiley)
[52] Cores Á, Clerigué J, Orocio-Rodríguez E and Menéndez J C 2022 Multicomponent reactions for the synthesis of active pharmaceutical ingredients *Pharmaceuticals* **15** 1009
[53] Mccray S B and Lyon D K 2012 Green drug delivery formulations *Green Techniques for Organic Synthesis and Medicinal Chemistry* (Wiley)
[54] Green Chemistry Challenge Winners | US EPA https://www.epa.gov/greenchemistry/green-chemistry-challenge-winners (accessed 3 March 2023)
[55] Fidler L, Green S and Wintemute K 2022 Pressurized metered-dose inhalers and their impact on climate change *Can. Med. Assoc. J.* **194** E460
[56] Pritchard J N 2020 The climate is changing for metered-dose inhalers and action is needed *Drug. Des. Devel. Ther.* **14** 3043–55
[57] Project Green MDI: Next Generation Metered Dose Inhalers: Promise for our Patients and the Planet https://www.rddonline.com/rdd/knowledge_space.php?id=21&sessionID=116 (accessed 1 May 2023) 2022
[58] ACS GCI Pharmaceutical Roundtable Portal *ACS GCI Pharmaceutical Roundtable Portal* https://www.acsgcipr.org/ (accessed 9 March 2023)
[59] Milanesi M, Runfola A and Guercini S 2020 Pharmaceutical industry riding the wave of sustainability: Review and opportunities for future research *J. Clean. Prod* **261** 121204
[60] Souza H, de O, Costa R, dos S, Quadra G R, Fernandez M A and dos S 2021 Pharmaceutical pollution and sustainable development goals: Going the right way? *Sustain. Chem. Pharm* **21** 100428
[61] Zhang W and Cue B W 2012 *Green Techniques for Organic Synthesis and Medicinal Chemistry* (Wiley)
[62] Sharma V 2015 *Applicability of Green Chemistry in Pharmaceutical Processes* (Pharma Bio World) https://www.piramalpharmasolutions.com/storage/app/uploads/public/5a1/6ca/80b/5a16ca80b33fa671899529.pdf (accessed 10 March 2023)
[63] Veleva V R, Cue B W and Todorova S 2018 Benchmarking green chemistry adoption by the global pharmaceutical supply chain *ACS Sustain. Chem. Eng* **6** 2–14
[64] Environmental Impact Considerations | FDA. https://www.fda.gov/animal-veterinary/development-approval-process/environmental-impact-considerations (accessed 10 March 2023)

[65] EUR-Lex-32001L0083—EN—EUR-Lex. https://eur-lex.europa.eu/legal-content/en/TXT/?uri=CELEX%3A32001L0083 (accessed 10 March 2023)
[66] National Pharmaceutical Strategy—Action Plan 2014—Government.se. https://www.government.se/reports/2014/06/national-pharmaceutical-strategy—action-plan-2014/ (accessed 10 March 2023)
[67] Summary of the Toxic Substances Control Act | US EPA. https://www.epa.gov/laws-regulations/summary-toxic-substances-control-act (accessed 10 March 2023)
[68] REACH—Chemicals—Environment—European Commission. https://ec.europa.eu/environment/chemicals/reach/reach_en.htm (accessed 10 March 2023)
[69] DeVito S C, Keenan C and Lazarus D 2015 Can pollutant release and transfer registers (PRTRs) be used to assess implementation and effectiveness of green chemistry practices? A case study involving the Toxics Release Inventory (TRI) and pharmaceutical manufacturers *Green Chem.* **17** 2679–92
[70] Veleva V and Cue B W 2017 Benchmarking green chemistry adoption by 'big pharma' and generics manufacturers *Benchmarking* **24** 1414–36
[71] Bennett J A, Campbell Z S and Abolhasani M 2019 Role of continuous flow processes in green manufacturing of pharmaceuticals and specialty chemicals *Curr Opin. Chem. Eng* **26** 9–19
[72] Continuous manufacturing builds on hype but adoption remains gradual. https://www.pharmaceutical-technology.com/features/continuous-manufacturing-builds-on-hype-but-adoption-remains-gradual/ (accessed 24 March 2023)
[73] Rogers L and Jensen K F 2019 Continuous manufacturing-the green chemistry promise? *Green Chem.* **21** 3481–98
[74] Poechlauer P, Colberg J, Fisher E, Jansen M, Johnson M D and Koenig S G *et al* 2013 Pharmaceutical roundtable study demonstrates the value of continuous manufacturing in the design of greener processes *Org. Process Res. Dev.* **17** 1472–8
[75] Proctor L, Dunn P, Hawkins J M, Wells A S and Williams M T 2010 Continuous processing in the pharmaceutical industry *Green Chemistry in the Pharmaceutical Industry* (Wiley)
[76] Green Chemistry & Commerce Council 2015 Advancing green chemistry: barriers to adoption & ways to accelerate green chemistry in supply chains *A Report for the Green Chemistry & Commerce Council About the Organizations* www.greenchemistryandcommerce.org (accessed 9 March 2023)
[77] Matus K J M, Clark W C, Anastas P T and Zimmerman J B 2012 Barriers to the implementation of green chemistry in the United States *Environ. Sci. Technol.* **46** 10892–9
[78] Veleva V R and Cue B W 2019 The role of drivers, barriers, and opportunities of green chemistry adoption in the major world markets *Curr. Opin. Green Sustain. Chem.* **19** 30–6
[79] Subramaniam S and Dugar S 2012 Outsourcing drug discovery to India and China: from surviving to thriving *Drug Discov. Today* **17** 1055–8
[80] Chaturvedi U, Sharma M, Dangayach G S and Sarkar P 2017 Evolution and adoption of sustainable practices in the pharmaceutical industry: an overview with an Indian perspective *J. Clean. Prod* **168** 1358–69
[81] Six barriers to implementation of green chemistry in India | Business Standard News. https://www.business-standard.com/content/b2b-chemicals/six-barriers-to-implementation-of-green-chemistry-in-india-114010600785_1.html (accessed 10 March 2023)
[82] Matus K J M, Xiao X and Zimmerman J B 2012 Green chemistry and green engineering in China: Drivers, policies and barriers to innovation *J. Clean. Prod.* **32** 193–203

[83] Wang M Y, Li X Y and He L N 2018 Green chemistry education and activity in China *Curr. Opin. Green Sustain. Chem.* **13** 123–9
[84] Savitskaya T, Kimlenka I, Lu Y, Hrynshpan D, Sarkisov V and Yu J *et al* 2021 Green Chemistry in China and Belarus *Green Chemistry* (Springer)
[85] Wilson M P and Schwarzman M 2009 Toward a new U.S. chemicals policy: Rebuilding the foundation to advance new science, green chemistry, and environmental health *Environ. Health Perspect* **117** 1202–9
[86] European Commission 2020 *Green Deal: Commission Adopts New Chemicals Strategy Towards a Toxic-Free Environment* (Press Release)
[87] Ratti R 2020 Industrial applications of green chemistry: status, challenges and prospects *SN Appl. Sci.* **2** 263
[88] Betts K 2015 How industrial applications in green chemistry are changing our world *American Chemical Society* 1–28
[89] Taber G P, Pfisterer D M and Colberg J C 2004 A new and simplified process for preparing N-[4-(3,4-dichlorophenyl)-3,4-dihydro-1(2H)-naphthalenylidene]methanamine and a telescoped process for the synthesis of (1S-cis)-4-(3,4-dichlorophenol)-1,2,3,4-tetrahydro-N-methyl-1-naphthalenamine mandelate: Key intermediates in the synthesis of sertraline hydrochloride *Org. Process Res. Dev.* **8** 385–8
[90] Dunn P J 2005 Synthesis of commercial phosphodiesterase(V) inhibitors *Org. Process Res. Dev.* **9** 88–97
[91] Savile C K, Janey J M, Mundorff E C, Moore J C, Tam S and Jarvis W R *et al* 2010 Biocatalytic asymmetric synthesis of chiral amines from ketones applied to sitagliptin manufacture *Science* **329** 305–9
[92] Cue B W, Berridge J and Manley J B 2009 PAT and green chemistry: The intersection of benign by design and quality by design *Pharm. Eng* **29** 8–20
[93] Tucker J L 2010 Green chemistry: Cresting a summit toward sustainability *Org. Process Res. Dev.* **14** 328–31
[94] Bystrzanowska M and Tobiszewski M 2018 How can analysts use multicriteria decision analysis? *TrAC—Trends Anal. Chem.* **105** 98–105
[95] Adverse Outcome Pathway (AOP) Research Brief | US EPA. https://www.epa.gov/chemical-research/adverse-outcome-pathway-aop-research-brief (accessed 5 April 2023)
[96] Administrator Wheeler Signs Memo to Reduce Animal Testing, Awards $4.25 Million to Advance Research on Alternative Methods to Animal Testing | US EPA. https://www.epa.gov/newsreleases/administrator-wheeler-signs-memo-reduce-animal-testing-awards-425-million-advance (accessed 5 April 2023)

Chapter 3

Ionic liquid technology for drug delivery applications

Sara A Abouelmagd and Sara A Hassan

Ionic liquids (ILs) are organic salts that melt below room temperature (or 100 °C). Thus, they mostly exist as liquids. Their formation is based on interaction between two oppositely charged bulky counter ions, hence, ILs possess great structural diversity per counter ions' structures. This imparts tunability to their properties. ILs have long been utilized for different applications in the fields of chemical synthesis and analysis. Only recently have ILs found their way into the area of pharmaceutical research. A significant portion of that research was devoted to the synthesis and investigation of active-pharmaceutical ingredient-ILs (API-ILs), where a drug is transformed into a molten salt with new physicochemical properties. Alternatively, ILs were employed to dissolve drugs and/or carry them across biological barriers, where they demonstrated excellent results for different classes of drugs. In this chapter, we discuss different aspects of IL utilization in the pharmaceutical field, including chemistry, application, translation potential and possible challenges.

3.1 Introduction

The process of developing a drug product is roughly divided into two stages: preformulation and formulation (figure 3.1). At preformulation stage, a collaborative effort takes place to study the physical and chemical properties of newly developed therapeutic molecules [1, 2]. Adapting the properties of these molecules for delivery, in suitable carriers, is not an easy task; formulation scientists are frequently challenged by molecules with poor solubility, high lipophilicity, and instability. Circumventing these unfavorable characters to render therapeutic molecules 'deliverable' paves the way for formulation scientists to package these molecules in vehicles and drug carriers suitable for the intended route of administration, required dosage and indication (figure 3.1). Hence, many strategies are being developed for overcoming delivery challenges and optimizing the therapeutic

doi:10.1088/978-0-7503-5613-8ch3

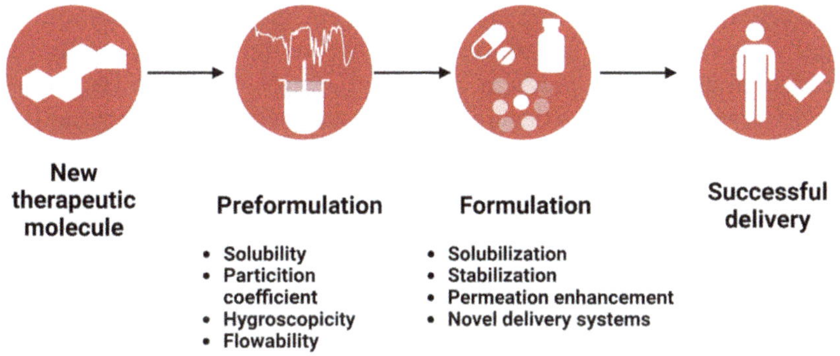

Figure 3.1. Tasks of preformulation and formulation research (created via bioRender.com).

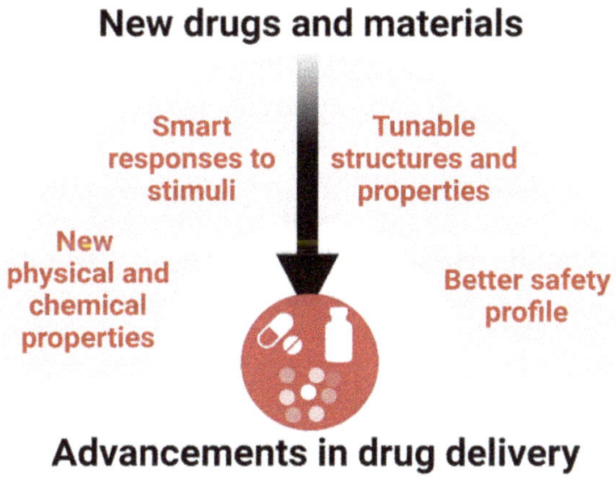

Figure 3.2. Different ways in which chemistry and materials science propel drug delivery (created via bioRender.com).

efficacy of delivered drugs. Based on preformulation studies of the drug, it may be transformed into a salt, chemically modified into a prodrug or reduced in particle size. The optimization of drugs' chemistry enables improvement of their physicochemical properties and biological effects. Over the years, newer generations of drugs with modified structures have demonstrated superior efficacy and reduced side effects [3].

At the formulation stage, poor physicochemical and pharmaceutical properties of the drugs are overcome by implementing suitable excipients and drug vehicles. Solubilizers, stabilizers, surface-active agents and permeation enhancers are among the excipients used [1, 2]. Hence, progress in drug delivery is driven by innovations accomplished in drug discovery, organic chemistry, and formulation, among other areas. Drug delivery science is built upon adapting physical and chemical sciences to achieve control over drug properties and behavior. Historically, innovations in chemistry and materials science have propelled the field of drug delivery [4, 5] (figure 3.2). Continuously, new materials with unique behavior, superior biodegradability and improved safety profiles are being introduced to replace old ones.

Drug delivery systems are being developed using greener solvents and methods. Additionally, development of stimuli-responsive materials enabled the design of smart delivery systems that overcome biological barriers [6]. Therefore, it is essential for drug delivery scientists to leverage advancements in chemistry and materials science to develop practical and effective solutions to delivery challenges.

In this chapter, we discuss different aspects of the development and implementation of IL technology in the pharmaceutical field. Specifically, we review ILs' physicochemical and pharmaceutical properties, focusing on their application as active-pharmaceutical ingredients and pharmaceutical vehicles. Moreover, we discuss their commercial applications and the industrial viewpoint.

3.2 Ionic liquids

3.2.1 Definition

An IL is an organic salt that melts below 100 °C, or at room temperature. To form an IL, two organic molecules carrying opposite charges are reacted, but as they fail to form an ordered crystalline structure, a low-melting point salt, i.e., a liquid, forms [7, 8]. The interaction between the two molecules is typically driven by ionic bonding, although hydrogen bonding and hydrophobic interactions significantly contribute to IL formation. Failure to form a solid is attributed to the molecules' bulky asymmetric structures and diffuse charge distribution [9, 10].

3.2.2 History and perspective

ILs were first introduced in the early 20th century, famously in 1914 by Paul Welden [11, 12]. Since then, ILs have been extensively researched and discussed, mostly, as solvents and extraction media due to their thermal stability and non-volatility. These ILs frequently contained salts of imidazolium, quaternary ammonium and phosphonium [13]. In the last three decades, new generations of ILs were introduced and the potential of ILs as tunable materials led to wider interest across different disciplines, with the term itself encompassing salts of different bioactive molecules [10, 11]. Modern IL research focuses on many aspects of their properties, most importantly tunability and biological effects. Tunability of ILs is attributable to the correlation between their properties and structures of the composing molecules (anions or cations) [10, 14]. Factors such as molecular weight, number of polar groups and chain length influence the melting point and the nature of the produced ILs [15]. Therefore, properties of a drug can be tailored by changing its counter ions' structure, resulting in ILs with tunable properties. Moreover, ILs' biological and therapeutic effects were studied [16]; inherently, an IL can acquire antibacterial effect when its functional groups are capable of interacting with bacteria and/or have membrane permeabilizing effects similar to those of detergents [17]. Additionally, the biological effects of drugs were transformed or enhanced upon their transformation into ILs, warranting research on the effects of IL formation on drugs' biological activities [18–20].

3.2.3 Chemistry of ILs

Understanding the chemistry and molecular interactions of ILs is essential for interpreting their actions and foreseeing their applications. Additionally, it is critical to understand how counter ions structures dictate whether an IL forms or not; molecules' charge, size and symmetry affect their ability to form ILs, as the strength of molecule–molecule interaction determines the melting point [14]. Ford *et al* (2020) listed structural features of ideal counter ions including: (i) high molecular weight and steric hindrance; (ii) diffuse charge; and (iii) reduced symmetry and higher conformational degrees of freedom [14]. Based on molecules' structures and functional groups, the IL produced can be: (i) protic IL; proton transfer occurs between Brønsted acid to Brønsted base, or (ii) aprotic IL; no proton transfer occurs and dissociable hydrogen exists [21, 22]. Protic ILs are easily prepared via acid-base neutralization, and have different ionization degrees based on proton transfer extent and hydrogen bond presence [23]. Their high ionicity requires high pK_a difference between the two compounds (up to 10) [22, 23]. Hence, using relatively weak acids can result in incomplete proton transfer and existence of neutral species within the liquid. On the other hand, ILs can be 'oligomeric,' i.e., contain oligomers of hydrogen-bonded counter ion molecules and therefore, the two counter ions exist in a non-stoichiometric ratio [24]. Overall, it is important to note that any IL is a summation of different intermolecular interactions involving ionizable and non-ionizable groups of the two compounds.

3.2.4 ILs versus deep eutectic solvents

Most literature uses the term IL to described organic salts composed of two oppositely charged molecules. For a true IL, at least by definition, an ionic bonding is essential, i.e., proton transfer occurs between the two molecules [25]. However, ILs exist with varying degrees of 'ionicity' per degree of proton transfer. Alternatively, a deep eutectic solvent (DES) is a structurally related type of liquid, where hydrogen bonding drives the association between two compounds. Therefore, the composing molecules are hydrogen bond donors and hydrogen bond acceptors, rather than anions and cations (figure 3.3). Many newly developed DESs for pharmaceutical applications contain compounds such as sugars, organic acids and amino acids [8]. DESs are frequently prepared via easier methods than those used for IL preparation. Grinding and heating can be sufficient for DES formation, unlike ILs which demand longer steps and product purification [26].

Regardless of driving interaction forces, both types of molecules, ILs and DESs, possess the same characteristics with respect to low vapor pressure, biodegradability and potential for drug properties modulation [28]. Distinguishing between the two can be challenging in some cases; more than one type of interaction may exist between the two molecules, and it can be analytically difficult to determine the dominant interaction type [29]. Moreover, hydrogen bonding can be strong enough to impart partial proton transfer and thus, partial ionization of the two molecules [30]. This prompted many researchers to use the term IL broadly in reference to the properties and applications of the liquid, where a low-melting point organic salt is

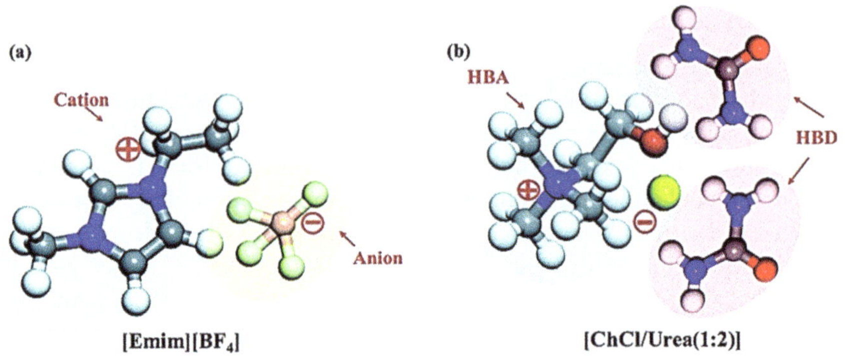

Figure 3.3. Examples of chemical structures for a typical IL = 1-ethyl-3-methylimidazolium tetrafluoroborate (a) and a typical DES = choline chloride and urea (b). Reprinted from [27], with permission from Royal Society of Chemistry.

formed of two oppositely charged molecules, regardless of the type of interaction [31, 32]. This is also warranted by the existence of complex systems with coexisting ionic and neutral species [33]. Other researchers regard DESs as a subclass of ILs or as IL analogs [27]. In the context of this chapter, we use the term IL to describe liquids that melt below 100 °C, where interaction is driven by ionic or hydrogen bonding, or both.

3.2.5 Pharmaceutical applications

In terms of pharmaceutical research, the growing interest in ILs is seen as a new take on how drug development and formulation is carried out. Capitalizing on what ILs have to offer has the potential to solve challenges encountered at the preformulation and formulation stages. There are two main directions for adapting ILs in the pharmaceutical research (figure 3.4). The first direction is to pair a drug molecule with a suitable counter ion to form an IL, i.e., an active-pharmaceutical ingredient IL (API-IL) [34]. The second direction is to use the IL as a drug carrier, or an ingredient of the formulation, acting to facilitate the solubilization or the permeation of a drug [35]. Throughout this chapter, we will discuss both approaches in detail, illustrating how each direction was investigated, and the most significant outcomes.

3.3 API-ILs

3.3.1 The need for API-ILs

Pharmaceutical companies depend primarily on solid crystal forms for drug delivery for many reasons including purity, thermal stability, ease of handling and manufacturing [36]. However, solid drug forms introduce their own problems, including polymorphic conversion, low solubility, poor bioavailability, and spontaneous crystallization of amorphous forms [36]. These problems are often overcome by developing a salt; almost 50% of available drugs are administered as salts [37]. Salt formation modulates drug's physicochemical properties, where bioavailability, effectiveness and safety are all significantly affected by the counter ion type.

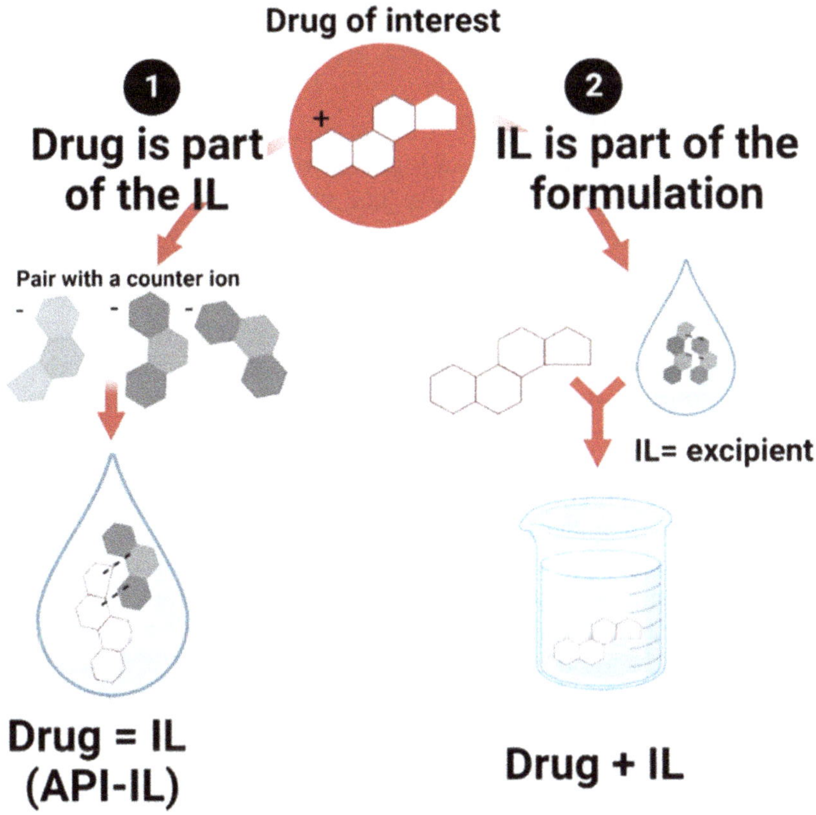

Figure 3.4. The two main approaches for utilization of ILs in pharmaceuticals (created via bioRender.com).

This is one of the reasons why regulatory agencies classify novel salts of registered APIs as new chemical entities [36]. Nonetheless, some problems remain unresolved by salt formation, including spontaneous interconversion of crystalline polymorphs, resulting in formation of polymorphs with different solubilities, efficacies and safety profiles [38]. Amorphous forms and co-crystals have also been developed to address such problems with varying degrees of success [39–41]. Therefore, there is a need for new solutions to ensure more APIs are developable and deliverable.

API-ILs represent a different type of solution to the aforementioned problems as they entirely evade the solid phase; ILs do not experience polymorphic conversions or any other solid state related problem [11]. It is envisioned that APIs can be screened for IL formation in early drug development stages in the same way as salt formation screening. By leveraging the tunability of API-ILs, more drugs can be developed as delivered. Moreover, older APIs and drug leads can be revisited and repurposed for new therapeutic purposes. Rogers and co-workers made the first attempt to prepare API-ILs [11]. They rationally combined different cationic and anionic drugs to modify their pharmaceutical properties including solubility, release rate, stability, and consequently improve their bioavailability and therapeutic effectiveness [11, 13, 42, 43]. In this section of the chapter, we will discuss how IL formation impacts API properties, and progress made in the literature towards their development.

3.3.2 API-ILs versus other drug forms

IL is a salt by definition; its formation is driven by ionic boding, but as discussed earlier, ionic interaction is not exclusive nor guaranteed in developed API-ILs; forces such as hydrogen bonding and hydrophobic interactions exist too. This has drawn several comparisons of API-ILs to other drug forms such as co-crystals and liquid crystals. A co-crystal is a combination of a drug and one or more co-formers, existing in a stoichiometric ratio, interacting via hydrogen bonding or different non-covalent or non-ionic interaction [39–41]. This prompted some researchers to refer to ILs where a proton is shared between the two molecules as liquid co-crystals [44]. Additionally, both ILs and co-crystals are formed by association of a drug and a counter molecule resulting in altered physicochemical properties. A co-crystal can have different melting point, dissolution rate and stability from the native drug [45]. Also, it is more likely to find a suitable co-former (counter molecule) for a drug, than a counter ion (in the case of salts), especially for weak or non-ionizable APIs [45]. However, one important distinction between ILs and co-crystals is the fact that co-crystal formation does not affect the bioactivity of the API.

On the other hand, liquid crystals (ionic liquid crystals; ILCs) are materials of liquid crystalline nature comprised of anion/cation combinations. Hence, unlike ILs, they have ordered structures with a degree of mobility [46]. On the molecular level, ILCs are composed of rigid units of organic molecules arranged in dynamic structures, thus existing as liquids. However, ILCs' applications in the pharmaceutical field are mostly limited to their occasional use as drug carrier materials [47].

3.3.3 Physicochemical and pharmaceutical properties

Diverse cation/anion combinations make it possible to create new APIs in the form of ILs with unique physicochemical and biological characteristics per desired application. Additionally, an API-IL can be composed of two active ingredients, resulting in a dual-active API-IL. The following are the key aspects of drug behavior impacted by API-IL formation, and a review of progress achieved in API-IL synthesis and characterization.

Melting temperature. Melting temperature is one of the key factors affecting drug processing and bioavailability [48]. Intermolecular forces (e.g., hydrogen bonding and van der Waals interactions), and crystal lattice symmetry affect the melting point of any given substance [49]. ILs are usually composed of counter ions with size, symmetry, or charge delocalization that frustrates the crystallization of the compound and consequently lowers its melting temperature [50–53]. Ford *et al* (2020) used three groups of alkyl sulphate counter ions and two model drugs, cinnarizine and lumefantrine, to study the impact of lipophilic counter ion on drugs' melting temperatures [14]. Results showed that long or branched-chain alkyl sulphate counter ions were more effective in increasing both drugs' solubility and lowering their melting points than those with shorter or straighter chains [14].

Thermal stability. Most ILs were reported to be thermally stable at temperatures up to 400°C [54]. The degree of thermal stability depends primarily on the characteristics of constituting counter ions, including coordinating nature, hydrophilicity and nucleophilicity. For example, increasing anions' hydrophilicity or decreasing their coordinating nature or nucleophilicity increased IL's thermal stability [55, 56]. IL's stability was also shown to be influenced by other factors, such as chain length, functionalization and the number of substituents in the cationic counter ion [57]; for example, imidazolium ILs were more thermally stable than piperidinium, pyridinium, and tetra-alkyl ammonium ILs [57, 58].

Viscosity. API-ILs can have an array of viscosities. Low mass transfer rates and difficult handling are two drawbacks of highly viscous ILs [56]. The glass transition temperature (T_g) and the cohesive energy strength were both related to viscosity of an IL; a lower T_g value indicates a reduction in cohesive forces and, consequently, a reduction in viscosity [59]. Hence, viscosity is influenced by drug/counter ion ratio, counter ion structure, and types of interactions that occur within an IL [56, 60, 61]. For instance, viscosities of ketoconazole ILs varied according to the ratios of tartaric and citric acids present as counter ions, where viscosity decreased upon increasing the molar ratio of the carboxylic acids reaching non-stoichiometric ratios (1:2.5 and 1:5; ketoconazole to acid) [60].

In terms of anion structure, symmetric and/or spherical anions were shown to increase the viscosity of ILs [56]. When lidocaine was paired with either ibuprofen or salicylic acid, lidocaine salicylic acid IL showed substantially greater viscosity because of the tighter packing of the smaller, more symmetric salicylate molecules (in comparison to ibuprofen) [62]. In another study, donepezil ILs of long chain unsaturated fatty acids, such as linoleic acid and oleic acid ILs showed lower T_g and viscosities than those of smaller docusate and ibuprofen anions [59]. When it comes to cation structure, long alkyl chains produce ILs with high viscosities, which is attributed to increased intermolecular interactions [56, 63, 64].

Solubility. One of the main purposes of creating API-ILs is to increase aqueous solubilities of native APIs. Counter ion structure as well as the manner with which the drug and counter ion interact determine net solubility. Solubilities of many poorly water-soluble drugs were shown to dramatically improve upon API-IL formation [65–67]. Methotrexate-based ILs prepared using different counter ions such as ammonium and cholinium ions exhibited aqueous solubility at least 5000 times that of native methotrexate [67]. Similarly, acyclovir ILs prepared using phosphonium, cholinium, ammonium and docusate counter ions demonstrated up to 400 times increase in its aqueous solubility [43]. In another study, pairing cholinium with acidic APIs including nalidixic acid, niflumic acid and 4-aminosalicylic acid improved their solubilities in water, gastric, and intestinal fluids [65]. Cholinium also helped increase the solubility of sulfasalazine 400 times in the form of IL [68]. Related results were reported with betulinic acid, etodolac, naproxen, ketoprofen, tolbutamide, ibuprofen, ampicillin and ketoconazole, where API-IL formation significantly enhanced their aqueous solubilities [60, 65, 66, 69–72]. Some examples of API-ILs with significantly improved solubilities are shown in figure 3.5.

Permeability. As API-IL formation impacts the size and lipophilicity of the API, API-ILs can be designed to enhance APIs' permeation through biological membranes

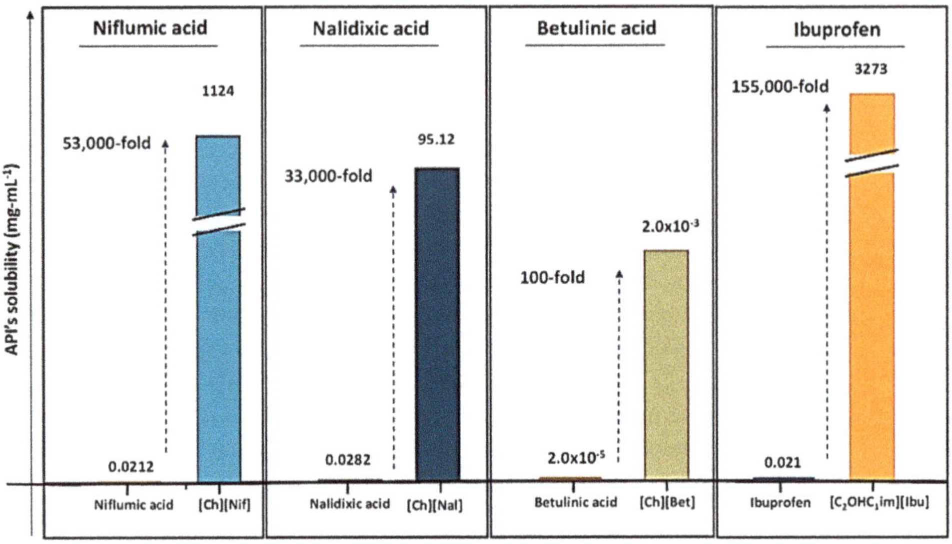

Figure 3.5. Examples illustrate how API-ILs of different APIs had much higher solubilities in aqueous medium in comparison to the parent APIs. Reproduced from [73]. CC BY 4.0.

via precise counter ion selection. Megwa *et al* (2010) paired salicylate anion with quaternary ammonium and alkyl ammonium cations resulting in significantly improved salicylate skin permeation [74]. Moreover, Rogers' group demonstrated that the membrane permeation of salicylate based ILs can be further improved by using PEGylated counter ions (i.e., addition of polyethylene glycol (PEG) to the counter ion) [75]. PEG was reacted with salicylate as a quaternary cationic PEG derivative (PEGylated tributylammonium; $[mPEG_3N_{444}]^+$). PEG's permeation enhancing effect was evident via 2.5-fold increase in salicylate transport across synthetic membrane (in comparison to non-PEGylated cations) [75]. Alternatively, more biocompatible counter ions were used for enhancing APIs' permeation in other reports [76]. Prolinium ethylester ibuprofenate IL showed 10-fold enhancement of ibuprofen's permeability through pig skin in comparison to pure drug in PBS/ethanol solution, without significant damage to fibroblast cells [76]. Another study revealed that hydrophobic molecular interaction between ibuprofen and alkyl chains in counter ions reinforced ionic association, ion pair formation, and hence, transdermal absorption [77].

3.3.4 Biological activity of API-ILs

Counter ion introduction via API-IL formation, does not only modulate the physicochemical properties of the API, but potentially impacts its biological activity. An API-IL can be developed to enhance or complement API's pharmacological actions. For example, lidocaine docusate IL enhanced the pharmacological properties of lidocaine [11]; it was shown to have longer and stronger antinociceptive effect, than native lidocaine, in two different mouse antinociception models. Moreover, at the cellular level, lidocaine docusate IL had a different mechanism of action from that of free lidocaine, as it suppressed neuritic outgrowth in pheochromocytoma (PC12) cells [11].

In another study, Ferraz *et al* (2014) demonstrated that ampicillin-based ILs have superior antibacterial activity against several Gram-negative resistant bacteria, demonstrating greater growth inhibition for several Gram-negative resistant bacteria and 10–1000 higher minimum inhibitory concentration (MIC) values [78]. Additionally, the anti-tumoral activity of these ampicillin-based ILs were investigated using different human cancer cell lines. It was found that 1-hydroxyethyl-3-methylimidazolium-ampicillin IL was the most pertinent ampicillin-based IL, with stronger antiproliferative efficacy and less cytotoxicity against healthy cells. In our own study, we reported the development an API-IL composed of anionic ketoprofen and cationic piperine (table 3.1) [34]. We demonstrated the effect of IL formation on the anti-inflammatory effect of ketoprofen and piperine. IL increased the *in vitro* inhibition of cyclooxygenase-2 and 15-lipooxygenase enzymes in comparison to physical mixture of ketoprofen and piperine. Additionally, when delivered transdermally, IL had 68% higher reduction of paw swelling than the physical mixture in a carrageenan-induced paw edema model.

3.3.5 Dual-active API-ILs

Dual API-ILs are ones where both composing molecules possess biological activity. A rational combination of two counter ions can be designed to induce synergism, provide additional therapeutic effect or counteract unfavorable side effects. Dual-active API-ILs have prompted numerous studies over the last few years. The most common examples of dual-active API-ILs are highlighted in table 3.1. In addition to modulated physicochemical effects, use of dual-functional API-ILs warrants coexistence of the two dissolved APIs together in body fluids at the same time [79]. This does not occur upon administration of APIs separately (in conventional forms) as each may dissolve at a completely different rate [79]. Reports show that ILs may be maintained as a nanostructured organization in aqueous media, rather than dissolving as separate ions [79].

3.4 ILs as part of pharmaceutical formulation

ILs have been employed to play different roles in dosage form design. This includes using IL as a vehicle or a formulation constituent (solvent, co-solvent, permeation enhancer, emulsifier, etc). The following is an overview of different ways in which ILs have been utilized in formulations.

3.4.1 IL as a solvent/vehicle

The pharmaceutical industry is one of the biggest consumers of the organic solvents [86]. Often, it is not possible to completely evade organic solvents' residues in the final pharmaceutical product even via various drying techniques [87]. Therefore, great efforts have been made to reduce the use of organic solvents and replace them with 'green' environmentally friendlier alternatives, such as ILs [87, 88]. Historically, ILs have long been investigated as solvents, co-solvents and hydrotropes for various drugs [89, 90]. This was first investigated by Jaitely *et al* (2010), where solubilization of penicillin V, progesterone and dexamethasone was studied using water-immiscible room temperature ILs (RTILs) [91]. While developed ILs were water immiscible,

Table 3.1. Examples of dual-active API-ILs.

Cationic API	Anionic API	Biological activity/ activities of the API-IL	References
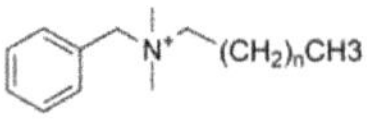 Benzalkonium	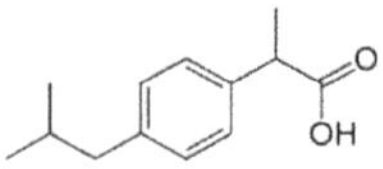 Ibuprofen	Antibacterial/anti-inflammatory	[80, 81]
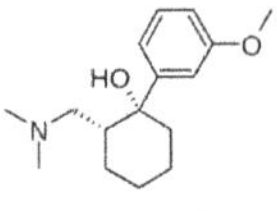 Tramadolium	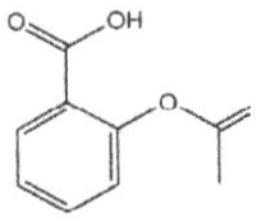 Aspirin	Dual anti-inflammatory effect	[82, 83]
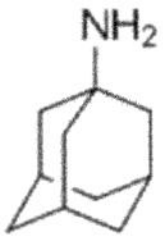 Amantadine	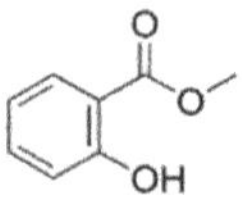 Salicylate	Antiviral/anti-inflammatory, analgesic and keratolytic	[23]
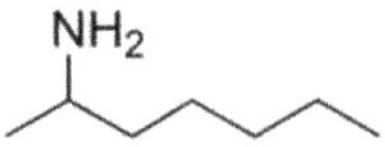 Tuaminoheptane	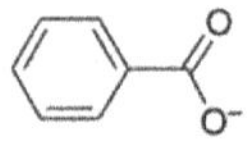 Benzoate	Vasoconstrictor/anti-inflammatory, analgesic and keratolytic	[23, 84]
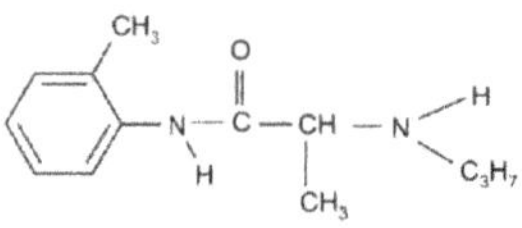 Prilocaine	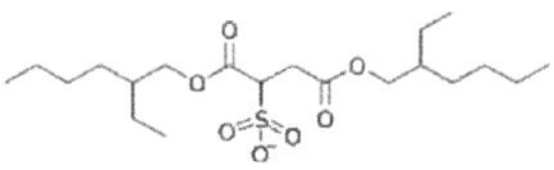 Docusate	Local anesthetics/ emollient	[85]
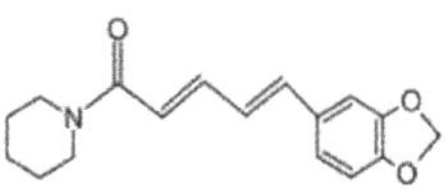 Piperine	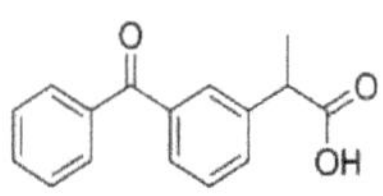 Ketoprofen	Dual anti-inflammatory effect	[34]
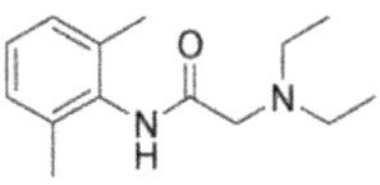 Lidocaine	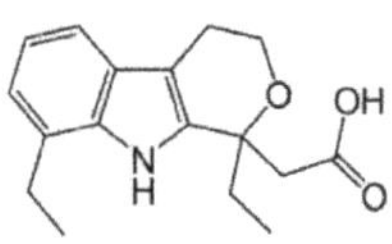 Etodolac	Local anesthetic/analgesic	[70]
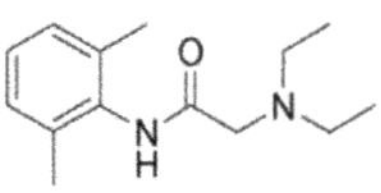 Lidocaine	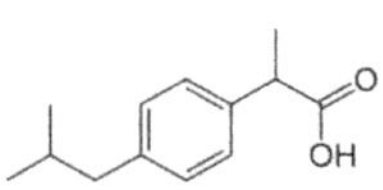 Ibuprofen 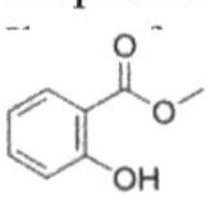 Salicylic acid	Local anesthetic/analgesic	[19, 30, 62]

they enhanced the release rates of these APIs into aqueous medium up to three-fold, where rates correlated with cation alkyl chain length [91]. McCrary and co-workers described the structural features of ILs required to solubilize amphiphilic poorly water soluble drugs, amphotericin B and itraconazole [92]; drugs' aqueous solubility were enhanced when using ILs with functional groups complementary to ion(s) of the API molecule, hence, disrupt inter/intramolecular hydrogen bonding and achieve optimal hydrophilic–lipophilic balance (HLB) [92].

Some studies employed experimental and molecular dynamics modelling to investigate the solubilization mechanisms of the cardiovascular drug, LASSBio-294, using imidazolium-based ILs [93, 94]. LASSBio-294 solubility was improved via formation of hydrogen bonding with IL, π–π interaction between IL's imidazolium cations and the drug's aromatic rings and van der Waals interaction [93, 94]. Figure 3.6 depicts the solvation mechanism for LASSBio-294; different structural features of the IL enabled its solubilizing effect on LASSBio-294. Furthermore, ILs were used as efficient solvents for a variety of biopolymers, including nucleic acids [95, 96], proteins [97, 98], and polysaccharides [96, 99]. They were also employed in their processing into films and micro- or nanoparticles.

It is noteworthy that ILs were frequently used as API solvents in microemulsions. IL-in-oil (IL/O) microemulsions approach was used to enhance transdermal

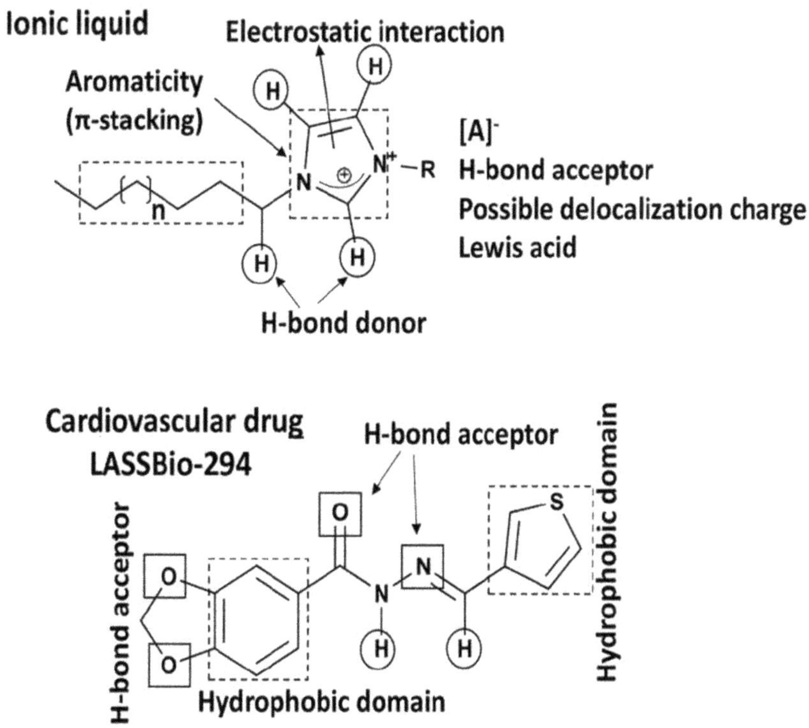

Figure 3.6. Schematic presentation of possible interactions between LASSBio-294 and solubilizing imidazolium-based ILs. Reprinted with permission from [94].Copyright (2014) American Chemical Society.

permeation of acyclovir. Acyclovir was dispersed in ILs droplets, then stabilized in a continuous oil phase via two non-ionic surfactants, tween-80, and span-20 (3:2 weight ratio) [100]. The ability of these carriers to solubilize three sparingly water soluble drugs, including acyclovir, methotrexate, and dantrolene sodium was investigated [101]. Different hydrophilic ILs were tested as dispersed phases and the results showed that ILs with coordinating anions (potent hydrogen bond acceptors) were the most successful ILs in generating microemulsion droplets [101].

3.4.2 IL as a permeation enhancer

IL can enhance membrane permeability via different mechanisms including disruption of cellular membrane, membrane fluidization, and development of diffusional pathways through extraction of lipids from the stratum corneum (SC) [102–104].

Disruption of cellular membrane; several studies were performed to illustrate the mechanism by which ILs interact with biological membranes [105, 106]. It was verified by neutron scattering that ILs decrease the lipid bilayer thickness and their cations accumulate between lipid's polar heads and hydrocarbon tails, thus altering lipid composition [107]. Later, using fluorescence imaging and x-ray scattering techniques, it was shown that amphiphilic ILs could be inserted into the lipid bilayer disrupting its packing [105]. This was further investigated by Dickinson *et al* (2016) using *Saccharomyces cerevisiae* yeast mitochondrial membrane; for imidazolium ILs, electrostatic interactions between cation's long side chains results in heterogeneous aggregation, while cation and anion's head groups space out evenly [108, 109]. This unique aggregation pattern disrupts self-assembled structure of the lipid bilayer increasing its permeability [109, 110]. In addition, the degree of hydrophobicity of the alkyl chains in the IL ions determines whether the membrane is disrupted or not [111].

Membrane fluidization; one study's experimental evidence shows that hydrophilic imidazolium-based ILs fluidize the cell membrane to open up channels for molecule diffusion [103]. Even though this study linked IL-enhanced cellular membrane permeability to cytotoxicity, it is conceivable that these processes should facilitate drug delivery to intended targets.

Development of diffusional pathways; Qi *et al* (2019) demonstrated that choline geranic acid ILs can form pores and transport pathways through the skin via extraction of lipids and proteins from the SC [112]. However, it is feasible to enhance the transdermal delivery of several APIs using ILs without affecting membrane integrity. This can be achieved by careful selection of IL ions, considering hydrophobic/hydrophilic balance, i.e., optimizing permeation across biological membranes as well as solubility in aqueous solutions [92, 113].

Several other factors should be considered when developing ILs as permeation enhancers, including chain length of the alkyl chains, IL electronic profile and degree of ionicity.

Chain length; Bhattacharya *et al* (2018) studied the effect of alkyl chain length on a model phospholipid membrane using two imidazolium-based ILs [109]. This study revealed that short chain ILs (ethyl hydrocarbon) interact less strongly, with lipid bilayers, than long chain ILs (butyl hydrocarbons), thus would be more diffusible through membranes. Other mechanisms were suggested by Almeida *et al* (2017) who investigated the effect of imidazolium-based ILs as a vehicle on permeation of two model drugs: caffeine and salicylic acid. For caffeine, skin permeation enhancement was related to ILs' alkyl chain length; the longer the alkyl chain the higher was the flux and diffusion through the skin [114]. This was attributed to the surface activity of longer alkyl chains as they disrupt skin membranes and thus increase drug flux. However, for salicylic acid, the alkyl chain length had a minor effect on the drug permeation [114]. In general, ILs with long alkyl chains have surfactant-like properties and hence are termed surface-active ILs (SAILs). SAILs were shown to have comparable (occasionally superior) surface activity to traditional surfactants [115]. SAILs have been investigated as drug carriers to develop transdermal, topical and even intravenous delivery systems [116, 117]. In transdermal drug delivery systems such as microemulsions, SAILs have been successfully used as substitutes for surfactants [118, 119].

The electronic profile; Zhang *et al* (2017) investigated 20 imidazolium ILs for enhancing transdermal delivery of testosterone using a quantitative structure–activity relationship (QSAR) model [120]. This study demonstrated ILs' skin permeation enhancement was dependent on their electronic properties, i.e., ionic composition.

Degree of ionicity; It was reported that partially ionized ILs can penetrate the membrane lipid bilayer (as hydrogen bond complex) more readily than fully ionized ILs mediated by optimal interactions with the lipid bilayers [23, 42, 84, 121].

3.5 IL-based drug delivery systems

The main difference between native API form and ILs is their liquid physical state. Whether they are used as API-ILs, or ILs are used to dissolve the API, IL-based delivery systems need to be approached differently from conventional solid drugs. Generally, ILs are either incorporated as part of a liquid or semisolid formulation or immobilized on a solid substrate. In this section, we will discuss different examples of delivery systems incorporating IL technology either as API-ILs, or as a part of the formulation. Key aspects of formulations designed for oral, dermal, or transdermal delivery are discussed, illustrating key findings and design aspects.

3.5.1 Oral drug delivery

For the development of an API-IL-based drug delivery system, one of the reported methods is loading API-ILs on high-surface area carrier material such as mesoporous silica [122]. Tetrabutylphosphonium-ibuprofenate and lidocainium-ibuprofenate ILs were loaded on silica to facilitate their handling and enable their rapid and complete release [122]. Importantly, it was found that the type of silica used, whether calcined or non-calcined, affects the IL release; calcined silica caused surface hydrophobication and thus, incomplete release of IL. Conversely, non-calcined silica had less hydrophobic surface and complete IL release. The type of medium used for *in vitro* release experiments was also found to affect the release rate with [122].

In another study, Zhang *et al* (2013) applied an all-in-one concept for preparation of API-IL vesicles; API-IL was used both as a carrier and a drug [123]. API-IL was produced by combining amitriptyline hydrochloride, a cationic drug, with sodium dodecyl sulphate, an anionic surfactant. Produced API-IL spontaneously self-assembled into ~342 nm vesicles when placed in an aqueous solution. Importantly, vesicles had high loading capacity of 57.7% and showed relative control of drug release in both acidic (pH 1.2) and neutral-pH (pH 7.4) medium [123]. When it comes to utilizing ILs as vehicles, Banerjee *et al* (2018) reported the use of cholinium geranate (CAGE) IL as a vehicle for insulin oral delivery. Insulin-CAGE were loaded into Eudragit L-100 enteric-coated tablets and administered to rats via oral gavage. Oral capsules were as effective as subcutaneously administered insulin but showed more prolonged effect. These effects were attributed to: (i) CAGE improving insulin paracellular transport; (ii) CAGE protecting insulin from enzymatic breakdown in the intestine; and (iii) CAGE-induced decrease in mucus layer thickness [124].

3.5.2 Dermal and transdermal drug delivery

ILs were mostly hailed in the literature for their ability to increase drug permeation through the skin and overcome the skin barrier. In proof-of-concept studies, these ILs were mostly used in their native form or after dispersion in a suitable vehicle. However, several IL-based drug delivery systems have been designed for skin application of ILs, including microemulsions [35, 125] patches/membranes [126, 127] and nanoparticles [128] and gels [129, 130].

Microemulsions. They represent one of the most studied systems for IL delivery. The use of ILs allowed introducing unique microemulsion systems designed to enhance permeation of drugs [113, 131]. Moreover, per IL nature, it can be incorporated in the microemulsion as a surface-active agent, oil phase or aqueous phase. Another advantage of the IL-microemulsion systems is the thermal stability of systems where aqueous phase is replaced by an IL [116].

In one study, imidazolium IL-based microemulsions were developed for topical drug delivery of dencichine, [132]. Dencichine is a hemostatic drug with a hydrophilic nature that hinders its permeability through skin's lipophilic surface. It was loaded into an IL-based microemulsion comprising 1-hydroxyethyl-3-methylimidazolium chloride ([HOEIM]Cl) and 1-butyl-3-methylimidazolium dodecanesulfate ([BMIM]$C_{12}SO_3$) within the hydrophilic and surfactant phases, respectively. Prepared microemulsion-incorporated isopropyl myristate and tween-80, had sub-100 nm droplets and increased dencichine skin permeation up to 10-fold. When applied *in vivo* to rat skin, it showed considerable hemostatic effect as demonstrated by bleeding time, with efficacy comparable to that of oral delivery [132].

Vesicles and nanoparticles. When ILs are employed to form vesicles, they are often highly stable, small in size with drug molecules adsorbed onto their surface. Importantly, they enhance the delivery of the drug across biological membranes. In one study, ILs composed of cationic diisopropanolamine or triisopropanolamine were combined with anionic octanoic or isostearic acid were used to form vesicles suspended in isopropyl myristate (figure 3.7). This system was tested for loading and

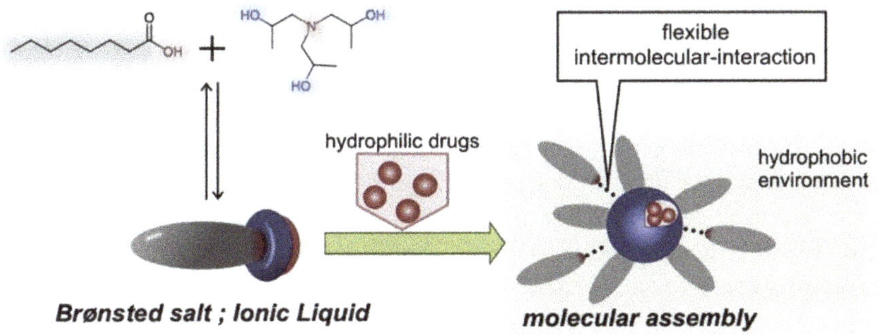

Figure 3.7. Schematic presentation of self-assembled IL aggregates designed for loading and delivery of hydrophilic drugs in the core; the alkyl chains of the carboxylic acid represent the hydrophobic region, while propanolamine derivative molecules arrangements represent the core. Excess acid was shown to enhance the performance of vesicles as drug carriers through the skin, due to hydrogen bonding with the vesicles, leading to superior skin penetration. Reprinted from [113], copyright (2016), with permission from Elsevier.

delivery of hydrophilic molecules; the system enabled skin permeation of phenol red at much higher amount than that observed with plain isopropyl myristate vehicle. Presence of excess carboxylic acid was found to contribute to the enhanced delivery, as IL forms hydrogen bonds with excess acid facilitating the transport of drug via the lipophilic skin barrier [113].

Mediated by intermolecular interactions, ILs were used to form stable and tunable polymeric nanoparticulate structures for a variety of applications [133]. IL-polymer nanoparticle hybrid systems were employed to overcome the low solubility of some drugs, including rutin [128]. Rutin-loaded poly(lactic-co-glycolic acid) (PLGA) nanoparticles, were prepared with the help of two amino-acid-based ILs; cholinium phenylalanine and cholinium L-glutamine. Considering the limited solubility of rutin, these systems were able to achieve high drug loading ranging from 51% to 76%. Nanoparticles were found to be nontoxic to keratinocytes [128].

Gels. One study reports the preparation of a self-polymerizing IL gel made from choline formate IL after mixing with 2-hydroxyethyl methacrylate, a known monomer of biocompatible polymers [134]. At room temperature, and different ratios of IL to the monomer, a viscous liquid, soft gel or hard gel can be produced due to radical polymerization. The tunability and biocompatibility of the components suggest the use of the gel for versatile biomedical applications. On the other hand, IL was successfully transformed to the form of an ionogel, which is a biphasic material consisting of a swollen silica-based network. In this approach, one-step nonaqueous sol-gel technique was employed to confine the IL within silica network (using either pure tetramethoxysilane or combined with methyltrimethoxysilane) [129, 130]. Ionogel of imidazolium ibuprofenate IL was shown to achieve ~50% drug loading, where the release kinetics were controlled via the properties of the silica network [129].

Patches. This is another approach where ILs are deposited on a solid support material to ease skin application. In one study, NSAID-cholinium-based ILs were incorporated into bacterial cellulose membranes [126]. ILs improved the solubility of NSAIDs, namely ibuprofen, naproxen, and ketoprofen, in aqueous medium by up to 100-fold. When bacterial cellulose membranes were impregnated with these ILs, the membranes' capacity to retain water was enhanced by up to 26-fold, enabling better absorption of inflammatory exudates. Moreover, 90% of the drugs were released in phosphate-buffered saline after 2 h of incubation [126]. Cholinium was also utilized in another study to prepare vitamin B ILs, including vitamins B3, B5 and B6. Prepared ILs had higher solubility than native vitamins. Upon incorporation into bacterial cellulose membranes, the ILs acted as plasticizers rendering the membrane less brittle and of 2.9 to 4.8-fold higher rehydration capacity. Hence, this system was proposed to be suitable for skin care applications [127].

3.6 Commercial application and industrial viewpoint

As discussed so far, ILs have proven their capability of solving challenges encountered at stages of drug development and pharmaceutical formulation. Whether they are used as APIs or part of the formulation, they were proven to make drugs easier to deliver, modulate their properties and enhance their therapeutic performance. Moreover, ILs have been explored at the stages of drug synthesis and manufacture. Figure 3.8 demonstrates the different aspects of IL use in the pharmaceutical field. Consequently, increased interest in pharmaceutical IL research brings up the discussions of translation potential and applicability. API-ILs have the potential to address challenges faced early on during the stages of lead development. As an application-driven technology, API-IL formation can make it into screening stage as an alternative approach to conventional salt formation. Unlike solid salts, API-ILs are not susceptible to polymorphic conversion and their solubility is not limited by a dissolution step [135]. Importantly, API-ILs tunability renders it possible to continuously tailor prepared ILs to obtain more favorable physicochemical properties [13].

On the other hand, ILs adapted for formulation and drug delivery applications possess many favorable characteristics as potential pharmaceutical excipients and solvents. These characteristics include their non-volatility and green nature [13]. ILs such as choline-geranic acid (CAGE) are undergoing development as a leading example of the next generation of delivery vehicles; CAGE's biocompatibility,

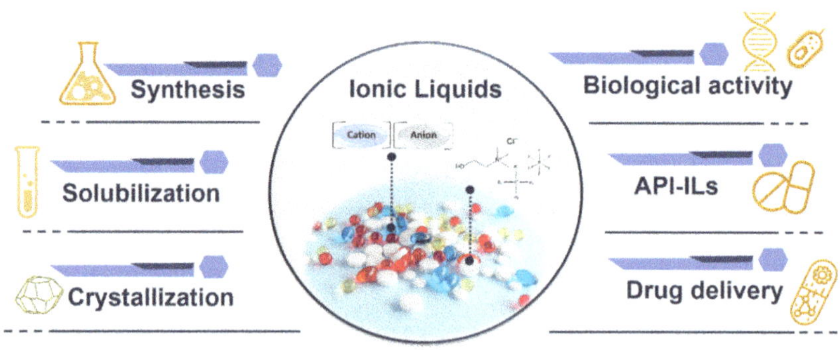

Figure 3.8. Applications of ILs in the pharmaceutical field. Reproduced from [73]. CC BY 4.0.

versatility, permeation enhancing effect and favorable antimicrobial effects set it as an example to what ILs can bring to the pharmaceutical industry [136].

While most of the interest in pharmaceutical ILs is recent, ILs found their way to pharmaceutical products many years ago. The first API-IL product to make its way as a commercial product is Flector® patch system which is the non-steroidal anti-inflammatory drug (NSAID) diclofenac in the form of epolamine, i.e., 1-(2-hydroxyethyl) pyrrolidinium, salt [9, 137, 138]. Diclofenac epolamine was shown to have higher solubility in 1-octanol, than other salts tested with mild detergent properties, accounting for its activity upon skin delivery [137]. Nonetheless, when Flector® was developed, less attention was directed to the nature of diclofenac salt, in comparison to its formulation and efficacy. Flector® is a 10 × 14 cm patch made of an adhesive material containing 1.3% diclofenac epolamine spread over a non-woven polyester felt packing and coated with a polypropylene film lining (https://www.flector.com/). Another set of products are currently under testing by MEDRx Inc., a company based in Japan developing transdermal and topical API-IL systems (https://www.medrx.co.jp/english/index.html). These systems include fentanyl patches for pain management (phase I), tizanidine patches for treatment of spasticity (phase II) and lidocaine patches for neuropathic pain (completed phase III) [139].

Regarding ILs used as vehicles and solvent systems, there is no mass application of ILs so far. However, CAGE stands out as one of the most studied IL/DES systems in the recent years with promising commercialization potential. Developed by the Mitragotri group, CAGE, which consists of choline and geranic acid (1:2, respectively) was extensively researched with interesting results reported regarding different aspects of its structure, formation, and performance [140, 141]. The group also showed a blueprint for IL clinical translation in seven stages, where CAGE synthesis, characterization and toxicological and clinical evaluation were described [142]. Industrially relevant scale-up processes were illustrated for economic and commercially applicable preparation, while clinical studies demonstrated its efficacy, when formulated as a gel (40%), for management of rosacea and facial redness (NCT04886739 and NCT04508660, respectively; https://clinicaltrials.gov/). Efficacy was attributed to a combination of inherent antimicrobial effect and deep dermal penetration [142].

One of the companies that is currently achieving progress in the area of pharmaceutical IL technology is i2O therapeutics (https://i2obio.com/). The company focuses on developing oral formulations of biologics. Such formulations are developed with a focus on protecting biologics from the GIT environment, reducing mucus viscosity, and enhancing intestinal absorption. These products aim to manage metabolic and inflammatory diseases efficiently and safely.

3.6.1 Translation and production challenges

Biological and toxic effects. Inherent biological effect of ILs is a double-edged sword; for API-ILs this frequently involves enhanced pharmacological effects or favorable complementary actions [88]. However, different ILs adapted as solvents and vehicles, comprising different counter ions' chemistries, have variable degrees of biologic and toxic effects [135]. These effects correlate to chemical structures of IL's composing ions. Choice of the counter ion structure will impact IL's biological and toxic effects; ions of biological origin and known safety will produce safer and more biocompatible ILs. Third-generation ILs are known for adapting materials such as amino acids and carbohydrates as counter ions with known biocompatibility and biodegradability [135]. On the other hand, commonly used imidazolium ions were shown to induce higher toxic effects when in IL form, in comparison to other cationic counter ions, unlike ILs composed of ammonium cations and carboxylic acid anions which were described to be safer [25, 135, 143]. Therefore, careful selection of precursors is necessary when designing new IL systems, and examination of possible biologic and toxic effects should be carried out to avoid any undesirable *in vivo* effects.

Regulatory aspects. API-ILs, by definition, are molten salts, hence, they will mostly be regarded by drug regulatory bodies as new entities or compounds, distinct from the native drug form. Nonetheless, the complexity sometimes encountered in defining API-IL systems can prove to be challenging with time. Systems comprising both hydrogen bonding and ionic interactions, such as oligomeric ILs and non-stoichiometric ILs, can be challenging to categorize using the same standards as solid crystalline APIs or co-crystals. For example, co-crystal systems where an API and co-former form a crystalline structure together, mostly driven by hydrogen bonding, are not considered new entities. The co-former is given an excipient status by the FDA and treated similarly to a polymorph [144, 145]. Specifically, the FDA identifies two conditions for such material to be considered a co-crystal when they have ionizable groups: (i) proof of absence of proton transfer between API and co-former (when $\Delta pK_a \geqslant 1$), and (ii) proof of API successful dissociation from the co-crystal before reaching site of action. Otherwise, it will be treated as a salt, i.e., a new entity by the FDA [144]. On the other hand, the fact that they are liquids is a major aspect of how they are set apart from conventional crystalline salts in terms of regulations [146]. Established FDA regulations are set for solids by default. A question arises of how flexible will the regulatory bodies be in terms of regulating API-ILs? The answer to the question will determine to how fast this technology can be adapted and whether real progress can be achieved on the commercial level.

Manufacture and scale-up. In terms of industrial IL preparation on the large scale, aspects such as good manufacturing process (GMP) regulations, cost, ease of manufacturing, materials availability and infrastructure are the most critical. Established FDA regulations and operating procedures were long set for solid APIs. Investing in establishing similar procedures and manufacturing processes is a relatively risky, but necessary process for pharmaceutical companies to undertake.

3.7 Future perspective

The use of ILs either as APIs or formulation component has great potential for overcoming the ongoing struggles of the pharmaceutical industry in terms of getting new therapies to the market. Even with expected challenges of IL regulations and manufacture, hallmark tunability of ILs renders these challenges beatable. Figure 3.9 depicts our SWOT analysis of pharmaceutical IL technology (strengths, weaknesses, opportunities, and challenges). Largely, the speed with which

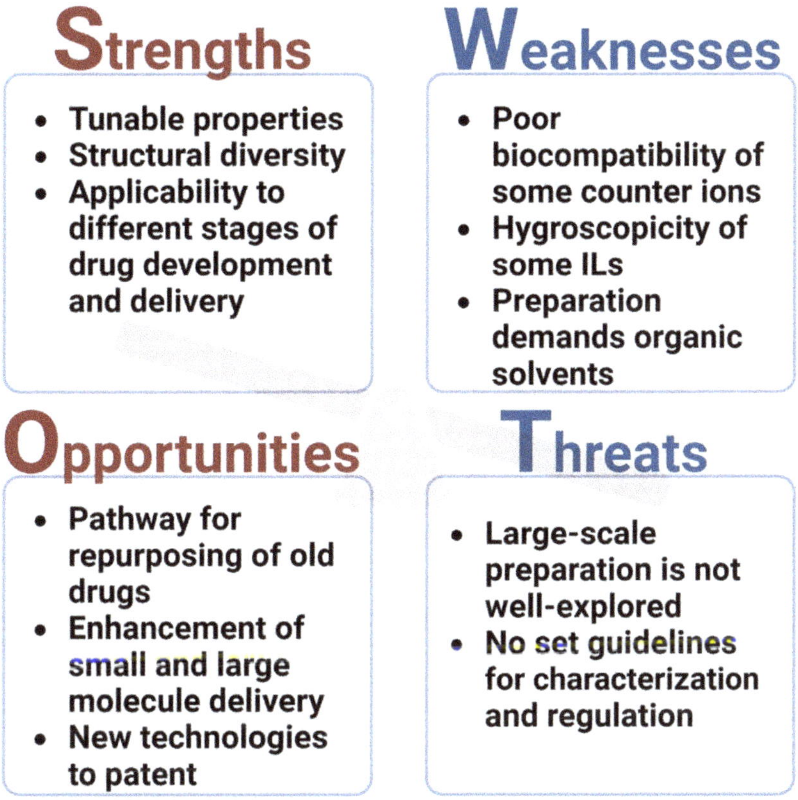

Figure 3.9. The strengths, weaknesses, opportunities, and threats (SWOT) analysis for use of ILs in pharmaceutical industry (created via bioRender.com).

pharmaceutical researchers can leverage IL potential is contingent upon the flexibility of regulatory authorities and audacity of the pharmaceutical industry. Regulatory bodies should set the stage for researchers to bring these technologies from the lab to the bed, which is attainable by setting clear and reasonable steps for characterizing and standardizing developed ILs. On the other hand, resourceful pharmaceutical companies can take the lead by investing in these technologies and: (i) incorporate screening for API-IL as a standard drug development process; (ii) develop facilities for large-scale manufacturing for these materials; (iii) push regulating bodies for standardization of IL manufacture and classification of API-ILs.

3.8 Conclusion

While still in their infancy, pharmaceutical IL technologies are beyond promising. Whether they are developed as unique and novel pharmaceutical excipients or new drug entities with superior properties, API-ILs demonstrate their potential as new drug forms with tunable structures and properties. Transforming a drug into an IL enables modulation of its solubility, permeability, and even stability. This opens the door for repurposing existing drugs with poor properties. On the other hand, leveraging ILs as permeation enhancers, vehicles, and solvents has already proven to be an efficient approach, showing impressive results with both small molecules and biologics. Importantly, understanding the molecular basis of ILs is necessary for their utilization. A multidisciplinary approach for the testing and application of pharmaceutical ILs is needed. Chemists and formulation scientists should work together to optimize IL preparation and implement the technology, which would in turn accelerate their development. Finally, it is up to regulatory agencies to keep up with the progress in this field to ensure new drugs and formulations have a clear path for characterization and approval.

References

[1] Pinak P 2019 *Preformulation Studies: An Integral Part of Formulation Design* ed A Usama and A Juber (Rijeka: IntechOpen) ch 1

[2] 2001 *Handbook of Modern Pharmaceutical Analysis* ed S Ahuja (Academic)

[3] Zhang Y, Chan H F and Leong K W 2013 Advanced materials and processing for drug delivery: the past and the future *Adv. Drug Deliv. Rev.* **65** 104–20

[4] Bae Y H and Park K 2020 Advanced drug delivery 2020 and beyond: perspectives on the future *Adv. Drug Delivery Rev.* **158** 4–16

[5] Elliott J and Hancock B 2006 Pharmaceutical materials science: an active new frontier in materials research *MRS Bull.* **31** 869–73

[6] Abouelmagd S A, Ellah N H A and Hamid B N A E 2019 *Temperature and pH Dual-Stimuli Responsive Polymeric Carriers for Drug Delivery* ed A S H Makhlouf and N Y Abu-Thabit (Woodhead Publishing) ch 3 pp 87–109

[7] Mangrule V, Pore Y and Disouza J 2017 Synthesis and physicochemical studies of fluconazole ionic liquids *J. Appl. Pharm. Sci.* **7** 84–9

[8] Zainal-Abidin M H, Hayyan M, Ngoh G C, Wong W F and Looi C Y 2019 Emerging frontiers of deep eutectic solvents in drug discovery and drug delivery systems *J. Control. Release* **316** 168–95

[9] Agatemor C, Ibsen K N, Tanner E E and Mitragotri S 2018 Ionic liquids for addressing unmet needs in healthcare *Bioeng. Transl. Med.* **3** 7–25

[10] Adawiyah N, Moniruzzaman M, Hawatulaila S and Goto M 2016 Ionic liquids as a potential tool for drug delivery systems *Med. Chem. Commun.* **7** 1881–97

[11] Hough W L, Smiglak M, Rodríguez H, Swatloski R P, Spear S K, Daly D T, Pernak J, Grisel J E, Carliss R D and Soutullo M D 2007 The third evolution of ionic liquids: active pharmaceutical ingredients *New J. Chem.* **31** 1429–36

[12] Walden P 1914 Molecular weights and electrical conductivity of several fused salts *Bull Acad. Imper. Sci.(St Petersburg)* **1800**

[13] Shamshina J L, Kelley S P, Gurau G and Rogers R D 2015 Chemistry: develop ionic liquid drugs *Nature News* **528** 188

[14] Ford L, Tay E, Nguyen T-H, Williams H D, Benameur H, Scammells P J and Porter C J 2020 API ionic liquids: probing the effect of counterion structure on physical form and lipid solubility *RSC Adv.* **10** 12788–99

[15] Sahbaz Y, Williams H D, Nguyen T-H, Saunders J, Ford L, Charman S A, Scammells P J and Porter C J H 2015 Transformation of poorly water-soluble drugs into lipophilic ionic liquids enhances oral drug exposure from lipid based formulations *Mol. Pharmaceutics* **12** 1980–91

[16] Ferraz R, Silva D, Dias A R, Dias V, Santos M M, Pinheiro L, Prudencio C, Noronha J P, Petrovski Z and Branco L C 2020 Synthesis and antibacterial activity of ionic liquids and organic salts based on Penicillin G and Amoxicillin hydrolysate derivatives against resistant bacteria *Pharmaceutics* **12** 221
[17] Yang D D, Paterna N J, Senetra A S, Casey K R, Trieu P D, Caputo G A, Vaden T D and Carone B R 2021 Synergistic interactions of ionic liquids and antimicrobials improve drug efficacy *iScience* **24** 101853
[18] Park H J and Prausnitz M 2015 Lidocaine-ibuprofen ionic liquid for dermal anesthesia *AlChE J.* **61** 2732–8
[19] Berton P, Di Bona K R, Yancey D, Rizvi S A A, Gray M, Gurau G, Shamshina J L, Rasco J F and Rogers R D 2017 Transdermal bioavailability in rats of lidocaine in the forms of ionic liquids, salts, and deep eutectic *ACS Med. Chem. Lett.* **8** 498–503
[20] Smith D J, Shah J K and Maginn E J 2015 Molecular dynamics simulation study of the association of lidocainium docusate and its derivatives in aqueous solution *Mol. Pharmaceutics* **12** 1893–901
[21] Yoshizawa M, Xu W and Angell C A 2003 Ionic liquids by proton transfer: vapor pressure, conductivity, and the relevance of ΔpKa from aqueous solutions *J. Am. Chem. Soc.* **125** 15411–9
[22] Koutsoukos S, Becker J, Dobre A, Fan Z, Othman F, Philippi F, Smith G J and Welton T 2022 Synthesis of aprotic ionic liquids *Nat. Rev. Methods Primers* **2** 49
[23] Stoimenovski J, Dean P M, Izgorodina E I and MacFarlane D 2012 Protic pharmaceutical ionic liquids and solids: aspects of protonics *Faraday Discuss.* **154** 335–52
[24] Kelley S P, Narita A, Holbrey J D, Green K D, Reichert W M and Rogers R D 2013 Understanding the effects of ionicity in salts, solvates, co-crystals, ionic co-crystals, and ionic liquids, rather than nomenclature, is critical to understanding their behavior *Cryst. Growth Des.* **13** 965–75
[25] Qader I B and Prasad K 2022 Recent developments on ionic liquids and deep eutectic solvents for drug delivery applications *Pharm. Res.* **39** 2367–77
[26] Płotka-Wasylka J, de la Guardia M, Andruch V and Vilková M 2020 Deep eutectic solvents vs ionic liquids: similarities and differences *Microchem. J.* **159** 105539
[27] Ma C, Laaksonen A, Liu C, Lu X and Ji X 2018 The peculiar effect of water on ionic liquids and deep eutectic solvents *Chem. Soc. Rev.* **47** 8685–720
[28] Wang J, Li M, Duan L, Lin Y, Cui X, Yang Y and Wang C 2022 Deep eutectic systems as novel vehicles for assisting drug transdermal delivery *Pharmaceutics* **14** 2265
[29] Bica K, Shamshina J, Hough W L, MacFarlane D R and Rogers R D 2011 Liquid forms of pharmaceutical co-crystals: exploring the boundaries of salt formation *Chem. Commun (Camb)* **47** 2267–9
[30] Wang H, Gurau G, Shamshina J, Cojocaru O A, Janikowski J, MacFarlane D R, Davis J H and Rogers R D 2014 Simultaneous membrane transport of two active pharmaceutical ingredients by charge assisted hydrogen bond complex formation *Chem. Sci.* **5** 3449–56
[31] Rogers R D and Gurau G 2018 Is 'choline and geranate' an ionic liquid or deep eutectic solvent system? *Proc. Natl Acad. Sci. USA* **115** E10999
[32] Banerjee A, Ibsen K, Brown T, Chen R, Agatemor C and Mitragotri S 2018 Reply to Rogers and Gurau: definitions of ionic liquids and deep eutectic solvents *Proc. Natl Acad. Sci. USA* **115** E11000–1

[33] Banerjee A, Ibsen K, Brown T, Chen R, Agatemor C and Mitragotri S 2018 Ionic liquids for oral insulin delivery *Proc. Natl Acad. Sci. USA* **115** 7296–301
[34] Hassan S A, Gad S F, Abdu-Allah H H M, Qayed W S, AbouElmagd S A and Ibrahim E A 2022 Ionic liquid of ketoprofen-piperine modulates the pharmaceutical and therapeutic characters of ketoprofen *Int. J. Pharm.* **620** 121724
[35] Zhou Z, Liu C, Wan X and Fang L 2020 Development of a w/o emulsion using ionic liquid strategy for transdermal delivery of anti-aging component α-lipoic acid: mechanism of different ionic liquids on skin retention and efficacy evaluation *Eur. J. Pharm. Sci.* **141** 105042
[36] Ferraz R, Branco L C, Prudencio C, Noronha J P and Petrovski Ž 2011 Ionic liquids as active pharmaceutical ingredients *Chem. Med. Chem.* **6** 975–85
[37] Bastin R J, Bowker M J and Slater B J 2000 Salt selection and optimisation procedures for pharmaceutical new chemical entities *Org. Process Res. Dev.* **4** 427–35
[38] Rodriguez H, Bica K and Rogers R D 2009 Ionic liquid technology: a potential new platform for the pharmaceutical industry *Trop. J. Pharm. Res.* **7** 1011–2
[39] Almarsson O and Zaworotko M J 2004 Crystal engineering of the composition of pharmaceutical phases. Do pharmaceutical co-crystals represent a new path to improved medicines? *Chem. Commun.* **2004** 1889–96
[40] Stanton M K and Bak A 2008 Physicochemical properties of pharmaceutical co-crystals: a case study of ten AMG 517 co-crystals *Cryst. Growth Des.* **8** 3856–62
[41] Aitipamula S, Banerjee R, Bansal A K, Biradha K, Cheney M L, Choudhury A R, Desiraju G R, Dikundwar A G, Dubey R and Duggirala N *et al* 2012 Polymorphs, salts, and cocrystals: what's in a name? *Cryst. Growth Des.* **12** 2147–52
[42] Bica K, Shamshina J, Hough W L, MacFarlane D R and Rogers R D 2011 Liquid forms of pharmaceutical co-crystals: exploring the boundaries of salt formation *Chem. Commun.* **47** 2267–9
[43] Shamshina J L, Cojocaru O A, Kelley S P, Bica K, Wallace S P, Gurau G and Rogers R D 2017 Acyclovir as an ionic liquid cation or anion can improve aqueous solubility *ACS Omega.* **2** 3483–93
[44] Pipkin L G, Copeland B C and Cojocaru O A 2022 Liquid co-crystals of dual-active phenothiazine-NSAID drugs: synthesis, spectroscopic, and thermal characterization *ACS Omega* **7** 16990–7001
[45] Jones W, Motherwell S and Trask A V 2006 Pharmaceutical cocrystals: an emerging approach to physical property enhancement *MRS Bull.* **31** 875–9
[46] Goossens K, Lava K, Bielawski C W and Binnemans K 2016 Ionic liquid crystals: versatile materials *Chem. Rev.* **116** 4643–807
[47] Rajak P, Nath L and Bhuyan B 2019 Liquid crystals: an approach in drug delivery *Indian J. Pharm. Sci.* **81** 11–21
[48] Black S N, Collier E A, Davey R J and Roberts R J 2007 Structure, solubility, screening, and synthesis of molecular salts *J. Pharm. Sci.* **96** 1053–68
[49] Marsh K N, Boxall J A and Lichtenthaler R 2004 Room temperature ionic liquids and their mixtures—a review *Fluid Phase Equilib.* **219** 93–8
[50] Hayes R, Warr G G and Atkin R 2015 Structure and nanostructure in ionic liquids *Chem. Rev.* **115** 6357–426
[51] Dean P M, Turanjanin J, Yoshizawa-Fujita M, MacFarlane D R and Scott J L 2009 Exploring an anti-crystal engineering approach to the preparation of pharmaceutically active ionic liquids *Cryst. Growth Des.* **9** 1137–45

[52] MacFarlane D R, Kar M and Pringle J M 2017 *Fundamentals of Ionic Liquids: From Chemistry to Applications* (New York: Wiley)

[53] Prakash A S 2011 The counter ion: expanding excipient functionality *J. Excip. Food Chem.* **2** 28–40

[54] Ghorbani M and Simone M I 2020 Developing new inexpensive room-temperature ionic liquids with high thermal stability and a greener synthetic profile *ACS Omega* **5** 12637–48

[55] Ngo H, LeCompte K, Hargens L and McEwen A 2000 Thermal properties of imidazolium ionic liquids *Thermochim. Acta* **357–358** 97–102

[56] Uddin M N, Basak D, Hopefl R and Minofar B 2020 Potential application of ionic liquids in pharmaceutical dosage forms for small molecule drug and vaccine delivery system *J. Pharm. Pharm. Sci.* **23** 158–76

[57] Cao Y and Mu T 2014 Comprehensive investigation on the thermal stability of 66 ionic liquids by thermogravimetric analysis *Ind. Eng. Chem. Res.* **53** 8651–64

[58] Tokuda H, Ishii K, Susan M A B H, Tsuzuki S, Hayamizu K and Watanabe M 2006 Physicochemical properties and structures of room-temperature ionic liquids. 3. Variation of cationic structures *J. Phys. Chem.* B **110** 2833–9

[59] Wu H, Fang F, Zheng L, Ji W, Qi M, Hong M and Ren G 2020 Ionic liquid form of donepezil: preparation, characterization and formulation development *J. Mol. Liq.* **300** 112308

[60] Keramatnia F, Jouyban A, Valizadeh H, Delazar A and Shayanfar A 2016 Ketoconazole ionic liquids with citric and tartaric acid: synthesis, characterization and solubility study *Fluid Phase Equilib.* **425** 108–3

[61] Wu X, Zhang H, He S, Yu Q, Lu Y, Wu W, Ding N, Zhu Q, Chen Z and Ma Y *et al* 2020 Improving dermal delivery of hyaluronic acid by ionic liquids for attenuating skin dehydration *Int. J. Biol. Macromol.* **150** 528–35

[62] Panić J, Tot A, Janković N, Drid P, Gadžurić S and Vraneš M 2020 Physicochemical and structural properties of lidocaine-based ionic liquids with anti-inflammatory anions *RSC Adv.* **10** 14089–98

[63] Dong K, Liu X, Dong H, Zhang X and Zhang S 2017 Multiscale studies on ionic liquids *Chem. Rev.* **117** 6636–95

[64] Tokuda H, Hayamizu K, Ishii K, Susan M A B H and Watanabe M 2005 Physicochemical properties and structures of room temperature ionic liquids. 2. Variation of alkyl chain length in imidazolium cation *J. Phys. Chem.* B **109** 6103–10

[65] Araújo J M M, Florindo C, Pereiro A B, Vieira N S M, Matias A A, Duarte C M M, Rebelo L P N and Marrucho I M 2014 Cholinium-based ionic liquids with pharmaceutically active anions *RSC Adv.* **4** 28126–32

[66] Florindo C, Araújo J M, Alves F, Matos C, Ferraz R, Prudêncio C, Noronha J P, Petrovski Ž, Branco L and Rebelo L P N 2013 Evaluation of solubility and partition properties of ampicillin-based ionic liquids *Int. J. Pharm.* **456** 553–9

[67] Moshikur R M, Chowdhury M R, Wakabayashi R, Tahara Y, Moniruzzaman M and Goto M 2019 Ionic liquids with methotrexate moieties as a potential anticancer prodrug: synthesis, characterization and solubility evaluation *J. Mol. Liq.* **278** 226–33

[68] Shadid M, Gurau G, Shamshina J, Chuang B-C, Hailu S, Guan E, Chowdhury S, Wu J-T, Rizvi S and Griffin R *et al* 2015 Sulfasalazine in ionic liquid form with improved solubility and exposure *MedChemComm* **6** 1837–41

[69] Zhao H, Holmes S S, Baker G A, Challa S, Bose H S and Song Z 2012 Ionic derivatives of betulinic acid as novel HIV-1 protease inhibitors *J. Enzyme Inhib. Med. Chem.* **27** 715–21
[70] Miwa Y, Hamamoto H and Ishida T 2016 Lidocaine self-sacrificially improves the skin permeation of the acidic and poorly water-soluble drug etodolac via its transformation into an ionic liquid *Eur. J. Pharm. Biopharm.* **102** 92–100
[71] Balk A, Wiest J, Widmer T, Galli B, Holzgrabe U and Meinel L 2015 Transformation of acidic poorly water soluble drugs into ionic liquids *Eur. J. Pharm. Biopharm.* **94** 73–82
[72] Viciosa M T, Santos G, Costa A, Danède F, Branco L C, Jordão N, Correia N T and Dionísio M 2015 Dipolar motions and ionic conduction in an ibuprofen derived ionic liquid *Phys. Chem. Chem. Phys.* **17** 24108–20
[73] Pedro S N, Freire R, Silvestre C S and Freire MG. A J 2020 The role of ionic liquids in the pharmaceutical field: an overview of relevant applications *Int. J. Mol. Sci.* **21** 8298
[74] Megwa S A, Cross S E, Benson H A E and Roberts M S 2010 Ion-pair formation as a strategy to enhance topical delivery of salicylic acid *J. Pharm. Pharmacol.* **52** 919–28
[75] Zavgorodnya O, Shamshina J L, Mittenthal M, McCrary P D, Rachiero G P, Titi H M and Rogers R D 2017 Polyethylene glycol derivatization of the non-active ion in active pharmaceutical ingredient ionic liquids enhances transdermal delivery *New J. Chem.* **41** 1499–508
[76] Furukawa S-Y, Hattori G, Sakai S and Kamiya N 2016 Highly efficient and low toxic skin penetrants composed of amino acid ionic liquids *RSC Adv.* **6** 87753–5
[77] Wu H, Deng Z, Zhou B, Qi M, Hong M and Ren G 2019 Improved transdermal permeability of ibuprofen by ionic liquid technology: correlation between counterion structure and the physicochemical and biological properties *J. Mol. Liq.* **283** 399–409
[78] Ferraz R, Teixeira V, Rodrigues D, Fernandes R, Prudêncio C, Noronha J P, Petrovski Ž and Branco L C 2014 Antibacterial activity of ionic liquids based on ampicillin against resistant bacteria *RSC Adv.* **4** 4301–7
[79] Stoimenovski J, MacFarlane D R, Bica K and Rogers R D 2010 Crystalline vs. ionic liquid salt forms of active pharmaceutical ingredients: a position paper *Pharm. Res.* **27** 521–6
[80] Hussan K S, Thayyil M S, Deshpande S, Jinitha T, Rajan V K and Ngai K 2016 Synthesis and molecular dynamics of double active pharmaceutical ingredient-benzalkonium ibuprofenate *J. Mol. Liq.* **223** 1333–9
[81] Hough W L and Rogers R D 2007 Ionic liquids then and now: from solvents to materials to active pharmaceutical ingredients *Bull. Chem. Soc. Jpn.* **80** 2262–9
[82] Pinto P C, Ribeiro D M, Azevedo A M, Justina V D, Cunha E, Bica K, Vasiloiu M, Reis S and Saraiva M L M 2013 Active pharmaceutical ingredients based on salicylate ionic liquids: insights into the evaluation of pharmaceutical profiles *New J. Chem.* **37** 4095–102
[83] Bica K, Rijksen C, Nieuwenhuyzen M and Rogers R D 2010 In search of pure liquid salt forms of aspirin: ionic liquid approaches with acetylsalicylic acid and salicylic acid *Phys. Chem. Chem. Phys.* **12** 2011–7
[84] Stoimenovski J and MacFarlane D 2011 Enhanced membrane transport of pharmaceutically active protic ionic liquids *Chem. Commun.* **47** 11429–31
[85] Moreira D N, Fresno N, Perez-Fernandez R, Frizzo C P, Goya P, Marco C, Martins M A and Elguero J 2015 Brønsted acid–base pairs of drugs as dual ionic liquids: NMR ionicity studies *Tetrahedron* **71** 676–85
[86] Slater C, Savelski M, Hesketh R and Frey E 2006 The selection and reduction of organic solvents in pharmaceutical manufacture *Proc. of the American Chemical Society 10th Green Chemistry and Engineering Conf. (Washington, DC)*

[87] Grodowska K and Parczewski A 2010 Organic solvents in the pharmaceutical industry *Acta Pol. Pharm.* **67** 3–12
[88] Egorova K S, Gordeev E G and Ananikov V P 2017 Biological activity of ionic liquids and their application in pharmaceutics and medicine *Chem. Rev.* **117** 7132–89
[89] Mizuuchi H, Jaitely V, Murdan S and Florence A T 2008 Room temperature ionic liquids and their mixtures: potential pharmaceutical solvents *Eur. J. Pharm. Sci.* **33** 326–31
[90] Moniruzzaman M and Goto M 2011 Ionic liquids: future solvents and reagents for pharmaceuticals *J. Chem. Eng. Jpn.* **44** 370–81
[91] Jaitely V, Mizuuchi H and Florence A T 2010 Current-stimulated release of solutes solubilized in water-immiscible room temperature ionic liquids (RTILs) *J. Drug Target.* **18** 787–93
[92] McCrary P D, Beasley P A, Gurau G, Narita A, Barber P S, Cojocaru O A and Rogers R D 2013 Drug specific, tuning of an ionic liquid's hydrophilic–lipophilic balance to improve water solubility of poorly soluble active pharmaceutical ingredients *New J. Chem.* **37** 2196–202
[93] Dasari S and Mallik B S 2020 Solubility and solvation free energy of a cardiovascular drug, LASSBio-294, in ionic liquids: a computational study *J. Mol. Liq.* **301** 112449
[94] Resende de Azevedo J, Letourneau J-J, Espitalier F and Ré M I 2014 Solubility of a new cardioactive prototype drug in ionic liquids *J. Chem. Eng. Data.* **59** 1766–73
[95] Pandey P K, Rawat K, Aswal V K, Kohlbrecher J and Bohidar H B 2017 DNA ionogel: structure and self-assembly *Phys. Chem. Chem. Phys.* **19** 804–12
[96] Rawat K, Aswal V K and Bohidar H B 2012 DNA–gelatin complex coacervation, UCST and first-order phase transition of coacervate to anisotropic ion gel in 1-Methyl-3-octylimidazolium chloride ionic liquid solutions *J. Phys. Chem.* B **116** 14805–16
[97] Meng Z, Zheng X, Tang K, Liu J, Ma Z and Zhao Q 2012 Dissolution and regeneration of collagen fibers using ionic liquid *Int. J. Biol. Macromol.* **51** 440–8
[98] de Carvalho R N L, Torres Lourenço N M, Gomes P M V and da Fonseca L J P 2013 Swelling behavior of gelatin-ionic liquid functional polymers *J. Polym. Sci., Part B: Polym. Phys.* **51** 817–25
[99] Murugesan S, Wiencek J M, Ren R X and Linhardt R J 2006 Benzoate-based room temperature ionic liquids—thermal properties and glycosaminoglycan dissolution *Carbohydr. Polym.* **63** 268–71
[100] Moniruzzaman M, Tahara Y, Tamura M, Kamiya N and Goto M 2010 Ionic liquid-assisted transdermal delivery of sparingly soluble drugs *Chem. Commun.* **46** 1452–4
[101] Moniruzzaman M, Kamiya N and Goto M 2010 Ionic liquid based microemulsion with pharmaceutically accepted components: formulation and potential applications *J. Colloid Interface Sci.* **352** 136–42
[102] Sidat Z, Marimuthu T, Kumar P, du Toit L C, Kondiah P P D, Choonara Y E and Pillay V 2019 Ionic liquids as potential and synergistic permeation enhancers for transdermal drug delivery *Pharmaceutics* **11** 96
[103] Kundu N, Roy S, Mukherjee D, Maiti T K and Sarkar N 2017 Unveiling the interaction between fatty-acid-modified membrane and hydrophilic imidazolium-based ionic liquid: understanding the mechanism of ionic liquid cytotoxicity *J. Phys. Chem.* B **121** 8162–70
[104] Zakrewsky M, Lovejoy K S, Kern T L, Miller T E, Le V, Nagy A, Goumas A M, Iyer R S, Del Sesto R E and Koppisch A T 2014 Ionic liquids as a class of materials for transdermal delivery and pathogen neutralization *Proc. Natl. Acad. Sci.* **111** 13313–8

[105] Jing B, Lan N, Qiu J and Zhu Y 2016 Interaction of ionic liquids with a lipid bilayer: a biophysical study of ionic liquid cytotoxicity *J. Phys. Chem.* B **120** 2781–9

[106] Benedetto A, Bingham R J and Ballone P 2015 Structure and dynamics of POPC bilayers in water solutions of room temperature ionic liquids *J. Chem. Phys.* **142** 124706

[107] Benedetto A, Heinrich F, Gonzalez M A, Fragneto G, Watkins E and Ballone P 2014 Structure and stability of phospholipid bilayers hydrated by a room-temperature ionic liquid/water solution: a neutron reflectometry study *J. Phys. Chem.* B **118** 12192–206

[108] Dickinson Q, Bottoms S, Hinchman L, McIlwain S, Li S, Myers C L, Boone C, Coon J J, Hebert A and Sato T K 2016 Mechanism of imidazolium ionic liquids toxicity in *Saccharomyces cerevisiae* and rational engineering of a tolerant, xylose-fermenting strain *Microb. Cell Fact.* **15** 17

[109] Bhattacharya G, Giri R, Dubey A, Mitra S, Priyadarshini R, Gupta A, Mukhopadhyay M and Ghosh S K 2018 Structural changes in cellular membranes induced by ionic liquids: from model to bacterial membranes *Chem. Phys. Lipids* **215** 1–10

[110] Yoo B, Jing B, Jones S E, Lamberti G A, Zhu Y, Shah J K and Maginn E J 2016 Molecular mechanisms of ionic liquid cytotoxicity probed by an integrated experimental and computational approach *Sci. Rep.* **6** 19889

[111] Shamshina J L, Barber P S and Rogers R D 2013 Ionic liquids in drug delivery *Expert Opin. Drug Deliv.* **10** 1367–81

[112] Qi Q M and Mitragotri S 2019 Mechanistic study of transdermal delivery of macromolecules assisted by ionic liquids *J. Control. Release* **311** 162–9

[113] Kubota K, Shibata A and Yamaguchi T 2016 The molecular assembly of the ionic liquid/aliphatic carboxylic acid/aliphatic amine as effective and safety transdermal permeation enhancers *Eur. J. Pharm. Sci.* **86** 75–83

[114] de Almeida T S, Julio A, Saraiva N, Fernandes A S, Araujo M E M, Baby A R, Rosado C and Mota J P 2017 Choline-versus imidazole-based ionic liquids as functional ingredients in topical delivery systems: cytotoxicity, solubility, and skin permeation studies *Drug Dev. Ind. Pharm.* **43** 1858–65

[115] Mahajan S, Sharma R and Mahajan R K 2012 An Investigation of drug binding ability of a surface active ionic liquid: micellization, electrochemical, and spectroscopic studies *Langmuir* **28** 17238–46

[116] Zech O, Thomaier S, Kolodziejski A, Touraud D, Grillo I and Kunz W 2010 Ionic liquids in microemulsions—a concept to extend the conventional thermal stability range of microemulsions *Chem. Eur. J.* **16** 783–6

[117] Bharmoria P, Singh T and Kumar A 2013 Complexation of chitosan with surfactant like ionic liquids: molecular interactions and preparation of chitosan nanoparticles *J. Colloid Interface Sci.* **407** 361–9

[118] Dobler D, Schmidts T, Klingenhöfer I and Runkel F 2013 Ionic liquids as ingredients in topical drug delivery systems *Int. J. Pharm.* **441** 620–7

[119] Islam M R, Chowdhury M R, Wakabayashi R, Kamiya N, Moniruzzaman M and Goto M 2020 Ionic liquid-in-oil microemulsions prepared with biocompatible choline carboxylic acids for improving the transdermal delivery of a sparingly soluble drug *Pharmaceutics* **12** 392

[120] Zhang D, Wang H-J, Cui X-M and Wang C-X 2017 Evaluations of imidazolium ionic liquids as novel skin permeation enhancers for drug transdermal delivery *Pharm. Dev. Technol.* **22** 511–20

[121] Tantishaiyakul V, Phadoongsombut N, Wongpuwarak W, Thungtiwachgul J, Faroongsarng D, Wiwattanawongsa K and Rojanasakul Y 2004 ATR-FTIR characterization of transport properties of benzoic acid ion-pairs in silicone membranes *Int. J. Pharm.* **283** 111–6

[122] Bica K, Rodríguez H, Gurau G, Cojocaru O A, Riisager A, Fehrmann R and Rogers R D 2012 Pharmaceutically active ionic liquids with solids handling, enhanced thermal stability, and fast release *Chem. Commun.* **48** 5422–4

[123] Zhang L, Liu J, Tian T, Gao Y, Ji X, Li Z and Luan Y 2013 Pharmaceutically active ionic liquid self-assembled vesicles for the application as an efficient drug delivery system *Chem. Phys. Chem.* **14** 3454–7

[124] Banerjee A, Ibsen K, Brown T, Chen R, Agatemor C and Mitragotri S 2018 Ionic liquids for oral insulin delivery *Proc. Natl. Acad. Sci.* **115** 7296–301

[125] Moniruzzaman M, Tamura M, Tahara Y, Kamiya N and Goto M 2010 Ionic liquid-in-oil microemulsion as a potential carrier of sparingly soluble drug: characterization and cytotoxicity evaluation *Int. J. Pharm.* **400** 243–50

[126] Chantereau G, Sharma M, Abednejad A, Vilela C, Costa E, Veiga M, Antunes F, Pintado M, Sèbe G and Coma V 2020 Bacterial nanocellulose membranes loaded with vitamin B-based ionic liquids for dermal care applications *J. Mol. Liq.* **302** 112547

[127] Chantereau G, Sharma M, Abednejad A, Neves B M, Sèbe G, Coma V, Freire M G, Freire C S and Silvestre A J 2019 Design of nonsteroidal anti-inflammatory drug-based ionic liquids with improved water solubility and drug delivery *ACS Sustain. Chem. Eng.* **7** 14126–34

[128] Júlio A, Caparica R, Costa Lima S A, Fernandes A S, Rosado C, Prazeres D M, Reis S, Santos de Almeida T and Fonte P 2019 Ionic liquid-polymer nanoparticle hybrid systems as new tools to deliver poorly soluble drugs *Nanomaterials* **9** 1148

[129] Viau L, Tourné-Péteilh C, Devoisselle J-M and Vioux A 2010 Ionogels as drug delivery system: one-step sol–gel synthesis using imidazolium ibuprofenate ionic liquid *Chem. Commun.* **46** 228–30

[130] Néouze M-A, Le Bideau J, Gaveau P, Bellayer S and Vioux A 2006 Ionogels, new materials arising from the confinement of ionic liquids within silica-derived networks *Chem. Mater.* **18** 3931–6

[131] Pal A and Yadav A 2016 Binding interactions of anesthetic drug with surface active ionic liquid *J. Mol. Liq.* **222** 471–9

[132] Wang C, Zhu J, Zhang D, Yang Y, Zheng L, Qu Y, Yang X and Cui X 2018 Ionic liquid—microemulsions assisting in the transdermal delivery of Dencichine: preparation, in-vitro and in-vivo evaluations, and investigation of the permeation mechanism *Int. J. Pharm.* **535** 120–31

[133] He Z and Alexandridis P 2017 Ionic liquid and nanoparticle hybrid systems: emerging applications *Adv. Colloid Interface Sci.* **244** 54–70

[134] Winther-Jensen O, Vijayaraghavan R, Sun J, Winther-Jensen B and MacFarlane D 2009 Self polymerising ionic liquid gel *Chem. Commun.* **2009** 3041–3

[135] Md Moshikur R, Chowdhury M R, Moniruzzaman M and Goto M 2020 Biocompatible ionic liquids and their applications in pharmaceutics *Green Chem.* **22** 8116–39

[136] Riaz M, Akhlaq M, Naz S and Uroos M 2022 An overview of biomedical applications of choline geranate (CAGE): a major breakthrough in drug delivery *RSC Adv.* **12** 25977–91

[137] Fini A, Fazio G and Rapaport I 1993 Diclofenac/N-(2-hydroxyethyl)pyrrolidine: a new salt for an old drug *Drugs Exp. Clin. Res.* **19** 81–8
[138] Petersen B and Rovati S 2009 Diclofenac epolamine (Flector®) patch *Clin. Drug Investig.* **29** 1–9
[139] MEDRx Pipeline 2023 https://www.medrx.co.jp/english/business/iltspipeline/index.html
[140] Banerjee A, Ibsen K, Iwao Y, Zakrewsky M and Mitragotri S 2017 Transdermal protein delivery using choline and geranate (CAGE) deep eutectic solvent *Adv Healthc Mater.* **6** 1601411
[141] Greene J R, Merrett K L, Heyert A J, Simmons L F, Migliori C M, Vogt K C, Castro R S, Phillips P D, Baker J L and Lindberg G E *et al* 2019 Scope and efficacy of the broad-spectrum topical antiseptic choline geranate *PLoS One* **14** e0222211
[142] Ko J, Mandal A, Dhawan S, Shevachman M, Mitragotri S and Joshi N 2021 Clinical translation of choline and geranic acid deep eutectic solvent *Bioeng. Transl. Med.* **6** e10191
[143] Jadhav N, Bhosale S, Bhosale S, Mali S, Toraskar P and Kadam T 2021 Ionic liquids: formulation avenues, drug delivery and therapeutic updates *J. Drug Delivery Sci. Technol.* **65** 102694
[144] *Research CfDEa. Regulatory Classification of Pharmaceutical Co-Crystals* 2018 ed Services USDoHaH
[145] Shamshina J L and Rogers R D 2014 Overcoming the problems of solid state drug formulations with ionic liquids *Ther. Deliv.* **5** 489–91
[146] Shamshina J L, Kelley S P, Gurau G and Rogers R D 2015 Chemistry: develop ionic liquid drugs *Nature* **528** 188–9

IOP Publishing

Advances in Drug Delivery Systems for Healthcare
From concept to clinic
Piyush Pradeep Mehta and Arpana Parihar

Chapter 4

Advances in drug delivery systems for healthcare—from theory to practice: 3D and 4D bioprinting—promises and realities

Cansu İlke Kuru*, **Fulden Ulucan-Karnak***, **M Batıkan Kandemir, Alperen Doğru and Mehmet Özgür Seydibeyoğlu**

Personalized medicine is becoming more and more common as it helps create better drugs with fewer adverse effects. To meet the needs of the patient, several dosages might be mixed into a single dose. To generate medicine according to patient demands, new additive manufacturing technology called three-dimensional (3D) bioprinting and 4D bioprinting is being used. They make use of controlled devices to layer-by-layer produce active pharmaceutical ingredients to create a suitable, customized drug transport structure using biological resourced inks. Contrary to three-dimensional printing, 4D bioprinting uses stimuli-sensitive biomaterials to mimic the dynamic nature of tissues. In this chapter, additive manufacturing printing technologies in the healthcare industry emphasized details in the concept of 3D and 4D bioprinting, especially for drug delivery applications. Also, this chapter includes the 'from idea to clinic' concept, which illustrates clearly the focus on the commercialization, market potential, industrial standpoint, and regulatory bodies' perspectives on developments in drug delivery systems.

4.1 Introduction

Manufacturing specific commodities via specific methods has been the focus of several technological advancements throughout human history. Manufacturing products with ease and low cost has been one of the main objectives of society since the beginning of the modern world. Within this concept, contrary to subtractive manufacturing, 'additive manufacturing (AM)' has been a very

* These authors contributed equally.

doi:10.1088/978-0-7503-5613-8ch4

important tool that enables manufacturers to make products in very sophisticated shapes and with endless material options [1–3]. AM was discovered in the 1980s but after the 2010s, the use of AM exploded, resulting in many commercial companies manufacturing machines and new materials with an infinite number of designs. These studies were not limited to industrial applications and there has been extensive research to use these technologies for medical purposes. One of the commercial uses of metallic material-based AM has been in the area of medical implants that are manufactured according to the needs of the patient. There are new approaches to top tint ceramic materials to be used as implants. Furthermore, bioprinting has been one of the most common areas in the medical field helping in many different disciplines [4, 5]. In this chapter, AM printing technologies in the healthcare industry are emphasized details in the concept of 3D and 4D bioprinting, especially for drug delivery applications. Also, this chapter includes the 'from idea to clinic' concept, which illustrates clearly the focus on the commercialization, market potential, industrial standpoint, and regulatory bodies' perspectives on developments in drug delivery systems.

4.2 Additive manufacturing printing in the healthcare industry

The AM process is introduced as a new technology that creates products in which materials are deposited in layers and 3D objects are generated. With the use of this technology, parts with a variety of structures and intricate geometries may be created from 3D model data utilizing a wide range of materials, including polymer, ceramic, metal, composite, etc. Today, AM is referred to by a variety of names, including 'solid freeform,' 'rapid tooling,' 'rapid casting,' 'rapid prototyping,' '3D printing,' and 'indirect AM.' In more detail, AM can be defined as 'printing' layers of materials using a Cartesian coordinate robot, much like an ink or laser printer does to deposit or fuse material layer by layer to generate objects in three dimensions [6, 7]. AM offers opportunities for customized production, freedom of design, portable manufacturing infrastructure, and recycling of used materials. In AM, a structure is formed from one to all. These processes offer opportunities for the controlled assembly of hybrid structures [8, 9].

AM technologies have made significant advances in producing medical devices and equipment, orthotic prostheses, medical modeling, and implants [10]. In parallel with the innovation potential, AM technologies are catalyzing the clinical impact of healthcare products with the latest advances in biomaterials. AM technologies are used by clinicians to fulfill a wide range of applications in health and medical requirements [11]. In the last few years, interest in AM has grown exponentially in the scientific community, especially in pharmaceutical and medical research. This is evidenced by the increase in the number of papers in this field over the years.

The three main medical uses of AM—dental implants, vascular grafts, and tendon replacement—were discussed in the study of Rodríguez-Salvador *et al* in 2018. The majority of medical devices, including hip, knee, and shoulder prostheses, jaw implants, and hip, knee, and shoulder prostheses, are primarily made of titanium and stainless steel metals which are expensive. AM presents a chance for innovation in the design of these medical products employing it, where the total cost and the manufacturing time could be markedly decreased [6].

In reality, AM offers the chance to produce specialized tools and equipment as well as specialized medical devices, such as implants, and will change the healthcare sector. Compared to conventional procedures that require multiple processes, this technology allows for a significantly shorter manufacturing time for implants. Additionally, implants can be created based on a patient's unique anatomy, ensuring a superior fit and lowering the likelihood of failure typical with mass-produced implants. For instance, images of the patient are acquired using x-ray, computed tomography (CT), or magnetic resonance imaging to design a prosthetic (MRI) [12, 13]. Some of the benefits of AM in the medical and dental fields can be summarized as cost and time savings, personalization, reduction of radiation exposure, enhanced accuracy, ease of use and design, a wide range of material applicability, and better stabilization [14].

4.2.1 3D printing

3D printing is a type of AM or layered manufacturing, a growing technology that works by depositing raw material layer upon layer to create 3D parts [12, 15]. In general, 3D printing strategies can be categorized under four headings: design, raw materials, production, and finishing.

Design is the digital creation of the design of the intended product. It is realized with computer-aided design software. By converting the design data into the relevant formats, different materials can be combined, with differentiated production in layers, customizations in geometry, and personalizations can be made.

Raw materials are used as powder, granules, filaments, or binder solutions to facilitate production. The form of the raw material varies depending on the AM technology used. The increase in the variety of materials that can be used in AM methods expands the usage areas of these production methods.

The production of the designed product is in layers in AM methods with the relevant production data using the specified raw materials. Unlike machining, AM enables the production of special drug geometries. AM methods can produce geometries that are impossible to produce with typical pharmaceutical manufacturing methods.

For finishing, the products are finalized with the processes performed. At this stage, processes such as coatings, subtracting, etc can be applied to give different features.

Figure 4.1 shows a flowchart of technical considerations for additive-manufactured medical devices. According to this guide prepared by the Food and Drug Administration (FDA), device design is first performed using models with predetermined standard dimensions or the patient's medical images. The device design is then converted into a digital file. The processed file is brought to a format

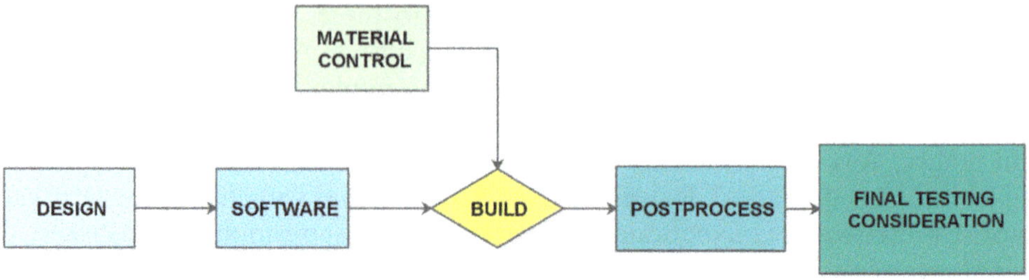

Figure 4.1. Flow chart of the AM process.

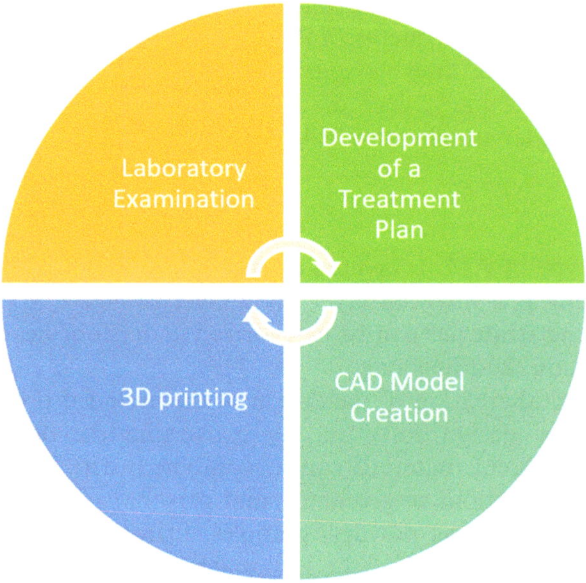

Figure 4.2. AM steps of a drug delivery systems.

compatible with the device and the printing parameters are optimized. After these processes, the printing process waits for the control process of the material to be used. The printing process is carried out with materials that meet the necessary conditions. After printing, device production is terminated by processes such as cleaning, annealing, post-printing machining, sterilization, packing, and labeling. The produced device becomes suitable for use after passing through characterization and tests [16].

In medical applications, there are numerous ways to administer a drug to a patient to treat some defects. The bodily part where the pharmacological components are administered determines how these treatments are commonly categorized. The selection of a drug delivery mechanism is influenced by a variety of elements, such as the disease, the desired outcome, the efficacy of the treatment's active ingredients, and in some situations, the preferences of the patient.

The drug distribution sector has been transformed from AM to personalized medicine. A typical AM drug delivery system begins with a laboratory examination that may include computed tomography (CT) or magnetic resonance imaging (MRI). This provides useful information about the patient's condition as well as the design requirements for achieving a patient-centered dosage form and a programmed release profile. This is followed by the development of a treatment plan, which may include the drugs to be administered and their desired release profile. AM technology is capable of not only providing personalized medication but also of delivering programmable drug release. Then, using computer-aided design (CAD), a digital model is created and 3D printing of the intended drug delivery system is achieved by drug loading onto the printed raw material (figure 4.2) [17, 18].

Taking all these factors into account, AM allows the production of orally degradable and highly porous structures. It improves drug efficacy and reduces side effects like unwanted undesirable effects that are possibly related to a drug and provides personalized dosing for developing children and potent drugs. Furthermore, drug-loaded implants can be designed according to the patient's anatomy [19, 20]. Potentials in design, customization, and on-site production are given in table 4.1.

AM technology has advanced quickly and has had a significant impact on patent applications. According to the report of Wohlers *et al* 2016, AM growth accelerated in 2014, increasing by 31.6% from 2013 to 2014 and 25.9% in 2015. Photopolymers were the most commonly used materials in AM by 2016, accounting for 45.5% of all

Table 4.1. The potential of AM for drug delivery systems.

Advantage categories	Potentials
Freedom of design	High porosity products Complex drug combination Combining different drugs and release mechanisms in single doses Ability to control drug release rate with variable filling and cavity structures Special forms of medicine for children
Customization	Dosing strong medicines Special dosing in budding children Drug-loaded implants suitable for patients' anatomy Reduced side effects Improving drug efficacy
On-site production	Medicines with a limited shelf life Fast time to market for new medicines

applications, followed by laser sintering polymer powders (24.9%), filaments (15.1%), and metals (11.5%). Such developments are increasing patent activity in the AM industry, which increased from 25 issued patents in 1995 to 668 in 2014 [21]. According to the report of Schubert *et al* in 2014, since 2009, intellectual property in the medical industry has expanded rather quickly, with companies rather than academic institutions taking the lead. In 2014, the AM business was valued at $700 million, but just 1.6% of that amount was spent in the healthcare sector, which is predicted to increase to 21% by 2024 [22].

4.2.2 4D printing

4D printing is the process of creating structures out of intelligent materials that enable the finished product to change its form, characteristics, or function in response to an outside stimulus like light, heat, or moisture over time. It is also suggested as the new technology for printing drug formulations in pharmaceutical technology. It offers faster growth, using smart materials, shape flexibility, and shape memory programming compared to 3D printing (figure 4.3) [23–26].

Shape differences in 4D materials are caused by many external stimuli, usually involving the expansion and contraction of the generated materials. Typically, the self-folding and self-activating effects of 4D manufactured materials are achieved with smart materials. Smart materials have two main features. These are shape change and shape memory. Deformable materials indicate the state of the material when exposed to discriminative stimuli. Shape memory is the place where the deformable material is not exposed to any stimulus. The material changes shape temporarily when exposed to an external stimulus [26, 27].

4.3 History of 3D printing technology for medical applications

Stereolithography (SLA), one of the first techniques of 3D printing, was invented by Chuck Hull in 1986 and inspired by the inkjet printer [28]. From the late 1980s to the early 1990s, tissue engineering emerged and the fused deposition modeling (FDM)

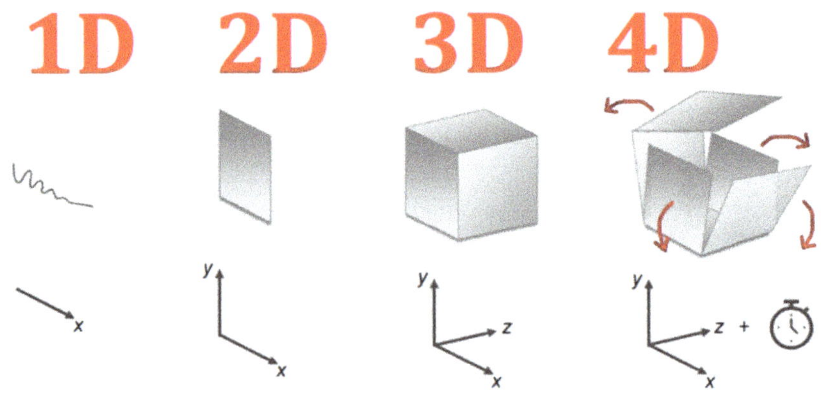

Figure 4.3. 4D printing approach.

technique was developed [29]. In the mid-1990s, microcontact printing was developed and organ enlargement, building scaffold production, dental implants, and prosthesis were carried out. In the late 1990s, the cells were written directly with a laser, and protein printing was developed.

At the beginning of the 2000s, scaffolds were produced for tissue engineering by the FDM technique, and inkjet printing of the cells was made. By the 2000s, working organs and dental implants began to be produced with 3D printing. In the late 2000s, prosthetics were made using 3D printing [30–32]. The first prosthetic leg transplant produced with a 3D printer was performed in 2008 [33], the first titanium jaw implant transplant produced with a 3D printer was performed in 2012 [34], and the first prosthetic eye transplant produced with a 3D printer was performed in 2021 [35].

Spritam®, the first pharmaceutical drug that was produced by AM methods, made a big splash with FDA approval in August 2015. The figures of Spritam can be found on the company's website (https://spritam.com/what-is-zipdose-technology/). This anti-epileptic orally disintegrating tablet (ODT) loaded with levetiracetam was manufactured by Aprecia Pharmaceuticals with the Massachusetts Institute of Technology patented Zip-Dose Technology [19, 36]. This ODT form (self-melting tablets), produced by AM, has a size (up to 1000 mg) and a highly porous structure that cannot be achieved by conventional manufacturing methods. Thanks to its porous structure, Spritam® has a wide contact area with saliva. It can disintegrate and dissolve within a few seconds after contact with saliva. This helps avoid the use of difficult-to-swallow pills in both elderly and young patients [37].

Small batch sizes and high drug loading flexibility are provided by 3D printing, which is essential for clinical investigations. As a result of a decrease in the amount of active pharmaceutical ingredients (APIs) needed and a shorter development period, expenditure is saved.

One of the largest lactose suppliers is DFE Pharma. Recently, DFE created lactose specifically for 3D printing (https://dfepharma.com/our-innovation-and-solutions/3d-printing/). The driving force behind this 3D printing discovery is DFE Pharma. To provide advice on the best lactose binder blends for 3D printing applications, they have screened more than 20 different lactose grades. They also make customized lactose-binder mixes. This expedites the development process and adds value to the formulation [38]. In the study of Korinde van den Heuvel, a product developer at DFE Pharma, it was investigated how varied lactose-starch base formulation particle size distributions affected crucial material properties such as wettability, consolidation, and flowability. It was discovered that a blend with fewer small particles allows the ink (liquid) to penetrate the powder bed more quickly. Using formulations including acetaminophen or diclofenac sodium, the effects of changing the print parameters or binder type on fundamental tablet qualities like hardness and dissolving were examined. It was discovered that because the base formulation and print settings are so tightly coupled, they must be optimized simultaneously. This work demonstrates in great detail how, while taking into account the formulation considerations mentioned, hydrophilic/hydrophobic APIs may be successfully formed into 3D printed tablets [39].

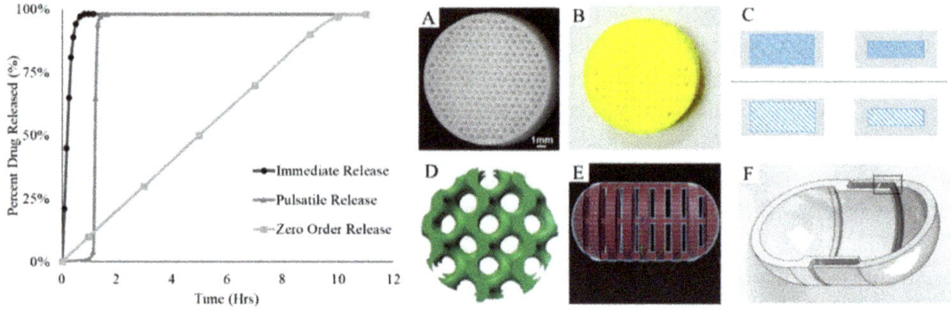

Figure 4.4. The products that are used for drugs delivery produced by AM methods. Reproduced from [46] CC BY 4.0.

With the impact of FDA approval, there has been a rapid increase in the number of studies and scientific research on AM technologies [40]. Although AM technologies have only recently been discovered to produce personalized drug delivery systems, these technologies have been used in various biomedical fields for many years, for example, custom prostheses, orthopedic implants and anatomical models, surgical instrumentation, etc.

Immediate release is desirable for fast-acting drugs such as pain relievers. Idealized release profiles for oral dosages produced by AM methods are in shown figure 4.4. With AM methods, the release profiles can be adjusted by filling percentage (A) [36]. The filling percentage of manufactured products can also be used for devices floating in the stomach (B) [41]. Erosion-related release profiles can be adjusted with shell designs of varying thicknesses or more complex geometries (C, D, E) [42–44]. In addition, pulsatile oscillation is possible by producing an outer shell of adjustable thickness, designed to be up to 600 microns (F) [45].

Patients' variability in age, fitness, gender, race, etc, and different health conditions is one of the problems encountered when administering medication to individuals. Intelligent and personalized drug delivery systems produced using novel approaches create significant opportunities. As a result, the advantages of AM have impressive implications for the range of products used in this field, particularly in the production of additives for drug delivery. Further advances in biomaterials are needed for the success and growth of AM technology in healthcare. AM technologies are showing promising results for pharmaceutical applications, pointing to the future of the healthcare industry.

4.4 3D Printing techniques for medical applications

Techniques such as forging and investment casting, which are frequently used in surgical implant production today, require costly additional processes such as machining (turning, milling, drilling) and finishing (grinding, polishing) due to the desired mechanical and aesthetic properties of the final product. In addition to their high cost, traditional production techniques are very demanding for personalized productions for medical purposes, due to time loss and high waste resulting from secondary processes. These additional processes may cause deterioration on the surfaces. For example, in titanium, chatter formation is observed during machining, due to its high strength, low elastic modulus, and low thermal conductivity (compared to steel and aluminum), which creates an irregular pattern on the spring back and surface [47, 48].

Personalized orthotic insoles, prosthetics, surgical guides, and one-off implants can be produced with 3D printing according to patient requests. Porous skeleton structures can be obtained by methods such as gas foaming, solvent casting, freeze-drying, and electrospinning, but in these techniques, it is difficult to control macro architecture because the 3D shape geometry is limited depending on the mold design. Thanks to advanced imaging techniques such as computer-aided drawing, magnetic resonance imaging, and computer tomography, patient-specific productions can be made by controlling both micro and macro architecture. In addition, AM eliminates the need for a coating process. Hip prostheses made of porous Ti, Ta metal, or calcium-phosphate-based ceramic coated Ti6A14V or CoCrM alloys used to improve bone tissue integration can be produced quickly and precisely with a single device without the need for additional processing by AM [48–50].

However, strength and fatigue are critical for load-bearing implants. During computer-aided design, the negative effect of porous structures on strength should be considered. Although the layer-by-layer printing process allows complex shape production, it may cause failure due to the formation of gaps and defects between layers. To prevent contamination and infection, the inside and outside environment of the 3D printing production platform should be hygienic. The surface properties of 3D-printed biomaterials affect their relationship with the surface texture. While rough surfaces with stair-stepped surface finish and material consolidation are beneficial for cell anchoring, proliferation, and integration, it is undesirable as it triggers foreign body reactions and causes particle release around the implant [48].

Studies now being conducted center on the use of 3D printing technology to manufacture pharmaceutical dosage forms, primarily solid oral dosage forms such as conventional and modified release tablets, implants, orodispersible tablets, and films. The extrusion process serves as the foundation for the majority of printing techniques (table 4.2). Tablets are currently the most used dose form. Despite this, it is stated that low patient compliance with medication delivery results in ineffective pharmacotherapy. The creation of various sizes, shapes, and designs of tablets could alter it [71, 72].

Orthopedic implants with lightweight, low volume, design flexibility, complex design, and cost-effectiveness can be produced by AM. However, difficulties continue in the production of human tissue and organs. Today, we aim to produce surgical tools by 3D printing with low risk in terms of human health, and after the developments in printing technology, it is foreseen that we will switch to patient-specific implant applications with high risk. For biomaterials to become widespread and standardized in the future with 3D printing, new sterilization, packaging, and transportation procedures similar to those used in medical devices need to be developed. 3D printing is slower and more costly for mass production compared to traditional manufacturing methods such as injection molding. Although the resolutions of printers are constantly improving (178 μm with FDM, 16 μm with

Table 4.2. Different dosage forms with some innovative 3D approaches.

3D printing method	Dosage form	Active ingredient	References
Fused deposition modeling	Caplet	Acetaminophen and caffeine	[51]
	Caplet	Budesonide	[52]
	Capsule	Acetaminophen	[53]
	Tablet	5-Aminosalicylic acid and 4-Aminosalicylic acid	[54]
	Tablet	Fluorescein sodium	[55]
	Implant	γ-Indomethacin	[56]
	T-shaped intrauterine systems	γ-Indomethacin	[56]
	Model of a nose adapted to the morphology of an individual	FPLA-salicylic acid and PCL salicylic acid	[57]
	Nanocapsules	Deflazacort	[58]
	Compartmentalized shells	Rifampicin (RIF) Isoniazid (ISO)	[59]
Pressure assisted syringe	Bilayer tablet	Guaifenesin	[60]
	Tablet polypill	Aspirin Hydrochlorothiazide and Atenolol and Pravastatin sodium and Ramipril and Captopril and Glipizide and Nifedipine	[61, 62]
	Tablet	Theophylline	[63]
Drop-on-solid deposition	Implant	Levofloxacin and Rifampicin and Isoniazid	[64, 65]
	Tablet	Chlorpheniramine maleate and Diclofenac sodium	[66]
	ODT	Acetaminophen and Levetiracetam	[67]
Drop-on-drop deposition	Mucosal thin films	Cetirizine hydrochloride Diphenhydramine hydrochloride Ibuprofen	[68]
Stereolithography (SLA)	Hydrogel	Ibuprofen and Riboflavin	[69]
	Biodegradable patch	5-fluorouracil	[70]

SLA, 80 μm with SLS), optimization and *in vitro* and *in vivo* studies are needed for the widespread production of biomaterials with these systems [48, 73].

Rapid prototyping, or 3D printing as it is commonly called, generally consists of three stages. These stages are modeling the product with the help of computer-aided drawing or medical imaging techniques (x-rays, CT scans), reducing the 3D model to two dimensions by slicing (voids, cantilever, undercuts are reduced to circles, lines, and points), the material is deposited layer by layer and the product takes its final form with post-printing (removing of support material and grinding,). Polymers, metals, and ceramics can be used as biomaterials in this 3D bioprinting. Mechanical-chemical properties, processing ability, cell-material interactions, and FDA approval are important parameters in the selection of these materials. There are a wide variety of printers depending on the material to be used and the print resolution [48]. The most common AM types used in biomedical applications are summarized in table 4.3. After this part, 3D printing techniques are given in detail, one from each main group given in figure 4.5.

4.4.1 Fused deposition modeling

Fused deposition modeling (FDM) is based on the principle of depositing the heated thermoplastic material layer by layer by flowing it through the extrusion head in a semi-liquid state. This technology was patented by S Scott Crump in 1992 [29]. In these devices, a single nozzle can be used, or multiple nozzles can be used to print more than one material. FDM printing resolution is around 100–150 μm. Melted materials (API and polymer blends) are stored in rolls that are arranged so that they pass through an extruder nozzle as the process progresses. Because the nozzle is above the material's melting point, the polymer–API mixture melts and deposits in the form of fine filaments that are immediately solidified, layer by layer (figure 4.6) [79]. Today, the FDM method is accepted as the most widely used 3D printing method due to its ease of use, free software support, wide design capability, and low cost [80]. Due to its capacity to produce complex pharmaceuticals with challenging geometries, it is the most widely utilized 3D printing technique currently being studied; however, quality and manufacturing efficiency must be improved before it can be employed in clinical settings [79].

The thermal and rheological behavior of the material is of critical importance for effective printing in FDM. The printing process usually takes place between ~110 °C and 140 °C. The printing temperature should be high enough to facilitate the adhesion of the layers and flow through the nozzle. Too high a viscosity will cause the nozzle to clog. Biocompatible rheological modifiers can be used to adjust viscosity, but high nozzle temperature may damage these agents and living cells. The build direction, layer thickness, raster angle, raster width, and infill density feed rate also affect the porosity and morphology of the scaffold to be printed. In addition, the use of support material for complex shapes causes limitations in the shape of the skeletal structure [73, 81].

The use of thermoplastics with a low melting temperature is ideal in FDM printers. Acrylonitrile butadiene styrene (ABS), polylactic acid (PLA), nylon, polycarbonate (PC), and polyvinyl alcohol (PVA) are the most used materials [82]. In the production of biomaterials with FDM, polycaprolactone (PCL) and poly (lactic-co-glycolic acid) (PLGA) derivatives are often used. PCL has features such as low melting temperature (~60 °C), low glass transition temperature (−60 °C), high

Table 4.3. A comparative table on solid, liquid, and powder techniques.

3D printing technique	Principle	Materials	Resolution	Advantages	Disadvantages	Medical applications
Solid (fused deposition Modeling)	Layer-by-layer deposition by directing material exiting a heated nozzle	Thermoplastics Ceramics Bioinks Hydrogels	100–200 μm [74]	Variety of colors, low cost, simple, widespread use, suitable for composite material use, open source design diversity	Slow, weak mechanical properties, support material need, anisotropy, low resolution, nozzles impart high shear forces on cells	Orthopedic implants, drug delivery systems, surgical sutures, and scaffolds for tissue engineering [75, 76]
Liquid (stereolithography)	Curing certain regions of the photopolymer resin layer (liquid at room temperature) with a point ultraviolet laser beam	Photopolymer Bio-resin	1.2–200 μm [74]	Quick, extremely good cell viability, high resolution, and nozzle-free	Toxicity, high cost, brittle structure, limited materials selection, possible harm to DNA by UV	Tablets, microneedles, biomedical scaffolds, dental prosthetics, medical devices [77]
Powder (selective laser sintering)	Sintering of binder powders with laser	Metal powder Thermoplastics ceramics	100–200 μm [74]	High strength, fast, no solvent and support structure required, numerous materials are available	For expensive raw powder material, post-processing required due to the rough surface	Tissue engineering scaffolds, drug/biomolecule delivery vehicles, biomedical prototypes, and devices [78]

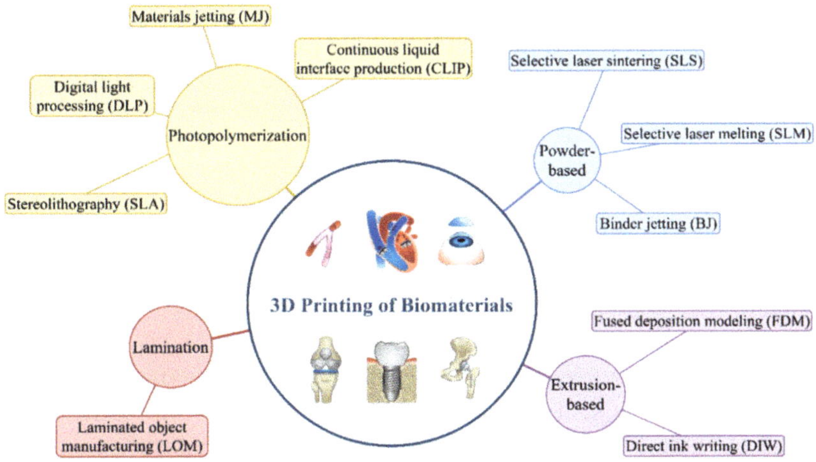

Figure 4.5. 3D printing techniques for use in medical applications.

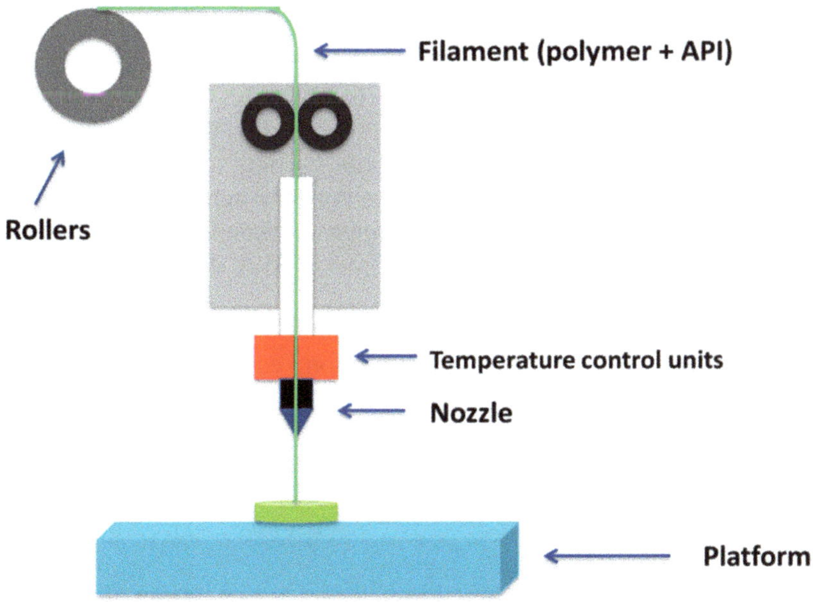

Figure 4.6. Schematic representation of fused deposition modeling. Reproduced from [79] CC BY 4.0.

thermal stability, moisture resistance, and bioresorbable and biocompatible at *in vitro* and *in vivo* conditions [83, 84]. With changes in the amount of monomer, features such as biocompatibility, biodegradability, and degradation rate can be adjusted. PLGA requires extrusion at high temperatures due to its high glass transition temperature (40 °C–60 °C). Thanks to the mobility of the extrusion head, the pore and channel sizes of the biocompatible skeleton structure can be adjusted. Since polymers such as ABS and thermoplastic polyurethane (TPU) are non-biocompatible, they are only used in implant and prosthetic prototyping [73, 85–88]. Biomaterials produced by FDM are used in tissue engineering, drug delivery systems for the fabrication of antimicrobial incorporated mesh, and biodegradable scaffold production for craniofacial anomalies solutions [89, 90].

4.4.2 Stereolithography

Stereolithography (SLA) is one of the first rapid prototyping techniques developed. It is a technology patented by Charles W Hull in 1986 [28]. This technique is based on the principle that the photocurable resin is cured and hardened by polymerization under the influence of an ultraviolet laser (figure 4.7). At the top of the bioink vat, where the biomaterial is exposed to light energy, polymerization takes place. The platform supporting the structure will be lowered into the vat after each layer is polymerized to allow for the photopolymerization of a new layer on top [91]. Each hardened layer descends into the liquid-filled tank below, a blade (sweeper) sweeps the layer flat, and the new layer begins to be processed. These processes are repeated until the 3D model is created. In the production of large parts, mask stereolithography (MSLA) is used because laser beam rasterization takes a lot of time [92]. MSLA uses an LCD to mask the UV light source by turning each pixel on or off, and the LCD acts as a stencil able to create the 2D shape for the UV light to shine through. In this technique, unlike SLA, after 3D printing, post-curing with UV light is required in a closed environment for ultimate strength and durability. The depth of polymerization varies depending on the power of the light source, scanning speed, monomer, and photoinitiators [93]. SL printing resolution is around 50–100 μm [80]. However, micro SLA (μ-SLA) and high-definition SLA devices can be reduced to single micrometer levels [94].

The advantages of the SLA technique are that complex shapes can be created in interior architecture, high printing resolution, easy resin evacuation, use of

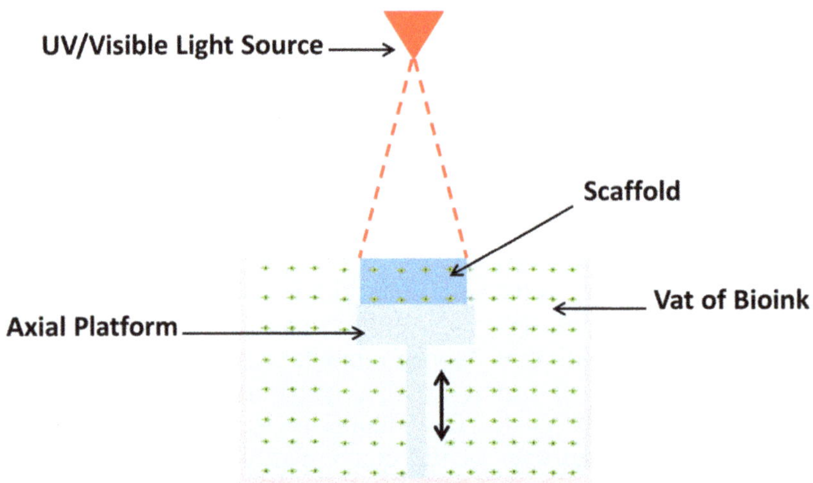

Figure 4.7. Schematic representation of stereolithography. Reproduced from [91] CC BY 4.0.

high-viscosity materials, and large-size model printing [73, 95]. However, this technique can only be applied to photopolymers [48]. UV light can damage biomolecules and cells. Oxygen inhibition can occur as the cured resin layer interacts directly with air. Thus, an irregular and sticky layer is formed on the surface, which is toxic, and resistant to mechanical forces. In addition, excessive curing causes increased brittleness [80]. The most common types of materials used in SLA printers are epoxy, thermoplastic elastomers, poly(ethylene glycol) (PEG)-based hydrogels, and acrylics. For medical applications, the amount of bio-containing, biodegradable, stable-size behavior during photopolymerization is very low. In addition, they do not have sufficient mechanical strength [73, 96]. Stereolithographic scaffolds with controlled microstructures can be produced with photocrosslinkable poly(propylene fumarate) (PPF) material by this technique. PPF is a non-toxic, biodegradable polymer with high mechanical properties used in the repair of bone defects. However, reactive diluents added to reduce the viscosity make the material non-degradable [96–98].

4.4.3 Selective laser sintering

The selective laser sintering (SLS) method is based on the principle of sintering powder layer by layer with a laser-based heat source. SLS was the first powder-based 3D printing technique and technology patented by Carl R Deckard in 1989 [99]. First, the powder is loaded into the supply container and digital instructions are programmed. The laser unit directs a high-powered beam to a reflective mirror. From there, a Galvo motor system steers the focused beam to the powder surface. Each layer of part geometry is then sintered by a heated bed of powder. The bed temperature is just below the melting point (0.5–1 Tm) of the material to prevent thermal distortion and facilitate the fusion of the sintered layer [73]. Pistons move the supply container up and the build chamber down while the roller moves across the bed to distribute the next layer of powder. Excess powder is captured in a collection container. The process is repeated layer by layer until the build is complete (figure 4.8). Unsintered powders are separated from the part by air jet, manually shaking or blowing method. SLS print resolution is around 50–100 μm [80].

The advantages of SLS are that the powder bed provides good support and that many types of materials can be used. However, high-resolution and high-intensity laser diodes are expensive, and laser printing system control is difficult [101]. Resolution may vary according to laser-beam diameter, the particle size of the powder, and scan line distance [48, 80]. In addition, laser properties affect the properties of the material to be sintered, such as mechanical properties, density, and surface texture [102].

The most commonly used material types in SLS printers are PC, nylon derivatives, acrylic, and PEEK powders [103]. CO_2 lasers with relatively high wavelengths are sufficient for sintering materials such as polymers with low melting temperatures. However, powerful Nd: YAG lasers with wavelengths approximately ten times lower than the CO_2 laser are used for metal and ceramic materials [102].

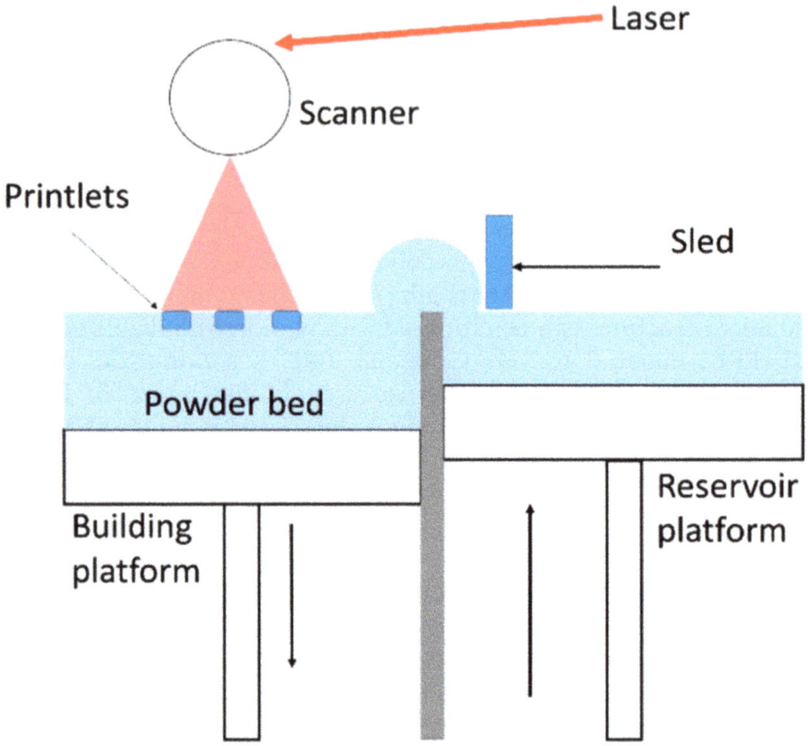

Figure 4.8. Schematic representation of selective laser sintering. Reproduced from [100] CC BY 4.0.

Materials such as bioceramic HA, tricalcium phosphate, and poly(3-hydroxybutyrate) are used in the medical applications of SLS. Due to its low melting temperature and high biocompatibility, scaffold production is made using PCL material with an SLS printer. Poly(vinyl alcohol) (PVA), poly(L-lactic acid) (PLLA), and PLGA are other scaffold production materials. Composites formed by blending bioceramics and biodegradable polymers are used in the production of bone tissue engineering scaffolds. SLS was utilized to create precise models of structures including the skull, mandible, and neuro network for surgical planning and simulation, especially in the disciplines of craniofacial and maxillofacial surgery, drug or biomolecule delivery vehicles, and neurosurgery [48, 102–104].

A brand-new chapter in 3D printing solid oral forms, specifically for personalized medicine, is selective laser sintering. Although both sintering parameters and material qualities demonstrate the capacity to change the internal structure of printouts, porosity stands out as the primary contribution of SLS technology. Thus, the most potential use of SLS in solid oral forms appears to be in orally disintegrating printouts. Also, earlier research on the SLS of drug-delivery systems aids in forecasting prospective pharmaceutical uses, such as controlled-release printouts. SLS may eventually prove to be a valuable tool for precision medicine, but there are still significant technological and governmental issues that need to be resolved [100].

4.4.4 Laminated object manufacturing

Laminated object manufacturing (LOM) is based on the principle of cutting solid-state sheets or bulk materials with a laser and joining them layer by layer with heat-sensitive adhesive. LOM is a technology patented by Michael Feygin *et al* in 1998 [105]. In this technique, first, materials are fed from the material supply roll, and with a hot roller, a heat-sensitive adhesive is activated. Lasers trace the prototype's required dimensions. By cutting the areas outside the drawn object into rectangles, a supporting structure is created for the lamination process and easy removal of the manufactured part from the total part is ensured. The layer-completed platform descends and moves out of the way. A new sheet of material is rolled into position. The platform descends into a fresh position to accept the subsequent layer (figure 4.9). The process is repeated until the model is finished. LOM print resolution is around 20–300 μm [80].

This technology allows large objects to be produced quickly and cost-effectively. Also, multicore or prototypes can be fabricated [82]. It does not contain toxic chemicals and complex chemical reactions [106]. The LOM technique is suitable for visual and aesthetic production, but it is not useful for structural production [107]. Its disadvantages are that it is not suitable for complex shape design, it is difficult to create a hollow structure in the model, low precision, and the amount of waste is high. In addition, post-fabrication processing may be required for dimensional stability [80].

The most commonly used materials are metal laminates, thermoplastic sheets such as polyvinyl caprolactam (PVC), and thin paper sheet [80, 82]. Automated fabrication of bioceramic non-resorbable bone implants is carried out with LOM [108].

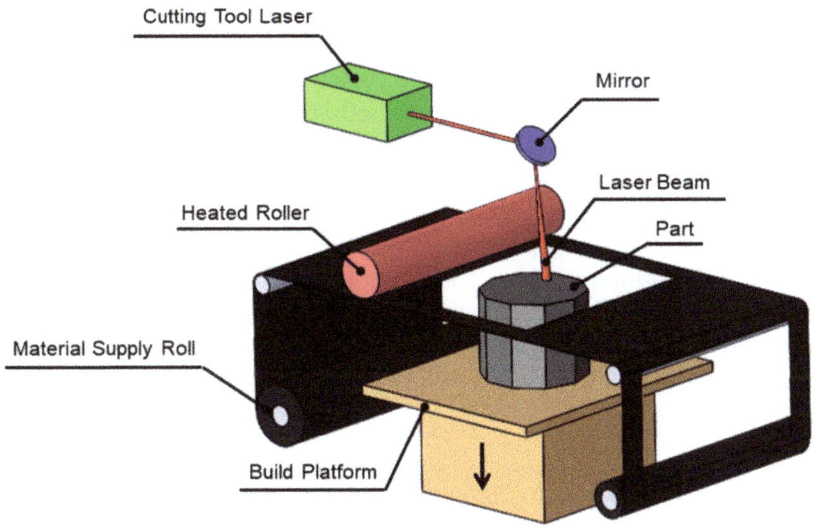

Figure 4.9. Schematic representation of laminated object manufacturing. Reproduced from [109] CC BY 4.0.

LOM technologies can be used for drug delivery applications using metals such as steel, titanium, and ceramics. It has a hybrid manufacturing advantage but requires tedious cleaning [110].

4.5 3D and 4D bioprinting

The health industry has enormous potential for cutting-edge technology known as AM, also known as computer-aided 3D printing. Dental, tissue, and organ fabrication; anatomical 3D models used for surgical training; medicines; and the development of patient-specific medical devices are now among its applications (such as prosthetics and implants). Moreover, 3D bioprinting is a leader in individualized therapy and improved drug delivery as opposed to mass-produced medications, which have low effectiveness in patients [111]. Although 3D printing might be cost-effective, there is a restriction in the lack of 3D-printable biomaterials for most applications. Developing economies may also be impacted by the loss of skilled workers needed to produce medical gadgets like prosthetic limbs and other devices. Customized 3D-printed organs and tissues for patients can do away with the costs of the donation procedure and guarantee that every transplant is accepted by the patient's body [112]. 3D bioprinting is the use of methods similar to 3D printing to mix cells, growth factors, and/or biomaterials to create biomedical parts, frequently to mimic the properties of natural tissue. In general, layer-by-layer 3D bioprinting can be used to deposit materials known as bioinks to produce tissue-like structures that are later utilized in many medical and tissue engineering sectors [113, 114].

Contrary to three-dimensional printing, 4D bioprinting uses stimuli-sensitive biomaterials to mimic the dynamic nature of tissues. 4D AM of biomaterials can be used for different approaches. 4D bioprinting is the application of 4D printing in medical sciences and technologies and is directly related to the maturation of assembled cells [115]. By introducing a fourth dimension—time—to 3D bioprinting, its theory advances the science. Its development is likely to be advantageous in fields including bioactuation, biosensing, and biorobotics [13]. Advances in wireless communication and data storage devices can help four-dimensional bioprinted constructions. To create a new generation of multifunctional and intelligent cellular-based structures for applications in tissue regeneration and drug release, these devices can be coupled with stimuli-responsive materials [116]. Here, the most crucial argument is that creating lower-dimensional, less complex objects would allow for simple, quick production of components at a reduced cost [117]. The manufacturing procedures for 4D are still difficult and expensive, in contrast to 3D bioprinting where costs are decreasing. Viable cells, tissues, and intelligent materials are still expensive and hardly used. To fully broaden the therapeutic possibilities, new smart-biomaterials that respond to various stimuli *in vivo* as well as a new set of bioinks for 4D bioprinting will be required in the future [118, 119].

4.5.1 Bioinks

Bioprinting is an emerging technology with various applications in the construction of functional tissue structures to replace injured or diseased tissues. It is a new approach that provides high reproducibility, precise control over fabricated structures and potentially enables highly efficient production. During the bioprinting process, a biomaterial solution or a mixture of several biomaterials, often in hydrogel form, often called bioink, is used to create tissue structures. This bioink can be crosslinked or stabilized during or immediately after bioprinting to create the final shape, structure, and architecture of the designed structure. Bioinks can be made from natural or synthetic biomaterials alone or a combination of the two as hybrid materials. In some cases, cell clusters without any additional biomaterials can also be adapted to be used as a bioink for bioprinting processes [120, 121]. For example, hydrogel-based bioprinting processes are advised for drug delivery investigations because the rate at which biopolymeric materials degrade can be a precisely adjustable factor in achieving controlled drug release [122, 123].

Some important properties of an ideal bioink material are bioprintability, high mechanical integrity and stability, insolubility in cell culture medium, biodegradability at a rate suitable for regenerating tissue, non-toxicity, and non-immunogenicity, and the ability to promote cell adhesion. In addition, bioink materials should be easily manufactured and processed, affordable, and commercially available [124, 125].

Many different biomaterials have been reported for use as bioinks in 3D printing. Polymers obtained from natural sources are called natural biomaterials in the biomedical field. These natural biomaterials have several advantages over synthetic materials, primarily related to biomimicry of extracellular matrix (ECM) composition or structure, self-assembly ability, biocompatibility, and biodegradation properties. However, synthetic polymers can be controlled by mechanical stability, photocrosslinking ability, pH and temperature responses, etc. This provides advantageous properties not found in natural polymers. Bioinks of natural origin can be based on biopolymers such as agarose, alginate (AL), collagen, hyaluronic acid, fibrin protein, albumin, elastin, protein class, keratin, laminarin, agarose, chondroitin sulfate, carrageenan, xanthan gum, glucan, heparin, fucoidan, guar gum, pectin, gellan gum, cellulose, silk protein, platelet lysates, and ECM. Synthetic bioinks can be based on pluronic, polyethyleneglycol (PEG), and methacrylate. It is also very common to use one or more materials in the composite form to obtain the desired properties in bioink production [126–129].

When a systematic review of the literature was examined, a total of 9720 studies were identified, including 58 using natural biomaterials, 26 using synthetic biomaterials, and 39 using a combination of biomaterials as bioinks. AL ($n = 50$) and PCL ($n = 33$) were the most commonly used bioinks, followed by gelatin ($n = 18$) and methacrylate gelatin (GelMA) ($n = 16$). In terms of bioprinting methods used, pneumatic extrusion bioprinting techniques are the most common ($n = 78$), followed by the piston ($n = 28$) bioprinting method. Most studies focus on the target tissue, most commonly bone, and cartilage, and are investigating bioinks with the most promising printability and biocompatibility properties [130].

AL can be used in knee cartilage repairs as a compound with good properties such as satisfactory mechanical properties and suitable compression modulus during the bioprinting process. AL transforms into a stable hydrogel through the ionic interaction between the AL's carboxyl groups and Ca^{2+}. The biocompatibility and controllable viscosity of AL improves scaffolding and bioprinting applications [131]. A variety of low molecular weight (M_w) medications can be delivered using AL structures. By adjusting the kind and method of the crosslinker, an AL-based biopolymer can be fine-tuned to control the rate at which cardiac medicines are released. The *in situ* gelling AL technology makes a superior medication delivery method for long-term use. AL is employed in drug delivery in the form of hydrogel, matrices, membranes, films, microspheres, and beads [132]. 3D bioprinting provides a rapid and robust approach to the production of functional tissues *in vitro*. To facilitate tissue formation, ALs have been widely used as bioinks to provide a matrix scaffold to guide specific 3D cell growth because they can potently form cell-compatible hydrogels in physiological conditions. In addition, they can be modified for a variety of tissue engineering applications, including bone, vascular, and adipose tissue engineering. However, natural AL is a bioinert material (lack of cell-adhesive parts) with limited biodegradation [133]. The naturally occurring biopolymer AL is cheaper and crosslinks with various salts such as $BaCl_2$, $CaCl_2$, and $ZnCl_2$, which shows good biocompatibility and compressibility, to form hydrogels [134]. It has been shown that AL-based bioinks can modulate important stem cell behaviors such as proliferation without affecting their printability and structural integrity after eight days in cell culture [135].

PCL is a biodegradable, biocompatible, and printable polymer with moderate mechanical strength that has been approved for use in medical devices by the FDA. Due to its non-toxicity, and outstanding flexibility, PCL is a polymer that can be used as a bioabsorbable suture and drug-delivery biomaterial [136]. PCL has drawbacks such as being hydrophobic and lacking support for cell adhesion [137]. According to reports, due to its exceptional properties, PCL, a semi-crystalline biocompatible polymer with a melting point of 60 °C that is easily soluble in organic solvents, is commonly employed in 3D printing applications. The goal, scaffold design, required mechanical qualities, and porosity must all be taken into account when choosing the printing method (extrusion versus inkjet), however, as PCL's molecular weight can range from 500 to 120 000 Da [138]. The most widely used 3D-printable biomaterial is PCL, which is especially suitable for 3D-printing a tracheal scaffold. PCL's hydrophobicity is bad for cell affinity and tracheal cartilage development. Due to its high hydrophilicity and role as the primary building block of cartilage tissue, collagen holds promise for overcoming PCL's disadvantages in composite materials. A PCL–collagen composite scaffold is anticipated to offer both cell affinity and mechanical stability based on the characteristics of both materials [139].

Gelatin (GE) is used as a bioink because it is a natural protein obtained by the hydrolysis of collagen and is widely used as a food ingredient. Therefore, it is biocompatible, degradable, and also contains arginine-glycine-aspartic acid (RGD) residues that promote cell adhesion, migration, and proliferation, thereby increasing its ability to mimic the *in vivo* microenvironment. It also contains a matrix metalloproteinase (MMP) sequence that supports cell enzymatic degradation. With this feature, it is widely used in tissue engineering [140, 141]. However, gelatin has poor thermostability (at temperatures above 37 °C, the gelatin will become a solution due to the breakdown of hydrogen bonds) and chemical crosslinks can affect the biocompatibility of gelatin, as some crosslinking reagents are toxic. Therefore, the application of gelling is limited by insufficient thermostability and the potential toxicity of chemical crosslinking. However, the side chains of gelatin have very large active groups, including –OH, –COOH, $-NH_2$, –SH, and so on. Therefore, it is possible to modify gelatin with certain groups to compensate for its shortcomings. The most commonly used modification is known as methacrylate gelatin (GelMA). Thanks to the methacrylate groups replacing the amino groups in the gelatin side chains, this modified gelatin is gelatin-like, and the solid–liquid transition is also affected by temperature. The water solution of the modified gelatin crosslinks leads to GelMA hydrogels with excellent thermostability. The GelMA hydrogel still can support cell behaviors as the RGD and MMP sequences are preserved, and the biocompatibility and degradation of gelatin are not affected. Moreover, the physical and chemical properties of GelMA hydrogels can be flexibly adjusted to meet the requirements of various applications [142]. Drug delivery is frequently integrated with hydrogel technologies to increase drug delivery effectiveness and decrease side effects to achieve superior tissue engineering performance. In a variety of ways, GelMA has been used as a medication delivery system. Due to an increase in hydrogel crosslinking density, the drug release is lowered when the GelMA ratio rises. One of the most efficient methods to regulate medication release is to alter the ratios of various hydrogels [143].

Nanocellulose can be used as an additive in the preparation of bioinks developed. Nanocellulose is a natural fiber that can be extracted from cellulose. It is the size of nanocellulose fiber that usually contains less than 100 nm in diameter and several micrometers in length. Nanocellulose is transparent and filled with a reactive surface of hydroxyl groups that can be functionalized to various surface properties [144]. Because of its significant specific surface area, high mechanical strength, stiffness, biocompatibility, and renewability, nanocellulose has recently received a lot of attention for its potential use in the drug delivery industry. These features make nanocellulose capable of having good drug loading and binding capacities. In the field of medication delivery, nanocellulose-based composite materials with better-designed architectures and multifunctions (e.g., pH or NIR responses) will surely be widely exploited [145]. In the context of biomedical hydrogels for tissue engineering, interest in nanocelluloses is mainly due to their structural similarity to ECMs, both in terms of porosity and interconnection framework, within the structural hydrogel and fibrous topography of cellulose fibrils, which are somewhat similar to collagen. They are also preferred for fibronectin in native ECM, as well as for their excellent biocompatibility to support important cellular activities, as has been suggested in numerous *in vitro* and *in vivo* studies. However, studies on the *in vivo* biodegradability and *in vivo* nanosafety validation of nanocellulose-based bioinks are still ongoing [146]. Due to their exceptional biocompatibility, biodegradability, and low cytotoxicity, nanocellulose-based materials have received extensive research and are regarded as promising for clinical and medical applications. Although nitrocellulose-based composites have a lot of potential in a range of biomedical and biotechnological applications, a thorough toxicological assessment of these materials is required before they are used in clinical settings [147].

Halloysite is also a great additive to bioinks development. Halloysite is a naturally occurring aluminosilicate mineral with the formula $Al_2Si_2O_5(OH)_4{\cdot}nH_2O$. This mineral is extracted from natural deposits in humid tropical regions in countries such as China, the USA, New Zealand, Australia, and Turkey. Halloysite nanotubes range in length from 200 to 2000 nm; outer and inner diameters are in the range of 50–70 and 10–20 nm, respectively. As a nanofiller, halloysite nanotubes significantly increase the compressive strength, compression modulus, and thermal stability of polymers. Halloysite by itself does not affect cell viability and may even promote cellular adhesion and proliferation. Halloysite nanotubes are a naturally occurring 'green' material that does not pose a significant biohazard. Halloysite nanoclay is a promising material for structuring biopolymer matrices. For tissue engineering and regenerative medicine, nanoclays hold promise as additive or bioactive agents as well as drug delivery vehicles. Their biocompatibility, low toxicity, simplicity of surface modification, material enhancing qualities, affordability, and capacity to encapsulate pharmaceuticals are the reasons for this. The use of clay nanomaterials enables the characterization of nanoparticles based on their size, solubility, surface charge, capacity for cationic exchange, dispersibility, and rate of drug release. The addition of halloysite, even at the rate of 3%–6% by weight, causes significant changes in the physicochemical properties of the obtained materials. The ability to sustain cell growth in scaffolds with extremely large amounts of nanotubes (up to 80%) can be exploited to create hard tissue substitutes such as bone. At the same time, the inclusion of nanotubes has no significant effect on the porosity of the materials, and at the same time, cell adhesion and proliferation are improved. Therefore, the high biocompatibility of halloysite-doped scaffolds and the ability to modulate the properties of matrices by modification of nanomaterials make polymer–halloysite composites a promising material for the fabrication of tissue-engineered scaffolds [148–150].

4.5.2 Cell source

Cells play an important role in tissue engineering approaches. Cells are seeded secondarily after the scaffold is built to construct during the printing process in bioprinting. The selection and supply of cells will have an impact on the success of both approaches [151]. Even though most drug delivery devices are acellular, choosing the right cells is crucial when building a drug screening platform to more accurately mimic the physiological state and pathological process of the tissue of interest. A 3D bioprinted cellular model is frequently produced using stem cells, cell lines, and primary cells as the three different types of cell sources [152]. The majority of *in vitro* platforms for disease modeling prefer using cells generated from human tissue to reduce the gap in biological responses caused by genetic differences between animals and humans [152, 153]. Regardless of the type of cell source, there is a significant likelihood of changes between batches. These variations can be attributable to several factors, including user technical proficiency, varying culture conditions, and variable cell differentiation potency. To eliminate discrepancies and differences between trials, it is crucial to define cells using a variety of tests and techniques [152, 154].

4.6 3D and 4D bioprinted drug delivery systems

Despite the difficulties of biocompatibility and resolution, 3D printing and 3D bioprinting are promising technologies for a wide range of healthcare applications, from cutting-edge tissue engineering therapies and regenerative medicine to pharmaceutical improvements [155].

The term 'personalized medicine' refers to medical care that is tailored to the patient. 3D printing is one method that could be used to implement personalized treatment. 4D printing is established while using materials that can be tweaked with stimulation. Several studies have been looking into a new field recently that blends medicines and 3D and 4D printing. As a result, numerous ideas for pharmaceutical products and formulas that may be customized and printed have emerged. Devices that can be made to deliver individualized medicine have drawn a lot of interest, ranging from oral formulations to drug-eluting implants [156]. Today, scientists may manufacture complete microneedle patches using a variety of 3D printing processes, or they can coat the printed patches with the desired medication solution. Inkjet bioprinting has mostly been used to make 2D patterns; it has not been fully investigated whether it may be utilized to produce sophisticated 3D structures. For transdermal insulin delivery, Ross *et al* (2015) coated metallic microneedle arrays with several layers of polymer holding insulin [157]. A drug-encapsulated microneedle patch system with an integrated 3D-printed microheater device was created by Yin *et al* (2019) to improve transdermal medication administration and develop a smart-sensor-assisted microneedle patch, applying heat to existing created microneedle patches may speed drug diffusion and help with regulated drug delivery. A 3D bioprinter from Cellink was used to create the microheater device [158].

Compared to conventional methods, 3D printing offers a lot more manufacturing flexibility for generating tablet medications. More options are now available than with simple tablet compression because of their ability to create complex tablets with instant release, delayed release, extended-release, pulsatory release, and the incorporation of numerous medications and multiple release profiles in one tablet [156]. A novel tablet design that increased the immediate drug release of 3D-printed tablets was recently displayed by Sadia *et al* (2018) the polymethacrylate tablets have internal channels with specified width, length, and configuration. These canals raise the surface-to-volume ratio of the tablet, enabling a quicker rapid drug release [159].

Stimulus-responsive implants for medication delivery have many uses. Several teams have developed implants that could serve as drug delivery devices using cutting-edge 4D printing technology. Stimulus-responsive implants for medication delivery have many uses. Several teams have developed implants that could serve as drug delivery devices using cutting-edge 4D printing technology. Melocchi *et al*'s (2019) research proved that it is possible to print a PVA-based intravesical medicine delivery system for bladder illnesses using 4D technology. Here, the team once more performed 3D printing with a composition containing a tracer using a Kloner 3D® 240 Twin fitted with a nozzle. In this drug delivery system, PVA demonstrated water-induced shape-memory behavior, which was regarded as the fourth dimension [160]. The exponential rise in the number of articles mentioning the phrase '3D printing drug delivery' suggests that studies using this phrase are still consistently being created. Although 3D and 4D bioprinting offers a new paradigm for medication administration, there is still a long way to go before either is routinely commercialized and used in clinical settings.

4.7 Promises and realities

Today, the main purpose of the drug development industry is to provide treatment by releasing the drug compatible with the body to the targeted area in a controlled and timely manner. The treatment of diseases is facilitated by the production of drug/protein-loaded biomaterials specifically for the patient by layered manufacturing. However, since the standardized dose and drug combinations used in the pharmaceutical industry are not suitable for every patient, treatments can be time-consuming and complex.

In this context, AM offers innovative solutions with superior features. With AM, drugs with different combinations and structures can be produced using a single device. Thus, the patient can easily use the tablets or pills he needs with a single drug at a time, in the right dose and easily. As a result, drug therapy with minimum toxicity is provided with the dosage appropriate for the metabolism of the patient [118, 161].

While tumor formation is prevented in cancer treatment with drug delivery systems produced with 3D bioprinting [162], tissue regeneration in the body can be facilitated with shape memory carriers produced with 4D bioprinting [118]. However, studies are needed to transform 3D and 4D bioprinting into industrial-scale, fast, trouble-free, and cost-effective production [163]. In particular, the high cost of viable cells, tissues, and smart materials is one of the biggest problems that needs to be solved with this technology [118]. In addition, the printing process needs optimization due to complex drug–material and drug–drug interactions [48]. Currently, there is no reliable computational model for the determination of mechanical properties such as the deformation of 4D bioprinting systems. The mechanical strength of soft materials such as biocompatible hydrogel used in printing is not at the desired level, and studies are needed to understand the behavior of materials *in vivo* conditions such as pH, and temperature [164, 165].

AM for drug delivery systems is expected to become popular in the future. It is an indisputable fact that studies will increase with the development of high-resolution and new stimulation systems on this research topic, which is located at the intersection of medicine, biomedical, biomaterials, and manufacturing. When it comes to human health, cross-industry studies will only be considered viable by regulatory authorities after they have been sensitively validated by their scientific evidence.

4.8 Current state-of-the-art and challenges in the market aspect of 3D–4D bioprinting drug delivery systems

Recent developments have enhanced 3D bioprinting technologies to the point where stakeholders now view them as the gold standard method for fabrication techniques. With the automated deposition of successive layers of biologically relevant and targetable materials, including biomaterials and nanomaterials, in a precise 3D space by potentially combining multiple methods, 3D bioprinting is undoubtedly emerging as a crucial biofabrication technology [166].

There are numerous recent book chapters and review articles that offer thorough analyses of 3D bioprinting. Presently, hundreds of businesses located in dozens of nations are working on 3D bioprinters, suitable bioinks, and add-ons [167]. Unsurprisingly, the phrase ‘bioprinting’ appears in a lot more patents than ‘biofabrication’ or other similar terms. However, the number of articles with the phrase ‘biofabrication’ in them is relatively similar to the number of articles with the term ‘bioprinting’; the term ‘biofabrication’ is also used in a variety of other contexts and senses [166].

The scientific and technological community is constantly being introduced to new 3D bioprinting technologies and procedures, and the biofabrication sector market is expanding quickly. It is possible that the need for smart materials, which can open up new avenues and dimensions for biofabrication processes and drive this change, will emerge as the next bioprinting trend. The first stimuli-responsive hierarchical self-morphing and active shape-changing biofabricated structures employing smart materials are now being demonstrated, in particular, via 4D bioprinting techniques [166, 168].

Although 3D printing in the pharmaceutical industry is still in its infancy, the medical device sector has achieved significant strides. The market for 3D printing is thought to be enormous overall and growing rapidly each year. According to estimates, the global market for 3D printing in healthcare will be worth US $3692 million by 2026, expanding at a Compound Annual Growth Rate (CAGR) of 18.2% from 2019 to 2026 [169].

Some pharmaceutical products produced with this technique began to attract worldwide attention. Regulatory agencies must also be prepared with complete awareness of the technological specifics and procedures for product evaluation to expedite product approval [169]. To further translate theory into practical and ground-breaking solutions, it is necessary to bridge the gaps between all stakeholders, including regulators, pharmaceutical makers, and researchers. To produce highly flexible and customized dose forms on demand, the study of the real-time safety and efficacy of 3D-printed items in clinical practice is also necessary [170].

Researchers should keep in mind device testing considerations before market submission of a device made using AM. Depending on the intended application, risk profile, and categorization and/or regulation for the device type, a substantial equivalence finding or clearance will require a different set of data, either in terms of type or quantity. The kind of information required for a device created via AM may also rely on some other criteria, such as whether the item is an implant, load-bearing, available in pre-specified standard sizes, or patient-matched. Given the range of devices that can be created by AM and the current AM technologies, not all of the concerns presented will apply to a single item. In figure 4.10, the steps of the device testing consideration process can be found [16].

4.9 Future remarks

Since 3D bioprinting is still in its early stages in the pharmaceutical industry, the transition to 4D bioprinting may occur sooner. The use of smart drugs can provide

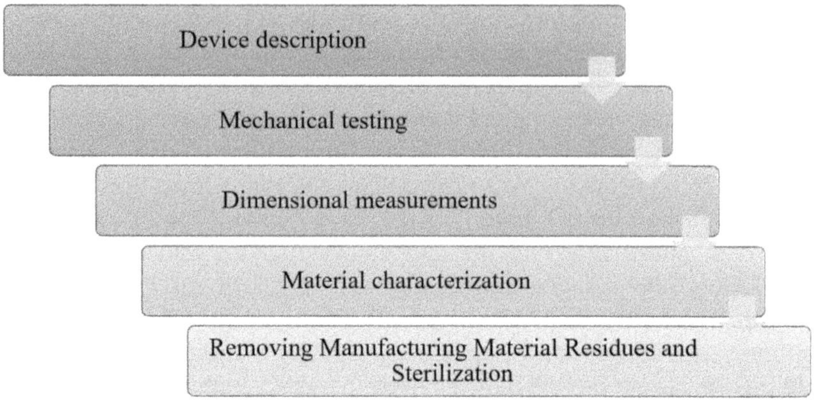

Figure 4.10. The steps of device testing consideration.

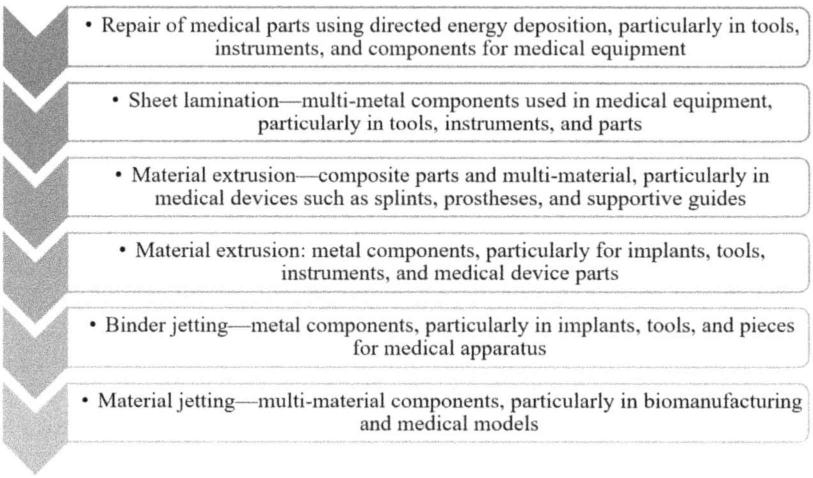

Figure 4.11. Areas of future research in medical AM using various processes [14].

more targeted therapy that can be tailored to the needs of each patient, ushering in a digital revolution in drug delivery and healthcare. It remains to be seen whether this approach is ultimately adopted, though the growing research and non-expert use of such drug delivery systems would suggest this will follow. Nonetheless, because the FDA supports the development of complex dosage forms and the use of innovative manufacturing approaches based on science and risk-based approaches, such innovative technologies may be adopted more quickly in healthcare. The main barriers to the widespread use of 3D printing at the moment are technical and quality control restrictions. It is projected that 3D printers could soon overtake pharmaceutical stores once the proper printing platform is built, ushering in a new era of digital health [24, 171] (figure 4.11).

4.10 Conclusions

While there are numerous benefits to incorporating AM techniques into healthcare, there are also some drawbacks. The first major roadblock is the approval of APIs in several currently available medicines. The second barrier is the printed polypills' economic feasibility in comparison to the currently used mass-manufactured medications. The third barrier is the requirement for newly established clinical guidelines to allow providers to prescribe for diseased states. For example, if the innovator company does not provide a legal license, the intellectual property protection of the therapeutic benefit of APIs in current medications and the chemical structure would legally prohibit sales. As a result, both patients and insurance companies prefer generic medications over brand medications. This method used by generic manufacturers could potentially be followed by generic medication polypills. To comply with the existing FDA regulations and guidelines, AM technology should be capable of reproducing pharmaceutical formulations that are bioequivalent to mass-manufactured tablets stably and consistently.

In comparison to traditional manufacturing technology, which includes 3D and 4D printing technologies, intelligent printing manufacturing is being developed as an advanced technology. Static structures can be created using 3D printing technology, and 4D printing which combines 3D printing with smart materials is thought to be a state-of-the-art technique. The structural reaction of 4D printing over time in response to environmental stimuli has recently come to light and attracted attention. Figure 4.12 shows the 3D and 4D printing technology's SWOT analysis, which is used to assess its advantages and prospects over the following few years.

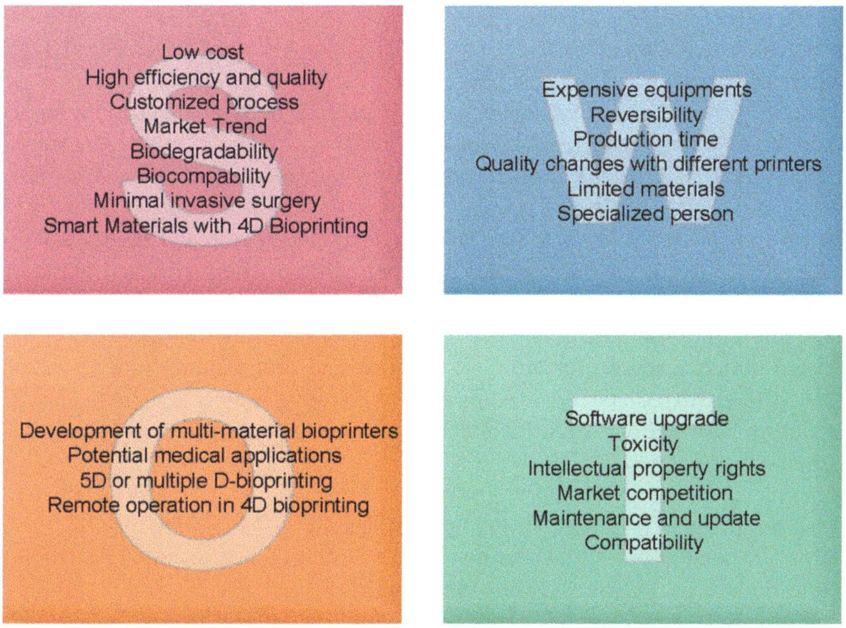

Figure 4.12. SWOT analysis to offer a situational assessment of the technology.

References

[1] Framinan J M, Perez-Gonzalez P and Fernandez-Viagas V 2023 An overview on the use of operations research in additive manufacturing *Ann. Oper. Res.* **322** 5–40

[2] Tofail S A M, Koumoulos E P, Bandyopadhyay A, Bose S, O'Donoghue L and Charitidis C 2018 Additive manufacturing: scientific and technological challenges, market uptake and opportunities *Mater. Today* **21** 22–37

[3] Lettori J, Raffaeli R, Peruzzini M, Schmidt J and Pellicciari M 2020 Additive manufacturing adoption in product design: an overview from literature and industry *Procedia Manuf.* **51** 655–62

[4] Wohlers T and Gornet T 2012 History of additive manufacturing Introduction of non-SL systems Introduction of low-cost 3D printers *Wohlers Rep.* **2012** 1–23

[5] Buj-Corral I, Tejo-Otero A and Fenollosa-Artés F 2020 Development of AM technologies for metals in the sector of medical implants *Metals (Basel)* **10** 686

[6] Rodríguez-Salvador M and Garcia-Garcia L A 2018 Additive manufacturing in healthcare *Foresight STI Gov.* **12** 47–55

[7] İyibilgin O and Gepek E 2021 Additive manufacturing technologies and its future in industrial applications *Int. J. Integr. Eng.* **13** 245–57

[8] Doğru A, Kandemir M B and Seydibeyoğlu M Ö 2022 3D nanoprinting in the aero-industries *Smart 3D Nanoprinting* (Boca Raton, FL: CRC Press) pp 23–41

[9] Gibson I, Rosen D and Stucker B 2015 *Additive Manufacturing Technologies* (New York: Springer)

[10] Gross B C, Erkal J L, Lockwood S Y, Chen C and Spence D M 2014 Evaluation of 3D printing and its potential impact on biotechnology and the chemical sciences *Anal. Chem.* **86** 3240–53

[11] Lee Ventola C 2014 Medical applications for 3D printing: current and projected uses *Pharm. Ther.* **39** 704–11

[12] Bozkurt Y and Karayel E 2021 3D printing technology; methods, biomedical applications, future opportunities and trends *J. Mater. Res. Technol.* **14** 1430–50

[13] Javaid M, Haleem A, Singh R P and Suman R 2022 3D printing applications for healthcare research and development *Glob. Heal. J.* **6** 217–26

[14] Salmi M 2021 Additive manufacturing processes in medical applications *Materials (Basel)* **14** 191

[15] Silva A L, Salvador G M, da S, Castro S V F, Carvalho N M F and Munoz R A A 2021 A 3D printer guide for the development and application of electrochemical cells and devices *Front. Chem.* **9** 684256

[16] Food and Drug Administration 2017 Technical considerations for additive manufactured medical devices:guidance for industry and food and drug administration staff document FDA-2016-D-1210 Center for Devices and Radiological Health 1–30 https://www.fda.gov/regulatory-information/search-fda-guidance-documents/technical-considerations-additive-manufactured-medical-devices

[17] Mohammed A, Elshaer A, Sareh P, Elsayed M and Hassanin H 2020 Additive manufacturing technologies for drug delivery applications *Int. J. Pharm.* **580** 119245

[18] Durga Prasad Reddy R and Sharma V 2020 Additive manufacturing in drug delivery applications: a review *Int. J. Pharm.* **589** 119820

[19] Maniruzzaman M 2019 *3D and 4D Printing in Biomedical Applications: Process Engineering and Additive Manufacturing* (Wiley)

[20] Norman J, Madurawe R D, Moore C M V, Khan M A and Khairuzzaman A 2017 A new chapter in pharmaceutical manufacturing: 3D-printed drug products *Adv. Drug Deliv. Rev.* **108** 39–50

[21] Wohlers, Wohlers T 2016 *Wohlers Report 2016* (Fort Collins, CO: Wohlers Associates. Inc.) https://worldcat.org/title/948549886 (accessed 17 January 2023)

[22] Schubert C, van Langeveld M C and Donoso L A 2014 Innovations in 3D printing: a 3D overview from optics to organs *Br. J. Ophthalmol.* **98** 159–61

[23] Bajpai A, Baigent A, Raghav S, Brádaigh C Ó, Koutsos V and Radacsi N 2020 4D printing: materials, technologies, and future applications in the biomedical field *Sustainability* **12** 10628

[24] Ahmed A, Arya S, Gupta V, Furukawa H and Khosla A 2021 4D printing: fundamentals, materials, applications and challenges *Polymer* **228** 123926

[25] Melocchi A, Uboldi M, Cerea M, Foppoli A, Maroni A and Moutaharrik S *et al* 2021 Shape memory materials and 4D printing in pharmaceutics *Adv. Drug Deliv. Rev.* **173** 216–37

[26] Subeshan B, Baddam Y and Asmatulu E 2021 Current progress of 4D-printing technology *Prog. Addit. Manuf.* **63** 495–516

[27] Kirillova A and Ionov L 2019 Shape-changing polymers for biomedical applications *J. Mater. Chem.* B **7** 1597–624

[28] Hull C 1986 Method and apparatus for production of three-dimensional objects by stereolithography *US Patent* 4999143A https://patents.google.com/patent/US4999143A/en

[29] Crump S S Apparatus and method for creating three-dimensional objects United States; 1989 https://patents.google.com/patent/US5121329A/en (accessed 22 February 2023)

[30] Prince J D 2014 3D printing: an industrial revolution *J. Electron. Resour. Med. Libr.* **11** 39–45

[31] Gross B C, Erkal J L, Lockwood S Y, Chen C and Spence D M 2014 Evaluation of 3D printing and its potential impact on biotechnology and the chemical sciences *Anal. Chem.* **86** 3240–53

[32] Melchels F P W, Domingos M A N, Klein T J, Malda J, Bartolo P J and Hutmacher D W 2012 Additive manufacturing of tissues and organs *Prog. Polym. Sci.* **37** 1079–104

[33] Sculpteo 2022 The History of 3D Printing: 3D Printing Technologies from the 80s to Today https://sculpteo.com/en/3d-learning-hub/basics-of-3d-printing/the-history-of-3d-printing/ (accessed 8 March 2023)

[34] Mandal A 2012 World's first 3D printed jaw transplant *News Medical* https://news-medical.net/news/20120207/Worlds-first-3D-printed-jaw-transplant.aspx (accessed 8 March 2023)

[35] British Man Receives the World's 3D-Printed Prosthetic Eye by Franhofer Technology — TechEBlog https://techeblog.com/first-3d-printed-prosthetic-eye/ (accessed 8 March 2023)

[36] Kyobula M, Adedeji A, Alexander M R, Saleh E, Wildman R and Ashcroft I *et al* 2017 3D inkjet printing of tablets exploiting bespoke complex geometries for controlled and tuneable drug release *J. Control. Release* **261** 207–15

[37] Kholgh Eshkalak S, Rezvani Ghomi E, Dai Y, Choudhury D and Ramakrishna S 2020 The role of three-dimensional printing in healthcare and medicine *Mater. Des.* **194** 108940

[38] 3D Printing https://dfepharma.com/our-innovation-and-solutions/3d-printing/

[39] van den Heuvel K A, Berardi A, Buijvoets L B and Dickhoff B H J 2022 3D-powder-bed-printed pharmaceutical drug product tablets for use in clinical studies *Pharmaceutics* **14** 2320

[40] Auriemma G, Tommasino C, Falcone G, Esposito T, Sardo C and Aquino R P 2022 Additive manufacturing strategies for personalized drug delivery systems and medical devices: fused filament fabrication and semi solid extrusion *Molecules* **27** 2784

[41] Li Q, Guan X, Cui M, Zhu Z, Chen K and Wen H *et al* 2018 Preparation and investigation of novel gastro-floating tablets with 3D extrusion-based printing *Int. J. Pharm.* **535** 325–32

[42] Arafat B, Wojsz M, Isreb A, Forbes R T, Isreb M and Ahmed W *et al* 2018 Tablet fragmentation without a disintegrant: a novel design approach for accelerating disintegration and drug release from 3D printed cellulosic tablets *Eur. J. Pharm. Sci.* **118** 191–9

[43] Fina F, Goyanes A, Madla C M, Awad A, Trenfield S J and Kuek J M *et al* 2018 3D printing of drug-loaded gyroid lattices using selective laser sintering *Int. J. Pharm.* **547** 44–52

[44] Zhang J, Yang W, Vo A Q, Feng X, Ye X and Kim D W *et al* 2017 Hydroxypropyl methylcellulose-based controlled release dosage by melt extrusion and 3D printing: structure and drug release correlation *Carbohydr. Polym* **177** 49–57

[45] Melocchi A, Parietti F, Loreti G, Maroni A, Gazzaniga A and Zema L 2015 3D printing by fused deposition modeling (FDM) of a swellable/erodible capsular device for oral pulsatile release of drugs *J. Drug Deliv. Sci. Technol.* **30** 360–7

[46] Kjar A and Huang Y 2019 Application of micro-scale 3D printing in pharmaceutics *Pharmaceutics* **11** 390

[47] Balazic M, Kopac J, Jackson M J and Ahmed W 2007 Review: titanium and titanium alloy applications in medicine *Int. J. Nano Biomater.* **1** 3–34

[48] Bandyopadhyay A, Bose S and Das S 2015 3D printing of biomaterials *MRS Bull.* **40** 108–14

[49] Colin A and Boire J Y 1997 A novel tool for rapid prototyping and development of simple 3D medical image processing applications on PCs *Comput. Methods Programs Biomed.* **53** 87–92

[50] Winder J and Bibb R 2005 Medical rapid prototyping technologies: state of the art and current limitations for application in oral and maxillofacial surgery *J. Oral Maxillofac. Surg.* **63** 1006–15

[51] Goyanes A, Wang J, Buanz A, Martínez-Pacheco R, Telford R and Gaisford S *et al* 2015 3D printing of medicines: engineering novel oral devices with unique design and drug release characteristics *Mol. Pharm.* **12** 4077–84

[52] Goyanes A, Chang H, Sedough D, Hatton G B, Wang J and Buanz A *et al* 2015 Fabrication of controlled-release budesonide tablets via desktop (FDM) 3D printing *Int. J. Pharm.* **496** 414–20

[53] Melocchi A, Parietti F, Loreti G, Maroni A, Gazzaniga A and Zema L 2015 3D printing by fused deposition modeling (FDM) of a swellable/erodible capsular device for oral pulsatile release of drugs *J. Drug Deliv. Sci. Technol.* **30** 360–7

[54] Goyanes A, Buanz A B M, Hatton G B, Gaisford S and Basit A W 2015 3D printing of modified-release aminosalicylate (4-ASA and 5-ASA) tablets *Eur. J. Pharm. Biopharm.* **89** 157–62

[55] Goyanes A, Robles Martinez P, Buanz A, Basit A W and Gaisford S 2015 Effect of geometry on drug release from 3D printed tablets *Int. J. Pharm.* **494** 657–63

[56] Genina N, Holländer J, Jukarainen H, Mäkilä E, Salonen J and Sandler N 2016 Ethylene vinyl acetate (EVA) as a new drug carrier for 3D printed medical drug delivery devices *Eur. J. Pharm. Sci.* **90** 53–63
[57] Goyanes A, Det-Amornrat U, Wang J, Basit A W and Gaisford S 2016 3D scanning and 3D printing as innovative technologies for fabricating personalized topical drug delivery systems *J. Control Release.* **234** 41–8
[58] Beck R C R, Chaves P S, Goyanes A, Vukosavljevic B, Buanz A and Windbergs M *et al* 2017 3D printed tablets loaded with polymeric nanocapsules: an innovative approach to produce customized drug delivery systems *Int. J. Pharm.* **528** 268–79
[59] Genina N, Boetker J P, Colombo S, Harmankaya N, Rantanen J and Bohr A 2017 Anti-tuberculosis drug combination for controlled oral delivery using 3D printed compartmental dosage forms: from drug product design to *in vivo* testing *J. Control Release.* **268** 40–8
[60] Khaled S A, Burley J C, Alexander M R and Roberts C J 2014 Desktop 3D printing of controlled release pharmaceutical bilayer tablets *Int. J. Pharm.* **461** 105–11
[61] Khaled S A, Burley J C, Alexander M R, Yang J and Roberts C J 2015 3D printing of five-in-one dose combination polypill with defined immediate and sustained release profiles *J. Control Release.* **217** 308–14
[62] Khaled S A, Burley J C, Alexander M R, Yang J and Roberts C J 2015 3D printing of tablets containing multiple drugs with defined release profiles *Int. J. Pharm.* **494** 643–50
[63] Pietrzak K, Isreb A and Alhnan M A 2015 A flexible-dose dispenser for immediate and extended release 3D printed tablets *Eur. J. Pharm. Biopharm.* **96** 380–7
[64] Huang W, Zheng Q, Sun W, Xu H and Yang X 2007 Levofloxacin implants with predefined microstructure fabricated by three-dimensional printing technique *Int. J. Pharm.* **339** 33–8
[65] Wu W, Zheng Q, Guo X, Sun J and Liu Y 2009 A programmed release multi-drug implant fabricated by three-dimensional printing technology for bone tuberculosis therapy *Biomed. Mater.* **4** 065005
[66] Rowe C, Katstra W, Palazzolo R, Giritlioglu B, Teung P and Cima M 2000 Multimechanism oral dosage forms fabricated by three dimensional printing™ *J. Control Release* **66** 11–7
[67] Yu D-G, Shen X-X, Branford-White C, Zhu L-M, White K and Yang X L 2009 Novel oral fast-disintegrating drug delivery devices with predefined inner structure fabricated by three-dimensional printing *J. Pharm. Pharmacol.* **61** 323–9
[68] Scoutaris N, Snowden M and Douroumis D 2015 Taste masked thin films printed by jet dispensing *Int. J. Pharm.* **494** 619–22
[69] Martinez P R, Goyanes A, Basit A W and Gaisford S 2017 Fabrication of drug-loaded hydrogels with stereolithographic 3D printing *Int. J. Pharm.* **532** 313–7
[70] Yi H-G, Choi Y-J, Kang K S, Hong J M, Pati R G and Park M N *et al* 2016 A 3D-printed local drug delivery patch for pancreatic cancer growth suppression *J. Control Release* **238** 231–41
[71] Jamróz W, Kurek M, Łyszczarz E, Brniak W and Jachowicz R 2017 Printing techniques: recent developments in pharmaceutical technology. acta pol pharm *Drug Res* **74** 753–63
[72] Horst D J 2018 3D printing of pharmaceutical drug delivery systems *Arch. Org. Inorg. Chem. Sci.* **1** 109
[73] Chia H N and Wu B M 2015 Recent advances in 3D printing of biomaterials *J. Biol. Eng* **9** 1–14

[74] Ahangar P, Cooke M E, Weber M H and Rosenzweig D H 2019 Current biomedical applications of 3D printing and additive manufacturing *Appl. Sci.* **9** 1713

[75] Chiulan I, Frone A, Brandabur C and Panaitescu D 2017 Recent advances in 3D printing of aliphatic polyesters *Bioengineering* **5** 2

[76] Xu W, Pranovich A, Uppstu P, Wang X, Kronlund D and Hemming J *et al* 2018 Novel biorenewable composite of wood polysaccharide and polylactic acid for three dimensional printing *Carbohydr. Polym.* **187** 51–8

[77] Lakkala P, Munnangi S R, Bandari S and Repka M 2023 Additive manufacturing technologies with emphasis on stereolithography 3D printing in pharmaceutical and medical applications: a review *Int. J. Pharm.* X **5** 100159

[78] Duan B and Wang M 2011 Selective laser sintering and its application in biomedical engineering *MRS Bull.* **36** 998–1005

[79] Konta A A, García-Piña M and Serrano D 2017 Personalised 3D printed medicines: which techniques and polymers are more successful? *Bioengineering.* **4** 79

[80] Lai J, Wang C and Wang M 2021 3D printing in biomedical engineering: processes, materials, and applications *Appl. Phys. Rev.* **8** 021322

[81] Wasti S and Adhikari S 2020 Use of biomaterials for 3D Printing by fused deposition modeling technique: a review *Front. Chem.* **8** 1–14

[82] Tappa K and Jammalamadaka U 2018 Novel biomaterials used in medical 3D printing techniques *J. Funct. Biomater* **9** 17

[83] Zein I, Hutmacher D W, Tan K C and Teoh S H 2002 Fused deposition modeling of novel scaffold architectures for tissue engineering applications *Biomaterials* **23** 1169–85

[84] Hutmacher D W, Schantz T, Zein I, Ng K W, Teoh S H and Tan K C 2001 Mechanical properties and cell cultural response of polycaprolactone scaffolds designed and fabricated via fused deposition modeling *J. Biomed. Mater. Res.* **55** 203–16

[85] Huang J J, Ren J A, Wang G F, Li Z A, Wu X W and Ren H J *et al* 2017 3D-printed 'fistula stent' designed for management of enterocutaneous fistula: an advanced strategy *World J. Gastroenterol.* **23** 7489–94

[86] Shen S, Wang H, Xue Y, Yuan L, Zhou X and Zhao Z *et al* 2017 Freeform fabrication of tissue-simulating phantom for potential use of surgical planning in conjoined twins separation surgery *Sci. Rep.* **7** 1–11

[87] Nair L S and Laurencin C T 2007 Biodegradable polymers as biomaterials *Prog. Polym. Sci. (Oxford)* **32** 762–98 www.elsevier.com/locate/ppolysci (accessed 20 February 2023)

[88] Park S H, Park D S, Shin J W, Kang Y G, Kim H K and Yoon T R *et al* 2012 Scaffolds for bone tissue engineering fabricated from two different materials by the rapid prototyping technique: PCL versus PLGA *J. Mater. Sci. Mater. Med.* **23** 2671–8

[89] Probst F A, Hutmacher D W, Müller D F, MacHens H G and Schantz J T 2010 Calvarial reconstruction by customized bioactive implant *Handchir. Mikrochir. Plast. Chir.* **42** 369–73

[90] Teo E Y, Ong S Y, Khoon Chong M S, Zhang Z, Lu J and Moochhala S *et al* 2011 Polycaprolactone-based fused deposition modeled mesh for delivery of antibacterial agents to infected wounds *Biomaterials* **32** 279–87

[91] Kačarević Ž, Rider P, Alkildani S, Retnasingh S, Smeets R and Jung O *et al* 2018 An introduction to 3D bioprinting: possibilities, challenges and future aspects *Materials (Basel)* **11** 2199

[92] Wang W L, Cheah C M, Fuh J Y H and Lu L 1996 Influence of process parameters on stereolithography part shrinkage *Mater. Design* **17** 205–13

[93] Heller C, Schwentenwein M, Russmueller G, Varga F, Stampfl J and Liska R 2009 Vinyl esters: low cytotoxicity monomers for the fabrication of biocompatible 3D scaffolds by lithography based additive manufacturing *J. Polym. Sci. Part A Polym. Chem.* **47** 6941–54

[94] Barry J J A, Evseev A V, Markov M A, Upton C E, Scotchford C A and Popov V K *et al* 2008 In vitro study of hydroxyapatite-based photocurable polymer composites prepared by laser stereolithography and supercritical fluid extraction *Acta Biomater.* **4** 1603–10

[95] Quan H, Zhang T, Xu H, Luo S, Nie J and Zhu X 2020 Photo-curing 3D printing technique and its challenges *Bioact. Mater.* **5** 110–5

[96] Lee K W, Wang S, Fox B C, Ritman E L, Yaszemski M J and Lu L 2007 Poly(propylene fumarate) bone tissue engineering scaffold fabrication using stereolithography: effects of resin formulations and laser parameters *Biomacromolecules* **8** 1077–84

[97] Jansen J, Melchels F P W, Grijpma D W and Feijen J 2009 Fumaric acid monoethyl ester-functionalized poly(D,L-Lactide)/N-vinyl-2—pyrrolidone resins for the preparation of tissue engineering scaffolds by stereolithography *Biomacromolecules* **10** 214–20

[98] Cheng L, Shoma Suresh K, He H, Rajput R S, Feng Q and Ramesh S *et al* 2021 3D printing of micro-and nanoscale bone substitutes: a review on technical and translational perspectives *Int. J. Nanomed.* **16** 4289–319

[99] Deckard C R 1986 Method and apparatus for producing parts by selective sintering *US Patent* US4863538A https://patents.google.com/patent/US4863538A/en

[100] Gueche Y A, Sanchez-Ballester N M, Cailleaux S, Bataille B and Soulairol I 2021 Selective laser sintering (SLS), a new chapter in the production of solid oral forms (SOFs) by 3D printing *Pharmaceutics* **13** 1212

[101] Mandrycky C, Wang Z, Kim K and Kim D H 2016 3D bioprinting for engineering complex tissues *Biotechnol. Adv.* **34** 422–34

[102] Pham D T and Dimov S S 2003 Rapid prototyping and rapid tooling—the key enablers for rapid manufacturing *Proc. Inst. Mech. Eng. Part C J. Mech. Eng. Sci.* **217** 1–24

[103] Duan B and Wang M 2011 Selective laser sintering and its application in biomedical engineering *MRS Bull.* **36** 998–1005

[104] Tan K H, Chua C K, Leong K F, Cheah C M, Gui W S and Tan W S *et al* 2005 Selective laser sintering of biocompatible polymers for applications in tissue engineering *Biomed. Mater Eng* **15** 113–24

[105] Feygin M, Shkolnik A, Diamond M N and Dvorskiy E 1996 Laminated object manufacturing system *US Patent* US5730817A https://patents.google.com/patent/US5730817A/en

[106] Dermeik B and Travitzky N 2020 Laminated object manufacturing of ceramic-based materials *Adv. Eng. Mater.* **22** 2000256

[107] Poomathi N, Singh S, Prakash C, Subramanian A, Sahay R and Cinappan A *et al* 2020 3D printing in tissue engineering: a state of the art review of technologies and biomaterials *Rapid Prototyp. J.* **26** 1313–34

[108] Klosterman D A *et al* 1999 *Development of a Curved Layer LOM Process for Monolithic Ceramics and Ceramic Matrix Composites* (Chemical and Materials Engineering Faculty Publications) 202 https://ecommons.udayton.edu/cme_fac_pub/202

[109] Razavykia A, Brusa E, Delprete C and Yavari R 2020 An overview of additive manufacturing technologies—a review to technical synthesis in numerical study of selective laser melting *Materials (Basel)* **13** 3895
[110] Phalke P, Balivada S and Murkute S 2022 Additive manufacturing technologies in tissue engineering and drug delivery system *Int. J. Health Technol. Innov.* **1** 14–23
[111] Thieringer F M, Honigmann P and Sharma N 2022 Medical additive manufacturing in surgery: translating innovation to the point of care *The Future of Healthcare* (Springer) pp 359–76
[112] Choonara Y E, du Toit L C, Kumar P, Kondiah P P D and Pillay V 2016 3D-printing and the effect on medical costs: a new era? *Expert. Rev. Pharmacoecon. Outcomes Res.* **16** 23–32
[113] Chimene D, Lennox K K, Kaunas R R and Gaharwar A K 2016 Advanced bioinks for 3D printing: a materials science perspective *Ann. Biomed. Eng.* **44** 2090–102
[114] Roche C D, Brereton R J L, Ashton A W, Jackson C and Gentile C 2020 Current challenges in three-dimensional bioprinting heart tissues for cardiac surgery *Eur. J. Cardio-Thoracic. Surg.* **58** 500–10
[115] Khoo Z X, Teoh J E M, Liu Y, Chua C K, Yang S and An J *et al* 2015 3D printing of smart materials: a review on recent progresses in 4D printing *Virtual Phys. Prototyping* **10** 103–22
[116] Ashammakhi N, Ahadian S, Zengjie F, Suthiwanich K, Lorestani F and Orive G *et al* 2018 Advances and future perspectives in 4D bioprinting *Biotechnol. J.* **13** 1800148
[117] Khan F A, Kursat Celik H, Oral O and Rennie A E W 2018 Short review on 4D printing *Int. J. 3D Print Technol. Digit. Ind* **2** 59–67
[118] Lukin I, Musquiz S, Erezuma I, Al-Tel T H, Golafshan N and Dolatshahi-Pirouz A *et al* 2019 Can 4D bioprinting revolutionize drug development? *Expert. Opin. Drug Discov.* **14** 953–6
[119] Wan Z, Zhang P, Liu Y, Lv L and Zhou Y 2020 Four-dimensional bioprinting: current developments and applications in bone tissue engineering *Acta. Biomater.* **101** 26–42
[120] Gungor-Ozkerim P S, Inci I, Zhang Y S, Khademhosseini A and Dokmeci M 2018 Bioinks for 3D bioprinting: an overview *Biomater. Sci.* **6** 915–46
[121] Gu Z, Fu J, Lin H and He Y 2020 Development of 3D bioprinting: from printing methods to biomedical applications *Asian J. Pharm. Sci.* **15** 529–57
[122] Tiwari A P, Thorat N D, Pricl S, Patil R M, Rohiwal S and Townley H 2021 Bioink: a 3D-bioprinting tool for anticancer drug discovery and cancer management *Drug Discov. Today* **26** 1574–90
[123] Fulden U-K 2021 3D bioprinting in medicine *Glob. J. Biotechnol. Biomater. Sci.* **7** 1–5
[124] Hospodiuk M, Dey M, Sosnoski D and Ozbolat I T 2017 The bioink: a comprehensive review on bioprintable materials *Biotechnol. Adv.* **35** 217–39
[125] Donderwinkel I, van Hest J C M and Cameron N R 2017 Bio-inks for 3D bioprinting: recent advances and future prospects *Polym. Chem.* **8** 4451–71
[126] Gopinathan J and Noh I 2018 Recent trends in bioinks for 3D printing *Biomater. Res.* **22** 11
[127] Can Y, Karaca R, Özbek F, Boz G, Yilmazer Aktuna A and Yilgör Huri P 2020 Bioinks for bioprinting tissues and organs *Nat. Appl. Sci. J.* **3** 13–33
[128] Benwood C, Chrenek J, Kirsch R L, Masri N Z, Richards H and Teetzen K *et al* 2021 Natural biomaterials and their use as bioinks for printing tissues *Bioengineering* **8** 27
[129] Su C, Chen Y, Tian S, Lu C and Lv Q 2022 Natural materials for 3D printing and their applications *Gels* **8** 748

[130] Tarassoli S P, Jessop Z M, Jovic T, Hawkins K and Whitaker I S 2021 Candidate bioinks for extrusion 3D bioprinting—a systematic review of the literature *Front. Bioeng. Biotechnol.* **9** 616753

[131] Roshangar Zineh B, Shabgard M R and Roshangar L 2018 An experimental study on the mechanical and biological properties of bio-printed alginate/halloysite nanotube/methylcellulose/russian olive-based scaffolds *Adv. Pharm. Bull.* **8** 643–55

[132] Pahlevanzadeh F, Mokhtari H, Bakhsheshi-Rad H R, Emadi R, Kharaziha M and Valiani A *et al* 2020 Recent trends in three-dimensional bioinks based on alginate for biomedical applications *Materials (Basel)* **13** 3980

[133] Jia J, Richards D J, Pollard S, Tan Y, Rodriguez J and Visconti R P *et al* 2014 Engineering alginate as bioink for bioprinting *Acta Biomater* **10** 4323–31

[134] Datta S, Barua R and Das J 2020 Importance of alginate bioink for 3D bioprinting in tissue engineering and regenerative medicine *Alginates—Recent Uses of This Natural Polymer* (IntechOpen) https://intechopen.com/books/alginates-recent-uses-of-this-natural-polymer/importance-of-alginate-bioink-for-3d-bioprinting-in-tissue-engineering-and-regenerative-medicine

[135] Gimble J M, Katz A J and Bunnell B A 2007 Adipose-derived stem cells for regenerative medicine *Circ. Res.* **100** 1249–60

[136] Yang Y, Wu H, Fu Q, Xie X, Song Y and Xu M *et al* 2022 3D-printed polycaprolactone-chitosan based drug delivery implants for personalized administration *Mater Des.* **214** 110394

[137] Mousavi Nejad Z, Zamanian A, Saeidifar M, Vanaei H R and Salar Amoli M 2021 3D bioprinting of polycaprolactone-based scaffolds for pulp-dentin regeneration: investigation of physicochemical and biological behavior *Polymers (Basel)* **13** 4442

[138] Vurat M and Parmaksiz M 2021 Mechanical evaluation of 3D printed poly(Caprolactone) scaffolds: effect of molecular weight *Int. J. 3D Print Technol. Digit. Ind.* **5** 251–8

[139] She Y, Fan Z, Wang L, Li Y, Sun W and Tang H *et al* 2021 3D printed biomimetic PCL scaffold as framework interspersed with collagen for long segment tracheal replacement *Front Cell Dev. Biol.* **9** 629796

[140] Indurkar A, Bangde P, Gore M, Reddy P, Jain R and Dandekar P 2020 Optimization of guar gum-gelatin bioink for 3D printing of mammalian cells *Bioprinting* **20** e00101

[141] Othman S A, Soon C F, Ma N L, Tee K S, Lim G P and Morsin M *et al* 2021 Alginate-gelatin bioink for bioprinting of hela spheroids in alginate-gelatin hexagon shaped scaffolds *Polym. Bull.* **78** 6115–35

[142] Vargas-Alfredo N, Munar-Bestard M, Ramis J M and Monjo M 2022 Synthesis and modification of gelatin methacryloyl (GelMA) with antibacterial quaternary groups and its potential for periodontal applications *Gels* **8** 630

[143] Piao Y, You H, Xu T, Bei H-P, Piwko I Z and Kwan Y Y *et al* 2021 Biomedical applications of gelatin methacryloyl hydrogels *Eng. Regen.* **2** 47–56

[144] Phanthong P, Reubroycharoen P, Hao X, Xu G, Abudula A and Guan G 2018 Nanocellulose: extraction and application *Carbon. Resour. Convers.* **1** 32–43

[145] Huo Y, Liu Y, Xia M, Du H, Lin Z and Li B *et al* 2022 Nanocellulose-based composite materials used in drug delivery systems *Polymers (Basel)* **14** 2648

[146] Wang X, Wang Q and Xu C 2020 Nanocellulose-based inks for 3D bioprinting: key aspects in research development and challenging perspectives in applications—a mini review *Bioengineering* **7** 40

[147] Patil T V, Patel D K, Dutta S D, Ganguly K, Santra T S and Lim K-T 2022 Nanocellulose, a versatile platform: from the delivery of active molecules to tissue engineering applications *Bioact. Mater.* **9** 566–89

[148] Naumenko E and Fakhrullin R 2019 Halloysite nanoclay/biopolymers composite materials in tissue engineering *Biotechnol. J.* **14** 1900055

[149] Biddeci G, Spinelli G, Colomba P and Di Blasi F 2022 Nanomaterials: a review about halloysite nanotubes, properties, and application in the biological field *Int. J. Mol. Sci.* **23** 11518

[150] Mobaraki M, Karnik S, Li Y and Mills D K 2021 Therapeutic applications of halloysite *Appl. Sci.* **12** 87

[151] Mani M P, Sadia M, Jaganathan S K, Khudzari A Z, Supriyanto E and Saidin S *et al* 2022 A review on 3D printing in tissue engineering applications *J. Polym. Eng.* **42** 243–65

[152] Gao G, Ahn M, Cho W-W, Kim B-S and Cho D-W 2021 3D printing of pharmaceutical application: drug screening and drug delivery *Pharmaceutics* **13** 1373

[153] Moysidou C-M, Barberio C and Owens R M 2021 Advances in engineering human tissue models *Front. Bioeng. Biotechnol.* **8** 620962

[154] Singh V K, Saini A, Kalsan M, Kumar N and Chandra R 2016 Describing the stem cell potency: the various methods of functional assessment and in silico diagnostics *Front. Cell. Dev. Biol.* **4** 134

[155] Osouli-Bostanabad K, Masalehdan T, Kapsa R M I, Quigley A, Lalatsa A and Bruggeman K F *et al* 2022 Traction of 3D and 4D printing in the healthcare industry: from drug delivery and analysis to regenerative medicine *ACS Biomater. Sci. Eng.* **8** 2764–97

[156] Willemen N G A, Morsink M A J, Veerman D, da Silva C F, Cardoso J C and Souto E B *et al* 2022 From oral formulations to drug-eluting implants: using 3D and 4D printing to develop drug delivery systems and personalized medicine *Bio-Design Manuf.* **5** 85–106

[157] Ross S, Scoutaris N, Lamprou D, Mallinson D and Douroumis D 2015 Inkjet printing of insulin microneedles for transdermal delivery *Drug Deliv. Transl. Res.* **5** 451–61

[158] Yin M, Xiao L, Liu Q, Kwon S, Zhang Y and Sharma P R *et al* 2019 3D printed microheater sensor-integrated, drug-encapsulated microneedle patch system for pain management *Adv. Healthc. Mater.* **8** 1901170

[159] Sadia M, Arafat B, Ahmed W, Forbes R T and Alhnan M A 2018 Channelled tablets: an innovative approach to accelerating drug release from 3D printed tablets *J. Control. Release* **269** 355–63

[160] Melocchi A, Uboldi M, Inverardi N, Briatico-Vangosa F, Baldi F and Pandini S *et al* 2019 Expandable drug delivery system for gastric retention based on shape memory polymers: development via 4D printing and extrusion *Int. J. Pharm.* **571** 118700

[161] Peng W, Datta P, Ayan B, Ozbolat V, Sosnoski D and Ozbolat I T 2017 3D bioprinting for drug discovery and development in pharmaceutics *Acta Biomater.* **57** 26–46

[162] Chircov C and Grumezescu A M 2019 *Three-Dimensional Bioprinting in Drug Delivery. Vol. 2, Materials for Biomedical Engineering: Nanomaterials-based Drug Delivery* (Amsterdam: Elsevier) pp 19–40

[163] Osouli-Bostanabad K, Masalehdan T, Kapsa R M I, Quigley A, Lalatsa A and Bruggeman K F *et al* 2022 Traction of 3D and 4D printing in the healthcare industry: from drug delivery and analysis to regenerative medicine *ACS Biomater. Sci. Eng* **8** 2764–97

[164] Yang Q, Gao B and Xu F 2020 Recent advances in 4D bioprinting *Biotechnol. J.* **15** 1900086

[165] Wan Z, Zhang P, Liu Y, Lv L and Zhou Y 2020 Four-dimensional bioprinting: current developments and applications in bone tissue engineering *Acta Biomater.* **101** 26–42
[166] Silva L P 2018 Current trends and challenges in biofabrication using biomaterials and nanomaterials: future perspectives for 3D/4D bioprinting *3D and 4D Printing in Biomedical Applications* (Weinheim: Wiley-VCH) pp 373–421
[167] Bicudo E, Faulkner A and Li P 2021 Sociotechnical alignment in biomedicine: the 3D bioprinting market beyond technology convergence *Technol. Soc.* **66** 101668
[168] Jamróz W, Szafraniec J, Kurek M and Jachowicz R 2018 3D Printing in pharmaceutical and medical applications—recent achievements and challenges *Pharm. Res.* **35** 176
[169] Beg S, Almalki W H, Malik A, Farhan M, Aatif M and Rahman Z *et al* 2020 3D printing for drug delivery and biomedical applications *Drug Discov. Today* **25** 1668–81
[170] Seoane-Viaño I, Trenfield S J, Basit A W and Goyanes A 2021 Translating 3D printed pharmaceuticals: from hype to real-world clinical applications *Adv. Drug Deliv. Rev.* **174** 553–75
[171] Trenfield S J, Awad A, Madla C M, Hatton G B, Firth J and Goyanes A *et al* 2019 Shaping the future: recent advances of 3D printing in drug delivery and healthcare *Expert. Opin. Drug Deliv.* **16** 1081–94

Chapter 5

Biomimicry in drug delivery: why, how, and what?

Deepak Kumar Sahel, Siddhanth Hejmady, Mahalaxmi Sharma, Tamanna Bhuyan, Surjendu Maity, Ankit Gangarade, Sudeep Pukale, Shahid Khan, Sangeeta Deka, Amanda Kirane and Saurabh Sharma

Biomimicry has emerged as a favorable strategy in advanced drug delivery, emulating the sophisticated design principles in naturally derived materials mimicking with a cellular component. This chapter examines the concept of biomimicry in drug delivery and delves into the employed rational design strategies. It highlights the necessity for inventive approaches that mimic biological systems for enhancing the therapeutic efficacy and resolve the toxicity issues. Also, it explores numerous biomimetic systems extensively, displaying the design principles and applications with the focus on the unique characteristics and the possibility for drug delivery. These mainly include cell membrane-based biomimetics inspired by bacteria, viruses, and eukaryotic cells, biomimetic polymeric micelles, liposomes, polymeric nanocarriers, hydrogels, etc. The targeting ability of biomimicry in drug delivery systems is a major focus with these systems harnessing biological targeting mechanisms to improve specificity along with higher efficacy and lower toxicity. Thus, this chapter explores the integration of biomimetic principles for the expansion of the domain of drug delivery.

5.1 Introduction

People have always suffered from debilitating diseases such as cancer, Alzheimer's, Parkinson, Stroke, Diabetes, and associated complications, etc. Although various treatments exist for the preliminary treatment of these diseases, such as classical drug therapy, radiotherapy, and surgery, these diseases are incurable due to a lack of conventional medicine. Various potent drugs have been discovered, repurposed, or involved in clinical therapy. However, they still have limitations or challenges in clinical use due to poor water solubility, low oral bioavailability, poor blood circulation, and poor cellular uptake, which overcome the therapeutic effect and

doi:10.1088/978-0-7503-5613-8ch5

raise new challenges such as systemic side effects, drug resistance, recurrence, and off-target effect [1].

A non-targeted delivery of any drug can damage/harm normal cells or organs beyond the site of interest. The development of a potential carrier that may increase the therapeutic efficacy of active pharmaceutical ingredient (API) at particular cells/tissue and minimize drug resistance/toxic effects by increasing the accumulation of drugs at the targeted site becomes an absolute need. Therefore, targeted pharmaceuticals have become a eye-catching and hot area for scientists to explore in drug delivery science [2]. Thus, the advanced drug delivery systems (ADDSs) with the potential to overcome the limitations mentioned above, protect drugs from inadequate metabolism, enhance drug accumulation at the target sites, and increase their safety are emerging as a crucial and rapidly growing field [3]. Following on from ADDSs, the biomimetic drug delivery system (BMDDS) is a unique drug delivery system that mimics biological structures or directly involves a complex biological process. The BMDDSs include albumin, erythrocytes, platelets, etc, with the benefits of non-toxicity and immunogenicity, inherent biocompatibility, massive drug loading, and excellent targeting [4] and can be employed for the treatment of various debilitating diseases. The BMDDSs could be classified into three important categories: biological, synthetic, or biohybrid systems. The most commonly used biomimetic materials in drug delivery include the cell membrane, lipoproteins, exosomes, viruses, proteins, and peptides. This chapter aims to overview the biological properties of these biomimetic DDSs and their importance and applications for managing debilitating diseases [5].

5.2 Biomimicry in drug delivery

In 1957, Otto Schmitt introduced the term 'biomimetic' to solve technological challenges based on the philosophy and practice of the biological sciences. Biomimetics has several synonyms, such as biomimesis, biomimicry, bionics, biognostics, and biologically influenced design (BIS) [6]. However, 'biomimetics' is the most recognized and significant of these words and is not so much a topic as a perspective. Conclusively, Biomimicry utilizes the philosophy and technology of the biological sciences to solve technological difficulties [7, 8]. In modern drug delivery systems, biomimetics develops intrinsic capacities in biomimetic drug carriers only via surface modification using amino acids, sugars, lipids etc. For this reason, the fundamental core materials, size, and type of drug carriers must mirror natural cell components to facilitate cellular internalization. In addition, targeted drug delivery into target cells may be achieved by biomimetic surface functionalizing of these nanocarriers with particular biological ligands or moieties that mimic the composition and functioning of exterior cell membranes. In addition, there are two primary types of biomimetic drug carriers based on the fundamental material: existing biological entities, such as inactivated viral vectors and bacterial vectors, and synthetic drug carriers, which are biomimetic-engineered nanoparticles (NPs) with similar properties to biological materials. The second category should be noted as safer for *in vivo* therapeutic uses.

5.3 Why biomimicry?

The application of biomimetics is a potential strategy for treating incurable diseases such as cancer. In recent investigations, scientists endeavored to get a detailed understanding of biological processes and systems. Understanding macromolecular structures and their complex processes at the cellular and subcellular level (such as the structure of proteins and their biological activities) enables scientists to imitate and replicate these natural processes for medicinal applications. Today, research on drug delivery systems is focused on targeted drug delivery, which might deliver the drug directly into the cytoplasm of specific cells without affecting healthy tissues or organs. Nanotechnology enabled the encapsulating of drugs in nanocarriers with ample advantages. Also, the challenges associated with insoluble, biodegradable therapeutic agents and drugs with high toxicity for biological systems have been substantially overcome. In addition, the NPs' modest size allowed them to diffuse across cells. However, these NPs were ineffective in targeting the release of drugs within particular cells. Attaching plasma proteins such as immunoglobulin G (IgG) and a stealth coating of polyethylene glycol (PEG) to the surface of the nanocarrier helps shield them from the immune system. It replicates the (enhanced permeation and retention) effect. However, because of unfavorable interactions between PEG and target cells and poor endosomal escape, cellular absorption of PEGylated NPs does not occur, and the loaded drugs get degradation in lysosomes. However, the surface modification of PEGylated NPs with proteins, vitamins, peptides, antibodies, and aptamers as functional ligands is one biomimetic strategy for overcoming the steric hindrance of PEGylated NPs. Based on target cell characteristics, such as the amount of overexpression of certain receptors on tumor cells, ligands with a high affinity for receptor-mediated attachment to target cells are identified. In the last 30 years, regulating drug release and using PEG for stealth effect to limit immune system activation have been key concerns. Recent research has focused on biomimetic processes, biomimetic drug carrier surface engineering, and bioinspiration from cellular communication signal pathways. Scientists strive to increase drug carrier half-life and reduce immunological activation. Sustained drug release through cellular internalization in target cells and reduced toxicity to healthy cells are other aims [9–12]. The biomimetic drug delivery methods include albumin, erythrocytes, exosomes, natural polymeric NPs, and platelets with the benefits of non-toxicity and immunogenicity, inherent biocompatibility, substantial drug loading, and excellent targeting would play a significant role in the treatment of disease. The following are the key advantages of biomimetic drug delivery systems.

5.3.1 Immunogenicity

To overcome the challenges of nano drug delivery systems to clinical translation, cell membrane cloaking has recently gained considerable interest to equip NPs with improved biocompatibility, reduced immunogenicity, and active targeting capabilities. For instance, platelets are blood components that assist in preventing bleeding after blood vessel damage. They escape phagocytic absorption by macrophages, target and attach to damaged vasculature, and exhibit increased binding to platelet-adhering pathogens. Platelet membrane biomimetic DDSs are anticipated to increase retention *in vivo*, evade absorption by macrophages, and minimize immunogenicity due to the CD47 membrane protein delivering 'don't eat me' signals to macrophages [13, 14]. Moreover, P-selectin is overexpressed on the platelet membrane (PLTM), allowing a PLTM-biomimetic DDS to preferentially bind to the CD44 receptors that are increased on the surface of cancer cells [15]. Gao *et al* (2017) developed a series of NPs by encapsulating perfluorocarbon in the biocompatible polymer poly(lactic-co-glycolic acid) (PLGA) and then coated them with a red blood cell membrane (RBCM). In comparison to uncoated particles, these NPs were able to extend blood circulation and provide excellent tumor penetration. This was ascribed to the CD47 protein on the RBCM controlling macrophage phagocytosis through interactions with signal regulatory protein (SIRP) [16, 17].

Wang *et al* (2019) developed PLTM-functionalized porous NPs to deliver bufalin to the tumor site. These PLGA-chitosan NPs loaded bufalin at 8.5%. PLTM coating led to pH-dependent sustained drug release for two days. The drug-loaded counterpart was biocompatible with H22 cells and could kill cancer cells *in vitro*. *In vivo* imaging demonstrated the accumulation of NPs in the tumor location, confirming their active targeting capabilities due to P-selectin binding to CD44 receptors overexpressed on H22 cells. The PLTM-coated NPs reduced tumor growth *in vivo* without harming critical organs. Novel PLTM-biomimetic formulations presented in this study offer anti-cancer drug carrier potential. Platelets selectively attach to wounded blood vessels. Therefore, PLTM-coated material might be utilized to deliver vascular-disrupting drugs or in combination with photothermal treatment to damage tumor blood vessels and boost anti-tumor action [18].

Mekuria *et al* (2016) compared two PAMAM dendrimers modified with two distinct targeting ligands (IL-6 and RGD) and used as drug carriers against cancer cells. Doxorubicin (DOX) was loaded into pH-sensitive PAMAM-IL-6 and PAMAM-RGD dendrimers for this purpose. *In vitro* tests demonstrated that the longer IL-6 ligand increased drug loading, intercellular uptake, and drug transfer through RME inside cancer cells [19].

5.4 Rationale design: how

It is intriguing to study how contemporary science has retraced the paths of Mother Nature to solve mysteries by adopting principles from living things. Significant advancements have been made in bio-inspired formulation preparation, formulation development, and therapeutic delivery. The delivery of active moieties has been made feasible by modifying or replicating the self-delivery cargo mechanism of microbes, cells, and organelles, which is very difficult to design using traditional nanoformulation owing to their architectural complexity. Numerous scientific studies have revealed that natural compounds and products structurally related to them play a crucial role in the medication discovery, design, development, and delivery processes [20–22].

5.5 Bio-inspired materials

Bio-inspired materials are synthetic materials that resemble the structure, features, or function of natural materials or biological components. Various delivery systems could be prepared using such bio-inspired material, as discussed below.

5.5.1 Natural polymer

The research area of targeted nanocarrier DDSs is increasing and to improve the biocompatibility of these nanocarriers, several researchers have been interested in biodegradable natural polymers such as malic acid, poly(malic acid), isolated from microorganisms or synthesized from malic, or aspartic acid was employed to generate water-soluble drug carriers or NPs in this context. Multiple research groups have shown the importance of such polyesters in drug delivery science [23].

5.5.1.1 Biomimetic lipids or hybrid lipids

Lipids are one of the most promising components in drug delivery science and they are interesting because the cell membrane is also made up of lipids. Therefore, lipids could be interesting biomimetic biomaterials. However, lipids and biopolymers may be arranged to form NPs to optimize drug loading. For evidence, there are distinct biomimetic NPs such as polystyrene sulfate NPs coated with one cationic dioctadecyl dimethylammonium bromide bilayer, which are loaded a antimicrobial peptide Gramicidin D for efficient delivery. Another example is silica NPs coated with one single bilayer of the antimicrobial cationic lipid DODAB. Another example is hybrid lipid/polymer indomethacin. These examples serve as a foundation for the development and characterization of innovative biomimetic NPs composed of lipids and/or biopolymers. Polymers and lipids in the hybrid NP composition may confer stability and/or bioactivity and/or offer suitable microenvironments for transporting bioactive medicines and biomolecules [23].

5.5.2 Cell membrane-based biomimetic

Cell membrane-containing drug delivery systems (CMDDSs) are now receiving considerable attention due to their ample advantages over conventional DDSs. The system is developed by extracting cell membranes from natural cells and covering NPs loaded with any drugs with cell membranes, which are the main materials for achieving various activities to increase the therapeutic effects. For example, glycans, sialic acid moieties, and CD47 have been attached to the surface of RBCms which led to improved circulation time of the NP. There are several cell membrane-based biomimetics systems, such as RBCMs, cancer cell membranes, PLTMs, stem cell membranes, macrophage membranes, and subcellular membranes, with several distinct benefits [24].

5.5.2.1 Red blood cell membranes

There are several limitations of the conventional DDS related to a clinical purpose, such as capturing and clearance by a mononuclear phagocytic system (MPS).

However, many strategies have been adopted to overcome the limitation, such as PEGylation and self-peptide decoration on the system surface, etc. Still, they could not escape from the MPS capturing and elimination from the body. There is some reported evidence that DiD-labelled RBCMs-coated NPs showed an improved half-life of 150% compared to the non-coated NP and were detected in the blood circulation after 72 h of injection. Moreover, the CD47 molecule was attached to the surface of the RBCMs, which helped prevent 'macrophages' capture [24]. Additionally, techniques were developed to stabilize the RBCMs carrier by inserting lipid and covalent conjugation, improving tumor suppression and metastasis elimination from the body [24]. Su *et al* (2017) reported RBC-mimetic vesicles coated on a hybrid polymeric NP loaded with paclitaxel into its core. Over it, tumor penetrating peptide was decorated, which improved by 5.8-fold the half-life compared to the non-decorated NP [25]. Conventionally, DOX is loaded into the liposomes, known as doxil formulation, but it can engulf immune cells. This limitation was overcome by loading DOX into an RBCM carrier due to itself having a natural lipid bilayer in its structure. Additionally, Zhang *et al* (2020) added cholesterol and ammonium sulfate to better stabilize the carrier system. This RBCM-DOX showed improvement in the median survival of mice for up to 39 days compared to the untreated control group having survival for up to 25.5 days for the orthotopic breast model [4]. Moreover, a nanodevice was developed to encapsulate DTX-Heparin sulfate conjugated micelles coated by an RBCM. The resulting system enhances cellular uptake and prolonged circulation profile of the drug as compared to the free drug.

5.5.2.2 Virus-like nanoparticles

The term viral nanoparticles (VNPs) refers to a wide range of naturally occurring nanomaterials generated from plant viruses, bacteriophages, and mammalian viruses. The use and development of VNPs and their genome-free variants, virus-like particles (VLPs), for nanomedicine are expanding at a fast rate. VLPs may contain various active substances and be genetically or chemically coupled to targeting ligands for tissue selectivity. VLPs are produced by scalable fermentation or molecular farming; the products are biocompatible and biodegradable. These features have led to various applications, including cancer medicines, immunotherapies, vaccines, antimicrobial therapies, cardiovascular therapies, gene therapies, imaging, and theranostic. The utilization of VLPs as drug delivery agents is developing, and enough research must be conducted consistently to convert these medicines into the clinic [26].

5.5.3 Biomimetic polymeric micelles

Polymeric micelles have recently appeared as promising alternative drug delivery carriers serving as potential platforms in cancer management [27, 28]. For getting maximum benefits from these type of DDSs they should hold numerous elementary properties required for accomplishing passive tumour targeting: (i) flexible inner hydrophobic core for proficiently incorporating and modulating the drug release profile; (ii) an outer hydrophilic shell imparting stealth properties resulting in delayed circulation time of drug; (iii) appropriate nano-size dimensions (10–100 nm) with a narrow polydispersity to circumvent fast renal clearance, thus leading to effective tumor accumulation via the enhanced permeation and retention (EPR) effect [29–31]. The major difference between these micelles and most of the other NPs is that the former are dynamic (spontaneous assembly at critical micelle concentration (cmc) and disassembly below cmc, whereas the latter are completely static in nature which doesn't involve the cmc concept.

Gongyan Liu *et al* (2016) synthesized self-assembled biomimetic polymeric micelles chemically constructed from an diblock copolymer i.e., poly(g-benzyl-L-glutamate)-block-poly(2-methacryloyloxyethyl phosphorylcholine) (PBLGb-PMPC), where PMPC acts as outer hydrophilic biomimetic shell (imparting stealth properties) and PBLG acts as inner hydrophobic biodegradable core (wherein a hydrophobic drug i.e., DOX was loaded). DOX-loaded PBLG-b-PMPC micelles demonstrated enhanced selective accumulation in tumour cells wherein these nanomaterials release drug very slowly at the intracellular level resulting in significant improvement in efficacy by inducing apoptosis along with lower systemic toxicities and enhanced circulation time, making this platform a very auspicious strategy in cancer treatment [32]. It was well evident that amino acid-based amphiphilic block copolymers exhibited excellent biocompatibility and biodegradation profile that made them very good alternative safe vehicles for delivering chemotherapeutics agents, resulting in higher cellular uptake and therapeutic efficacy [33]. Pukale *et al* (2021) proved the potential advantages of bifunctional peptide-based metallodendrimer for wound healing and acne management applications wherein the authors have synthesized a polylysine based peptide metallodendrimer coordinately complexed with zinc [34]. The potential anti-cancer properties of octenidine are well established on various cell lines but owing to its cationic nature, its therapeutic applications are hindered due to toxicity concern on surrounding healthy cells. Kashapova *et al* (2020) developed biomimetic vesicular systems based on amphiphilic calix [4] resorcinols functionalized with acetate groups and octenidine. The resultant nanosystems exhibited high cytotoxicity ($IC_{50} = 0.4$ μM) and selectivity (selectivity index >20) toward the HuTu 80 cell line, making them promising alternatives [35]. Genexol PM, a marketed polymeric micelle comprising pegylated polylactic acid copolymer loaded with paclitaxel, is one of the very good examples of biomimetic polymeric micelle used for treating several types of cancers [36].

5.5.4 Biomimetic liposomes

Liposomes are minute artificial vesicles that are spherical in shape with a bilayer formed via the self-assembly of phospholipids and cholesterol in an aqueous medium. The similarity between the cell membrane in humans and the lipid bilayer makes liposomes a possible carrier in drug delivery. Also, liposomes are biocompatible, biodegradable, and non-toxic with the ability to hold both hydrophilic and hydrophobic compounds in the interior aqueous section and the phospholipids, respectively [37, 38]. Besides, liposomes may be prepared via employing the methodology to mimic the biological behavior of cells through different biomimetic strategies. Also, biomimetic liposomes may be targeted with specific ligands to attain the intracellular delivery of biomolecules/drugs. Additionally, the controlled release of the loaded drugs either in a passive or active manner could be achieved by biomimetic liposomes against distinct stimuli present in a cellular microenvironment [38].

Furthermore, Song *et al* (2005) established hybrid biomimetic liposomes via fusion with PLTMs (P-Lipo) to achieve atherosclerosis targeting. This study employed an extrusion method for forming hybrid nanovesicles by fusing artificial lipid membranes and natural PLTMs. These hybrid biomimetic liposomes were expected to display retention of the physicochemical and pharmaceutical characteristics of the liposomes as well as the targeted capability of platelets. Also, the similarity of these biomimetic liposomes to existing liposomal technology along with the enhanced utilization effectiveness of PLTM may result in successful clinical translation as well as personalized medicine [38]. Moreover, Li and group constructed an active targeting biomimetic liposome via the conjugation of elemene (ELE) and cabazitaxel (CTX) with transferrin (Tf) and fixing glioma cell membrane proteins (CMP) onto the liposome (Tf-ELE/CTX@ BLIP) using extrusion approach. This nanocarrier was designed for the enhancement of transport across the blood-brain barrier (BBB), improvement of homotypic targeting in glioma tumor-bearing mice, and delivery of drugs against the glioma site [39].

Besides, Loureiro *et al* (2018) have worked toward the evaluation of the performance of liposomes and micelles as two biomimetic models. Here, 1,2-dimyristoyl-sn-glycero-3-phosphorylcholine (DMPC) was utilized to prepare biomimetic liposomes via classical thin-film hydration with DMPC serving as a typical phospholipid of natural membranes. DMPC has two hydrophobic chains with 14 carbon atoms and unilamellar vesicles of this lipid with a diameter greater than 100 nm were used here. The study concluded that liposomes served as the best biomimetic models to assess the lipophilicity of active agents by way of determining the partition coefficients (log K_p) [40]. Also, Xiong and group aimed for the application of biomaterials in the phototherapy of echinococcosis and constructed a phototheranostic system employing a Lipo-ICG i.e., liposomes of the neutrophil-membrane-camouflaged indocyanine green type. This nanosystem was developed to attain active targeting for the near-infrared fluorescence diagnosis as well as photothermal treatment of echinococcosis. The lipo-ICG was formulated using 1,2-distearoyl-sn-glycero-3-phosphoethanolamine-N-[amino(polyethylene glycol)-2000] (DSPE-PEG2000) and 1,2-dioleoyl-sn-glycero-3-phosphocholine (DOPC) in the thin-film strategy. These biomaterials have been approved by the U.S. Food and Drug Administration showcasing high biocompatibility with the biomimetic liposomes displaying biosafety and non-toxicity in the *in vivo* system. Additionally, Liu *et al* (2022) loaded platinum NPs (nano-Pt) in liposomes with nano-Pt acting as a catalase-like nanoenzyme that could lead to an enhancement of photodynamic therapy (PDT) via the supply of catalytic oxygen. Reverse phase evaporation was utilized for nano-Pt encapsulation as opposed to thin-film hydration, that can result in high aqueous loading in the interior, particularly for compounds that are soluble in water. The lipid bilayer was loaded with verteporfin (VP), the clinical photosensitizer to offer PDT action, and murine macrophage cell membranes were hybridized in the membrane of the liposomes to offer targeting and biomimetic characteristics [40]. Also, biomimetic liposomes were prepared by He *et al* (2018) to ensure the dietary absorption and oral delivery of biomacromolecules through the interactions of vitamin ligands and the respective receptors. Niacin and thiamine were conjugated with stearamine and used for the decoration of liposomes loaded with insulin, which was prepared by modified reversed-phase evaporation [41]. Thus, the biomimetic alteration of the liposomal surface along with the biomimetic techniques of formulating liposomes improve the targeting capacities of therapeutic liposomes in drug delivery.

5.5.5 Biomimetic polymeric nanoparticles

These includes nanoscale structures of biodegradable polymers (such as polylactic acid (PLA), poly(lactic-co-glycolic acid (PLGA), polycaprolactone (PCL) etc) with suitable surface functionalization for improving their biomimetic properties functioning as advanced biomaterials having great scope in the field of pharmaceuticals and tissue engineering. Liu *et al* (2012) carried out biomimetic modification of paclitaxel-loaded poly(lactic-co-glycolic acid) NPs using endogenous pulmonary surfactants wherein two anionic phospholipids (dipalmitoylphosphatidylserine (DPPS) and dipalmitoylphosphatidylglycerol (DPPG),) and two neutral phospholipids (dipalmitoylphosphatidylamine (DPPE) and dipalmitoylphosphatidylcholine (DPPC)) at various molar ratios were evaluated for their *in vivo* fate in pulmonary drug delivery w.r.t. mucous penetration and mucoadhesive properties. Results demonstrated that NPs whose modification was carried out by DPPS increased the mucus permeability, whereas DPPE, DPPC, and DPPG enhanced mucoadhesion, of the NPs. Biomodification with anionic phospholipids (DPPG and DPPS) significantly enhanced uptake by alveolar macrophages compared to that of neutral phospholipids (DPPE and DPPC). All these biomodified NPs exhibited improved uptake and retention of drug by lung epithelial cells [42]

Recently, Pukale *et al* (2021) synthesized biomimetic NanoBrids-based platform technology for topical delivery of clobetasol propionate (super potent corticosteroid) for ameliorating imiquimod-induced psoriasis-like inflammatory skin condition in Swiss albino mice. These platforms comprised of monolithic lipid-polymer hybrid NPs developed using polyethylene glycol-polylactic acid (PEG-PLA) (polymer), glyceryl monostearate and Precirol® ATO (solid lipid), and linoleic acid and oleic acid (oil or liquid lipid). These novel nanosystems demonstrated significant improvement in delivering the drug into deeper dermal layers with good skin retentive capabilities without any systemic leakage of active ingredient that results in most of the side effects associated with corticosteroids such as HPA-axis suppression. Further, these systems proved to be very effective compared to the conventional marketed product (Clobetamos®) [43]. Further, this platform was explored for topical delivery of other hydrophobic drugs such as cholecalciferol and coenzyme Q10, respectively, demonstrating significantly improved anti-psoriatic therapeutic efficacy [44, 45]. Sharma and his colleagues recently developed biodegradable and biomimetic lipopolymeric NPs for the co-delivery of a hydrophobic small molecule (docetaxel; DTX) and hydrophilic biological macromolecule (miRNA-34a) for breast cancer treatment. Results showed that the nanoplexes possessed very high (94.8%) encapsulation efficiency of DTX, imparting sustained drug release profile up to 2 days with significantly high transfection efficiency in 4T1 and MDA-MB-231 breast cancer cell line employing majorly clathrin and lipid-raft mediated endocytic uptake mechanisms. Further, these nanosystems displayed enhanced apoptosis (~1.6–2.0 folds), cytotoxicity (~3.5–5 folds), and ~4–7 folds change in expression of apoptotic genes compared to the free treatment group in breast cancer cells. *In vivo*, pharmacokinetic data showed a greater half-life of both therapeutic agents compared to free forms with no potential toxicity signs [46].

Recently, cell-based drug delivery systems have gained focus for their versatile applications in treating several disease conditions wherein the NPs are coated with endogenous cellular membranes for improvising the biomimetic features. In one attempt authors had developed dimethyl fumarate-loaded platelet-based NPs for improving brain distribution, which was a major challenge that was of significant importance in treating disease such as multiple sclerosis [47]. In other reports, erythrocyte membrane-camouflaged polymeric NPs, where surfaces of NPs are coated with erythrocyte cell membranes served as potential biomimetic drug delivery platforms that provide several advantages such as improved drug residence in the body by overcoming systemic clearance imparting stealth properties [48]. Alginates polysaccharide-based scaffolds provide several advantages in drug delivery and tissue engineering due to their appealing biological properties, which can be very easily modulated by chemical cross-linking and ionic combination of other suitable polymers [49]. ABRAXANE® is a good example of a biomimetic polymeric NP, a marketed product comprising paclitaxel-coated with albumin protein used to treat several types of cancer [50].

Polymeric nanocarriers have also been explored for the *in vitro* and *in vivo* delivery of nucleic acid, specifically CRISPR/Cas9 components [51, 52]. For example, Sahel *et al* (2022) reported lipopolymeric nanoplexes containing CRISPR/Cas9 ribonucleoprotein (RNPs) for *in vitro* gene editing in HEK293T cells. As per the reports, the lipopolymeric nanoplexes were able to transfect ~80% of the cell with >50% of gene editing. Additionally, the lipopolymeric nanoplexes were found stable under *in vivo* conditions and able to transfect muscle tissue after intramuscular injection [53].

5.5.6 Biomimetic nanohydrogel

Biomimetic nanohydrogels are materials that mimic the properties of natural hydrogels found in the body and can be used for drug delivery [7]. Hydrogels are gel-like materials that are composed of crosslinked polymers and can hold large amounts of water [54, 55]. They are attractive for drug delivery because they can be designed to release drugs in a controlled manner over an extended period of time [56, 57]. Biomimetic nanohydrogels are designed to mimic the properties of natural hydrogels in the body, such as those in the extracellular matrix (ECM). They can be synthesized using a variety of polymers, such as proteins, polysaccharides, or synthetic polymers [57]. Biomimetic nanohydrogels have several potential advantages for drug delivery [58]. They can be designed to control the release of drugs by incorporating certain chemical or physical properties that allow for the controlled release of the drug over a specific period of time. Some ways in which drug release can be controlled in biomimetic nanohydrogels include using pH-sensitive groups in the hydrogel: these groups can be designed to release the drug when the pH changes, such as when the drug is in an acidic environment like the stomach [59]. By incorporating enzymes or other catalysts into the hydrogel, these catalysts can be used to break down the hydrogel matrix and release the drug over time [60]. By using temperature-sensitive groups in the hydrogel, these groups can be designed to release the drug when the temperature changes, such as when the drug is exposed to body heat [54]. By incorporating swelling agents into the hydrogel, these agents can cause the hydrogel to swell or shrink in response to different stimuli, which can affect the release rate of the drug [54]. By using stimuli-responsive polymers in the hydrogel, these polymers can be designed to respond to specific stimuli, such as light or magnetic fields, which can be used to trigger drug release [61]. By designing biomimetic nanohydrogels with these properties, it is possible to control the release rate of drugs and improve their therapeutic effectiveness (figure 5.1).

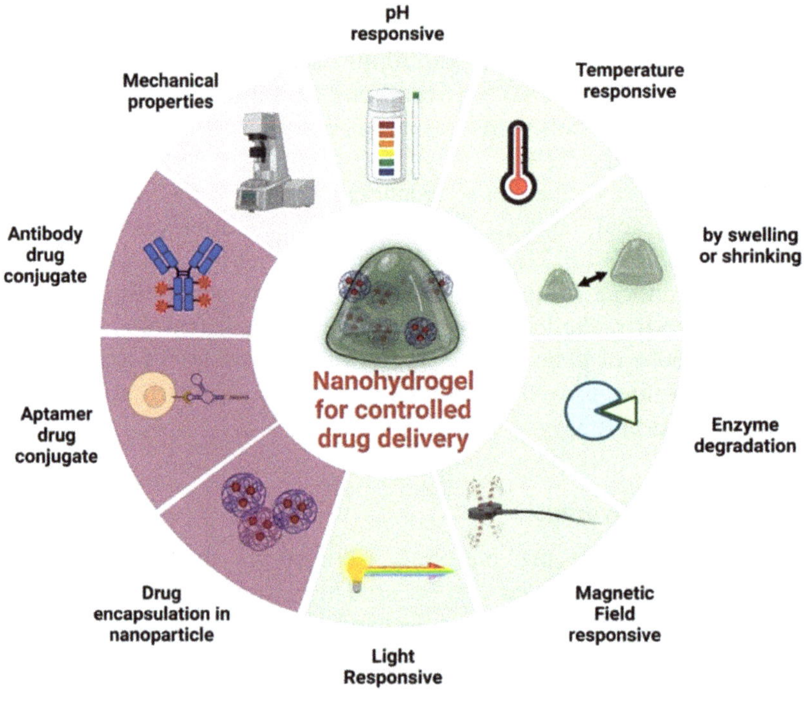

Figure 5.1. The advantages of using nanohydrogel in controlled drug delivery application.

Biomimetic nanohydrogels can be designed to target specific cells or tissues in a number of ways, which can help to reduce unwanted side effects of drugs. Some strategies that can be used include using specific ligands or targeting moieties. These molecules can be incorporated into the hydrogel and can bind to specific receptors on the surface of targeted cells or tissues [54]. This can help to increase the specificity and selectivity of drug delivery. Using physical or chemical properties of the hydrogel, the size, shape, and surface properties of the hydrogel can be designed to facilitate specific interactions with targeted cells or tissues. For example, hydrogels with a size and shape similar to that of red blood cells can be used to target the vasculature [62]. Using stimuli-responsive polymers, polymers that respond to specific stimuli, such as pH or temperature, can be incorporated into the hydrogel [54]. This can allow the hydrogel to release the drug only in specific environments or in the presence of specific signaling molecules. Using imaging agents, imaging agents, such as fluorescent dyes or radioisotopes, can be incorporated into the hydrogel. These agents can be used to track the movement of the hydrogel and confirm that it is reaching the desired target [63]. By designing biomimetic nanohydrogels with these properties, it is possible to increase the specificity and selectivity of drug delivery and reduce the risk of unwanted side effects.

Additionally, the mechanical properties of biomimetic nanohydrogels can play a significant role in drug delivery (figure 5.1) [64]. These properties can affect how the hydrogel behaves and interacts with the surrounding environment, which can in turn impact the release rate and distribution of the drug. For example, the mechanical stiffness of the hydrogel can influence its ability to deform and conform to the shape of the targeted tissue [65]. Hydrogels that are too stiff may not be able to effectively deliver drugs to certain tissues, while hydrogels that are too soft may not be able to sustain their shape and may not be suitable for certain drug delivery applications [65]. The swelling behavior of the hydrogel can also affect drug delivery. Hydrogels that swell excessively may burst and release the drug too quickly, while hydrogels that do not swell enough may not release the drug at an appropriate rate [66]. The mechanical properties of biomimetic nanohydrogels can also influence the drug release rate by affecting the diffusion of the drug through the hydrogel matrix. Hydrogels with a more porous structure may allow for faster drug diffusion, while hydrogels with a more compact structure may slow down drug diffusion [67]. Overall, the mechanical properties of biomimetic nanohydrogels can significantly impact their performance as drug delivery systems, and it is important to carefully consider and optimize these properties in the design of these systems. Overall, biomimetic nanohydrogels have the potential to be useful for drug delivery, although more research is needed to fully understand their properties and optimize their use in drug delivery applications.

5.5.7 Biomimetic exosome

Various small molecules, inorganic substances, and biomacromolecules are used to treat disease, but these naked medications face low stability and poor pharmacokinetic behavior issues, affecting their therapeutic effects. Nowadays, exogenous and endogenous nanomaterials have been gaining scientific attention as drug delivery vehicles, and out of this, exosomes showed promising impacts due to their biocompatibility, low immunogenicity, low toxicity, and ability to cross biological barriers. Biomimetic exosomes are specifically designed lipids, proteins, and RNA, which have similar structures to liposomes or natural exosomes. However, exosome employment as drug delivery vehicles is constrained by considerable difficulties, including poor homogeneity, complicated contents, and low yields.

To overcome these limitations, several methods have been used to create engineered exosomes or biomimetic exosomes, which can be prepared by three strategies such as: top-down, in which materials are prepared by the breakdown of large materials into the nanoscale structure such that cells are used as bulk materials in this case, and its cell membrane is ruptured to get small vesicles; bottom-up strategy, in which small molecules dissolve in an organic solvent precipitated with anti-solvent in the presence of the stabilizer. This technique is mainly used to prepare liposomes conjugated with peptides, antibodies, NPs embedded with protein, liposomes modified with membrane proteins, and entirely synthesized nanovesicles and biological approaches in which the virus could act as vehicles for gene therapy to a package of nucleic acids and exosomes will facilitate the uptake of virus-host to the target cells, but this type of approach could initiate immunogenicity. In recent years, biomimetic exosomes have been used to deliver small molecule therapeutic agents, such as hydrophobic moieties that can be encapsulated in phospholipid vesicles and hydrophilic moiety in the core of artificial exosomes, which some targeting moieties on the surface of the artificial exosomes could also fabricate. PLTMs could also be used as vectors to escape the immune response into the body. siRNA, shRNA, miRNA, antisense oligonucleotide (ASO), CRISPR/Cas9 system, plasmid DNA, and mRNA could be delivered to the target cell via biomimetic exosome for the treatment of the disease. Further, clinical studies of biomimetic exosomes have just recently started, and synthetic biomimetic materials have not yet been employed for clinical transformation. The greatest obstacle is the lack of standardized procedures for preparation, characterization, and biocompatibility-related issues. In addition, synthesizing biomimetic exosomes requires a completely automated purification procedure. Fully developed biomimetic exosomes are portable, and the alteration of antibodies and other functional groups may aid in regulating the release of biomimetic exosomes [68].

5.5.8 Biomimetic nanorobots

The principle of biomimetics focuses on Nature as a model to create systems that resemble biological systems for solving human problems. Specifically, biomimicry principles have greatly influenced the field of nanorobotics by allowing us to comprehend fundamental concepts, thus paving the way to practical nanotechnology [37, 38, 69].

Biomimetic nanorobots are dynamic nanoscale structure (between 1 and 100 nm in size) with enhanced sensing, operation, swarm intelligence, actuation, and cooperative behaviour. The various aspects of biomimetic nanorobotics encapsulate two mimetic principles, including: (a) 'machine nanomimetics', which creates nanomachine components inspired by macro-scale machines; and (b) 'bionanomimetics,' where biological entities are employed to create the nanomachine components [37, 38, 69]. These biocompatible intelligent nanorobotic systems are capable of self-assembly, collision avoidance, localized drug delivery, information processing, and nanorobot excretion via self-closing machinery [70].

Interestingly, several biologically inspired materials have been employed to engineer the organic nanobots with negligible toxicity. The fabrication of medical nanorobots with biological sensors and propulsion equipment has gained significant attention for delivering accurate drug doses to the desired location [69, 71, 72]. Further, the convergence of robotic technology with micro- and nano-electromechanical systems has revolutionized the field of medical robotics for therapeutic purposes. These intelligent nanobots can communicate with physicians via signals at wave frequencies of 1–100 MHz to achieve motion control [69, 72, 73]. Besides, the motion of nanorobots is principally categorized as self-propulsion, external stimuli-based propulsion, and biohybrid-based propulsion [69, 74]. Unlike traditional drug delivery systems, which rely on blood flow to reach the target, the designed medical nanorobots can deliver therapeutics to difficult-to-reach areas through autonomous motion. The propulsion of nanobots is driven by endogenous power using chemical reaction energy in the presence of fuel. The exogenous propulsion of nanorobots can be supported by the introduction of external magnetic fields, light energy, acoustic fields, and electric fields [74–77].

5.5.8.1 Types of engineered biomimetic nanorobots

The different types of biomimetic nanorobots based on different biological materials are represented in figure 5.2. They areas follows. (a) Mammalian cell-based biomimetic nanorobots, which typically consist of a synthetic NP core encapsulated in a cell membrane layer [69]. For example, a PLTM-camouflaged nanorobot was developed to enhance the delivery of a drug, bortezomib, to treat multiple myeloma [78]. Interestingly, the engineering of sperm cells in robots can carry therapeutics other than assistance in artificial insemination procedures [79]. (b) Pathogen-based biomimetic nanorobots exploit the novel structures of viruses, bacteria, and fungi to enhance targeted drug delivery. For instance, cationic NPs coated with bacterial vectors (Salmonella) were designed for effective delivery of an oral DNA vaccine [69, 80]. (c) Biomolecular-based biomimetic systems employ biological molecules like lipids, proteins, polysaccharides, DNA, cofactors, and enzymes for designing nanorobots. For instance, Liang *et al* (2020) engineered H-ferritin nanocaged NPs as an effective drug delivery nanosysytem in cancer [81]. Further, a lipid-based therapeutic nanorobot was manufactured to deliver siRNA to cancer cells [82]. Li *et al* (2018) engineered DNA origami nanorobots to distribute thrombin to the targeted location for cancer therapy [83].

5.5.8.2 Nanorobots for targeted drug delivery

Medical nanorobots must mimic the innate intelligence of their biological entities (i.e., bacteria, RBCs, or stem cells) in terms of their operational stability, collective

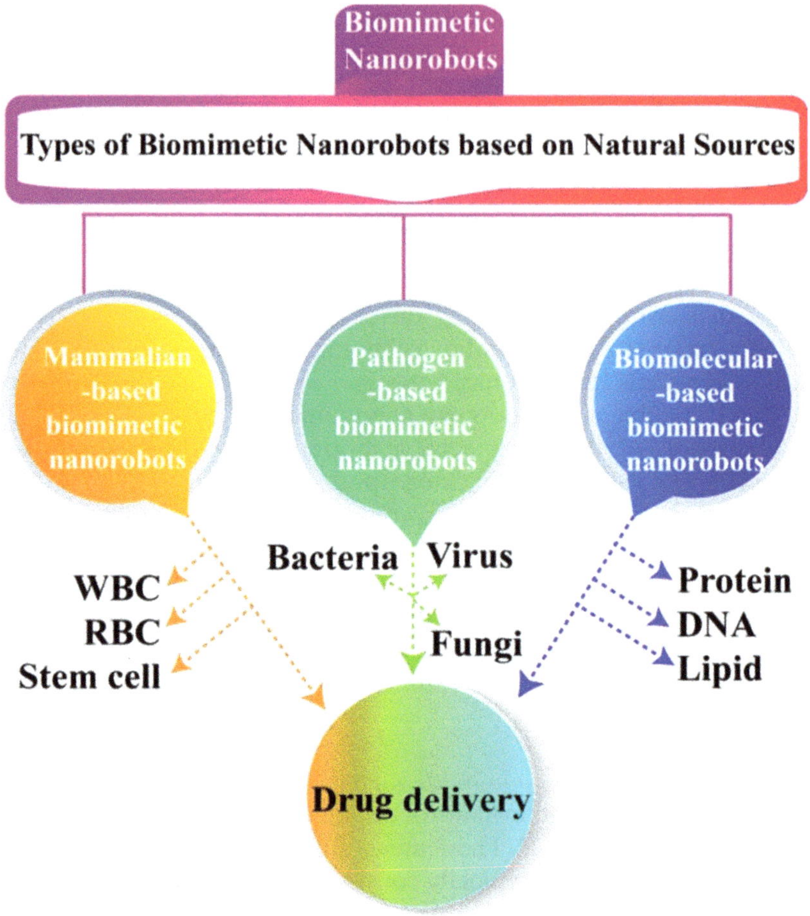

Figure 5.2. Schematic representation of various types of biomimetic nanorobots based on natural sources.

motion, and functionality. Such cell-based nanorobots are considered effective and biocompatible for targeted drug delivery owing to the presence of a good immune escape mechanism. The cell-based nanobots achieve precision therapeutic efficacy by rapidly delivering payloads to the affected regions, thus reducing the local and systemic adverse effects of drug toxicity [76, 84]. For instance, a magnetically controlled cell robot drug carrier was developed by mimicking macrophages for targeted killing of tumors [85]. Shao *et al* (2017) fabricated biohybrid nanobots by precoating *Escherichia coli* on the surface of mesoporous silica NPs (MSNs) and neutrophils [86]. In another study, therapeutic nanobots were designed by embedding magnetic NPs (MNPs) inside RBCs, loaded with DOX and quantum dots (QDs). The movement of RBC nanobots was guided by a magnetic and acoustic field, resulting in a prolonged release of DOX with three times less cytotoxicity [84]. Felfoul *et al* (2016) presented the coupling of a magneto-aerotactic bacteria (Magnetococcus marinus strain MC-1) with drug-containing nanoliposomes to penetrate the hypoxic areas of tumors and facilitate targeted drug delivery in the affected regions [87]. Fascinatingly, synthetic ciliary bands were activated by ultrasound and could mimic the ciliary bands of starfish larva [88]. Furthermore, ultrasound-driven nanowire motors were designed for rapid release of drugs to cancer cells stimulated by light [89].

The main advantage of these therapeutic nanorobots is their site-specific drug delivery capability with improved reproducibility and intracellular imaging, which can be demonstrated from the increase in doctor–patient acceptance ratio [90]. However, nanorobotic systems are still in their early stages, and further research is needed to explore their dependability for targeted drug delivery in physiological environments. The transition from theory to practice is fraught with challenges, including enhanced therapeutic efficacy, biocompatibility, intracellular localization, excretion from the body, Brownian motion, and aggregation [91]. Efforts should be coordinated on nanorobotic systems to investigate their long-term effects and to verify *in vivo* drug delivery by real-time tracking [91, 92].

5.6 Targeting ability of biomimetic drug delivery system

The biomimetic drug delivery systems (BDDSs) have self-targeting ability with cancers, also called passive targeting, through EPR [93]. It is now well known that rapidly growing tumors recruit new blood vessels in response to hypoxia, which are leaky and allow for enhanced selective permeation of macromolecules larger than 40 kDa and nanosystems into the tumor stroma. Moreover, the immature lymphatic drainage helps the nanocarrier system to be retained in the tumor tissues.

However, the BDDSs can also be modified with moieties possessing specific targeting functions for particular cells, such as neuropilin-1-targeting peptides, folic acid, neurotensin peptide, c(RGDyK)-peptides, antibodies, transferrin, galactose, and aptamers [93]. This strategy will increase the affinities of nanocarriers for the surface of cancer cells, increasing drug penetration at higer cost. The first evidence of this phenomenon was proposed in 1980 with antibodies grafted on the surface of liposomes. Other ligands, such as peptides, nucleic acids, and aptamers, were quickly screened after this [94]. We have summarized different kinds of active targeting moieties in table 5.1 and figure 5.3 shows a SWOT analysis of a biometric DDS.

5.7 Conclusions

As per the ongoing preclinical and clinical research, it is now fully discovered that biomimetic DDSs could provide highly efficient and targeted delivery of therapeutic micro and macromolecules. Moreover, the biomimetic DDS possesses immense advantages, such as high payload efficiency, better cellular uptake, modified circulation time, *in vivo* stability, non-toxicity, and tissue-specific delivery. However, the rationale design and development of these nanocarrier systems could provide a sustainable and biologically responsive release of medicament *in vivo*. Moreover, the scalability of these nanocarriers is another advantage that makes them a potential candidate for clinical translation. This area is rapidly growing, and the pharmaceutical industries are investing huge capital in these delivery systems.

Table 5.1. Different active targeting moieties to improve the efficiency of BDDSs.

Category	Moiety	Binding affinity	Pros	Cons
Small molecules [93]	Galactose	Glycoprotein receptors	Low cost, Low Mol. Wt and easy to conjugate	Low circulation half-life
	Folate	Folate receptors		
Antibodies [9–12]	Herceptin Rituxan	Her2	High binding affinity, approved for clinical applications	High cost, immunogenicity
	CD19	CD20 and CD19 antigen		
	Bevacizumab	VEGF receptors		
Peptides [9–12]	cRGD	Integrins receptors	High affinity	Low circulation half-life
	GE11	EGFR		
Proteins [39]	Transferrin	Transferrin receptor	Clinically approved	High cost
Aptamers [9–12]	Pegaptanib	VEGF receptors	It could be designed for any biological target	High cost

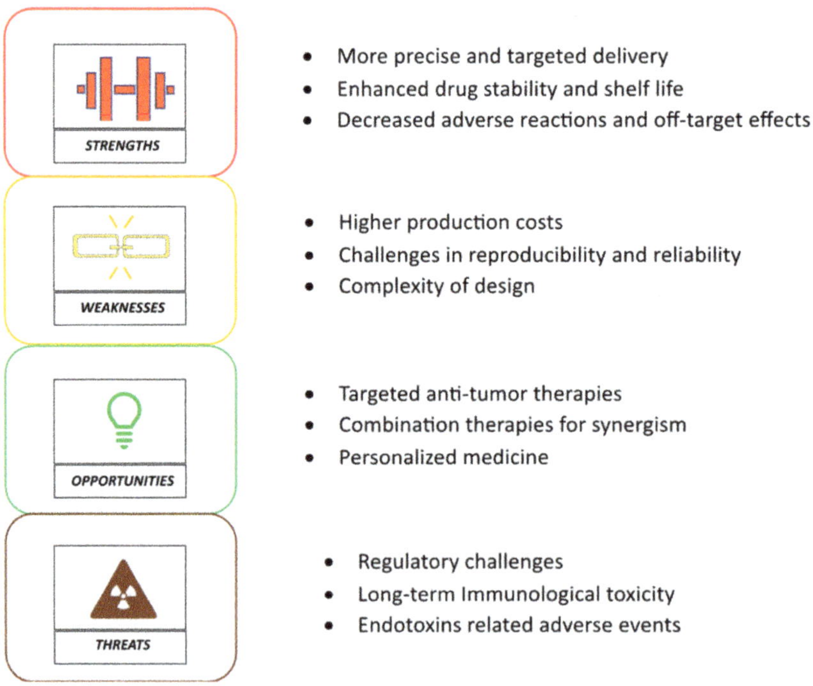

Figure 5.3. SWOT analysis of a biomimetic DDS [95].

Therefore, it will be interesting to see how the biomimetic DDSs will grow in terms of their clinical applications.

Conflict of interest

The authors declare no conflict of interest

References

[1] Islam M S, Renner F, Foster K, Oderinde M S, Stefanski K and Mitra S 2022 Enhanced aqueous dissolution of hydrophobic apixaban via direct incorporation of hydrophilic nanographene oxide *Colloids Surf.,* B **216** 112512

[2] Din F U, Aman W, Ullah I, Qureshi O S, Mustapha O, Shafique S and Zeb A 2017 Effective use of nanocarriers as drug delivery systems for the treatment of selected tumors *Int. J. Nanomed.* **12** 7291–309

[3] Wen H, Jung H and Li X 2015 Drug delivery approaches in addressing clinical pharmacology-related issues: opportunities and challenges *AAPS J.* **17** 1327–40

[4] Zhang M, Du Y, Wang S and Chen B 2020 A review of biomimetic nanoparticle drug delivery systems based on cell membranes *Drug Design Dev. Ther.* **14** 5495–503

[5] Chen Y X, Wei C X, Lyu Y Q, Chen H Z, Jiang G and Gao X L 2020 Biomimetic drug-delivery systems for the management of brain diseases *Biomater. Sci.* **8** 1073–88

[6] Vincent J F, Bogatyreva O A, Bogatyrev N R, Bowyer A and Pahl A K 2006 Biomimetics: its practice and theory *J. R. Soc. Interface* **3** 471–82

[7] Sheikhpour M, Barani L and Kasaeian A 2017 Biomimetics in drug delivery systems: a critical review *J. Control. Release* **253** 97–109

[8] Vincent J F 2009 Biomimetics—a review *Proc. Inst. Mech. Eng. Part H, J. Eng. Med.* **223** 919–39

[9] Venkatesh S, Byrne M E, Peppas N A and Hilt J Z 2005 Applications of biomimetic systems in drug delivery *Expert Opin. Drug Deliv.* **2** 1085–96

[10] Gong Y K and Winnik F M 2012 Strategies in biomimetic surface engineering of nanoparticles for biomedical applications *Nanoscale* **4** 360–8

[11] Balmert S C and Little S R 2012 Biomimetic delivery with micro- and nanoparticles *Adv. Mater. (Deerfield Beach, Fla.)* **24** 3757–78

[12] Peppas N A 2004 Intelligent therapeutics: biomimetic systems and nanotechnology in drug delivery *Adv. Drug Deliv. Rev.* **56** 1529–31

[13] Rao L, Bu L L, Meng Q F, Cai B, Deng W W, Li A, Li K, Guo S S, Zhang W F and Liu W 2017 Antitumor platelet-mimicking magnetic nanoparticles *Adv. Funct. Mater.* **27** 1604774

[14] Ye L, Ma S, Robinson B W and Creaney J 2019 Immunotherapy strategies for mesothelioma–the role of tumor specific neoantigens in a new era of precision medicine *Expert Rev. Respir. Med.* **13** 181–92

[15] Hu Q, Sun W, Qian C, Wang C, Bomba H N and Gu Z 2015 Anticancer platelet-mimicking nanovehicles *Adv Mater. (Deerfield Beach, Fla.)* **27** 7043–50

[16] Gao M, Liang C, Song X, Chen Q, Jin Q, Wang C and Liu Z 2017 Erythrocyte-membrane-enveloped perfluorocarbon as nanoscale artificial red blood cells to relieve tumor hypoxia and enhance cancer radiotherapy *Adv. Mater. (Deerfield Beach, Fla.)* **29** 1701429

[17] Martinez J O *et al* 2018 Biomimetic nanoparticles with enhanced affinity towards activated endothelium as versatile tools for theranostic drug delivery *Theranostics* **8** 1131–45

[18] Wang H, Wu J, Williams G R, Fan Q, Niu S, Wu J, Xie X and Zhu L M 2019 Platelet-membrane-biomimetic nanoparticles for targeted antitumor drug delivery *J. Nanobiotechnol.* **17** 60

[19] Mekuria S L, Debele T A, Chou H Y and Tsai H C 2016 IL-6 antibody and RGD peptide conjugated poly(amidoamine) dendrimer for targeted drug delivery of hela cells *J. Phys. Chem.* B **120** 123–30

[20] Timko B P and Kohane D S 2012 Materials to clinical devices: technologies for remotely triggered drug delivery *Clin. Ther.* **34** S25–35

[21] Ranney D F 2000 Biomimetic transport and rational drug delivery *Biochem. Pharmacol.* **59** 105–14

[22] Rashid M and Rahman M 2021 Importance and prospects of bioinspired and biomimetic materials for drug delivery *Bioinspired and Biomimetic Materials for Drug Delivery* ed M Nurunnabi (Woodhead Publishing) ch 1 pp 1–14

[23] Loyer P and Cammas-Marion S 2014 Natural and synthetic poly(malic acid)-based derivates: a family of versatile biopolymers for the design of drug nanocarriers *J. Drug Target.* **22** 556–75

[24] Lang T, Yin Q and Li Y 2018 Progress of cell-derived biomimetic drug delivery systems for cancer therapy *Adv. Ther.* **1** 1800053

[25] Su J, Sun H, Meng Q, Zhang P, Yin Q and Li Y 2017 Enhanced blood suspensibility and laser-activated tumor-specific drug release of theranostic mesoporous silica nanoparticles by functionalizing with erythrocyte membranes *Theranostics* **7** 523–37

[26] Chung Y H, Cai H and Steinmetz N F 2020 Viral nanoparticles for drug delivery, imaging, immunotherapy, and theranostic applications *Adv. Drug Deliv. Rev.* **156** 214–35

[27] Cabral H and Kataoka K 2014 Progress of drug-loaded polymeric micelles into clinical studies *J. Control. Release* **190** 465–76

[28] Miyata K, Christie R J and Kataoka K 2011 Polymeric micelles for nano-scale drug delivery *React. Funct. Polym.* **71** 227–34

[29] Duncan R 2003 The dawning era of polymer therapeutics *Nat. Rev. Drug Discov.* **2** 347–60

[30] Kataoka K, Harada A and Nagasaki Y 2001 Block copolymer micelles for drug delivery: design, characterization and biological significance *Adv. Drug Deliv. Rev.* **47** 113–31

[31] Davis M E, Chen Z and Shin D M 2008 Nanoparticle therapeutics: an emerging treatment modality for cancer *Nat. Rev. Drug Discov.* **7** 771–82

[32] Liu G, Zhuang W, Chen X, Yin A, Nie Y and Wang Y 2016 Drug carrier system self-assembled from biomimetic polyphosphorycholine and biodegradable polypeptide based diblock copolymers *Polymer* **100** 45–55

[33] Feng W, Huang Z, Kang X, Zhao D, Li H, Li G, Xu J and Wang X 2021 Self-assembled nanosized vehicles from amino acid-based amphiphilic polymers with pendent carboxyl groups for efficient drug delivery *Biomacromolecules* **22** 4871–82

[34] Pukale S, Pandya A and Patravale V 2021 Synthesis, characterization and topical application of novel bifunctional peptide metallodendrimer *J. Drug Deliv. Sci. Technol.* **66** 102925

[35] Kashapova N E, Kashapov R R, Ziganshina A Y, Amerhanova S K, Lyubina A P, Voloshina A D, Salnikov V V and Zakharova L Y 2022 Self-assembling nanoparticles based on acetate derivatives of calix[4]resorcinol and octenidine dihydrochloride for tuning selectivity in cancer cells *Colloids Surf.,* A **654** 130087

[36] Werner M E, Cummings N D, Sethi M, Wang E C, Sukumar R, Moore D T and Wang A Z 2013 Preclinical evaluation of Genexol-PM, a nanoparticle formulation of paclitaxel, as a

novel radiosensitizer for the treatment of non-small cell lung cancer *Inter. J. Radiat. Oncol. Biol. Phys.* **86** 463–8

[37] Hwang J, Jeong Y, Park J M, Lee K H, Hong J W and Choi J 2015 Biomimetics: forecasting the future of science, engineering, and medicine *Int. J. Nanomed.* **10** 5701–13

[38] Bar-Cohen Y 2005 *Biomimetics: Biologically Inspired Technologies* (Boca Raton, FL: CRC Press)

[39] Li J, Zeng H, You Y, Wang R, Tan T, Wang W, Yin L, Zeng Z, Zeng Y and Xie T 2021 Active targeting of orthotopic glioma using biomimetic liposomes co-loaded elemene and cabazitaxel modified by transferritin *J. Nanobiotechnol.* **19** 1–19

[40] Loureiro D R, Soares J X, Lopes D, Macedo T, Yordanova D, Jakobtorweihen S, Nunes C, Reis S, Pinto M M and Afonso C M 2018 Accessing lipophilicity of drugs with biomimetic models: a comparative study using liposomes and micelles *Eur. J. Pharm. Sci.* **115** 369–80

[41] He H, Lu Y, Qi J, Zhao W, Dong X and Wu W 2018 Biomimetic thiamine-and niacin-decorated liposomes for enhanced oral delivery of insulin *Acta Pharm. Sinica* B **8** 97–105

[42] Liu Q, Xue J, Zhang X, Chai J, Qin L, Guan J, Zhang X and Mao S 2022 The influence of a biomimetic pulmonary surfactant modification on the *in vivo* fate of nanoparticles in the lung *Acta Biomater.* **147** 391–402

[43] Pukale S S, Sharma S, Dalela M, Singh A K, Mohanty S, Mittal A and Chitkara D 2020 Multi-component clobetasol-loaded monolithic lipid-polymer hybrid nanoparticles ameliorate imiquimod-induced psoriasis like skin inflammation in Swiss albino mice *Acta Biomater.* **115** 393–409

[44] Pukale S S, Mittal A and Chitkara D 2021 Topical application of vitamin D(3)-loaded hybrid nanosystem to offset imiquimod-induced psoriasis *AAPS Pharm. Sci.Tech.* **22** 238

[45] Pukale S S, Sahel D K, Mittal A and Chitkara D 2022 Coenzyme Q10 loaded lipid-polymer hybrid nanoparticles in gel for the treatment of psoriasis like skin condition *J. Drug Deliv. Sci. Technol.* **76** 103672

[46] Sharma S, Pukale S, Sahel D K, Singh P, Mittal A and Chitkara D 2021 Folate targeted hybrid lipo-polymeric nanoplexes containing docetaxel and miRNA-34a for breast cancer treatment *Mater. Sci. Eng.* C **128** 112305

[47] Mehdi-alamdarlou S, Ahmadi F, Azadi A, Shahbazi M-A, Heidari R and Ashrafi H 2022 A cell-mimicking platelet-based drug delivery system as a potential carrier of dimethyl fumarate for multiple sclerosis *Int. J. Pharm.* **625** 122084

[48] Hu C-MJ, Zhang L, Aryal S, Cheung C, Fang R H and Zhang L 2011 Erythrocyte membrane-camouflaged polymeric nanoparticles as a biomimetic delivery platform *Proc. Natl. Acad. Sci.* **108** 10980–5

[49] Aguero L, Alpdagtas S, Ilhan E, Zaldivar-Silva D and Gunduz O 2021 Functional role of crosslinking in alginate scaffold for drug delivery and tissue engineering: a review *Eur. Polym. J.* **160** 110807

[50] Zhao M, Lei C, Yang Y, Bu X, Ma H, Gong H, Liu J, Fang X, Hu Z and Fang Q 2015 Abraxane, the nanoparticle formulation of paclitaxel can induce drug resistance by up-regulation of P-gp *PLoS One* **10** e0131429

[51] Lohia A, Sahel D K, Salman M, Singh V, Mariappan I, Mittal A and Chitkara D 2022 Delivery strategies for CRISPR/Cas genome editing tool for retinal dystrophies: challenges and opportunities *Asian J. Pharm. Sci.* **17** 153–76

[52] Sahel D K, Mittal A and Chitkara D 2019 CRISPR/cas system for genome editing: progress and prospects as a therapeutic tool *The J. Pharm. Exper. Ther.* **370** 725–35

[53] Sahel D K, Salman M, Azhar M, Goswami S G, Singh V, Dalela M, Mohanty S, Mittal A, Ramalingam S and Chitkara D 2022 Cationic lipopolymeric nanoplexes containing the CRISPR/Cas9 ribonucleoprotein for genome surgery *J. Mater. Chem.* B **10** 7634–49
[54] Gangrade A, Gawali B, Jadi P K, Naidu V G M and Mandal B B 2020 Photo-electro active nanocomposite silk hydrogel for spatiotemporal controlled release of chemotherapeutics: an *in vivo* approach toward suppressing solid tumor growth *ACS Appl. Mater. Interfaces* **12** 27905–16
[55] Gangrade A and Mandal B B 2019 Injectable carbon nanotube impregnated silk based multifunctional hydrogel for localized targeted and on-demand anticancer drug delivery *ACS Biomater. Sci. Eng.* **5** 2365–81
[56] Janani G, Kumar M, Chouhan D, Moses J C, Gangrade A, Bhattacharjee S and Mandal B B 2019 Insight into silk-based biomaterials: from physicochemical attributes to recent biomedical applications *ACS Appl. Bio. Mater.* **2** 5460–91
[57] Gangrade A and Mandal B B 2020 Drug delivery of anticancer drugs from injectable 3D porous silk scaffold for prevention of gastric cancer growth and recurrence *ACS Biomater. Sci. Eng.* **6** 6195–206
[58] Dalwadi C and Patel G 2015 Application of nanohydrogels in drug delivery systems: recent patents review *Recent Pat. Nanotechnol.* **9** 17–25
[59] Rizwan M, Yahya R, Hassan A, Yar M, Azzahari A D, Selvanathan V, Sonsudin F and Abouloula C N 2017 pH sensitive hydrogels in drug delivery: brief history, properties, swelling, and release mechanism, material selection and applications *Polymers* **9** 225
[60] Chandrawati R 2016 Enzyme-responsive polymer hydrogels for therapeutic delivery *Exper. Biol. Med. (Maywood, N.J.)* **241** 972–9
[61] Zhao W, Odelius K, Edlund U, Zhao C and Albertsson A-C 2015 *In situ* synthesis of magnetic field-responsive hemicellulose hydrogels for drug delivery *Biomacromolecules* **16** 2522–8
[62] Kozlovskaya V, Alexander J F, Wang Y, Kuncewicz T, Liu X, Godin B and Kharlampieva E 2014 Internalization of red blood cell-mimicking hydrogel capsules with pH-triggered shape responses *ACS Nano* **8** 5725–37
[63] Wang H, Mao D, Wang Y, Wang K, Yi X, Kong D, Yang Z, Liu Q and Ding D 2015 Biocompatible fluorescent supramolecular nanofibrous hydrogel for long-term cell tracking and tumor imaging applications *Sci. Rep.* **5** 1–10
[64] Li J and Mooney D J 2016 Designing hydrogels for controlled drug delivery *Nat. Rev. Mater.* **1** 1–17
[65] Mantha S, Pillai S, Khayambashi P, Upadhyay A, Zhang Y, Tao O, Pham H M and Tran S D 2019 Smart hydrogels in tissue engineering and regenerative medicine *Materials* **12** 3323
[66] Lee P I 1985 Kinetics of drug release from hydrogel matrices *J. Control. Release* **2** 277–88
[67] Raja I S and Fathima N N 2014 Porosity and dielectric properties as tools to predict drug release trends from hydrogels *SpringerPlus* **3** 1–10
[68] Wang X, Zhao X, Zhong Y, Shen J and An W 2022 biomimetic exosomes: a new generation of drug delivery system *Front. Bioeng. Biotechnol.* **10** 865682
[69] Nehru S, Misra R and Bhaswant M 2022 Multifaceted engineered biomimetic nanorobots toward cancer management *ACS Biomater. Sci. Eng.* **8** 444–59
[70] Kumar R, Baghel O, Sidar S K, Sen P K and Bohidar S K 2014 Applications of nanorobotics *Int. J. Sci. Res. Eng. Technol* **3** 1131–7

[71] Mavroidis C and Ferreira A 2013 Nanorobotics: past, present, and future *Nanorobotics: Current Approaches and Techniques* (Springer) pp 3–27
[72] Vega Baudrit J R, Gutierrez B, Villalobos Bermúdez C, Corrales Ureña Y R and Vargas Chacón S 2017 Nanobots: development and future *Int. J. Biosens. Bioelectron.* **2** 146–51
[73] Li J, Esteban-Fernández de Ávila B, Gao W, Zhang L and Wang J 2017 Micro/nanorobots for biomedicine: delivery, surgery, sensing, and detoxification *Sci. Robot.* **2** eaam6431
[74] Wu R, Zhu Y, Cai X, Wu S, Xu L and Yu T 2022 Recent process in microrobots: from propulsion to swarming for biomedical applications *Micromachines* **13** 1473
[75] Chen X Z, Jang B, Ahmed D, Hu C, De Marco C, Hoop M, Mushtaq F, Nelson B J and Pané S 2018 Small-scale machines driven by external power sources *Adv. Mater.* **30** 1705061
[76] Medina-Sánchez M, Xu H and Schmidt O G 2018 Micro- and nano-motors: the new generation of drug carriers *Ther. Deliv.* **9** 303–16
[77] Kumar S, Nasim B and Abraham E 2018 Nanorobots a future device for diagnosis and treatment *J. Pharm. Pharm.* **5** 44–9
[78] Yoo J-W, Irvine D J, Discher D E and Mitragotri S 2011 Bio-inspired, bioengineered and biomimetic drug delivery carriers *Nat. Rev. Drug Discov.* **10** 521–35
[79] Xu H, Medina-Sánchez M, Magdanz V, Schwarz L, Hebenstreit F and Schmidt O G 2018 Sperm-hybrid micromotor for targeted drug delivery *ACS Nano* **12** 327–37
[80] Hu Q, Wu M, Fang C, Cheng C, Zhao M, Fang W, Chu P K, Ping Y and Tang G 2015 Engineering nanoparticle-coated bacteria as oral DNA vaccines for cancer immunotherapy *Nano Lett.* **15** 2732–9
[81] Meng X, Gao L, Fan K and Yan X 2020 Nanozyme-based tumor theranostics *Nanozymology: Connecting Biology and Nanotechnology* (Springer) pp 425–57
[82] Kenny G D, Kamaly N, Kalber T L, Brody L P, Sahuri M, Shamsaei E, Miller A D and Bell J D 2011 Novel multifunctional nanoparticle mediates siRNA tumour delivery, visualisation and therapeutic tumour reduction *in vivo J. Control. Release* **149** 111–6
[83] Li S, Jiang Q, Liu S, Zhang Y, Tian Y, Song C, Wang J, Zou Y, Anderson G J and Han J-Y 2018 A DNA nanorobot functions as a cancer therapeutic in response to a molecular trigger *in vivo Nat. Biotechnol.* **36** 258–64
[84] Suhail M, Khan A, Rahim M A, Naeem A, Fahad M, Badshah S F, Jabar A and Janakiraman A K 2022 Micro and nanorobot-based drug delivery: an overview *J. Drug Target.* **30** 349–58
[85] Dai Y, Bai X, Jia L, Sun H, Feng Y, Wang L, Zhang C, Chen Y, Ji Y and Zhang D 2021 Precise control of customized macrophage cell robot for targeted therapy of solid tumors with minimal invasion *Small* **17** 2103986
[86] Shao J, Xuan M, Zhang H, Lin X, Wu Z and He Q 2017 Chemotaxis-guided hybrid neutrophil micromotors for targeted drug transport *Angew. Chem.* **129** 13115–9
[87] Felfoul O, Mohammadi M, Taherkhani S, De Lanauze D, Zhong Xu Y, Loghin D, Essa S, Jancik S, Houle D and Lafleur M 2016 Magneto-aerotactic bacteria deliver drug-containing nanoliposomes to tumour hypoxic regions *Nat. Nanotechnol.* **11** 941–7
[88] Dillinger C, Nama N and Ahmed D 2021 Ultrasound-activated ciliary bands for microrobotic systems inspired by starfish *Nat. Commun.* **12** 6455
[89] Garcia-Gradilla V, Sattayasamitsathit S, Soto F, Kuralay F, Yardımcı C, Wiitala D, Galarnyk M and Wang J 2014 Ultrasound-propelled nanoporous gold wire for efficient drug loading and release *Small* **10** 4154–9

[90] Soto F, Wang J, Ahmed R and Demirci U 2020 Medical micro/nanorobots in precision medicine *Adv. Sci.* **7** 2002203
[91] Hu M, Ge X, Chen X, Mao W, Qian X and Yuan W-E 2020 Micro/nanorobot: a promising targeted drug delivery system *Pharmaceutics* **12** 665
[92] Giri G, Maddahi Y and Zareinia K 2021 A brief review on challenges in design and development of nanorobots for medical applications *Appl. Sci.* **11** 10385
[93] Attia M F, Anton N, Wallyn J, Omran Z and Vandamme T F 2019 An overview of active and passive targeting strategies to improve the nanocarriers efficiency to tumour sites *J. Pharm. Pharmacol.* **71** 1185–98
[94] Leserman L D, Barbet J, Kourilsky F and Weinstein J N 1980 Targeting to cells of fluorescent liposomes covalently coupled with monoclonal antibody or protein A *Nature* **288** 602–4
[95] Sheikhpour M, Barani L and Kasaeian A 2017 Biomimetics in drug delivery systems: a critical review *J. Control. Release* **253** 97–109

Chapter 6

Personalized healthcare: advances and avenues

Amitava Basu, Punita Aggarwal, Sugato Banerjee, Amalendu Samanta and Subhamay Panda

Personalizing healthcare is meant to improve health, prevent sickness, and tailor treatment to each person's unique needs to improve the overall health of the population. By quantifying disease patterns and predicting health hazards, this could help in designing interventions and suggest possible treatment strategies to individuals within certain populations. Here we discuss the role of advanced diagnostic tools, genetic screening, 3D printing, AI-based instrumentations, targeted drug delivery and digital health information systems in personalized healthcare. We also discuss the financial and logistic challenges of implementing personalized medicine for all, especially in developing economies, and future opportunities.

6.1 Introduction

The focus of personalizing healthcare is on taking important factors into account, such as enhancing health, preventing sickness, and tailoring treatment to each person's unique needs. By quantifying disease patterns and predicting health hazards, this could enhance our ability to tailor treatment interventions to the needs of the person. From the early 19th century to the 21st century, medicine has transformed beyond the imagination from the treatment and myth used earlier to the modern and artificial intelligence (AI) used today with surgery to targeted drug delivery. Both the utilization of x-rays for diagnostic imaging and the manufacture of particular medicines were made possible by the application of physics and chemistry, respectively. Targeted therapy is now feasible due to a greater understanding of the molecular route and signalling. With the use of chemical synthesis and nanoscale drug delivery, precise treatment strategies with lower adverse effects are becoming available [1]. The medical field is much more concerned with promoting personalized healthcare strategies. An innovative and strategic approach to healthcare, personalized healthcare is backed by instruments for individualized treatment and custom health planning that have been made possible by advances in

doi:10.1088/978-0-7503-5613-8ch6

science and technology [2]. These methods enhance our ability to identify and quantify illness patterns, identify potential health risks, and customize therapeutic interventions.

6.2 Brief understanding of health and healthcare

The right to the best possible level of health is a universal human right. This is the primary cornerstone of healthcare. To efficiently organize and enhance national health systems and bring services for health and wellbeing closer to communities, primary healthcare takes a holistic approach for the entire society. It comprises three parts: (1) integrated healthcare to address individuals' requirements for health throughout their lives; (2) enabling people, families, and communities to take control of their own health; (3) addressing the larger determinants of health through multisector policy and action. The dynamics that are covered under health of an individual include physical wellness, emotional wellness, social wellness, intellectual wellness, environmental wellness, spiritual wellness, vocational wellness and financial wellness. Types of services that can be covered under healthcare include health and medicine, counselling and therapy, nursing and nutrition, which broadly vary based on the economy of the country. Various other dynamics that are covered under healthcare include: ambulatory surgical centres, blood banks, birth centres, medical and clinical offices, diabetics, hospitals, imaging and radiology centres, mental health and addiction centres, nursing homes, telephonic health services and senior citizen care services [3, 4].

With the completion of the Human Genome Project in the year 2003, the focus toward the genome and genomic driven human health has increased. The genomic application in practice and prevention program was established by CDC (Centres for Disease Control and Prevention) in 2005 that further encourages genetic testing and genomic technology in healthcare [1]. Even after two decades, the idea of healthcare and personalization at the genomics level is still a far held dream for most developing nations [4]. For electronic health records (EHRs), the scenario varies between the developed and developing nations. While most developed nations have successfully developed the system of archiving and accessibility to healthcare records, the developing nations require more resources and efforts for implementation [5].

6.3 WHO and healthcare

The World Health Organization (WHO) is focusing on the quality of healthcare to introduce effectiveness, safety, equity, efficacy and integration. The old definition of healthcare in the system was—'any of the activity with its primary purpose to promote, restore, or maintain health', the fundamentals of which lie in the hands of the government, whether it is developing or in its developed state [2, 4]. The approach of personalized healthcare care is tailored, predictive, preventive, and participative. It incorporates the ideas of systems biology to medicine. When it comes to personalized healthcare the goal is to provide proper treatment to the patient, at the proper dose, and at the right time by targeting the right factors which are responsible for the condition. Factors that come into the picture range from literacy rate, technology advancement, economy, population and many more that shape healthcare in the developed and developing countries. The primary principles of healthcare are accessibility, health promotion, public participation, appropriate skills/technology (AI support) [5], and intersectoral cooperation. To bring advancement in personalized healthcare systems, development is needed in various sectors, including biomarker identification, recording long-term disease/treatment history and analysis, dietary needs/genetics, lifestyle and environmental make-up.

6.4 Healthcare status in developed and developing nations

According to the available data, integrating personalized medicine/health (PM) into patient care practices offers a significant potential to raise healthcare quality at a reduced cost. Different reimbursement models, the anticipated need for quick and precise genomic information on critically ill hospital patients, and the need for a framework to enable consistent and coherent information sharing between community health services and hospitals—could make it challenging for PM even though it has promising health outcomes. Although the significance of the private sector in delivering healthcare in developing nations is now well accepted, thorough cross-country comparisons have been hampered by the lack of information on various types of providers [6]. Advanced diagnostic tools have replaced basic staining protocols like hematoxylin and eosin (H&E) tissue staining in high income countries. The development of customized medicine is the result of development in fundamental research [7]. Various developing countries are coming up with potential for cost-effective innovations to help personalized medication [8]. Various programs like the UNICEF (United Nations International Children's Emergency Fund) Power Program [9] are taking steps for assistance in the welfare of developing countries. When there is more proof of the effectiveness of personalized health technologies, governments with legal and constitutional obligations to enhance the health of their populace can assist their development and offer them through state-funded programmes. It is crucial to strike a balance between addressing equality issues among various communities and enhancing healthcare effectiveness. In underdeveloped nations, the adoption of PM is still in its early stages [10]. The international Clinical Pharmacogenetics Implementation Consortium was most recently founded by the Pharmacogenomics Knowledgebase and the Pharmacogenomics Research Network to support the creation of new pharmacogenomics clinical practice guidelines [11]. As a result of their frequent independence, programmes for personalized medicine are unable to benefit from the lessons learned by other healthcare delivery systems. To address issues in these areas, both short-term tactics to introduce straightforward programmes that can provide remedies and long-term strategies to encourage structural and cultural change will likely be required [13] (figure 6.1).

6.5 Personalized healthcare: present status

6.5.1 DNA-based screening in personalized healthcare

A highly effective and accurate DNA tool has been developed along with methylation biomarkers that gives an alternative screening options such as the methylation of SDC2 in DNA from stool samples for early detection of colorectal cancer [13]. Other DNA-based screening is included with testing of hepatocellular carcinoma, when

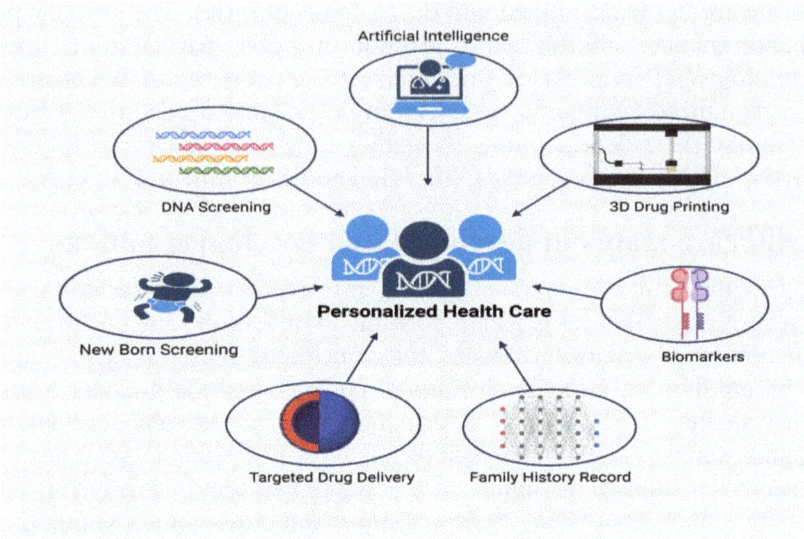

Figure 6.1. Representation of various advances to support personalized healthcare.

compared to the serum alpha-fetoprotein (AFP) and the GALAD score, the HelioLiver Test performed better in detecting Hepatocellular carcinoma (HCC) suggesting its importance in HCC surveillance settings [14]. With the development of DNA-based nanotechnology, the nanodevices using DNA have been introduced that construct the DNA-based biosensors. Various strategies included DNA amplification, enzyme dependent strategies as well as enzyme free strategies [15, 16], e.g., interconnection between Warfarin drug and CYP2C9 or VKORC1 gene variant [17, 18]. Cancer screening using genes—BRCA1, BRCA2, HNPCC, TP53, PTEN and CAD screening: 9p21. Genetic virulence, antibiotic, and heavy metal resistance all seem to be determined through analysis using molecular DNA-based approaches [19].

6.5.2 Personalized healthcare with artificial intelligence

The usage of AI in medicine spans a wide range, from the completely virtual (such as deep-learning-based health information management systems and active physician treatment decision-making) to the cyber-physical (e.g., robots used to assist the attending surgeon and targeted nanorobots for drug delivery) [20]. Quick access to diagnostic and early delivery of medical support can be provided using home monitoring as well as wearable devices [21], e.g. in characterization and detection of polyps in colonoscopy [22]. By employing massive data sets to train AI methods and validate AI models before deploying the methods on individual patients, many of the problems affecting personalized medicine today could be resolved. AI has already been used to identify blood sugar, cardiac activity, several cancers, including breast, liver, and colorectal cancer, using radio genomic correlations [23]. Another study involved use of AI to predict and analyse the conditions in critically ill patients who require prolonged mechanical ventilation (PMV) [24]. AI-assisted monitoring may

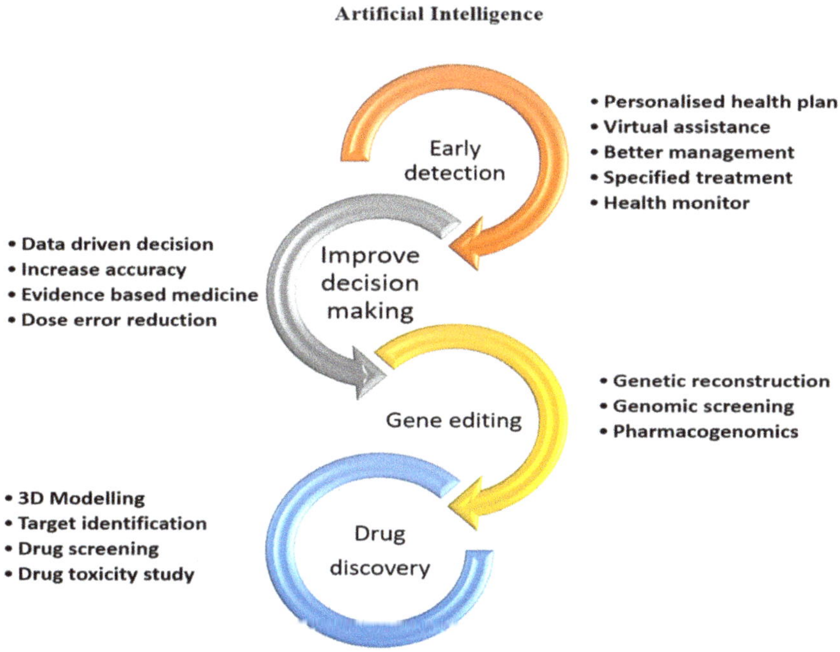

Figure 6.2. Representation of AI in personalized healthcare.

also be used in real time to evaluate the likelihood of intrapartum stress during labour and guide the decision between a caesarean section and a typical vaginal delivery in an effort to decrease perinatal issues and stillbirths [25] (figure 6.2).

6.5.3 Liquid biopsy

In the area of biomarker research, liquid biopsies (LBs) represent a revolutionary opportunity. Liquid biopsies, particularly those of circulating cell-free DNA (cfDNA), are significantly less likely to result in morbidity due to their minimally invasive nature and can be scheduled more frequently to provide a distinct view of the disease at various points in time [26]. Recently, digital PCR has developed into a sensitive technique for detecting cfDNA point mutations [27]. A simple and regular cfDNA test can also be used to monitor any changes that occur during treatment, serving as a precursor to metastasis, resistance, or recurrence. cfDNA most likely reflects the genetic make-up of all cancer subclones, in contrast to tissue biopsy, which ignores tumour heterogeneity [28]. The isolation of CTCs, ctDNA, and EVs from the blood of patients with various malignancies is one of the more recent LB techniques. LB offers molecular tumour information that can enable early tumour burden diagnosis and possible therapeutic interventions [29].

6.5.4 Healthcare digitalization and records on family history

Personal digital assistants (PDAs) have the potential to change how healthcare is delivered in the future since they attempt to combine and integrate the capabilities into a single versatile, adaptable, and portable device [30]. Maintaining the family history and

Table 6.1. List of popular databases used for digitalization of personalized healthcare.

Sr. No.	Database	Remark	References
1.	Epic Systems Software	Designed for documentation of perfusion activities as part of the patient electronic medical record.	[34]
2.	Health Facts® (HF)	A leading EHR vendor, maintains one of the largest vendor-specific EHR databases.	[35]
3.	MedHost	EHR based on Clinical Emergency Data Registry.	[36]
4.	Netsmart Technology	EHR based on facilitating data exchange.	[37]
5.	Athenahealth	A cloud-based service for maintaining EHR.	[38]

patients disease record are done using databases like ARCH Corpus, medicaid services and EHR-HL7 [31]. Numerous studies have demonstrated the value of PDA-based medication references, including drug interaction monitoring and parenteral nutrition, blood products, and chemotherapy [32]. Various databases involving IT support are being used e.g., medical database, health database and bio bank [33] (table 6.1).

6.5.5 New-born screening

One of the country's most effective public health programmes in the era of individualized medicine is new-born screening. With early detection, families might be able to avoid a time-consuming and difficult 'diagnostic procedure.' By having the ability to thoroughly genotype DNA extracted from dried blood spot samples used in new-born screening programmes, new avenues in new-born screening as well as for the study of the genetic influence of many complex disorders have become possible [39, 40]. Three key areas are covered by the new-born screening programme: hearing loss, serious cardiac problems, and a variety of metabolic, hematologic, endocrine, and other inheritable diseases [41]. The pulse oximetry screening test has a sensitivity of about 75% for critical congestive heart defects (CCHDs) [42], while the hearing screening has a high sensitivity of 92% [43]. According to recent data, around 3400 infants receive early intervention for disorders detected by universal new-born screening for four million infants that undergo screening each year [44]. The number of tests increased fivefold after tandem mass spectrometry (MS/MS) was recently included [45], which shows that the screening is moving in the right direction for new-born screening and will help the development of the era of genomic medicine.

6.5.6 3D printing

The capacity to customize dosage forms for specific individuals is one of 3D printing's significant advantages in the pharmaceutical industry. It is proven that several 3D printing technologies may provide cancer-specific medications for tumours of the breast, liver, thyroid, and kidney. The use of cancer model research for diagnosis and treatment has been significantly impacted by three-dimensional printing [46]. Pharmaceutical dosage forms with a wide range of shapes, release profiles, and medication combinations can be created via 3D printing [47]. Various printing technologies used by pharmaceutical industries are inkjet printing method used for colour modelling [48], stereolithography used in bone and dental model [49], multiJet modelling used in dental casts [49], fused deposition modelling used in medical instruments and rapid prototyping exoskeleton [50]. Other printers commercially used for 3D printing include continuous inkjet printer, drop-on-demand inkjet printer, thermal inkjet printer, and binder jet printer [47]. The available marketed product example i.e., Spritam® technology is approved as one the effective 3D printed drug products for the treatment of epilepsy, utilizing the zip dose technique. Another example of 3D printing medical material is DENTCA and OsteoFab™ is a patient specific cranial device [51].

6.5.7 Biomarkers-assisted diagnosis in relation to drug–diagnostic co-development

Biomarkers are used to identify individuals with a particular disease subtype or to detect or confirm the presence of an illness or condition of interest. It can be used in terms of diagnosis, monitoring, prediction, progression, safety and response [52]. Various biomarkers currently being used are HLA allele (HLA-B5701) to identify hypersensitivity reactions caused by abacavir therapy [53], TRACERx analysis to identify earlier circulating tumour DNA [54], sweat chloride for detection of cystic fibrosis [55], monoclonal protein (M Protein) for detection of monoclonal gammopathy leading to blood cancer [56], Apolipoprotein E (APOE) gene variations for analysing the risk of Alzheimer's disease [57] and serum creatinine that can be used to monitor nephrotoxicity [58]. Circulating cancer biomarker development is a rapidly growing field. Recent evidence suggests a real clinical value for the use of biomarkers [59] (table 6.2).

6.5.8 Nanocarrier therapy for treating invasive tumours

This includes using lipid-based nanoparticles, metal-based nanoparticles, inhibiting efflux transporters [72]. Lipid-based nanoparticles can be lBNP CPT-11 (Phase I)/ Lactoferrin- and RGD-commodified, temozolomide and vincristine-coloaded nanostructured lipid carriers for gliomatosis cerebri combination. Multifunctional targeting daunorubicin plus quinacrine liposomes are modified by wheat germ agglutinin and tamoxifen, for treating brain glioma and glioma stem cells. Paclitaxel is delivered using positively-charged solid lipid nanoparticles in the treatment of glioblastoma. Gold nanoparticles used with cisplatin, doxorubicin (DOX), L-aspartate TMZ, and iron oxide nanoparticles used with chlorotoxin, gemcitabine, PTX, 5-fluorouracil, DOX are examples of metal-based nanoparticles. Rats bearing glioma xenografts live longer when magnetic nanoparticles are combined with magnetic paclitaxel nanoparticles. PEGylated-poly (L-lactic co-glycolic acid), polybutylcyanoacrylate, and poly (-amino ester) are examples of polymer-based nanoparticles [73, 74].

Table 6.2. Representation of biomarkers for various cancers.

Sr. No.	Biomarkers	Remark	References
1.	pANCAs (Antineutrophil cytoplasmic antibodies)ASCAs (Anti-Saccharomyces cerevisiae antibodies)	Biomarkers for Crohn's disease and ulcerative colitis	[60]
2.	CA 19–9 (Carbohydrate antigen marker)	Biomarkers for pancreatic monitoring therapy	[61]
3.	tCECs (tumour-associated circulating endothelial cells)	New diagnostic marker for prostate cancer	[62]
4.	MT2(Melatonin receptor), peripheral blood mononuclear cells (PBMCs) and programmed cell death ligand-1	Serving as prognostic marker for non-small cell lung cancer (NSCLC)	[63–65]
5.	Tissue polypeptide-specific antigen (TPS)	Serves as prognostic marker for breast cancer	[66]
6.	Serum alpha fetoprotein (AFP), des-gamma-carboxy prothrombin (DCP) TSGF (tumour-specific growth factor)	Serum tumour markers for detection of hepatocellular carcinoma	[67, 68]
7.	NMP 22 (nuclear matrix protein)	Marker for detecting bladder cancer	[69]
8.	MSI (microsatellite instability)	Predictive biomarkers for metastatic solid tumours	[65]
9.	BCR-ABL1 marker	Marker for detection of chronic myeloid leukemia (CML)	[70]
10.	TPS	Biomarkers for colorectal cancer	[71]

6.5.9 Digital inhaler devices

Digital inhaler devices are another AI-based device that helps to manage and treat respiratory disorders including asthma and chronic obstructive pulmonary disease (COPD), digital inhaler devices—also referred to as smart inhalers or connected inhalers—combine traditional inhalers with digital technology. These tools are designed to improve drug adherence, track usage patterns, offer individualized insights, and give patients the power to take charge of their respiratory health. Digital inhalers can include capabilities like environmental monitoring in addition to medication adherence and data insights. Some devices are capable of detecting environmental elements that may have an impact on respiratory symptoms, such as pollen counts and air quality. By avoiding triggers or modifying their treatment plans appropriately, patients can benefit from proactive management of their diseases thanks to this information [75, 76].

6.6 Challenges in the personalized healthcare field

To analyze the barriers and hazards of a particular healthcare system, it is urgently necessary to analyze the fundamental features of that particular healthcare system and its components. Personalized healthcare, which involves tailoring medical treatments to individual patients based on their unique genetic, environmental, and lifestyle factors, is a key area in the healthcare system. Healthcare treatments and practices, especially in the area of personalized healthcare, often differ across countries and even across different regions, peoples of different income groups of the same country. Most of the developed countries of the world largely depend on the conventional medicine healthcare model which uses different professionally qualified medical stakeholders to deliver medical advice and other ailments to make people and the nation healthier. However, in developing nations, apart from the conventional medicine healthcare model, naturopathic medicine is significantly important in the holistic wellness of the people. For example, in the conventional model, the doctor might prescribe a medicine to normalize blood pressure and sugar. In the naturopathic model, a medical advisor may suggest herbs, diet, and exercise as remedies [77]. The major differences behind the application of different healthcare models between developed and developing nations are traditional knowledge, people's perception, education, resources, and health infrastructure. Different health indices have been developed by researchers around the world to gauge the standards and deficiencies of healthcare systems in different countries of the world and in different parts of a particular country. The WHO also provides different statistical data related to health issues of different countries. Recently, WHO published World Health Report, 2022 [78] which amply feeds researchers with necessary information for making comparisons, detecting the lacunae and making policy recommendations to improve overall and personalized healthcare systems. Besides this, some other notable indices like Global Wellness Index developed by investment firm Letter One, Bloomberg's Healthiest Country Index, Universal Health Coverage Index by WHO, Euro health consumer index (EHCI) by Health Consumer Power House, Roche's FutureProofing Personalized Healthcare Index etc also provide relevant information for the research and analysis on this area.

From the overall analysis of different reports and indices it may be observed that in many countries the established healthcare system requires revolutionary changes due to the inadequacy of current health systems in meeting the diverse healthcare needs of people, coupled with the escalating costs of healthcare delivery. This has resulted in an uneven distribution of healthcare services, leading to unjust outcomes, reduced wellbeing, and diminished economic productivity. The central objective of healthcare should be personalized care, which serves to fortify health systems and enhance the overall wellbeing of our society. The COVID-19 pandemic also highlighted the need for a personalized and data-driven approach to healthcare. It is clear that there is no single solution that fits everyone's needs when it comes to health. Whether it's prevention, treatment, or rehabilitation, we must tailor our approach to our unique circumstances. This includes being proactive in managing our risk factors and overall health, rather than waiting until we become sick. The pandemic has raised awareness of the importance of taking preventative measures and using data to make informed decisions about our health [79]. Hence personalized healthcare has become an area of budding interest and investment in healthcare sectors across the globe. Though it has the potential to revolutionize the healthcare industry, there are several logistic and financial obstacles that must be addressed before it can become widely available to the people. In this article, we will explore these limitations and discuss some potential solutions to overcome them. Now in order to find out these obstacles and limitations, if we can analyze the components or parameters described in various health indices, then we will be able to reach our goal much faster. One of the health indices we mentioned earlier is the FutureProofing Personalized Healthcare Index [80]. Several studies have been conducted based on this personalized healthcare index to address different social, legal and economic issues on healthcare and for the holistic development of personalized healthcare systems [81–83]. Many of its components have been adopted from indicators considered by WHO and other organizations. Here, primarily four important metrics have been used viz. health information, health services, personalized technologies and policy context. Each primary metric contains several parameters in terms of which the performance and personalized healthcare status of different countries of the world have been measured. The metric health information includes cancer registries, data infrastructure, national EHR strategy and its uses, patient data control, patient right to access data, regional cross-border data-sharing system, regulatory frameworks for the provision of e-health services etc. The second primary metric health services consider parameters like academic articles on personalized medicine, equity in terms of GINI Coefficient, genomic testing, integrated care initiatives, number of practicing physicians per 1000 people, expenditure on R&D as percentage of GDP, level of implementation of telemedicine etc. The third primary metric personalized technologies comprise the share of the adult population who would use a connected health device, decision support systems in mobile-health (M-health) technology, availability of CAR-T therapy, genetic disease screening, telemedicine penetration in hospitals, share of population with wearable healthcare devices etc. Finally, the fourth metric policy context which covers polities, frameworks, partnerships, people, and drivers that will facilitate personalized healthcare include access to digital education, access to data for research, total number of bio banks, civic participation in sharing personal data, consideration of AI and genomics ethics, digitalization of public services, policy concerning the use of genomics in healthcare or health services, extent of internet access, national AI initiatives, existence of public–private partnership (PPP) legislation and number of PPP projects in the healthcare sector, rural–urban internet usage gap etc.

We have noticed a lot of obstacles, problems, and difficulties when critically analyzing various writings and reflections of health indices. There are also variations in the level, trend, spread, etc of the problems. After all, in many cases the problems are interrelated and related to the problems in different social and economic contexts. While it is not possible to analyze all the problems on this small scale, some important financial and logistic obstacles that we can mention are as follows.

6.6.1 Economical obstacles allied with personalized healthcare

(a) **Treatment cost:** Personalized healthcare is expensive, as it requires specialized technologies and treatments that may not be covered by insurance and not bearable by poorer strata of population. This can limit access to personalized healthcare for patients who cannot afford it. Especially in developing economies due to huge inequality of income and wealth, treatment cost is a significant burden for the underprivileged class of people.
(b) **Investment in health infrastructure, research and development:** Huge investment is required for development in health infrastructure, especially in underdeveloped countries. Besides improvement in health infrastructure, significant investment is required in R&D activities for improving personalized healthcare systems. R&D expenditure as percentage of GDP is significantly low in developed as well as in developing nations.
(c) **Public expenditure on the health sector:** Increase in public expenditure on health is one of the most important factors for equal accessibility of personal healthcare facilities for the majority of people in most parts of the world. However, in the context of increasing trends in fiscal deficit, increasing public expenditure on health sector is a major challenge facing all countries of the world.
(d) **Economic inequality:** Huge income inequality as reflected through the GINI coefficient, especially in developing nations, makes many personalized healthcare benefits, such as use of wearables, M-Health technology, bio banks etc, mere daydreams for a significant portion of population.
(e) **Insurance coverage:** Insurance coverage is very important in the context of personalized healthcare. In many parts of the world insurance coverage for personalized healthcare treatments is limited or nonexistent. This creates a financial burden for patients who require these treatments but cannot afford them. Reimbursement of insurance coverage is also a burning problem in personalized healthcare. In many cases insured persons are not reimbursed for the full cost of personalized healthcare treatments. This creates financial disincentives for the people adopting these treatments.

6.6.2 Logistic complications associated with personalized healthcare

(a) **Data collection and analysis:** Personalized healthcare relies on the collection and analysis of large amounts of patient data. This requires a robust and secure data infrastructure, and also requires advanced analytics and machine learning capabilities to process and interpret the data.
(b) **Inadequacy of number of qualified doctors and trained supporting staff:** In many parts of the world qualified medical professionals are inadequate compared to their requirements for having a sound personalized healthcare system. Besides this, physicians need to be educated on how to use and interpret personalized healthcare data. This will require additional training and resources to ensure that they are able to incorporate this data into their clinical decision-making.

(c) **Regulatory approval:** New personalized healthcare treatments and technologies require regulatory approval before they can be implemented in a clinical setting. This can be a time-consuming and expensive process that may delay the availability of these treatments to patients.
(d) **Privacy concerns:** With so much sensitive data being collected, privacy concerns can arise. There is a risk of data breaches, which can have serious consequences for patients and healthcare providers.
(e) **Infrastructure:** Personalized healthcare requires advanced infrastructure to support data processing, storage, and analysis. This can be a major barrier for smaller healthcare providers who may not have the resources to invest in these technologies.

6.7 Personalized healthcare—futuristic possibilities

Personalized healthcare is a rapidly growing field that holds immense potential for revolutionizing healthcare delivery across the globe. The main pillars in the future of personalized healthcare are access, affordability and equality. Although difficult trade-offs are inevitable, there are opportunities to simultaneously improve access, affordability, and equity [84]. The key objective is to develop novel, tailored, data-driven, and resilient health systems that are equipped for the future. This approach has the potential to improve patient outcomes and reduce healthcare costs by targeting the underlying causes of disease and providing more effective treatments. To achieve this, there is a need for extensive collaboration across different sectors and borders, holistic utilization of data, and the integration of emerging digital technologies to build better, sustainable, and personalized healthcare systems. As we look to the future, there are several exciting possibilities for personalized healthcare that could transform the way we think about personalized healthcare. The following are some of the futuristic possibilities:

- **Cost reduction:** Healthcare providers and manufacturers should take necessary steps to reduce the cost of healthcare products and services. This can be achieved through increased competition, the development of generic drugs and medical devices, and the negotiation of lower prices with insurance providers. For example, HDFC Ergo Health Insurance offers a 'no claim bonus' feature, which rewards customers with a discount on their premium if they do not make any claims during the policy period. Apollo Munich Health Insurance offers a 'restore benefit,' which restores the entire sum insured if the customer exhausts their coverage during the policy period. They also offer discounts for purchasing policies online and for long-term policies etc. In future, more such offers will enrich the personalized healthcare system. The government should also provide necessary support and government agencies should keep strict vigilance on these endeavors.
- **Expansion of insurance coverage:** Insurance providers should be encouraged to expand coverage for alternative therapies and preventive care. By covering a broader range of healthcare products and services, insurance providers can help to improve patients' access to care and reduce the financial burden of

healthcare. For example, United Healthcare (USA) offers discounts for customers who participate in wellness programs, quit smoking, or achieve certain health milestones; ICICI Lombard Health Insurance offers coverage for alternative therapies like Ayurveda, yoga, and naturopathy under their Wellness Program. They also cover preventive health checkups for policyholders; Blue Cross Blue Shield (USA) offers coverage for acupuncture, naturopathy under their Alternative Medicine policy. They also cover preventive care services like annual physicals and mammograms. In future, other alternative and preventive therapies will also be covered by personalized healthcare service providers. Necessary legislations should be enacted through insurance regulatory and development authorities.

- **Genomic and personalized medicine:** The field of genomics has made significant progress in recent years, with the cost of sequencing a genome dropping significantly. This has led to the development of personalized genomic medicine, which involves using a patient's genetic information to diagnose and treat disease [85]. With the increasing availability of genetic testing, we can expect to see a rise in personalized treatments that are tailored to a patient's unique genetic profile. For example, genetic testing can be used to identify patients who are at higher risk for certain diseases and recommend early interventions, genomic sequencing enables doctors to identify genetic variations that may affect drug metabolism, efficacy, or side effects. This information can be used to customize drug doses or select alternative drugs that are more effective for the patient.
- **Wearable technology:** Wearable technology is already a growing trend in healthcare, with devices like Fitbit and Apple Watch tracking activity levels, heart rate, and other health metrics [86]. Besides these, Biostrap is a wearable device that tracks physical activity and monitors vital signs like heart rate and blood oxygen levels. The device also includes a sleep tracker that provides detailed insights into sleep quality and duration, allowing users to make adjustments to their sleep habits for better health. Lumen is another wearable device that analyzes users' breath to determine their metabolic rate and provide personalized nutrition recommendations. However, the next wave of wearable technology is likely to be even more sophisticated, with devices that can monitor blood glucose levels, detect early signs of disease, and provide personalized feedback on lifestyle and diet.
- **Artificial intelligence:** AI has the potential to transform healthcare delivery by enabling more accurate and timely diagnosis and treatment [87]. With the help of AI, doctors can analyze large amounts of medical data to identify patterns and predict outcomes, which can lead to more effective treatments and better patient outcomes. For example, Babylon Health is a mobile app that uses AI-powered chatbots to provide users with medical advice and guidance. The app can help users manage chronic conditions, order prescriptions, and access healthcare providers via video chat. Path AI is a digital pathology platform that uses AI algorithms to analyze medical images and help pathologists diagnose diseases like cancer. Ada Health is an AI-powered

health assessment tool that helps users identify potential health issues and receive personalized health advice. The app uses machine learning algorithms to analyze user data and provide personalized recommendations for improving health and wellness. In future, these AI-based health platforms will play a more important role in personalized healthcare.

- **Telemedicine:** The COVID-19 pandemic has accelerated the adoption of telemedicine, with more patients opting for virtual consultations rather than in-person appointments. As technology continues to improve, we can expect to see even more sophisticated telemedicine platforms that enable patients to receive personalized care from anywhere in the world. For example, Teladoc, Doctor on Demand, Amwell, MDLIVE etc are telemedicine platforms that allow users to consult with healthcare providers via video, phone, or messaging. The platform offers a range of services, including primary care, mental health, and dermatology consultations, as well as chronic care management.
- **Improvement in EHR:** Healthcare providers should work to improve the coordination and accessibility of patient information. This can be achieved through the adoption of common EHR systems and the development of standards for sharing patient data. By improving the exchange of information, healthcare providers can ensure that patients receive the most effective and appropriate care. For example, Epic Systems Corporation's EHR platform, called EpicCare, enables healthcare providers to manage patient information, track medical histories, and coordinate care across different specialties and settings, Cerner Corporation's EHR platform, called Power Chart, provides healthcare providers with tools for managing patient information, tracking medical histories, and coordinating care across different settings, Allscripts' Sunrise is also an EHR platform which offers a range of tools for managing patient information, tracking medical histories, and coordinating care across different specialties and settings.
- **Blockchain technology:** Blockchain technology has the potential to transform healthcare by enabling secure, decentralized sharing of medical data. With blockchain, patients can maintain control over their medical records, and doctors can access real-time medical information from anywhere in the world [88]. This can lead to more accurate diagnoses and more personalized treatments. For example, medical chain, Burst IQ, Simply Vital Health etc are blockchain-based platforms that allow patients to control and share their medical records with healthcare providers securely. These platforms provide patients with a digital wallet that stores their medical records and allows them to grant or revoke access to healthcare providers as needed.

The futuristic possibilities of personalized healthcare, analyzing its potential strengths, weaknesses, opportunities and threats (SWOT) in the context of the broader healthcare landscape may be presented with the help of the following diagram (figure 6.3).

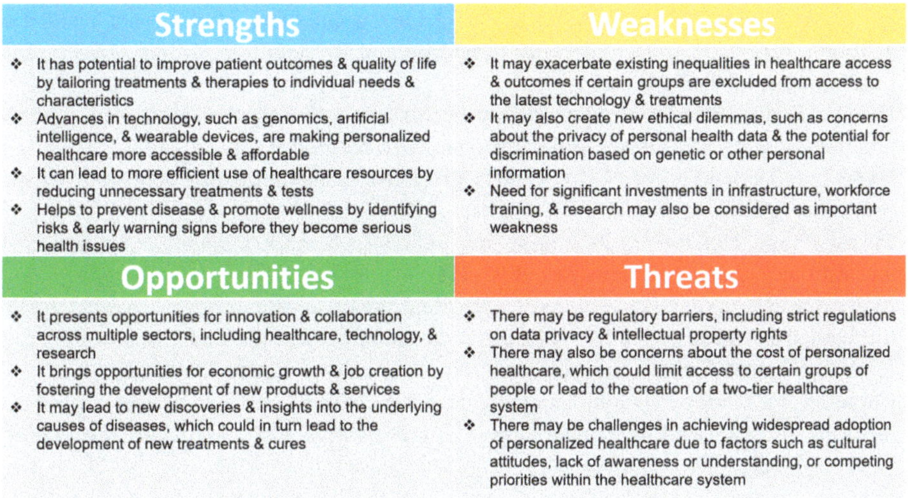

Figure 6.3. The SWOT analysis for personalized healthcare.

6.8 Conclusion

There have been ground-breaking advances in personalised healthcare including DNA-based screening, introduction of AI in healthcare, liquid biopsy, healthcare digitalization, new born screening, 3D printing, nanocarrier based therapy, digital inhaler devices. However, personal healthcare is confronted with significant financial and logistical obstacles, yet there are numerous opportunities to improve the system over its present status. The system can be enriched by reducing the cost of healthcare products and services, expanding insurance coverage, and improving the coordination of patient information. There are limitless possibilities for personalized healthcare, and with the continuous evolution of technology, we can expect even more innovative solutions that offer patients timely and effective care. However, new technologies also bring challenges, such as privacy concerns, data security, and regulatory oversight. In conclusion, the future of personalized healthcare is promising, and with the right investments in technology and innovation, we can establish a healthcare system that is personalized, efficient, and accessible to all.

References

[1] Evans J and Khoury M J 2007 Evidence based medicine meets genomic medicine *Genetics Med.* **9** 799–800

[2] Spaulding A *et al* 2017 Organizational capacity for change in health care: development and validation of a scale *Health Care Manage. Rev.* **42** 151–61

[3] Neves A L and Burgers J 2022 Digital technologies in primary care: implications for patient care and future research *Eur. J. Gen. Pract* **28** 203–8

[4] Pritchard D E *et al* 2017 Strategies for integrating personalized medicine into healthcare practice *Per. Med.* **14** 141–52

[5] Al-Aswad A M *et al* 2013 A review paper of the current status of electronic health records adoption worldwide: the gap between developed and developing countries *J. Health Inform. Dev. Countries* **7** 153–64

[6] Hanson K and Berman P 1998 Private health care provision in developing countries: a preliminary analysis of levels and composition *Health Policy Plan.* **13** 195–211

[7] Hood L and Friend S H J N R C O 2011 Predictive, personalized, preventive, participatory (P4) cancer medicine *Nat. Rev. Clin. Oncol.* **8** 184–7

[8] Tiwari R and Herstatt C 2012 Assessing india's lead market potential for cost-effective innovations *J. Indian Business Res.* **4** 97–115

[9] Malone KJTIJoCsR 2015 Children's rights and the crisis of rapid urbanisation: Exploring the United Nations post 2015 sustainable development agenda and the potential role for UNICEF's child friendly cities initiative *Int. J. Children's Rights* **23** 405–24

[10] Chong H Y, Allotey P A and Chaiyakunapruk N 2018 Current landscape of personalized medicine adoption and implementation in Southeast Asia *BMC Med. Genomics* **11** 94

[11] Saito YClinical Pharmacogenetics Implementation Consortium *et al* 2016 Clinical Pharmacogenetics Implementation Consortium (CPIC) guidelines for human leukocyte antigen B (HLA-B) genotype and allopurinol dosing: 2015 update *Clin. Pharmacol. Ther.* **99** 36–7

[12] Pritchard D E *et al* 2017 Strategies for integrating personalized medicine into healthcare practice *Pers Med.* **14** 141–52

[13] Oh T J *et al* 2017 Feasibility of quantifying SDC2 methylation in stool DNA for early detection of colorectal cancer *Clin. Epigen.* **9** 126

[14] Lin N *et al* 2022 A multi-analyte cell-free DNA-based blood test for early detection of hepatocellular carcinoma *Hepatol. Commun.* **6** 1753–63

[15] Jung C, Allen P B and Ellington A D J N 2016 A stochastic DNA Walker that traverses a microparticle surface *Nat. Nanotechnol.* **11** 157–63

[16] Wang Q *et al* 2022 Development of the DNA-based biosensors for high performance in detection of molecular biomarkers: more rapid, sensitive, and universal *Biosens. Bioelectron.* **197** 113739

[17] Schwarz U I *et al* 2008 Genetic determinants of response to warfarin during initial anticoagulation *New Engl. J. Med.* **358** 999–1008

[18] Vetsch J *et al* 2018 Cancer-related genetic testing and personalized medicine for adolescents: a narrative review of impact and understanding *J. Adolesc. Young Adult Oncol.* **7** 259–62

[19] Dweba C C, Zishiri O T and El Zowalaty M E 2019 Isolation and molecular identification of virulence, antimicrobial and heavy metal resistance genes in livestock-associated methicillin-resistant staphylococcus aureus *Pathogens* **8** 79

[20] Hamet P and Tremblay J J 2017 Artificial intelligence in medicine *Matabolism* **69** S36–40

[21] Johnson K B *et al* 2021 Precision medicine, AI, and the future of personalized health care *Clin. Transl. Sci.* **14** 86–93

[22] Kudo S E *et al* 2019 Artificial intelligence and colonoscopy: current status and future perspectives *Digest. Endosc.* **31** 363–71

[23] Bibault J-E *et al* 2018 Deep learning and radiomics predict complete response after neo-adjuvant chemoradiation for locally advanced rectal cancer *Sci. Rep.* **8** 12611

[24] Parreco J *et al* 2018 Using artificial intelligence to predict prolonged mechanical ventilation and tracheostomy placement *J. Surg. Res.* **228** 179–87

[25] Fergus P, Hussain A J B E O, Al-Jumeily Obe D, Huang D-S and Bouguila N 2017 Classification of Caesarean section and normal vaginal deliveries using foetal heart rate signals and advanced machine learning algorithms *BioMed. Eng. OnLine* **16** 89
[26] Han X, Wang J and Sun Y 2017 Circulating tumor DNA as biomarkers for cancer detection *Genom. Proteom. Bioinform.* **15** 59–72
[27] Di Meo A *et al* 2017 Liquid biopsy: a step forward towards precision medicine in urologic malignancies *Mol. Cancer* **16** 80
[28] Wan J *et al* 2017 Liquid biopsies come of age: towards implementation of circulating tumour *DNA* **17** 223–38
[29] Lone S N *et al* 2022 Liquid biopsy: a step closer to transform diagnosis, prognosis and future of cancer treatments *Mol. Cancer* **21** 79
[30] Baumgart D C 2005 Personal digital assistants in health care: experienced clinicians in the palm of your hand? *Lancet* **366** 1210–22
[31] Medicare C f and Medicaid Services H J F r 2010 Medicare and medicaid programs; electronic health record incentive program *Final Rule* **75** 44313–588
[32] Enders S J, Enders J M and Holstad S G 2002 Drug-information software for Palm operating system personal digital assistants: breadth, clinical dependability, and ease of use *Pharmacotherapy* **22** 1036–40
[33] Schmidt M *et al* 2019 The Danish health care system and epidemiological research: from health care contacts to database records *Clin. Epidemiol.* **11** 563–91
[34] Steffens T G, Gunser J M and Saviello G M 2015 Perfusion electronic record documentation using epic systems software *J. Extra. Corpor. Technol* **47** 237–41
[35] DeShazo J P and Hoffman M A 2015 A comparison of a multistate inpatient EHR database to the HCUP Nationwide Inpatient Sample *BMC Health Serv. Res.* **15** 384
[36] Taylor A *et al* 2022 Development and testing of data infrastructure in the American college of emergency physicians' clinical emergency data registry for opioid-related research *J. Am. Coll. Emerg. Physicians Open* **3** e12816
[37] Scalia K 2009 Facilitating data exchange *Behav. Healthc.* **29** 30–1
[38] Santillana M *et al* 2016 Cloud-based electronic health records for real-time, region-specific influenza surveillance *Sci. Rep.* **6** 25732
[39] Yang L, Chen J and Shen B 2017 Newborn screening in the era of precision medicine *Adv. Exp. Med. Biol.* **1005** 47–61
[40] Pitt J J 2010 Newborn screening *Clin. Biochem. Rev.* **31** 57–68
[41] McCandless S E and Wright E J 2020 Mandatory newborn screening in the United States: History, current status, and existential challenges *Birth Defects Res.* **112** 350–66
[42] Thangaratinam S *et al* 2012 Pulse oximetry screening for critical congenital heart defects in asymptomatic newborn babies: a systematic review and meta-analysis *Lancet* **379** 2459–64
[43] US Preventive Services Task Force 2008 Universal screening for hearing loss in newborns: US Preventive Services Task Force recommendation statement *Pediatrics* **122** 143–8
[44] 2011 Ten great public health achievements--United States, 2001–2010 *MMWR Morb. Mortal Wkly. Rep.* **60** 619–23
[45] McCabe L L and McCabe E R B 2008 Expanded newborn screening: implications for genomic medicine *Ann. Rev. Med.* **59** 163–75
[46] Bhuskute H, Shende P and Prabhakar B 2021 3D printed personalized medicine for cancer: applications for betterment of diagnosis, prognosis and treatment *AAPS Pharm. Sci. Tech.* **23** 8

[47] Vaz V M and Kumar L 2021 3D printing as a promising tool in personalized medicine *AAPS Pharm. Sci. Tech.* **22** 49

[48] Aimar A, Palermo A and Innocenti B 2019 The role of 3D printing in medical applications: a state of the art *J. Healthc. Eng.* **2019** 5340616

[49] Cohen A *et al* 2009 Mandibular reconstruction using stereolithographic 3-dimensional printing modeling technology *Oral Maxillofacial Surg.* **108** 661–6

[50] Tanaka K S and Lightdale-Miric N J J 2016 Advances in 3D-printed pediatric prostheses for upper extremity differences *J. Bone Joint Surg.* **98** 1320–6

[51] Prasad L K and Smyth H 2016 3D Printing technologies for drug delivery: a review *Drug Dev. Ind. Pharm.* **42** 1019–31

[52] Gromova M *et al* 2020 Biomarkers: opportunities and challenges for drug development in the current regulatory landscape *Biomark. Insights* **15** 1177271920974652

[53] Phillips E and Mallal S 2009 Successful translation of pharmacogenetics into the clinic: the abacavir example *Mol. Diagn. Ther.* **13** 1–9

[54] Jamal-Hanjani M *et al* 2014 Tracking genomic cancer evolution for precision medicine: the lung TRACERx study *PLoS Biol.* **12** e1001906

[55] Farrell P M *et al* 2008 Guidelines for diagnosis of cystic fibrosis in newborns through older adults: Cystic Fibrosis Foundation Consensus Report *J. Pediat.* **153** S4–S14

[56] Kyle R A *et al* 2002 A long-term study of prognosis in monoclonal gammopathy of undetermined significance *New Engl. J. Med.* **346** 564–9

[57] Chartier-Hariln M-C *et al* 1994 Apolipoprotein E, ε4 allele as a major risk factor for sporadic early and late-onset forms of Alzheimer's disease: analysis of the 19q13 2 chromosomal region *Hum. Mol. Genetics* **3** 569–74

[58] Wasung M E, Chawla L S and Madero M J 2015 Biomarkers of renal function, which and when? *Clin. Chim. Acta* **438** 350–7

[59] Ruwali M *et al* 2021 Updates in pharmacogenetics of non-small cell lung cancer *Pharmacogenetics* ed I A Khalil (InTech Open)

[60] Viennois E, Zhao Y and Merlin D 2015 Biomarkers of inflammatory bowel disease: from classical laboratory tools to personalized medicine *Inflamm. Bowel. Dis.* **21** 2467–74

[61] Ludwig J A and Weinstein J N J N R C 2005 Biomarkers in cancer staging, prognosis and treatment selection *Nat. Rev. Cancer* **5** 845–56

[62] Bhakdi S C *et al* 2019 Accuracy of tumour-associated circulating endothelial cells as a screening biomarker for clinically significant prostate cancer *Cancers* **11** 1064

[63] Jablonska K *et al* 2019 Prognostic impact of melatonin receptors MT1 and MT2 in non-small cell lung cancer (NSCLC) *Cancers* **11** 1001

[64] Noé G *et al* 2019 Differential kinase activation in peripheral blood mononuclear cells from non-small-cell lung cancer patients treated with nivolumab *Cancers* **11** 762

[65] Wang Y *et al* 2021 FDA-approved and emerging next generation predictive biomarkers for immune checkpoint inhibitors in cancer patients *Front. Oncol.* **11** 683419

[66] Ahn S K and Jung S Y 2021 Current biomarkers for precision medicine in breast cancer *Adv. Exp. Med. Biol.* **1187** 363–79

[67] Zhou L, Liu J and Luo F 2006 Serum tumor markers for detection of hepatocellular carcinoma *World J. Gastroenterol* **12** 1175–81

[68] Behne T and Copur M S 2012 Biomarkers for hepatocellular carcinoma *Inter. J. Hepatol.* **2012** 859076

[69] Wang Z *et al* 2017 Evaluation of the NMP22 bladderchek test for detecting bladder cancer: a systematic review and meta-analysis *Oncotarget* **8** 100648–56
[70] Quintás-Cardama A and Cortes J 2009 Molecular biology of bcr-abl1-positive chronic myeloid leukemia *Blood* **113** 1619–30
[71] Lech G *et al* 2016 Colorectal cancer tumour markers and biomarkers: recent therapeutic advances *World J. Gastroenterol.* **22** 1745–55
[72] Upton D H *et al* 2022 Challenges and opportunities to penetrate the blood-brain barrier for brain cancer therapy *Theranostics* **12** 4734–52
[73] Martinelli C, Pucci C and Ciofani G 2019 Nanostructured carriers as innovative tools for cancer diagnosis and therapy *APL Bioeng.* **3** 011502
[74] Wei Q Y, Xu Y M and Lau A T Y 2020 Recent progress of nanocarrier-based therapy for solid malignancies *Cancers (Basel)* **12**
[75] Mehta P P 2021 Dry powder inhalers: a concise summary of the electronic monitoring devices *Ther. Deliv.* **12** 1–6
[76] Henriet A C *et al* 2010 Respimat®, first Soft Mist™ inhaler: new perspectives in the management of COPD *Rev. Mal. Respir* **27** 1141–9
[77] Tauziaq J 2021 Healthcare in developing vs. developed countries Study.com https://study.com/academy/lesson/healthcare-in-developing-vs-developed-countries.html
[78] World health statistics 2022 Monitoring health for the SDGs, sustainable development goals https://who.int/publications/i/item/9789240051157
[79] Atzmon S 2022 A personalized approach and focus on prevention will transform healthcare management in India *Health News* https://health.economictimes.indiatimes.com/news/industry/a-personalized-approach-and-focus-on-prevention-will-transform-healthcare-management-in-india/90800485
[80] Roche Futureproofing Healthcare. Personalised Health Index. https://futureproofinghealthcare.com/en
[81] Horgan D, Borisch B and Richer E *et al* 2020 Propelling health care into the twenties *Biomed. Hub.* **5** 15–67
[82] Błoński M 2019 Legal and economic aspects of healthcare systems in the Netherlands and Luxembourg *IusNovum* **13** 14–34
[83] Orlinski R and Macuda M 2022 Management crisis in health care system in COVID-19 conditions *Eur. Res. Studies J.* **25** 52–61
[84] Shrank W H, DeParle N A, Gottlieb S, Jain S H, Orszag P and Powers B W *et al* 2021Feb1 Health costs and financing: challenges and strategies for a new administration *Health Affairs (Millwood)* **40** 235–42
[85] Ginsburg G S and Willard H F 2009 Genomic and personalized medicine: foundations and applications *Transl. Res.* **154** 277–87
[86] Smuck M, Odonkor C A and Wilt J K *et al* 2021 The emerging clinical role of wearables: factors for successful implementation in healthcare *Npj Digit. Med.* **4** 45
[87] Bajwa J, Munir U, Nori A and Williams B 2021 Artificial intelligence in healthcare: transforming the practice of medicine *Future Healthcare J.* **8** e188–94
[88] Saeed H, Malik H, Bashir U, Ahmad A, Riaz S and Ilyas M *et al* 2022 Blockchain technology in healthcare: a systematic review *PLoS One* **17** e0266462

IOP Publishing

Advances in Drug Delivery Systems for Healthcare
From concept to clinic
Piyush Pradeep Mehta and Arpana Parihar

Chapter 7

Advances and future trends in medical inhalers

Nani Kadrichu

This chapter provides a brief background of orally inhaled therapy and its potential benefits compared to oral gastrointestinal delivery, then comprehensively reviews the four groups of medical inhalers: pressurized metered dose inhalers (pMDIs), dry powder inhalers (DPIs), nebulizers, and soft mist inhalers (SMIs). For each group, the narrative presents high level operating principles, shortcomings, and mitigating improvements. The story of well-designed inhalers used in some failed clinical trials is also discussed. The author presents how advances in pMDI design have addressed patient coordination and dose variability issues. Scrutiny of propellant use has driven efforts to develop more environmentally friendly options. The chapter follows with a discussion of DPIs, presenting single-dose and multi-dose inhalers followed by the Open-Inhale-Close concept. The author also elaborates on some of the first DPIs used to deliver systemic therapies through the lungs. Attention is drawn to common misconceptions surrounding high resistance inhalers and how better understanding can facilitate future DPI designs. New DPI design approaches are also presented. Next, the history of nebulizers is reviewed starting from low efficiency jet nebulizers to the introduction of vibrating mesh nebulizers to improve efficiency. Optimized nebulizers with breath-actuated capabilities are discussed, and the role of nebulizers in critical care is presented. The applications of the final group, SMIs, are then related along with a focus on their reusability. It is the hope of the author that the story of medical inhalers is better understood by reading this chapter.

7.1 Overview of medical inhalers

7.1.1 Why inhalation?

Medication has been aerosolized and delivered directly to the lungs by oral inhalation for thousands of years [1]. It was recognized early on that direct delivery of some locally acting drugs such as corticosteroids and β_2-agonists to the lungs achieved a rapid onset of action and provided fast relief to asthma patients. Local delivery of anti-infective medications such as tobramycin to treat pulmonary

doi:10.1088/978-0-7503-5613-8ch7

infections was also found to enable high therapeutic doses while avoiding side effects resulting from systemic administration. Pulmonary delivery of small and large systemically acting molecules such as levodopa and insulin has been evaluated as a means of bypassing first-pass metabolism, avoiding the discomfort associated with injection, and improving the onset of action.

Delivery by oral inhalation is performed using a medical device known as an inhaler, which is designed to produce an aerosol that consists of small particles or droplets to be breathed in by the patient. These particles should ideally be within a respirable size range to facilitate delivery of the aerosol to the lungs when the medication is properly inhaled. The aerosol itself is produced from a solution, suspension, or dry powder containing the drug substance and excipients as needed to meet target stability and performance criteria. Because of the many factors that must be considered to enable delivery of a sufficient dose of medication to the desired location in the lungs, inhalers have proven very challenging to design. As a result, there are continuing opportunities for improvement of existing inhalers and development of new inhaler approaches.

Even though the first consideration for selection of inhalation as the delivery route of a new medicine is the benefit to the patient, there are also business reasons for pursuing this product form such as market exclusivity. Inhaled products have historically been difficult to develop, require market authorization as combination products, are challenging to administer correctly, and can suffer from poor patient compliance. In contrast, oral pharmaceutical products such as tablets dominate the United States Food and Drug Administration (FDA) approved drug space because they are relatively straightforward to develop, easy to administer, and enjoy high patient compliance. Because the development pathway for inhaled products is very complex, time consuming, and expensive, there is a high barrier to entry of generic competitors for these products as compared to oral products.

A recent example of the difficulty that generic manufacturers face in inhaled product development was the race to market a generic version of Advair Diskus® (GlaxoSmithKline, UK), a fluticasone/salmeterol multi-dose dry powder inhaler (DPI) for asthma therapy. Although the GSK patent for the combination product expired in 2010 and the last patent for the Diskus® DPI device expired in 2016, the first generic competitor (Wixela™ Inhub™, Mylan/Viatris) was not approved until 2019. Other potential competitors were not as successful: Despite investing $442M on their own Advair generic product, Novartis abandoned development in 2020 after receiving a Complete Response Letter from FDA in 2018 [2]. As shown by Zhong [3], oral delivery remains the primary route for registration of new drugs with 62% of total FDA approvals versus 1.2% for inhalation (figure 7.1(A)) over the time frame of 1980 to 2017. Generic drug companies are therefore more likely to pursue registration of oral agents, with the recent percentage of generic drugs registered as orals exceeding 60% (figure 7.1(B)).

As described by Zhong *et al* (2018), companies willing to invest the extra effort in developing and marketing inhaled products are able to enjoy longer market exclusivity for these products when compared to oral drugs. Zhong *et al* calculated a ratio of generic drug approvals to new drug approvals to reflect the technical barriers to generic drug entry for different routes of administration, with the higher

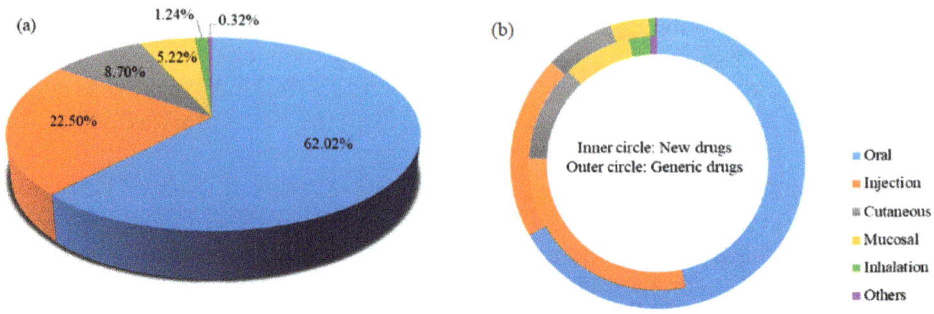

Figure 7.1. (A) The overall distribution of administration route of FDA-approval pharmaceutical products. (B) The proportion of administration route. Inner circle represents drugs; outer circle represents generic drugs. Reproduced from [3] CC BY 4.0.

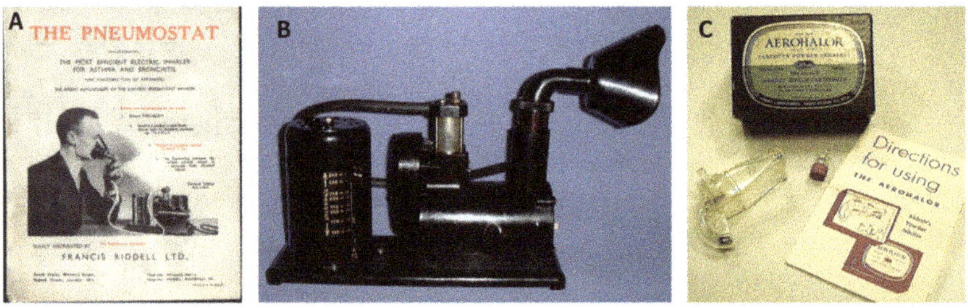

Figure 7.2. A patient using The Pneumostat and a close-up image of The Pneumostat (A and B) and Aerohalor™ (Abbott Laboratories) for isoetharine bronchodilator and penicillin, patented by Mack Fields (C) (courtesy of The Inhalatorium—Mark Sanders).

number corresponding to a lower technical barrier. The oral route presents the lowest technical barrier to entry of a generic drug (ratio of 4.69) while the inhalation route shows the highest technical barrier to entry (ratio of 0.97). Zhong *et al* present these ratios as evidence that oral innovator drugs are much more likely than inhaled innovator drugs to experience generic competition after patent expiry [3].

7.1.2 Where have we been and where are we going?

Modern inhalation devices began to take shape in the 1800s [1]. Continued improvements in their simplicity and efficiency coupled with parallel advances in drug discovery eventually led to significant increases in the number of marketed inhalation products by the mid-20th century. The desire to aerosolize liquids to provide a therapeutic effect resulted in development of early nebulizers including the Pneumostat™ [1] (figures 7.2(A) and (B)), while the use of dry powders to relieve asthma symptoms or congestion led to design of the first DPIs such as the Aerohalor (figure 7.2(C)), the 'first truly commercially successful DPI', approved in 1948 [1]. Inspired by Susie's question *'Daddy, why can't they put my asthma medicine in a spray-can like they do hair spray?'*, Riker's Laboratories drove the development of the first pMDIs for acute asthma therapy in 1956 [1]. Further advances in nebulizer and DPI designs have occurred due to the uptake of these types of inhalers in treatment of other diseases such as cystic fibrosis, for which delivery of large doses of antibiotics to treat local lung infections is required. These inhalers enable delivery of medications to the site of action to achieve a higher local dose than would be possible via systemic exposure due to the concomitant side effects. In 2003, the soft mist inhaler (SMI) was introduced as a propellant-free alternative for delivery of low dose medications [4]. Additional DPI and nebulizer designs have been introduced as the number of molecules considered for delivery by inhalation and their associated therapeutic areas and patient groups continue to expand. For those interested in more details, an entertaining review of the history of inhalers is provided by Stein and Thiel [1]. Other reviews on medical inhalers can be found elsewhere [5–8].

The state of the inhaled therapeutics field circa 2010 was discussed at the 1000 Years of Pharmaceutical Aerosols Conference. One particular session of the conference reviewed the limitations of existing aerosol delivery devices whilst considering opportunities and goals for their continued evolution [6]. This session focused on the pMDI as the primary example of an aerosol device due to its extensive use history, but also touched on DPIs and nebulizers. In proposing sustaining changes that would drive continued evolution of the device space and provide benefit to patients, patient compliance and product efficacy were defined as the areas most in need of continued improvement. Regarding compliance, the authors noted that patients tend to better follow a dosing regimen if they feel that the drug is working, and therefore that the time and effort spent in using the inhaler have been worthwhile. As to efficacy, it was thought that reducing dose variability through new approaches to formulation and device development would lead to improved shot-to-shot content uniformity and total dose delivered for multi-dose inhalers such as pMDI and better unit-to-unit consistency for single-use inhalers such as some DPIs. More reliable and reproducible dosing would then result in better product efficacy, especially for drugs with narrow therapeutic windows. Inhaler design and particle engineering as part of combination product development are examples of sustaining approaches that have been taken to address these requirements.

As anyone who has conducted a human factors study can attest, the user experience is far from consistent and is challenging to accommodate through design only, thus requiring well-tested instructions for use (IFU). As shown in figure 7.3, patient compliance and adherence for inhalers tends to decline more significantly than for other dosage forms, probably reflecting the greater challenges patients face in using inhalers [7]. An inhaler that is intuitive to patients and insensitive to variations in patient physiology and use, while also being safe and inexpensive, was thought to be key to positively affecting patient compliance. Smith *et al* (2010) called for a simple 'open-inhale-close' inhaler design that requires minimal manipulation and ideally provides reliable performance independent of patient inhalation [6]. A dose counter on a pMDI exemplifies the incremental, sustaining improvements that have been made to improve compliance; in this case, through helping the user to know how many doses remain in the pMDI cartridge. An additional example is perhaps the multi-dose DPI, which obviates the need of the patient to open the device to insert a capsule or other powder container to administer every dose.

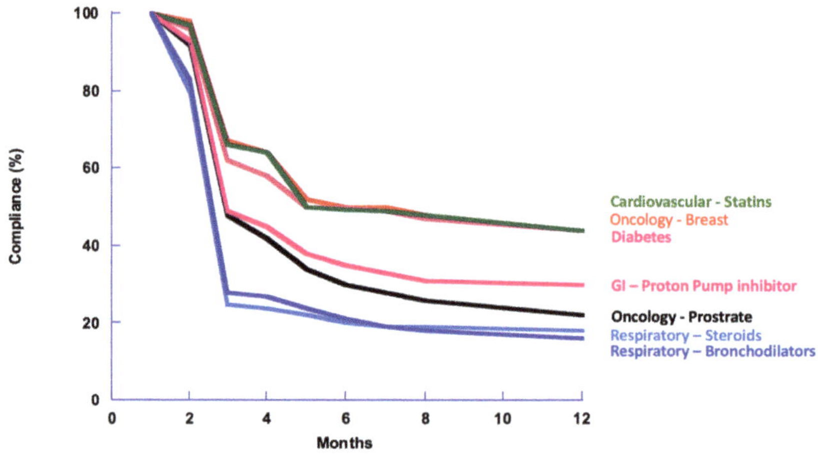

Figure 7.3. Higher reduction in patient compliance for respiratory drug delivery relative to other dosage forms. Adapted from [7] CC BY 4.0.

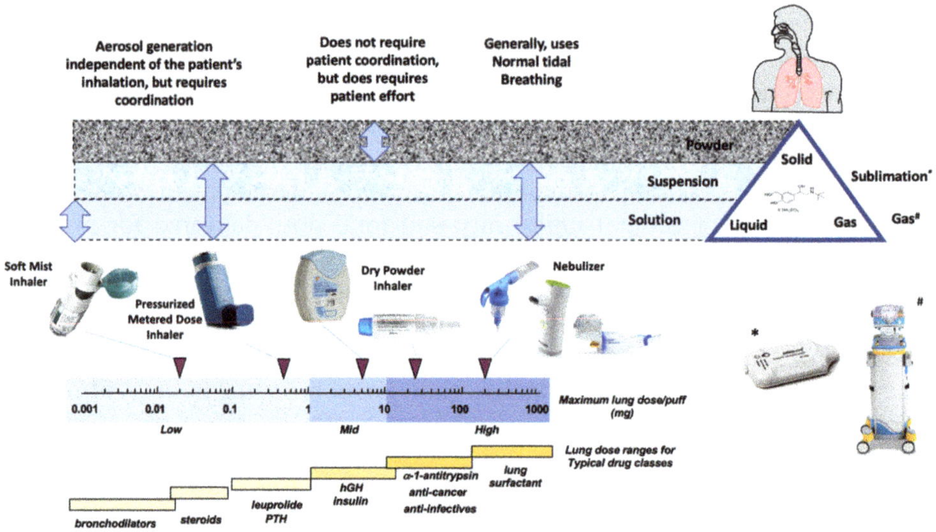

Figure 7.4. Different inhalers for major inhaled drug classes covering different dose requirements (drug form, patient inhalation technique). Adapted from [7] CC BY 4.0.

As predicted, there have been incremental improvements in patient compliance and product efficacy since 2010. Clark (2022) reviewed recent advances and ongoing limitations of the four major aerosol device categories (i.e., pMDI, DPI, nebulizer, and SMI) against the different drug product classes they address and described ways in which these inhalers continue to be developed to better serve these drug classes [7]. For example, advances in particle engineering have enabled design of DPIs with lower pressure drops that can achieve higher fine particle fractions (FPFs) of these powders to improve compliance by reducing patient discomfort and enhancing product efficacy by increasing lung deposition. Also, as described in figure 7.4, as the respiratory disease field has evolved, it has been found that different drugs will require specific aerosol devices depending on their dosing requirements. The pMDIs can only be used for low-dose drugs due to their limited metered volume, while nebulizers are capable of longer delivery time of several milliliters of drug solution. Further device design improvements can thus be targeted to specific disease classes, drug doses, and/or patient populations. In the context of the global pulmonary therapeutics market and opportunities, current formulation strategies, and patient adherence and compliance, this chapter will carefully review the basic operations and current state of the art of the different inhaler types, provide some specific guidance regarding their design and performance, and present a brief overview of some upcoming medical inhalers.

7.2 Pressurized metered dose inhalers (pMDIs)

The pMDI is designed to rapidly aerosolize a small volume of volatile liquid propellant in which a drug substance is either dissolved or dispersed (figure 7.5). In solution pMDIs, the API is either dissolved directly in the propellant or dissolved in ethanol that is then mixed with the propellant. Surfactants may sometimes be used to facilitate drug dissolution or, in the case of suspension pMDIs, to retard particle aggregation and improve dose uniformity. The drug solution or suspension is filled into a canister such that the propellant is placed under pressure. The canister includes a small dosing valve on one end, which when actuated allows a metered dose of the canister contents to flow into the valve. The propellant rapidly undergoes an adiabatic expansion due to drop in pressure, resulting in a two-phase gas/liquid air-blast that forms a dispersion of liquid droplets [8]. pMDIs can deliver a maximum lung dose of approximately 0.5 mg per puff. The canister containing the drug product fits into a holder that is configured to direct the atomized material through a mouthpiece at a high velocity imparted by rapid evaporation of the propellant. The spray duration of a pMDI is typically about 100–200 ms as compared to patient inhalation of several seconds [8]. Therefore, failure to

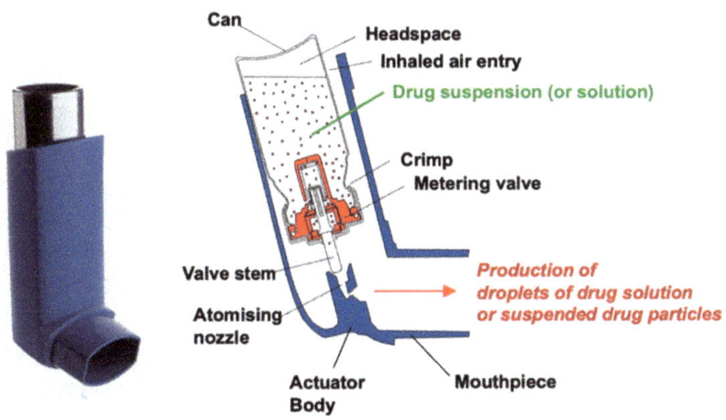

Figure 7.5. A pMDI and its inner workings. (Courtesy of Andy Clark.)

synchronize between the instantaneous spray duration and the start of patient inhalation is known to be the most common error patients have with pMDIs [9]. Several factors affect the properties of the pMDI plume, such as propellant, formulation, valve volume, and spray orifice diameter. These parameters have been well characterized theoretically [10, 11]. Recently, Myatt *et al* (2022) suggested that the influence of valve orifice diameter on oropharyngeal deposition should also be considered since plume force was observed to depend on valve orifice diameter in a pMDI system [12].

The high, ballistic velocity of the emitted aerosol can be mitigated using a spacer device, which when attached to the pMDI mouthpiece provides distance and time for the spray velocity to decay. The spacer helps the patient to inhale the dose more gently, which assists in reducing oropharyngeal deposition. Spacers can also reduce the occurrence of thrush, a fungal infection of the mouth and throat by corticosteroids [13, 14]. There are various types of spacers (with or without a one-way inspiratory valve). Large spacers tend to transport higher amounts of small-sized aerosols more effectively than small spacers. Some spacers are available with antistatic coatings to reduce deposition on the chamber wall due to electrostatic charge; if not, they should be primed or washed with ionic detergent prior to use.

Because pMDIs are limited to delivery of small quantities of drug per dose, they are primarily used to administer potent compounds such as anticholinergics, corticosteroids, and β_2-agonists for the treatment of asthma and chronic obstructive pulmonary disease (COPD). pMDIs are, as a result, the most-prescribed inhalation devices, with 55 million pMDI devices sold in the United States in 2019 alone (approximately 75% of the inhaler market as compared to 25% for DPIs) [15]. The market distribution is similar in the United Kingdom. Parts of the European Union, however, greatly prefer DPIs to MDIs; for example, in Sweden DPIs garner 85% of the market in 2017 as compared to 13% for pMDIs [16].

There are many issues surrounding the efficiency and ease-of-use of pMDIs that have driven ongoing improvements to these devices. It is difficult for patients to coordinate their inhalation maneuver with actuation of the pMDI device, and lack of coordination can result in high dose-to-dose variability and lower efficacy. Because of this issue, breath-actuated and breath-coordinated pMDIs have been developed with the intent of synchronizing patient inhalation with release of drug product from the metering valve. Breath-actuated pMDIs have been shown to improve coordination as compared to standard pMDI for patients with poor inhalation technique [17], and asthma control was improved when a breath-actuated pMDI was used [18]. Examples of breath-actuated pMDIs are Autohaler™ by 3M and Easi-Breathe by Baker Norton, which rely on patient inhalation to trigger atomization. A breath-coordinated pMDI (Tempo, MAP Pharmaceuticals) allows the patient to comfortably actuate the inhaler to improve coordination and ensure a precise dose. Training devices such as Flo-Tone and Clip-Tone, which provide an audible cue upon inhaler actuation, have also been implemented to reduce inhalation errors. Flo-Tone or Clip-Tone connected to a smartphone app along with verbal counseling has been shown to reduce errors and improve lung function relative to traditional verbal counseling alone [19, 20]. It is expected that caregivers and patients will focus on proper education and continuous training via the use of digital apps connected to pMDIs [21, 22].

7.2.1 Environmental impact

An ongoing issue surrounding the use of pMDIs is their environmental impact. pMDIs were initially developed using chlorofluorocarbon (CFC) propellants such as Freon-11 and Freon-12 that were found to contribute to global warming as ozone-depleting agents and were eventually banned in 1987 through the Montreal Protocol, which called for the elimination of CFC propellants by 1996. Two hydrofluoroalkanes (HFA), HFA-134a and HFA-227, were approved by the FDA in 1994 to replace CFCs. According to a recent scientific assessment, after 40 years these reduction efforts have proven successful, and the ozone layer is on its way to recovery by 2066. A non-exhaustive list of pMDI products containing these HFA propellants that are currently marketed in the United States is provided in table 7.1 [15]. Although HFAs have been successfully used as alternatives to ozone-depleting substances, their role as global warming agents has become of greater concern. The expanding use of HFAs in large-scale applications such as refrigeration drove the adoption of the Kigali Amendments to the Montreal Protocol in 2016, which directed the phase down of HFAs by more than 80% in 30 years and replacement with more environmentally friendly alternatives. The reduction of fluorine-containing gas uses (including HFAs—table 7.2) is expected to cause significant price increases due to the decline in demand of and accompanying supply issues with the propellants. As a result, regulatory bodies are directing elimination of HFA propellants and are seeking the next generation even though HFA emissions associated with pMDI use only contributed an estimated of <0.1% to the total amount of global warming gases in 2014 [16, 23].

How can the pharmaceutical industry address concerns regarding environmentally friendly propellant use? One approach might be to replace pMDIs with DPIs to reduce their carbon footprint. The global economic impact of switching to DPIs was assessed using asthma/COPD prescription data from IQVIA database. While the assessment showed that the transition to DPIs is feasible for long-acting drugs, this is not the case for relief medication (short acting beta agonist, SABA), for which prescribed doses dominate globally (>50%). The price would increase by up to 5× in almost all countries when SABAs are switched to a DPI [25].

Further factors that prevent the switch for relief medication (SABA) from pMDIs to DPIs may include the inability of patients requiring rescue therapy to breath effectively. Also, patients have been observed to suffer negative consequences when switching from their established inhaler [28] without proper training and education [29]. Approximately 3.7% of patients have experienced an exacerbation due to switching to a DPI [30]. It is well known that switching inhalers can present regulatory challenges due to the lack of clarity regarding comparability and clinical data requirements. In addition, the total environmental impact beyond just that of the propellant over the inhaler lifecycle should also be considered [31]. Alternative inhalers such as SMIs that can address potential concerns around patient breathing

Table 7.1. Manufacturers of currently available HFA MDIs for use in the United States. Adapted from [15, 24] with permission.

Manufacturer	MDI product name	Active ingredient	FDA approval date
HFA-227ea			
AstraZeneca	Symbicort®	Budesonide, formoterol fumarate dihydrate	7/21/2006
Merck Sharp and Dohme	Asmanex® HFA	Mometasone furoate	4/25/2014
Merck Sharp and Dohme	Dulera®	Mometasone furoate; Formoterol fumarate dihydrate	6/22/2010
HFA-134a			
Sunovian Pharmaceuticals Inc	Xopenex®	Levalbuterol tartrate	03/11/2005
AstraZeneca	Bevespi Aerosphere®	Formoterol fumarate, glycopyrrolate	04/25/2016
AstraZeneca	Breztri Aerosphere®	Budesonide; formoterol fumarate; glycopyrrolate	07/23/2020
Boehirnger Ingelheim	Atrovent®	Ipratropium bromide	11/17/2004
Covis Pharma B.V.	Alvesco®	Ciclesonide	01/10/2008
GlaxoSmithKline	Advair®	Fluticasone propionate; salmeterol xinafoate	06/08/2006
GlaxoSmithKline	Flovent®	Fluticasone propionate	05/14/2004
GlaxoSmithKline	Ventolin®	Albuterol sulfate	04/19/2001
Kindeva Drug Delivery LP	Proventil® HFA	Albuterol sulfate	08/15/1996
Teva	ProAir®	Albuterol sulfate	10/29/2004
Norton Waterford LTD	QVAR® Redihaler™	Beclomethasone dipropionate	08/03/2017
Armstrong Pharmaceuticals Inc.	Primatene Mist	Epinephrine	11/07/2018
Cipla Pvt Ltd	Generic Albuterol Sulfate	Albuterol sulfate	04/08/2020
Lupin Inc	Generic Albuterol Sulfate	Albuterol sulfate	08/24/0202
Perrigo Pharmaceuticals Co	Generic Albuterol Sulfate	Albuterol sulfate	02/24/2020

effort are being evaluated by several companies including Boehringer Ingelheim, Merxin, Pharmaero, and Well-Bridge. However, any switch is likely to be costly. For rescue therapy, patients relying on pMDIs for rescue therapy are advised to

Table 7.2. Environmental characteristics of propellants in MDIs. Adapted from [25–27] with permission.

Propellant	Formula (MW)	GWP ($CO2 = 1$)	Atmospheric lifetime (Years)	Boiling point (°C)	Density at 20 °C (g/mL)	Solubility of water in propellant (ppm)	Dipole moment (Debye)
CFC-11[1]	$CFCl_3$ (137.4)	4660	55	23.7	1.49	100	0.45
CFC-12[1]	CF_2Cl_2 (120.9)	10 800	113	−29.3	1.33	90	0.51
HFA-134a	CF_3-CFH_2 (102.0)	1300	14	−26.2	1.23	2200	2.06
HFA-227a	CF_3-CFH-CF_3 (170.0)	3350	31–42	−16.5	1.41	610	1.46
HFA-152a	CF_2H-CH_3 (66.1)	138	1.5	−24.7	0.91	2200	2.26
HFO-1234ze	$CF_3CH{=}CHF$ (114.0)	<1	18 days	−18.9	1.29	225	1.44

choose the most appropriate device for their treatment, and for caregivers to prioritize patient wellbeing first over the environment.

Future developments in pMDI acceptability have focused on identification of new propellants with lower global warming potential (GWP) such as HFA-152a (Koura Global Boston, USA) and HFO-1234ze (Honeywell, North Carolina, USA). Use of these new propellants is projected to reduce the carbon footprint by up to 92%. HFO-1234ze is currently preferred over HFA-152a since it is less flammable with a narrow flammability range and presents a lower GWP. HFA-152a is considered flammable but can be managed in a GMP manufacturing environment [25]. Manufacturing capability for medical grade HFA-152a has been completed (Koura Global). HFA-152a administered via inhalation to healthy volunteers was shown to be well tolerated and rapidly cleared from the blood [32]. At least three companies (Chiesi, AstraZeneca, and GSK) have committed to invest in new low GWP propellants by 2025. In the meantime, development studies continue to progress to assess container closure systems for compatibility with formulations incorporating HFA-152a [33].

7.3 Dry powder inhalers (DPIs)

A DPI is a small portable inhaler that can be used to aerosolize drug powder without the need for a propellant and is less reliant on patient breath coordination during the inhalation maneuver. The first modern DPI, Spinhaler® (Fisons, UK) was launched in 1967 and since then there have been many advances in DPI design [1]. This section will discuss the types of DPIs that are currently available in the market or in development including those that are not available for use. Some others have also provided reviews on DPIs [6, 7, 16, 34–39].

7.3.1 Passive and active DPIs

Most marketed DPIs are passive, in that they rely on patient inhalation to dispense and disperse a powder formulation into an aerosol with a particle size suitable for transport into the lungs. Because no powder is emitted until the patient inhales, the coordination issues experienced with pMDIs are largely eliminated when using a DPI. While it is an advantage of DPIs that no propellant or external power source is required to provide energy for powder dispersion, at the same time this reliance on the patient's inspiratory pressure to empty the powder from the dosage unit and deagglomerate it can be a source of both inhaled dose and lung dose variability. This is especially true for first-generation DPI products, such as Intal Spinhaler® (Fisons, UK) and Ventolin® Rotahaler® (GSK, UK), which were developed to administer drugs formulated in powders using micronized lactose carrier blends (LBs). The same is also true with the spheronized (SPH) powder technology (e.g., Pulmicort® Turbuhaler®, AstraZeneca, UK) DPI.

LBs consisting of adhesive mixtures of fine drug particles adhered to coarse lactose particles by blending are the most common dry powder formulation for inhalation. The powder is typically filled into capsules or blisters for insertion into the inhaler, or in a reservoir that is part of the inhaler itself. Prior to inhalation, the inhaler is manipulated to open the package (e.g., capsule) to expose the powder. To effectively separate drug from carrier particles during aerosolization of an LB or

SPH formulation, the balance between drug/carrier adhesion and detachment needs to be considered because coarse agglomerates from which the drug does not detach are primarily deposited in the upper respiratory tract (URT). Unfortunately, for binary adhesive LB mixtures and SPH formulations most current DPIs do not generate sufficient dispersion energy to produce good drug/carrier separation, leading to incomplete detachment of drug and carrier particles and only a small fraction of the nominal dose reaching the lungs due to its bimodal distribution [39]. Consequently, binary adhesive LB mixtures often exhibit low total lung deposition (TLD) [36, 38]. Improved dispersibility has been shown with new LB powders consisting of ternary mixtures of fine and coarse lactose with magnesium stearate as a force control agent (FCA) [40, 41]. However, since coarse lactose is still present, URT deposition can still be significant.

Engineered powders with corrugated surfaces, lower density, increased drag force, and reduced interparticle cohesive forces do not require blending with large or non-respirable carrier particles as compared to LB. These powders display lower URT and higher lung deposition due to their characteristics of smaller aerodynamic size [39] unlike LB and SPH formulations. Other engineered powders are listed in table 7.3. Another marketed DPI which does not rely on powder deagglomeration includes Adasuve® Staccato (Alexza), which uses thermal energy to vaporize its drug and delivers condensed loxapine droplets to patients.

In contrast to passive DPIs, active DPIs do not rely on patient inhalation for powder dispersion. Instead, they utilize energy from compressed air or other sources to disperse the powder in a more consistent manner for the patient to inhale. While the particle size of the dispersed powder is independent of patient inhalation, the TLD still is still affected by the patient inhalation flow rate (Q). In this case, the particle size generated by these types of devices is constant, as it is pre-dispersed by the inhaler, and therefore as Q increases the TLD is expected to decrease due to increasing URT deposition. Some examples of active DPIs include the PDS device used in Exubera® which uses compressed air and was briefly marketed (Pfizer), and Spiros® device which uses a small motor and rotating blade to disperse the powder which was in development by Dura Pharmaceuticals but never made it to market. A non-exhaustive list of recently approved DPIs is provided in table 7.4, which

Table 7.3. Examples of approved engineered powders.

Technology	Brand name/company	Drug	Status
PulmoSphere™	TOBI® Podhaler®/Vietris	Tobramycin	Approved
Aerospheres®	Bevespi Aerosphere/ AstraZeneca	Glycopyrrolate/Formoterol/ Fumarate	Approved
Technospheres®	Alfrezza®/Mannkind Corporation	Insulin	Approved
ARCUS®	Inbrija®/Acorda Therapeutics	Levodopa	Approved
PRINT®	Yutrepia/Liquidia Corporation	Treprostinil	Approved

Table 7.4. Some of the recent FDA approved DPIs. Adapted from [15, 34] CC BY 4.0.

FDA approval year	Product name	Active ingredient	Formulation technology	Dose configuration	Image, webpage and/or current status
2022	Tyvaso DPI®	Treprostinil	Technosphere technology (fumaryl diketopi perazine carrier)	Single dose (cartridge)	https://www.tyvaso.com/dpi/
2020	ArmonAir® Digihaler®	Fluticasone propionate	Lactose-based formulation	Multi-dose (reservoir)	https://www.digihaler.com/inhalers/armonair
2019	AirDuo® Digihaler®	Fluticasone propionate; salmeterol xinafoate	Lactose-based formulation	Multi-dose (reservoir)	https://www.digihaler.com/inhalers/airduo
2019	Duaklir® Pressair®	Aclidinium bromide; Formoterol fumarate	Lactose-based formulation	Multi-dose (reservoir)	
2019	Wixela Inhub®	Fluticasone propionate; salmeterol xinafoate	Lactose-based formulation	Multi-dose (blister)	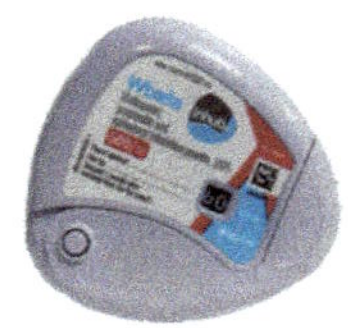 https://www.wixela.com/
2018	Inbrija®	Levodopa	Spray dried powder	Single dose (capsule)	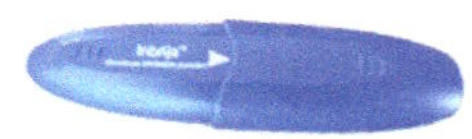 https://www.acorda.com/products/products/inbrija
2018	ProAir® Digihaler®	Albuterol sulfate	Lactose-based formulation	Multi-dose (reservoir)	https://www.digihaler.com/inhalers/proair

(Continued)

Table 7.4. (*Continued*)

FDA approval year	Product name	Active ingredient	Formulation technology	Dose configuration	Image, webpage and/or current status
2017	Trelegy Ellipta	Fluticasone furoate; umeclidinium bromide; vilanterol trifenatate	Lactose- and magnesium stearate-based formulation	Multi-dose (blister) Available in 2 strengths: 100/62.5/25 and 200/62.5/25 mcg	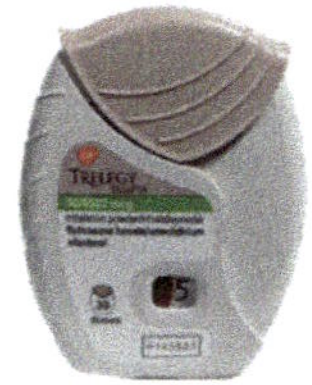 https://www.trelegy.com/
2017	ArmonAir® RespiClick®	Fluticasone Propionate	Lactose-based formulation	Multi-dose (reservoir)	Discontinued in 2017
2017	AirDuo® RespiClick®	Fluticasone propionate; salmeterol xinafoate	Lactose-based formulation	Multi-dose (reservoir)	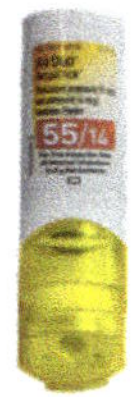
2015	Seebri™ Neohaler®	Glycopyrrolate	Lactose- and magnesium stearate-based formulation	Single dose (capsule)	Discontinued in 2020
2015	Ultibron™ Neohaler®	Indacaterol and glycopyrrolate	Lactose- and magnesium stearate-based formulation	Single dose (capsule)	Discontinued in 2020
2014	Arnuity Ellipta	Fluticasone furoate	Lactose-based formulation	Multi-dose (blister) Available in 3 strengths: 50, 100 and 200 mcg	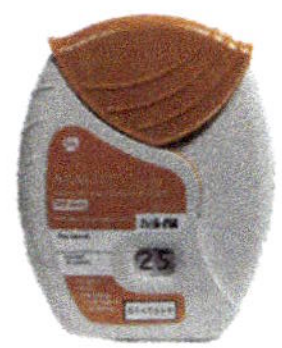 https://arnuity.com/

2013	Breo Ellipta	Fluticasone furoate; Vilanterol trifenatate	Lactose- and magnesium stearate-based formulation	Multi-dose (Blister) Available in 2 strengths: 100/25 and 200/25 mcg	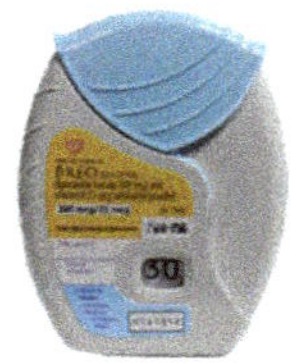 https://www.mybreo.com/
2015	ProAir® RespiClick®	Albuterol sulfate	Lactose-based formulation	Multi-dose (reservoir)	https://hcp.proair.com/about-respiclick-bai
2014	Afrezza® Dreamboat®	Insulin	Technosphere technology (fumaryl diketopiperazine carrier)	Single dose	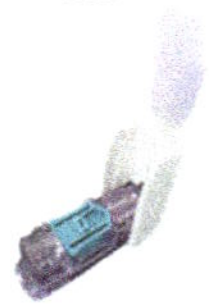 https://afrezza.com/
2014	Incruse Ellipta	Umeclidinium bromide	Lactose- and magnesium stearate-based formulation	Multi-dose (blister)	https://incruse.com/
2013	Anoro Ellipta	Umeclidinium bromide and vilanterol	Lactose- and magnesium stearate-based formulation	Multi-dose (blister)	https://www.anoro.com/
2013	TOBI Podhaler®	Tobramycin	PulmoSphere™ Technology (small, low-density, porous particles)	Single dose (Capsule)	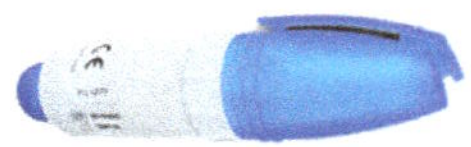 https://www.tobipodhaler.com/en
2012	Fostair NEXThaler®	Beclometasone dipropionate, formoterol fumarate dihydrate	Lactose- and magnesium stearate-based formulation	Multi-dose (reservoir)	https://www.chiesiair.co.uk/patient/fostair-nexthaler/

(*Continued*)

Table 7.4. *(Continued)*

FDA approval year	Product name	Active ingredient	Formulation technology	Dose configuration	Image, webpage and/or current status
2012	Tudorza® Pressair®	Aclidinium Bromide	Lactose-based formulation	Multi-dose (reservoir)	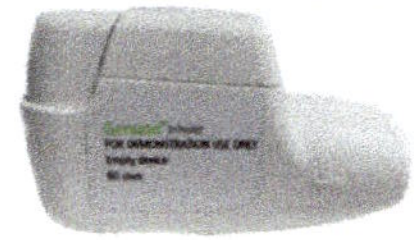 https://www.tudorza.us/
2012	Adasuve® Staccato	Loxapine	Staccato® OBT™ system (Rapid vaporization = Rapid absorption = Rapid onset of action)	Single dose (contains a thin film of excipient-free drug on substrate)	https://www.adasuve.com/ (Not considered a 'true' DPI since it does not rely on deagglomeration process, but with sublimation of drug vapor)
2011	Arcapta™ Neohaler®	Indacaterol	Lactose-based formulation	Single dose (capsule)	Discontinued in 2020
2006	Exubera®	Insulin	Spray dried powder	Single dose (blister)	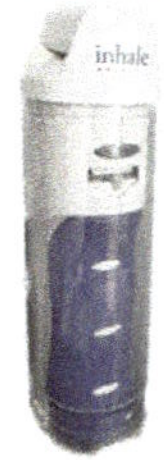 Discontinued in 2007
2006	Symbicort® Turbuhaler®	Budesonide/ formoterol fumarate	Lactose-based formulation	Multi-dose (reservoir)	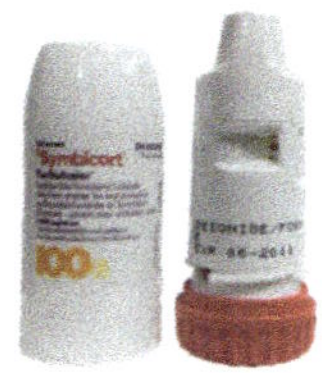

2006	Pulmicort™ Flexhaler™	Budesonide	Spheronized particles	Multi-dose (reservoir)	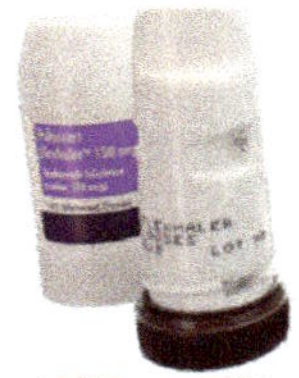
2005	Asmanex® Twisthaler®	Mometasone furoate	Spheronized particles	Multi-dose (reservoir) (0.22 mg/puff) 2008 (0.11 mg/puff)	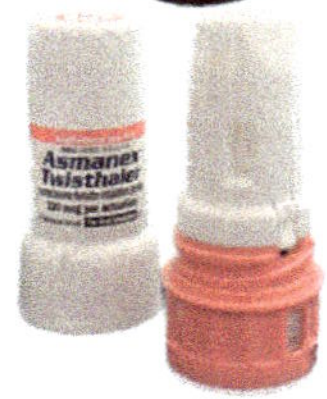 https://www.asmanex.com/asmanex-twisthaler/
2000	Flovent® Diskus®	Fluticasone propionate	Lactose-based formulation	Multi-dose (Blister)	
2000	Advair® Diskus®	Fluticasone propionate; salmeterol xinafoate	Lactose-based formulation	Multi-dose (blister)	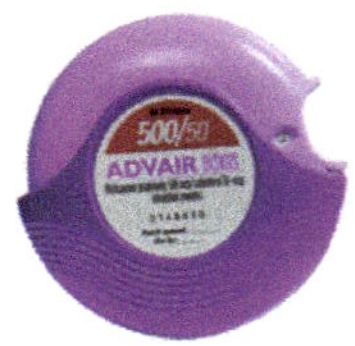 https://www.advair.com/

includes such key properties as dosing configuration (i.e., single or multi-dose), formulation technologies, and powder container (e.g., capsule, reservoir, etc).

7.3.2 Essential performance attribute: d_a^2Q

In discussing passive DPI performance, it is important to describe an impaction parameter (d_a^2Q). It is a crucial factor in understanding respiratory deposition. It is a parameter residing in the Stokes number (Stk), a dimensionless number that defines the ratio of the particle inertia to the viscous drag acting on the particle and is influenced by particle size, density, and fluid velocity (equation 7.1) [42].

$$Stk = \frac{\rho_p d_p^2 u}{18\eta D} \quad \frac{d_a^2 Q C_c}{18\eta D} \tag{7.1}$$

where ρ_p, d_p, u, η, and D are the particle density, particle size, linear velocity, dynamic viscosity of air, and characteristic diameter of an obstacle, respectively. Q, Cc, and d_a are the volumetric flow rate, Cunningham slip correction factor, and aerodynamic diameter, respectively. d_a^2Q is a parameter which controls the URT deposition [31, 33, 34]. When d_a^2Q is high, it signifies that the inertial forces dominate. High flow rates and large particles increase the impaction parameter and promote deposition in the URT [43]. In this case, larger particles with higher velocity are less likely to follow the air flow streamlines, cannot make the sharp turns and are filtered in the URT. For a dry powder formulation, d_a^2Q is a better *in vitro* indicator of *in vivo* lung delivery than merely d_a or $FPD_{<3.3\mu m}$ (fine particle dose) since respiratory deposition relies on both d_a and Q. Both d_a and $FPD_{<3.3\mu m}$ are generally derived from a cascade impactor (e.g., next-generation impactor, NGI) and they are common attributes used in quality control for product performance. However, it is incorrect to use them while neglecting Q to assess flow rate independent *in vivo*. In fact, flow rate independent can only be considered when d_a^2Q is relatively constant across Q. It is also important to note that an NGI classifies particles by different stages with approximately a constant d_a^2Q. Another performance attribute worth noting is stage grouping (e.g., Stage 3—filter), which is outside the scope of this section. A more detailed explanation on d_a^2Q is provided elsewhere [44].

The relationship between d_a^2Q and URT deposition is presented in figure 7.6, which is based on a compilation of clinical data by Stahlhofen *et al* (1989) [45]. This figure demonstrates a trend of increasing URT deposition with increasing d_a^2Q. It is important to note that the highest variability in URT deposition and thus high variability in TLD occurs when d_a^2Q is between approximately 1500 and 5000. This high variability has been attributed to subject-to-subject variations in URT physiology. Unfortunately, most marketed passive DPIs generally operate in this region. In contrast, low d_a^2Q (<= 100) tends to result in the lowest URT deposition and highest lung deposition (figure 7.6).

To facilitate effective lung delivery, passive DPIs should be designed to achieve a low impaction parameter d_a^2Q (with units of μm^2 l min^{-1}). Note that both d_a and Q serve as competing parameters since in most passive DPIs d_a decreases (i.e., powder dispersion improves) with increasing Q. However, increasing Q leads to higher drug losses in the URT region due to impaction and consequently lower TLD. A positive dependence of TLD on Q is achieved when dispersion dominates (e.g., Budesonide Turbuhaler®), while a negative flow rate dependence of TLD is observed when impaction dominates (Albuterol Spiros®) [39]. Based on the reviewed literature, dispersion tends to dominate over impaction losses in the URT [7, 39] for most but not all DPIs using LB formulations. For engineered powders, the dispersion and impaction effects are more balanced with the consequence that flow-rate independent performance can be achieved, in that d_a^2Q is relatively constant as Q varies (i.e., d_a decreases by just the right amount to offset increases in Q). The competition between dispersion and impaction becomes an important aspect of passive DPIs for delivery of LB formulations. Understanding of these effects can guide engineers to better design DPIs in properly budgeting components needed for deagglomeration, or DPI resistance (see section 4.4).

The degree of URT deposition was explained by the variability in TLD by Borgström *et al* (2006) [46]. In general, low URT deposition leads to high TLD with low variability and that high URT deposition leads to low TLD with high variability. Therefore, it is critical that an inhaler should be designed to reduce URT deposition and therefore variability in order to achieve high and consistent drug delivery to the lungs [46], ideally by minimizing URT deposition or by bypassing the URT completely. This has been shown as possible for carrier-free formulations comprised of low-density porous particles [39]. In general, first-generation passive DPIs with large d_a^2Q tend to exhibit higher flow rate dependence and correspondingly higher TLD deposition with increasing Q. Active DPIs, such as Exubera® and Spiro®, on the other hand, can never be categorized as flow-rate independent since the deposition of the constant pre-dispersed particle size increases with increasing Q.

7.3.3 Essential component of DPI: dispersion engines

Various DPI dispersion engines have been used to generate the necessary air flow and turbulence within an inhaler to achieve sufficient powder deagglomeration. Some common engines include rotating disk, particle collisions, cyclone chamber, orifice, and venturi. A dispersion engine is used in an inhaler to significantly increase particle velocity and improve dispersion. Most dispersion engines work based on the principle of a narrowing pathway that accelerates the air flow, creating a pressure drop and generating turbulence for powder dispersion (i.e., Bernoulli effect). Some devices, such as Twisthaler™ (Merck, US) use a rotating disk mechanism to disperse the powder, while a swirl chamber uses a tangential air flow to create a vortex-like motion to disperse dry powder particles. The dispersion engine is typically positioned between the drug chamber and the inhaler mouthpiece and is part of the air flow path within the DPI. It is an essential design feature because it contributes to the device resistance by affecting the air flow rate and the patient's ability to effectively inhale the medication.

The starting point of the air flow path is an inlet through which the air enters when the patient inhales. The geometry of the inlet channel or pathway contributes to the overall inhaler resistance. The channel directs the air flow into the drug chamber, where

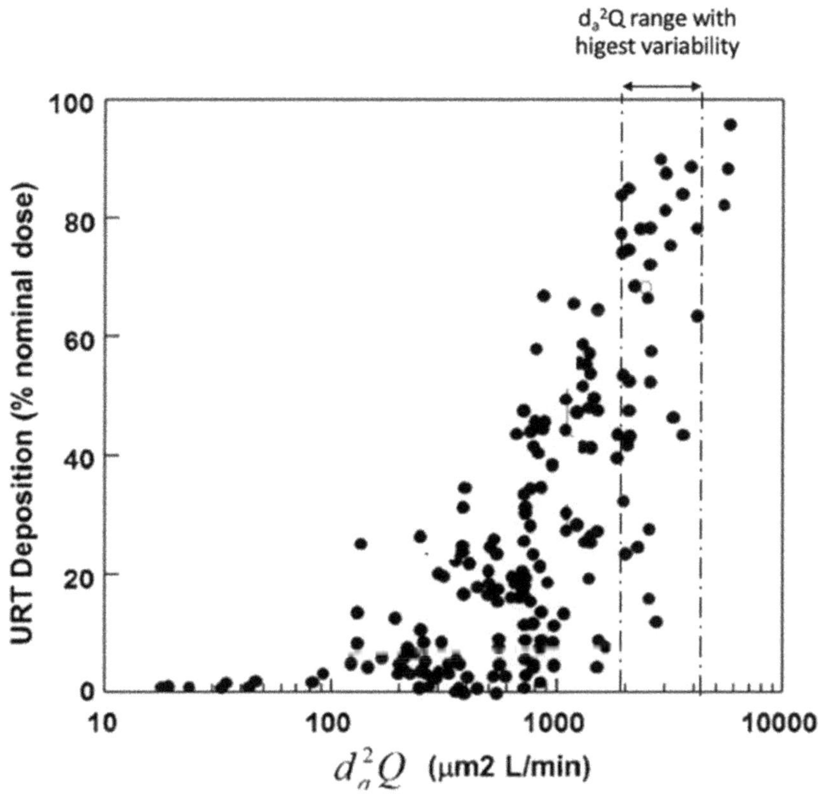

Figure 7.6. % URT deposition as a function of inertial impaction parameter, d_a^2Q for monodisperse aerosols. Adapted from [7] (CC BY 4.0) using data presented by Stahlhofen [45].

the dry powder is contained in a capsule, blister, or reservoir. Prior to inhalation, the inhaler is manipulated to pierce or otherwise open the package to expose the powder. The holes in the capsule or blister can then serve as another narrowing pathway. In the case of a capsule DPI, when the air enters the drug chamber it creates turbulent flow that causes the capsule to shake or rotate and empty the powder from the chamber. Deagglomeration of the powder occurs due to the high-speed rotation of the capsule and the ejection of the powder through the tiny, pierced holes. The air flow passes through the chamber and entrains the powder, which then exits the dispersion engine into the DPI mouthpiece. A multi-dose DPI operates in an analogous manner, though in addition to the above the patient advances the device to the next dose to be dispersed. Multi-dose DPIs, which initially entered the market around 1990, can consist of a wheel of blisters, a reservoir and holding chamber, or another configuration.

Most DPIs use a simple dispersion engine to deagglomerate the powder. It was originally thought that the pressure drop created by this dispersion engine would effectively disperse powder in a passive DPI, especially for LB formulations. Efforts to further improve powder dispersion in LB formulations have led to development of a more involved dispersion engine device known as AOS™ (Respira Therapeutics, USA) which is based on the RS01 DPI (Plastiape S.p.A, Italy). The dispersion mechanisms in

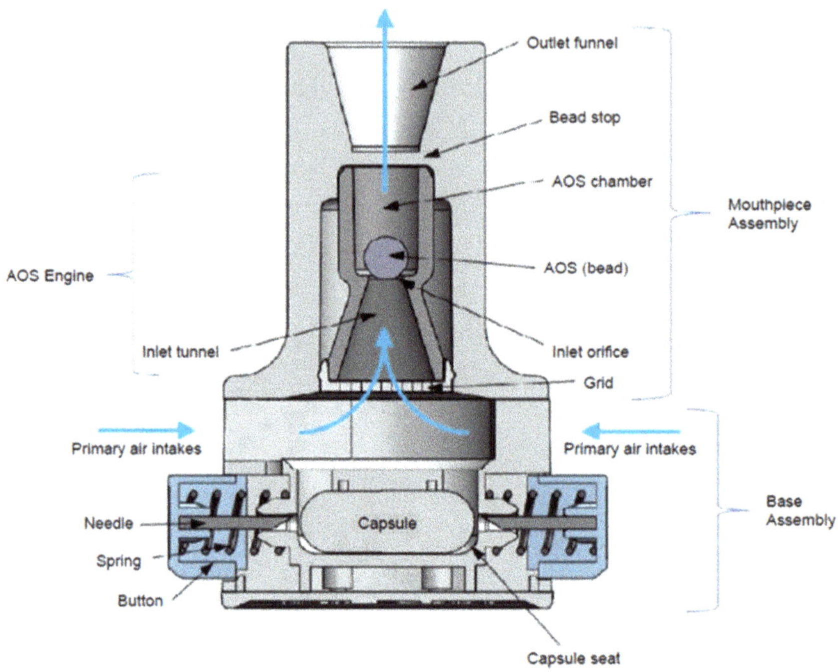

Figure 7.7. Cross-sectional view of the AOS DPI showing the added powder dispersion mechanism, AOS Engine, within the mouthpiece (Reproduced with permission from *Respiratory Drug Delivery* 2020, Virginia Commonwealth University).

the AOS are designed in series starting with particle collisions with the walls and rotation of the capsule followed by an accelerated flow through an orifice and collisions with a bead inside the mouthpiece assembly (figure 7.7) [47, 48]. The AOS is currently in clinical development for treatment of pulmonary hypertension. A double dispersion engine known as Aspire® was developed at Novartis Pharmaceuticals with two parallel venturis. This inhaler is discussed in section 4.7.

7.3.4 Inhaler resistance

Passive DPIs are typically categorized as low, medium, or high resistance as directed by their pressure drops and flow rates. The device resistance is defined by the internal geometry of the inhaler, the air flow paths or channels within the inhaler, and the size, shape, and characteristics of the drug chamber. The resistance of an inhaler contributes to its pressure drop and flow rate characteristics. The resistance and flow rate of various DPIs can be found in Clark and Hollingworth [49]. Due to geometry, inhaler resistance is typically much higher than human conducting airway resistance. Low-resistance devices have been classified as achieving flow rates >90 l min^{-1} at a pressure drop of 4 kPa, while high-resistance devices would achieve flow rates <50 l min^{-1} at the same pressure drop. The flow rates for medium-resistance devices lie in between the high and low resistance inhalers. The dependence of patient inhalation rate (Q) on pressure drop (ΔP) has been established as follows [49]:

$$Q = \frac{\sqrt{\Delta P}}{R} \tag{7.2}$$

where Q = inhalation flow rate, ΔP = pressure drop, and R = inhaler resistance. In practice, inhaler resistance typically ranges from 0.01 to 0.06 $\text{kPa}^{1/2}\ \text{l}^{-1}\ \text{min}^{-1}$. Each inhaler exhibits a different value of Q derived from equation 7.2 for a standard ΔP, usually set at 4 kPa for *in vitro* testing. Therefore, inhalers with different resistances should not be compared using the same value of Q. Higher pressure drops are typically reached at lower flow rates when patients breathe through high resistance inhalers due to their greater inspiratory pressure requirements. In contrast, patients tend to achieve their highest flow rates when using low resistance inhalers [38, 39].

7.3.5 Which is more important: inspiratory pressure or peak inspiratory flow rate?

Each DPI has its own unique resistance; therefore, peak inspiratory flow rate (PIFR) should not be used as a metric to select a DPI. The ability of a patient to inhale through a DPI, coupled with misconceptions regarding the usefulness of PIFR, have been discussed extensively [50]. Maximum mouth pressure drop, which in turn depends on the respiratory muscle health, gender, and age of the patient, has been suggested as a more suitable metric to assess a patient's ability to use a passive DPI. Women, young children, and the elderly tend to have weaker respiratory muscles, which supports clinical observations of such patients lacking the ability to achieve the flows and pressure drops needed for efficacious use of many DPIs. This dependence is less likely for some modern dry powder formulations that can be easily deagglomerated at very low pressure drops.

Based on *in vivo* and *in vitro* data from commercially available DPIs, a pressure drop of 1 kPa has been proposed as that below which a decline in performance for bronchodilators might be expected [50]. This limit is proposed instead of a suggested 60 l min^{-1} cutoff for comparing inhalers using the In-Check DIAL device. The remedy would be to convert the PIFR obtained by In-Check to pressure drop using equation (7.2) in order to determine whether the cutoff of 1 kPa can be achieved. Otherwise, the most appropriate way to check patient ability to use the inhaler is by measuring the PIFR with the inhaler in line and calculate the pressure drop to ensure that it is above 1 kPa. In most cases, the ability of a patient to use an inhaler correctly also relies on proper training and how well they follow instructions.

7.3.6 Essential device design features: exit velocities and turbulent flows

Even though passive DPIs are classified by their resistance as mentioned above, such classifications have led to misinterpretation regarding their performance. Due to the lower patient air flow rates typically attained when using high-resistance devices, it has been assumed that delivery using these devices results in higher lung deposition with lower variability because aerosolized particles can more easily follow the lower-velocity flow into the deep lung with minimal impaction losses in the URT region. However, this may not necessarily apply to all high resistance devices (see example below). Despite its lower inspiratory flow rate, a high resistance device does not

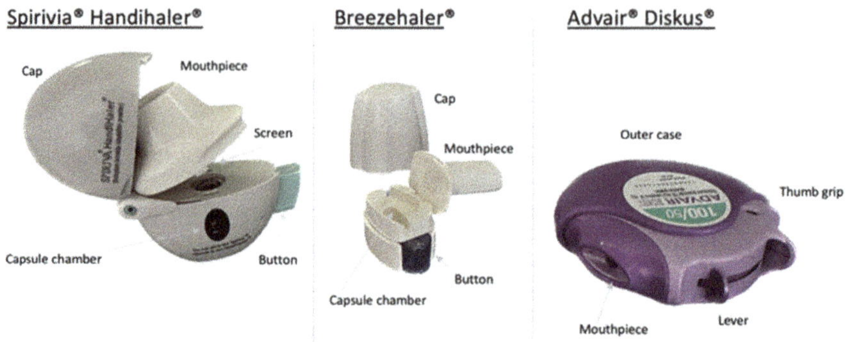

Figure 7.8. Spiriva w/HandiHaler, Seebri® w/Breezhaler, Advair Diskus.

necessarily ensure reduced URT deposition. In contrast, the higher-velocity air that passes through a low resistance inhaler designed to improve deagglomeration (e.g., Breezehaler®) can result in a lower d_a^2Q and reduced URT deposition [39]. It is important that the high velocity generated in a low resistance inhaler be dissipated prior to exiting the mouthpiece so that drug loss in URT region can be reduced.

Cardwell *et al* (2014) used photon image velocimetry (PIV) to measure flow velocities at 4 kPa exiting the mouthpieces of three DPIs (figure 7.8) and showed that Breezhaler®, with the lowest resistance ($R = 0.019$ kPa^{½} min l^{-1}, 103 l min^{-1}), also exhibited the lowest exit velocity and turbulence due to the presence of an extended mouthpiece which effectively slowed the velocity [51]. In contrast, another low–medium resistance device, the Diskus® ($R = 0.025$ kPa^{½} min l^{-1}, 81 l min^{-1}), displayed 3× higher maximum exit velocities (~60 m s^{-1}) due to its lack of an extended mouthpiece. The higher velocities resulted in greater losses in the URT and lower TLD. HandiHaler®, a high-resistance device ($R = 0.05$ kPa^{½} min l^{-1}, 39 l min^{-1}), was expected to exhibit a lower exit velocity than Breezhaler®, but data measured at the mouthpiece exit by PIV showed that the actual exit velocity of HandiHaler® was twice as large as that of Breezhaler® (~40 m s^{-1} versus ~20 m s^{-1}). Like Diskus®, this was likely due to its more complex inhaler geometry and the lack of an extended mouthpiece. The prevailing wisdom that high-resistance devices have low variability leads to many ignoring the options for low-resistance devices with low exit velocities. Overall, Cardwell *et al* (2014) demonstrated that robust device design and selection should include experimental characterization and consideration of flow fields at the exit of the mouthpiece in addition to device resistance, as the ability to predict device performance from resistance and mouthpiece exit area alone is limited [51].

Harris (2018) described *in silico* work demonstrating the effect of inlet velocity and dispersion engine resistance on deagglomeration of lactose blends [52]. Using model swirl chambers representing high, medium, and low resistance inhalers (i.e., HandiHaler®, Advair Diskus®, and Cyclohaler®, respectively), it was shown that higher resistance can promote high swirl chamber air velocities at low patient inspiratory air flow rates, theoretically leading to more efficient deagglomeration of drug and carrier particles. It was concluded that high swirl chamber resistance improved DPI performance and consistency between different patient groups because high velocities (Mach 0.4) for deagglomeration were achieved at lower air flow rates. This approach could be an advantage for lactose blend formulations as long as the exit flow velocity is dissipated prior to inhalation. In contrast, carrier-free engineered powder formulations with corrugated morphology and hydrophobic surfaces, such as PulmoSphere™ [53] can achieve high TLD from low resistance devices without requiring high deagglomeration velocities [54].

7.3.7 Open-inhale-close DPIs

The design and performance aspects of current DPIs as described above have informed development of Open-inhale-close inhalers as advocated during the 1000 Years of Pharmaceutical Aerosols Conference in 2010 [6]. These inhalers would ideally facilitate patient ease-of-use and improve compliance due to their simplicity. The Ellipta® device manufactured by GlaxoSmithKline, an example of such an inhaler, is available in configurations that use either a single strip of 30 unit-dose blisters (Arnuity Ellipta®) for monotherapy or two strips of 30 unit-dose blisters (Breo Ellipta®) for combination therapy and has been approved in multiple countries for use in a number of asthma and COPD products. Since it comes with several brand name products, mix ups in its use have been reported [55]. Its design, functionality, and aerosol performance have been described in detail elsewhere [56]. Another open-inhale-close inhaler is the ProAir Digihaler® (Teva Pharmaceutical Industries, Israel), which is a multi-dose (200 doses) DPI developed with patient compliance in mind. Its built-in electronics and pressure sensor measure and record the patient's use and breathing technique, which can be transmitted to the healthcare provider via Bluetooth connectivity [57]. Since this inhaler is an open-inhale-close system, like Ellipta®, the dose is prepared as the patient opens the cap and potential errors leading to drug waste could occur if the patient does not inhale upon opening the cap. Further, drug is also wasted if the patient inadvertently exhales into or shakes the device. The inhaler is discarded upon completion of the last dose [39].

Dosing errors can be overcome by inclusion of breath actuation as in NEXThaler® and Aspire (developed by Novartis San Carlos). The NEXThaler® DPI (Chiesi) is also an open-inhale-close multi-dose breath-actuated inhaler for asthma use (R = 0.036 kPa$^{1/2}$ min l^{-1}; 55 l min^{-1} at 4 kPa) in which actuation is automatically triggered at a patient flow rate of 35 l min^{-1} (or 1.6 kPa). Since the powder only aerosolizes upon patient inhalation, the dose is not wasted if the patient does not inhale. The dose counter only advances after dose delivery. The design of the NEXThaler also prevents unnecessary exposure of powder to moisture. However, the inhaler lacks dosing monitoring and any feedback mechanism capability. The inhaler is designed to generate extra-fine (mass median aerodynamic diameter <2 μm) aerosols [58]. Images of both Ellipta® and NEXThaler® are provided in igure 7.9.

Aspire (formerly referred to as USSC-03), a modular breath-actuated multi-dose DPI with telehealth capability was developed to meet the 'open-inhale-close' concept [59]. Features of this inhaler included a replaceable cartridge of 31 doses in blister format (i.e., one cartridge per month), and a use life of one year (figure 7.10). The inhaler

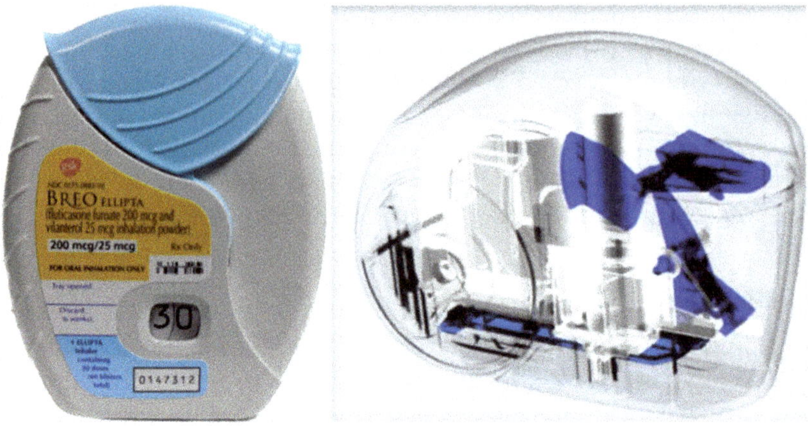

Figure 7.9. Pictorial representation Breo Ellipta® (100/25) device and NEXThaler inhaler device (Source NEXThaler®: DDL 2015 [117], with permission from DDL/The Aerosol Society).

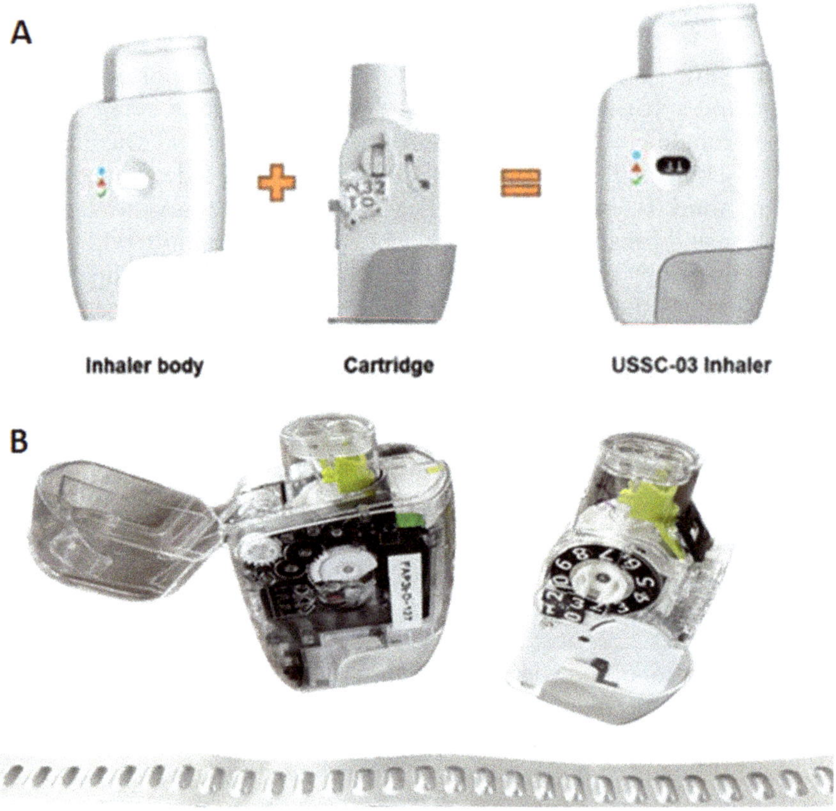

Figure 7.10. Photograph of Aspire or USSC-03 inhaler (A). Reproduced from [59] with permission from *Respiratory Drug Delivery* 2016, Virginia Commonwealth University. Transparent view of Aspire inhaler (B).

operates as follows. When patient inhalation reaches ~1.5 kPa, the blister is pierced and the powder in the blister is dispersed to form an aerosol bolus that is inhaled by the patient. Since the blister is not pierced until the patient inhales, this approach reduces potential errors due to the patient exhaling into the device, minimizes ramping effects on blister emptying, and minimizes drug waste [39]. The dispersion engine of the Aspire inhaler consists of two venturis in parallel, and since powder only passes through one or the other at a time there is no significant impact on inhaler resistance. The inhaler generates particle velocities of Mach 0.4 and reaches a much lower mouthpiece exit velocity than would be observed with a single venturi. Aspire is a truly mechanical inhaler that also has a capability to be connected by Bluetooth to monitor patient use parameters including time, date, and breathing profile. Aspire was designed to facilitate adherence because the patient is not required to perform exhalation prior to inhalation and no breath-hold is needed at the end of inhalation. Therefore, with Aspire, potential errors associated with these steps that are seen with other DPIs are avoided. Aspire also presented excellent aerosol performance data (TLD of 80%) [60, 61]. However, this DPI is not currently available commercially.

7.3.8 High payload DPIs

Most DPIs for asthma and COPD patients deliver small doses (<1 mg) per actuation along with the mass of adhesive mixture (in mg) in the powder container (e.g., blister or capsule). Other DPIs (figure 7.11) have been designed to administer large doses of drugs such as antibiotics using multiple inhalations; for instance, the target dose of tobramycin delivered using the TOBI® Podhaler® requires four capsules BID of approximately 55 mg of powder per capsule. Twincer™ has been used to administer approximately 50 mg of powder containing the antibiotic colistimethate sodium (colistin) per actuation to cystic fibrosis (CF) patients in compassionate use programs in the Netherlands since 2015 [62, 63]. The RS01 (Plastiape S.p.A) is a DPI that can accommodate larger quantities of powder by allowing a range of capsule sizes depending on the capsule volume cavity needed to hold the powder load.

Colobreathe® (PH&T, Italy) and Inbrija® (Acorda, USA) are other marketed high-dose drugs delivered using DPIs. Colobreathe (colistimethate sodium) is administered as a 125 mg dose BID in at least three inhalations per dose using the Turbospin® inhaler and is approved in Europe for treatment of chronic *Pseudomonas aeruginosa* infections for CF patients aged >6 years [65]. Inbrija® is provided as two size 00 capsules each containing 42 mg of levodopa powder, a low-density engineered powder, thus requiring inhalations of the content of two capsules to achieve an 84 mg nominal dose. Inbrija® can be dosed up to five times per day as needed for patients with Parkinson's disease. Parts of the Inbrija® combination product package and inhaler are shown in figure 7.12. Other clinical evaluations of high-dose DPIs have included ciprofloxacin inhalation powder (Bayer/Novartis), in which a 50 mg powder mass (32.5 mg dose) was administered in a single inhalation [66].

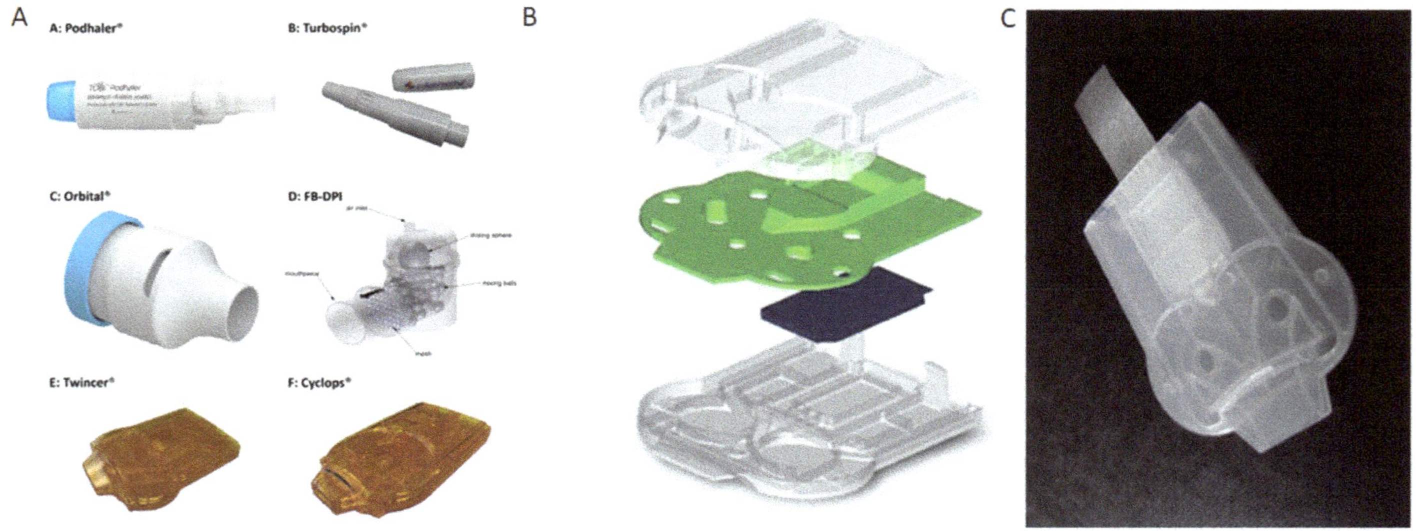

Figure 7.11. Six DPIs capable of high dose delivery: (a) Podhaler (Novartis AG); (b) Colobreathe (PH&T, Italy); (c) Orbital (Pharmaxis Ltd); (d) FO-DPI (VCU); (e) Twincer (Univ. Groningen); (f) Cyclops (Univ. Groningen) (A) [64] CC BY 4.0. Twincer (exploded) consisting of three plate-like parts and a blister as dose compartment (B) and Twincer transparent first injection-molded prototype (C) (reprinted from [118] by permission of Oxford University Press on behalf of the Royal Pharmaceutical Society).

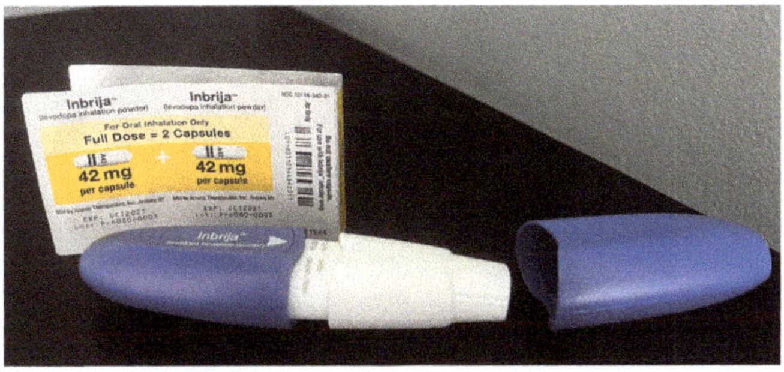

Figure 7.12. Parts of Inbrija® package and inhaler.

7.3.9 DPIs for systemic delivery

As with pMDIs, DPIs were initially applied to treatment of asthma and COPD but have expanded into other therapeutic areas such as antibiotics for cystic fibrosis. They have also been applied to delivery of systemically acting small and large molecule drugs such as levodopa (Inbrija®) and insulin, respectively. DPIs are attractive for oral inhalation because they usually require a short time to administer a single dose. Also, since the drug product is a solid, for the most part DPIs do not rely on cold chain storage to maintain drug stability nor is the powder required to be sterile.

The Exubera® (Pfizer/Nektar) combination product for inhalation delivery of insulin powder was approved for use by FDA in early 2006 but was removed from the market by Pfizer in 2007 due to poor sales (figure 7.13). Competitor products in development at that time, including by Aradigm/Novo Nordisk and Alkermes/Eli Lilly, were also terminated shortly thereafter. Only MannKind continued with development and eventual commercialization of Afrezza®, which was approved in 2014 and is still on the market even though its sales are very low.

7.3.10 Future DPI trend

7.3.10.1 Dry Powder Nebulizer

Dry Powder Nebulizer is a prototype novel inhaler developed by Moraga-Espinoza *et al* (2022). It is a hand-held device that uses the motion of magnets to disperse and fluidize powder for inhalation through a mesh screen (figure 7.14). A study was conducted that showed a high respirable fraction of the emitted powder mass (ca. 75%) for budesonide powders. Unfortunately, information on the nominal mass was not provided in the paper [67].

7.3.10.2 CLIPhaler©, a one-component inhaler

The CLIPhaler© is a single-dose blister DPI designed with only one component (figure 7.15). The design is adaptable for reuse or disposal after use. However, only minimal performance data are available at this point [68].

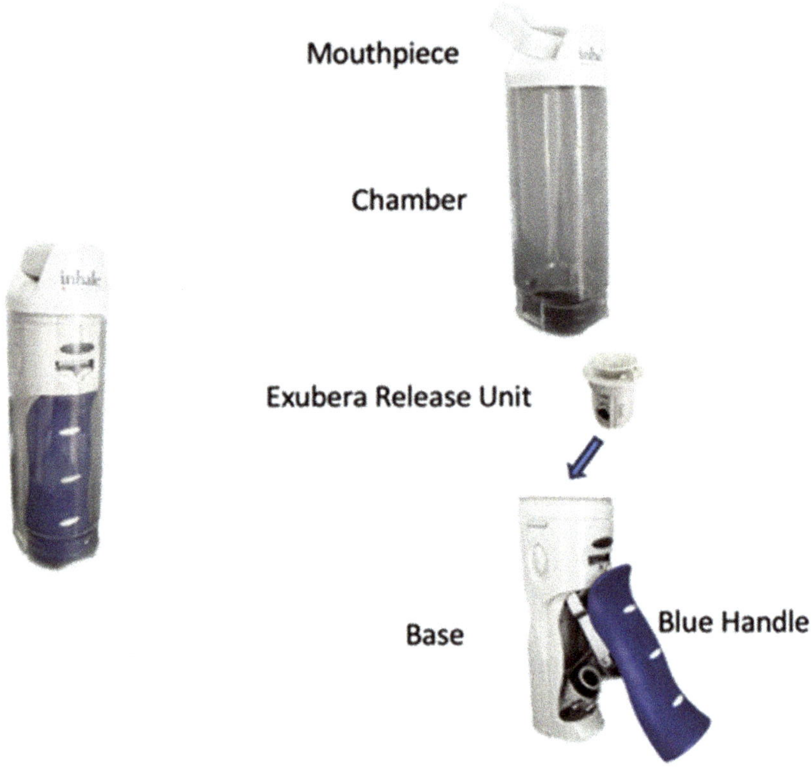

Figure 7.13. Exubera® Pulmonary Delivery System and its main components.

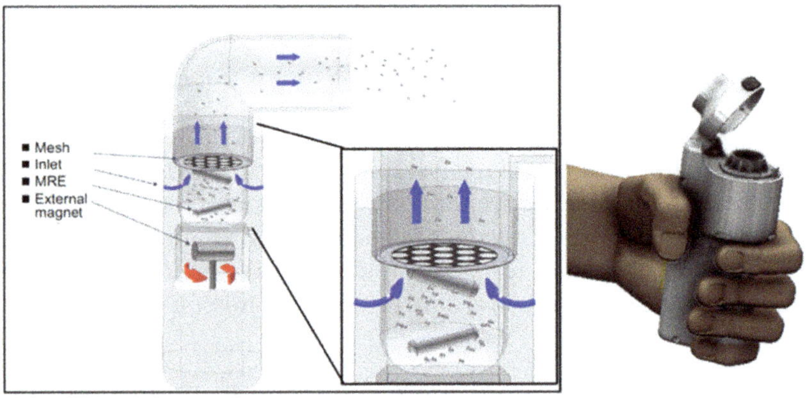

Figure 7.14. Dry powder nebulizer (reproduced from [67] with permission from *Respiratory Drug Delivery* 2022, RDD Online).

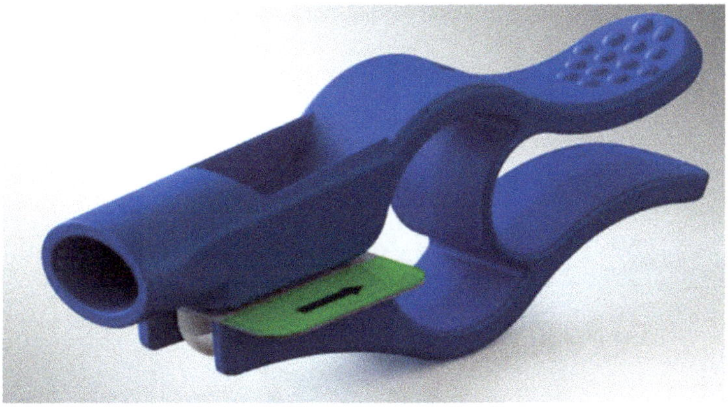

Figure 7.15. CLIPhaler with a blister inserted (courtesy of Klaus-Deiter Beller).

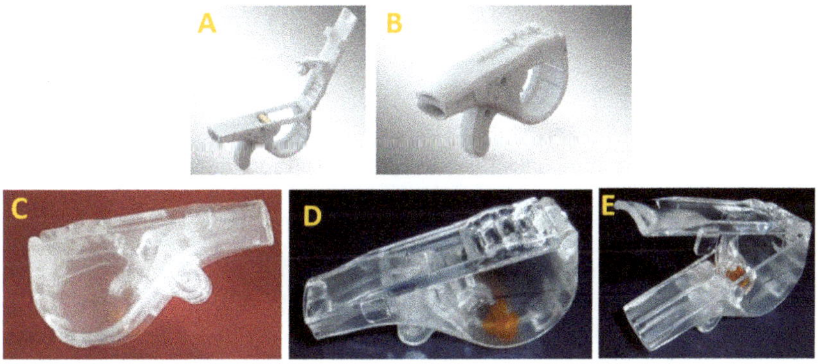

Figure 7.16. Top rows—Whistle open (A) and close (B); Bottom row—Whistle transparent (C), Whistle with capsule inserted (D) and Whistle closed with capsule pierced (E) (courtesy of Klaus-Deiter Beller).

7.3.10.3 Whistle

A reusable three-piece single-dose capsule DPI, Whistle, has also been designed by the inventor of CLIPHaler to deliver medium to large doses of powder in three simple steps [69]. Whistle is a patent protected device (figure 7.16). Both the CLIPhaler and Whistle DPIs are designed for fully automated assembly and low-cost manufacturing.

7.4 Nebulizers

7.4.1 Jet, ultrasonic, and vibrating mesh nebulizers

Nebulization of a liquid to form an aerosol for inhalation is the oldest means of pulmonary delivery. While this approach has been followed for millennia, the first modern configuration known as the jet nebulizer has only been commercially available since the 1930s. The jet nebulizer uses compressed air to aerosolize a drug solution or suspension via the venturi effect. When a compressed air stream is fed through a nozzle inside the nebulizer body, a negative pressure is created at the

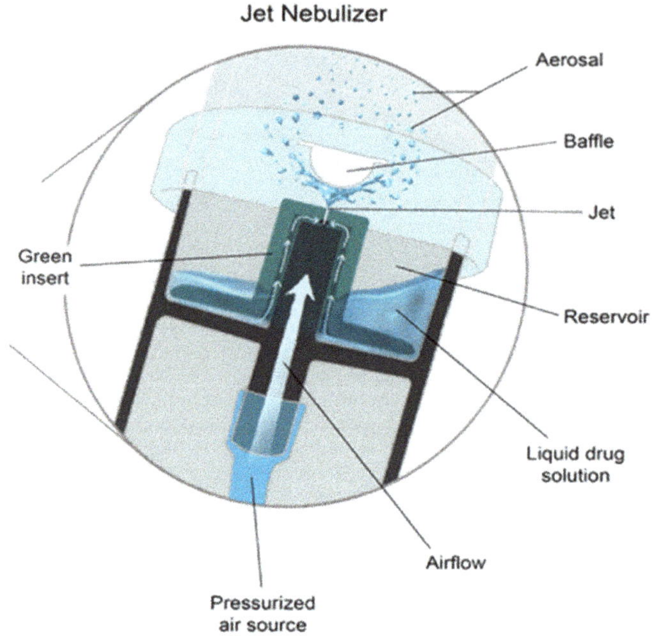

Figure 7.17. Jet nebulizer and main components. Reproduced with permission from Elsevier [70], copyright (2023).

nozzle outlet (Bernoulli effect) that pulls liquid from a reservoir into the air stream and in the process disperses the liquid into droplets. A size-selective baffle placed above the nozzle removes large droplets and allows only fine droplets to be entrained in the air stream, while the large droplets rain back into the reservoir (figure 7.17). The air stream with entrained droplets then exits the inhaler through a mouthpiece for inhalation by the patient [70]. By the end of dosing, only about 20% of the nominal solution volume will have been delivered to the patient with up to 50% retained in the device as residual volume.

Nebulizers generate an aerosol that can be easily inhaled without requiring patients to coordinate their breathing with device actuation. However, several minutes may be needed to administer a large-volume dose, which can result in some loss of compliance due to patient discomfort and patience. For young children, use of a facemask is often required. Problems associated with facemasks include loss of drug on the surface of the facemask due to impaction, and leakage of drug due to a poor seal around the face. Consequently, a reduction in dose of up to 85% can occur with children [71]. Also, unlike DPIs, nebulizers may require cleaning and/or disinfection and are not always particularly portable. The drug product, usually contained in form-fill-seal ampoules or vials, may require refrigeration during storage to prevent chemical degradation and must be sterile to ensure no biological growth during storage. Nonetheless, there has been a noticeable increase in the use of nebulization therapy in clinical trials conducted over the period 2000 to 2021 [98].

The droplet size distribution (DSD) generated by a jet nebulizer depends on the velocity of the air stream and the nebulizer geometry, while the total administration time is determined by the air flow rate and the amount of liquid to be nebulized. Liquid viscosity does not strongly affect the performance of a jet nebulizer, possibly because its effect is masked by the presence of the baffle. However, the droplet size tends to decrease as viscosity increases, while the effect of surface tension is less obvious. As the air inside the nebulizer becomes saturated with vapor, evaporation of the solution causes its temperature to decrease by up to 15 °C, which may affect solution viscosity and drug solubility. As nebulization continues, the drug concentration in the remaining solution may also increase due to evaporation [72].

In its simplest and most common configuration, a jet nebulizer will continuously emit aerosol until the volume of liquid in the reservoir is too small to be effectively taken up by the air stream. This liquid is also part of the residual volume and is considered waste. Additional drug solution is lost because the nebulizer continues to generate aerosol during patient exhalation. Improvements in jet nebulizer design to reduce drug loss during nebulization have included breath-enhanced features such as a one-way valve that allows for increased air flow during inhalation and minimizes drug loss by diverting patient exhalation or breath-actuated capabilities that allow aerosol generation only during patient inhalation.

The only breath-actuated jet nebulizer currently marketed is Aero Eclipse® II BAN™ (Trudell Monaghan Medical Co.). Vectura Group also offers a means of synchronizing a nebulizer and enabling slow, deep patient inhalation through use of the AKITA® system, a smart nebulization technology, which guides inhalation to improve drug delivery to the lungs (figure 7.18). This system enables aerosolization only during the inhalation cycle, thus approximating breath actuation. It can be adapted for use with a jet nebulizer, but it is not portable.

Ultrasonic and vibrating mesh nebulizers are more recent types of inhalers that were introduced commercially in the 1960s and 1990s, respectively. Ultrasonic nebulizers use a piezoelectric crystal vibrating at a high frequency (>1 MHz) to disrupt the surface of a liquid reservoir and cause cavitation, thereby generating droplets for inhalation. As in a jet nebulizer, a baffle is also present to remove large droplets. They do not require compressed air for operation and can in theory be turned on or off easily in response to patient inhalation or exhalation. The drawbacks of ultrasonic nebulizers are that the energy input can increase the reservoir solution temperature by up to 15 °C which may degrade the drug, they have long nebulization times, and they can still exhibit significant drug losses due to large residual volumes. Additionally, higher solution viscosity provides more resistance to cavitation and therefore reduces the output rate. McCallion *et al* (1995) evaluated jet and ultrasonic nebulizer performance using liquids with a wide range of viscosities and surface tensions and found that ultrasonic nebulizers were more sensitive than jet nebulizers to increasing viscosity [73]. In addition, ultrasonic nebulizers cannot nebulize suspension formulations. However, ultrasonic nebulizers are quieter than jet nebulizers.

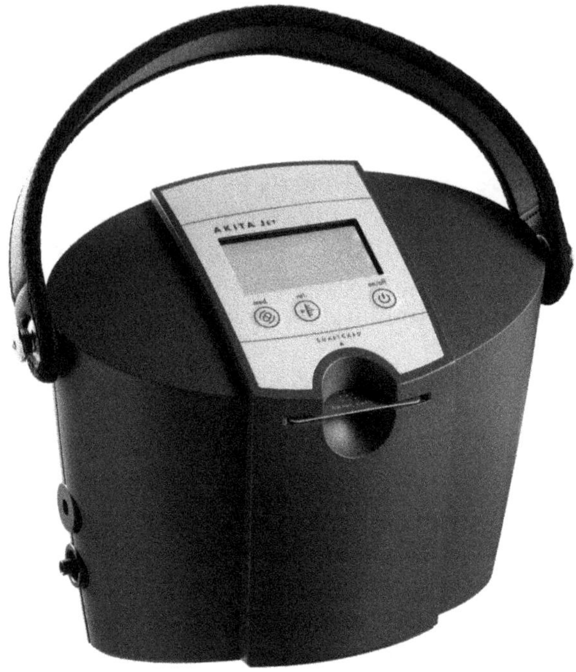

Figure 7.18. AKITA system, a smart nebulization technology (courtesy of Vectura Group Ltd).

Vibrating mesh nebulizers also use a piezoelectric crystal but in this case the crystal vibrates a membrane that is filled with a large number of small almost identically sized and spaced holes. Vibration of the mesh causes the drug solution, which is in contact with the membrane, to be extruded through the holes to generate an aerosol for inhalation. Since the liquid reservoir is in direct contact with the plate the device can be designed to achieve a very low residual volume. The DSD of the generated aerosol is controlled primarily by the hole size, while vibration rate controls delivery rate. Liquid properties such as viscosity and surface tension are secondary. Also, because the formulation is extruded directly through the holes in the mesh, a baffle is not needed to screen out large droplets. The shear forces generated on the drug solution during the extrusion process are expected to be less than seen with jet nebulizers, which may result in less degradation of shear-sensitive drugs such as biologics. Further, the drug formulation passes only once through the mesh, rather than the repeated passes that may take place in a jet nebulizer. The output rate of a vibrating mesh nebulizer may be compromised when dealing with higher-viscosity formulations (i.e., around 2 cPa) making vibrating mesh nebulizers more sensitive to viscosity than jet nebulizers. Vibrating mesh nebulizers are more portable and quieter than jet nebulizers and have demonstrated shorter overall administration time [74, 75]. The higher efficiency of vibrating mesh nebulizers relative to jet nebulizers has been demonstrated in many *in vivo* studies and has made vibrating mesh nebulizers ideal for use in administering expensive drugs. Although

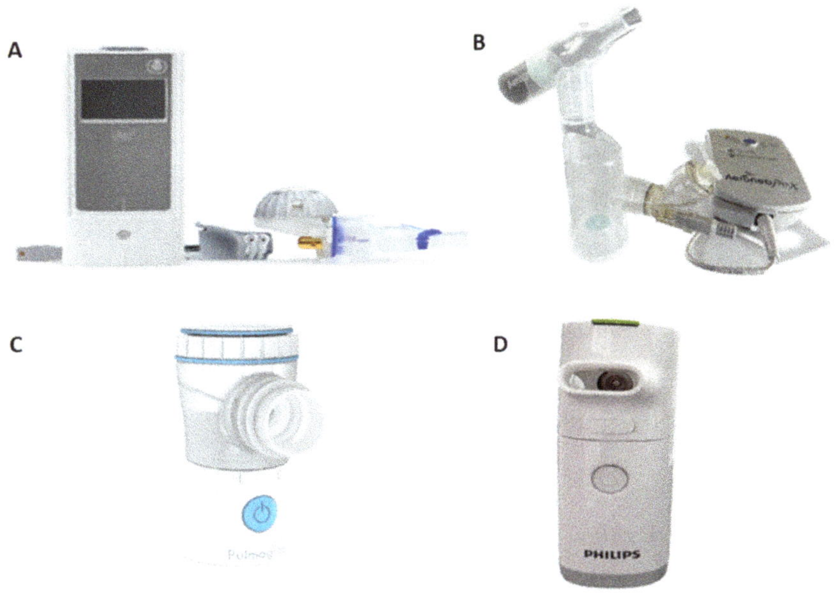

Figure 7.19. Pictorial representation of eFlow® rapid nebulizer system [A] (courtesy of PARI Pharma GmbH), Aeroneb Solo with Aeroneb Pro-X Controller [B], HCmed Pulmogine™ mesh nebulizer [C] (courtesy of HCMed) and Philips InnoSpire Go [D].

vibrating mesh nebulizers have higher efficiency, clogging has been reported to occur after repeat use and/or when nebulizing suspensions which may lead to the need for timely replacement [76, 77]. Some examples of vibrating mesh nebulizers include the PARI e-Flow™, Pulmogine/Deepro and Philips Respironics InnoSpire Go (figure 7.19). These nebulizers are available for home use. The Aerogen® Solo device, which is commonly used in a critical care hospital setting, is often paired with an Aerogen® Ultra Chamber to capture aerosol during exhalation to boost delivery efficiency (figure 7.19**B**).

Omron introduced the first portable vibrating mesh nebulizer (NE-UO3) in the 1990s and improved upon it with the introduction of the MicroAir® nebulizer in the 2000s. These nebulizers use energy from activation of a piezoelectric crystal to vibrate a transducer horn, which in turn pushes liquid through a mesh to generate droplets. Omron supplies their mesh design to Profile Therapeutics (acquired by Respironics) which later launched the i-neb® Adaptive Aerosol Delivery (AAD®) System. The i-neb ADD is a breath-actuated nebulizer referred to as an 'intelligent' nebulizer for its ability to provide precise dosing to patients via two different breathing profiles (tidal and slow-deep) and to log patient and device use for downloading to a monitoring station. The i-Neb AAD is approved for use with inhaled iloprost in the US and as a multipurpose nebulizer in Europe (figure 7.20). Its *in vitro* performance has been evaluated thoroughly as described elsewhere [78, 79]. However, its high cost, cleaning regimen, and challenging user interface quickly became limitations.

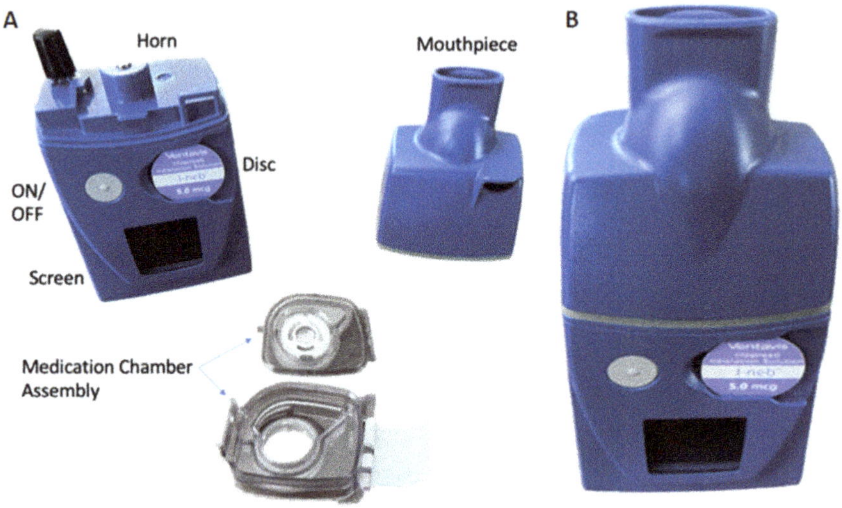

Figure 7.20. Pictorial representation of I-neb ADD components (A) and complete assembled I-neb ADD device (B).

Two major manufacturers of vibrating mesh nebulizers are PARI GmbH and Aerogen Ltd. PARI uses a stainless-steel mesh with holes manufactured using a precision laser drilling technique provided by The Technology Partnership, while Aerogen uses a Pd/Ni alloy mesh with holes manufactured using electroplating to form tapered nozzles. SEM images of the hole structures for both meshes (figure 7.21) show the differences in their appearance. The Aerogen mesh technology is also used in the InnoSpire Go nebulizer, which was launched in 2016 by Philips to expand their home care portfolio while Aerogen continued to focus on nebulizer use in the hospital setting. Because these nebulizers all operate in a continuous mode, drug losses can occur during patient exhalation.

Recent drug-device combination approvals that incorporate the PARI mesh include Arikayce® (Insmed Inc., US), which uses an optimized e-Flow device (the Lamira® Nebulizer System—igure 7.22(A)) for delivery of amikacin liposomal inhalation suspension, 590 mg/8.4 ml vial, and Lonhala® Magnair® (Sunovion Pharmaceuticals Inc.), which uses the closed Magnair® e-Flow system (figure 7.22(B) and (C)) to deliver 25 μg glycopyrrolate twice daily for treatment of airway obstruction in COPD patients. The Lamira® system is an open design wherein the patient pours the contents of a vial into the nebulizer reservoir for administration, while in the Magnair® system the patient inserts an ampoule of solution that is pierced and emptied when the device is closed. This approach is used to deter off-label use of the Magnair device. Both products were approved by FDA in 2018. Other, older approvals of e-Flow containing products for treatment of infections related to CF include Cayston® (Gilead Sciences Inc.), approved by FDA in 2010, which uses the custom Altera e-Flow system to deliver 75 mg aztreonam lysine three times daily, and Quinsair® (Chiesi), approved in EU in 2015, which uses

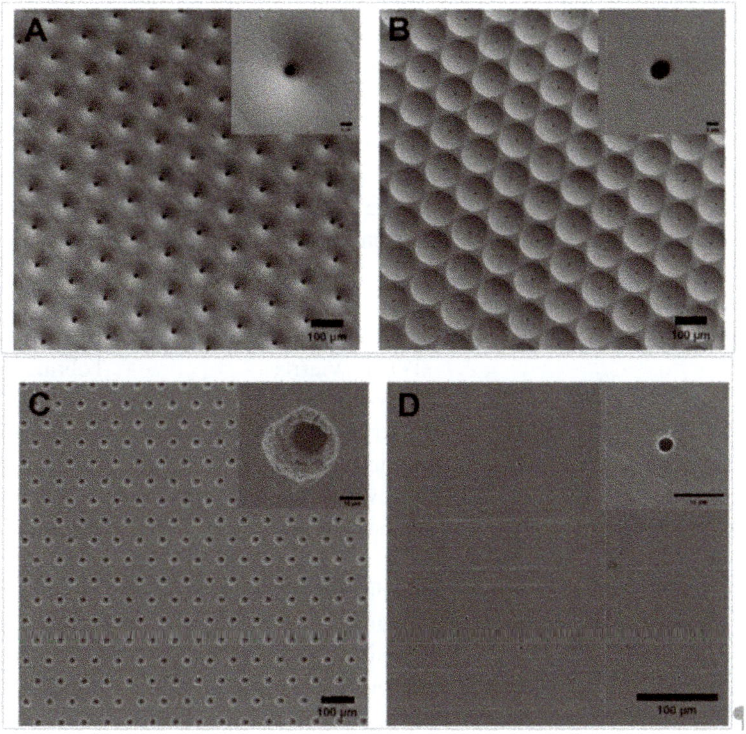

Figure 7.21. SEM images of Aeroneb® Pro (A and B) and eFlow® Rapid (C and D); Reservoir side (A and C) and Outlet side (B and D). Reprinted from [119], copyright (2014) with permission from Elsevier.

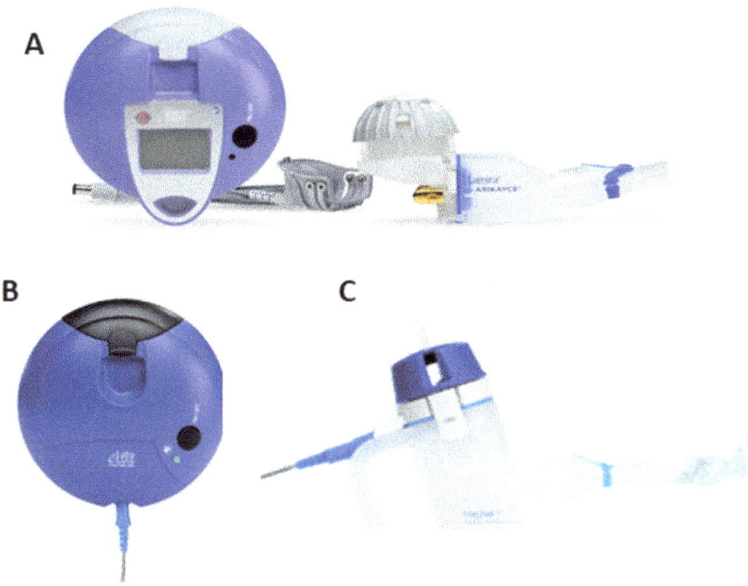

Figure 7.22. Lamira® Nebulizer System (A) and Magnair® eFlow system (B) and (C) (courtesy of PARI Pharma GmbH). Magnair was discontinued in June, 2023.

Table 7.5. Approved nebulized products.

Technology	Brand name/company	Drug
Jet nebulizers (Pari LC Jet Plus®; Hudson® T Up-Draft II) PARI eFlow®	Pulmozyme® rhDNase/ Roche	rhDNase
I-neb AAD® Fox® Nebulizer	Ventavis®/Philips/ Respironics Breelib™	Iloprost
Ultrasonic nebulizer	Tyvaso®/Tyvaso	Treprostinil
Jet nebulizer	TOBI®/Viatris	Tobramycin
Jet nebulizer	Coly-mycin® M	Colistimethate sodium
eFlow®	Altera® Cayston®/Gilead	Aztreonam lysinate
SPAG-2 Jet nebulizer	Virazole®	Ribavirin
eFlow®	eFlow® rapid for Colfinair®	Colistimethate sodium
Respirgard® II Jet Nebulizer	Nebupent[v]	Pentamidine isethionate
eFlow®	Zirela® for Quinsair®[a]	Levofloxacin
eFlow®	Magnair™ for Lonhala[b]	Glycopyrrolate
eFlow®	Lamira® for ARIKAYCE®	Amikacin sulfate
eFlow®	Tolero® for Vantobra®[1]	Tobramycin

[a] Ex-US.
[b] Discontinued in June, 2023.

the Zirela® e-Flow system to administer 240 mg levofloxacin (2.4 ml) BID. PARI provides customized chambers to capture aerosols during exhalation and can modify the mesh configuration and electronics to improve performance for each application. Some approved nebulized products are included in table 7.5.

Additional mesh-type nebulizers have entered the inhaler market in recent years, including the FOX® Inhalation System introduced by Vectura in 2014. This is a hand-held breath-actuated system that features a nickel mesh. It incorporates a regulated flow/volume system to provide slow and deep inhalation to target deep lungs during aerosol delivery. Vectura is collaborating with Aerami to support the development of inhaled imatinib (VR325) using the FOX® Inhalation System (figure 7.23) for the treatment of pulmonary arterial hypertension. Afina™ (Aerami) is also a portable breath-actuated vibrating mesh nebulizer designed to aerosolize insulin (figure 7.24). It has a visual indicator to inform the patient to inhale properly and a Bluetooth connection to enable data collection. Another breath-actuated vibrating mesh nebulizer currently in development is the AdheResp® (HCmed Innovations Co. Ltd, Taiwan) (figure 7.25). This nebulizer incorporates a pressure sensor to allow aerosolization during inhalation only and Bluetooth connectivity for monitoring of patient use. Unlike the Pulmogine nebulizer, the AdheResp mesh is oriented in a horizontal position underneath the drug solution to minimize the residual volume in the reservoir. Other mesh nebulizers include those from HCMed, AireHealth,

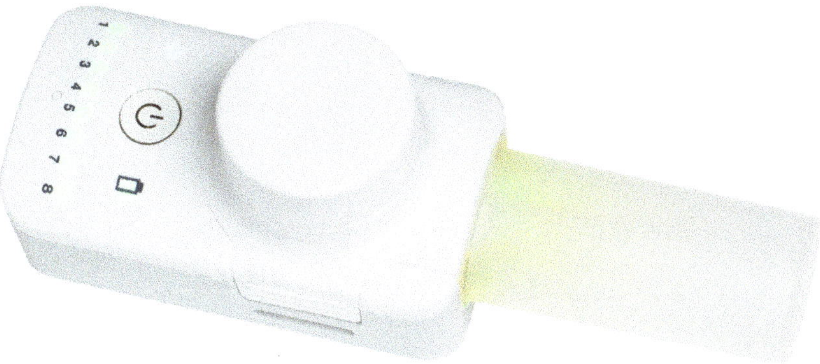

Figure 7.23. Picture of FOX® Inhalation System (courtesy of Vectura Group Ltd).

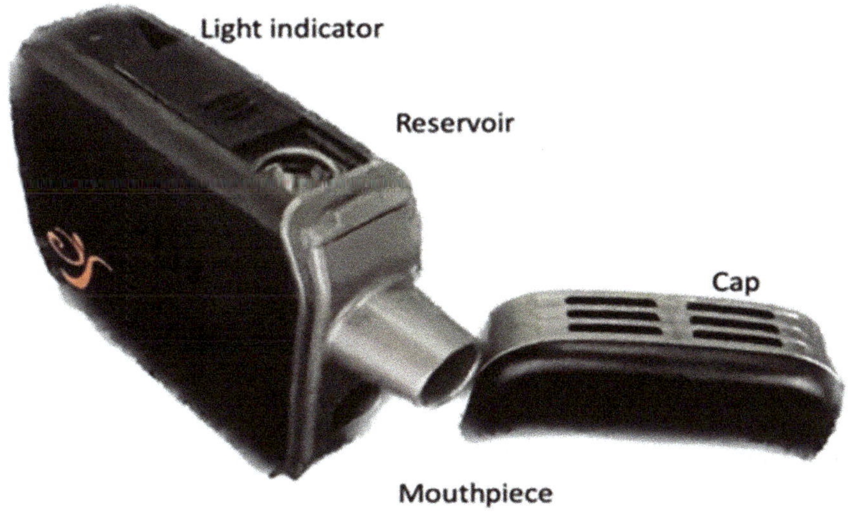

Figure 7.24. Picture of Aerami's proprietary breath-actuated nebulizer i.e., AFINA™ inhaler.

Microbase®, FeelLife, and Kolibri (Pulmotree). All these nebulizers (except for Kolibri) have recently obtained 510(k) clearance from FDA.

7.4.2 Nebulizers used in critical care

Nebulizers and pMDIs are commonly used in a hospital setting to deliver drugs to invasive and non-invasive mechanically ventilated patients. Nebulizers are preferentially used to deliver high doses of medication. Jet nebulizers are considered the standard and least expensive care for this delivery; however, the limitations of the jet nebulizer include its low efficiency (i.e., 10%–15%) and the need for a compressed air source for aerosol generation. Additional adjustment of the ventilator settings is also needed when adding the volume of compressed air to the circuit. Vibrating mesh nebulizers have been shown to be superior to jet nebulizers in this setting due to their

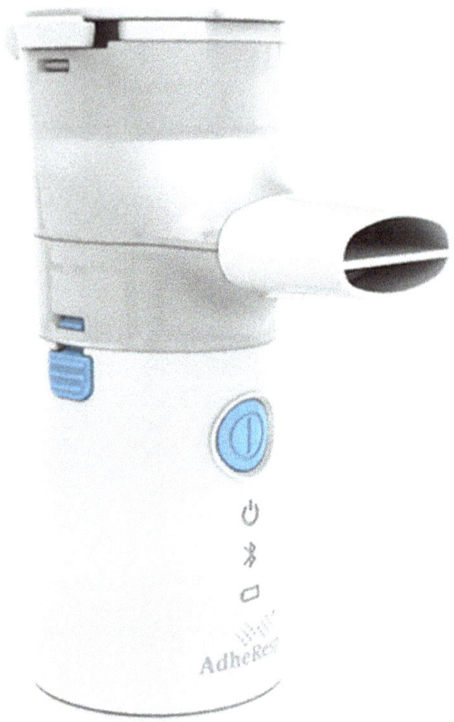

Figure 7.25. AdheResp, a breath-actuated nebulizer by HCMed (courtesy of HCMed).

portability, low noise, and higher efficiency. The residual volume of vibrating mesh nebulizers is typically <10% of the nominal dose, while that of jet nebulizers and ultrasonic nebulizers were 30% and 50%, respectively. Furthermore, vibrating mesh nebulizers do not require an external air source to generate droplets. These nebulizers have also demonstrated better clinical outcomes (i.e., shorter ICU or Emergency Department stays) in critical care patients [80–83]. Because of these positive attributes, the vibrating mesh nebulizer has become the leading choice for use in critical care units. A more comprehensive review on aerosol delivery in pulmonary critical care is provided elsewhere [84–86]

Aerogen Ltd developed the industry standard mesh nebulizer for delivery of antibiotics, vaccines, and proteins in the critical care space. In clinical trials conducted between 2000 and 2016 that included the use of mechanical ventilators, 76% of reported trials used Aerogen nebulizers while 14% used PARI nebulizers and 10% used other jet nebulizers [87]. Aerogen Pharma, the drug development arm of Aerogen Ltd, has also developed the photo defined aperture plate (PDAP™), which is a new technology with a shower head concept that includes 15,600 pre-formed nozzles (figure 7.26). The PDAP has been used to generate smaller droplets at higher output rates than the other Aerogen mesh nebulizers. This technology is currently being used in a nasal delivery system in clinical trials for treatment of respiratory distress syndrome in premature infants. *In vitro* comparisons between PDAP and

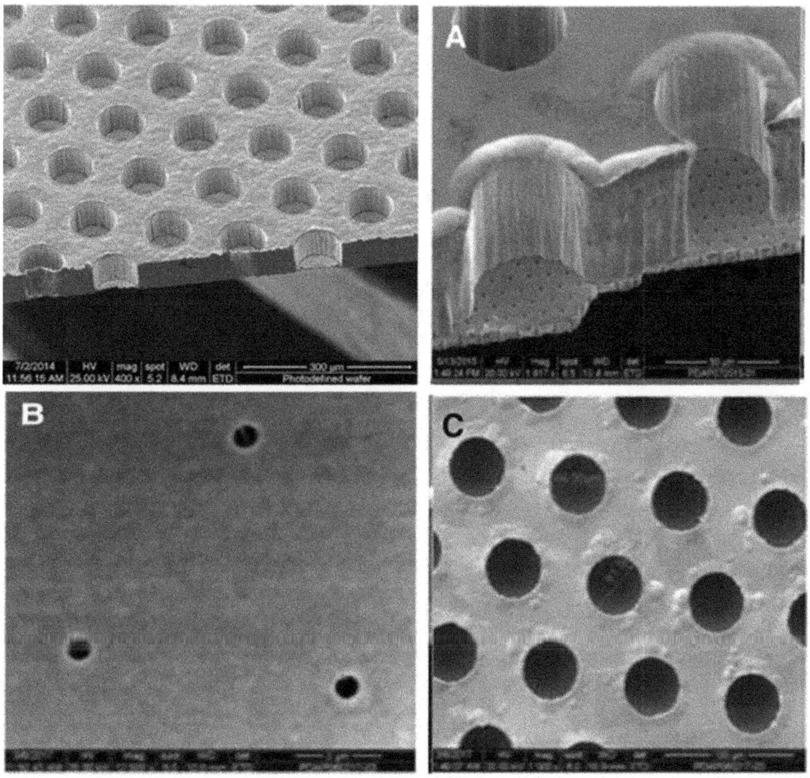

Figure 7.26. Scanning Electron Microscope (SEM) image of PDAP mesh magnification 400× [Left] (courtesy of Aerogen Pharma—Andy Clark. General perspective view of reservoir wells on a thick support layer overlaid on a thin outlet layer as captured by SEM magnification 817× (A), Reservoir image of the PDAP (photo defined aperture plate) device as captured by SEM (B) and Outlet holes of the PDAP device aperture plate as captured by SEM (C), reproduced from [88] CC BY 4.0.

Aerogen Solo showed that PDAP achieved higher efficiency (25%) versus Solo (18%) when tested during mechanical ventilation [88]. Additional information on critical care delivery to infants can be found elsewhere [35]. PARI also offers a variant of the eFlow mesh technology for use with mechanically ventilated patients in critical care settings (figure 7.27). It is a drug-specific device with a removable reservoir to prevent off-label use. The nebulizer is controlled using an electronic ePort® control module. This device was evaluated by Cardeas Pharma in a Phase 3 clinical trial of an amikacin/phosphomycin combination solution for treatment of CF patients [89].

An example of another device for which development was completed but the product was never commercialized is the proprietary pulmonary drug delivery system (PDDS®). This is a high-efficiency breath-actuated vibrating mesh that was developed by Nektar/Bayer to deliver amikacin inhalation solution to mechanically ventilated patients presenting gram-negative pneumonia [90]. The aerosol delivery was synchronized with the inhalation cycle of the mechanical ventilator such that aerosolization occurred during 75% of the inhalation cycle and chase air was

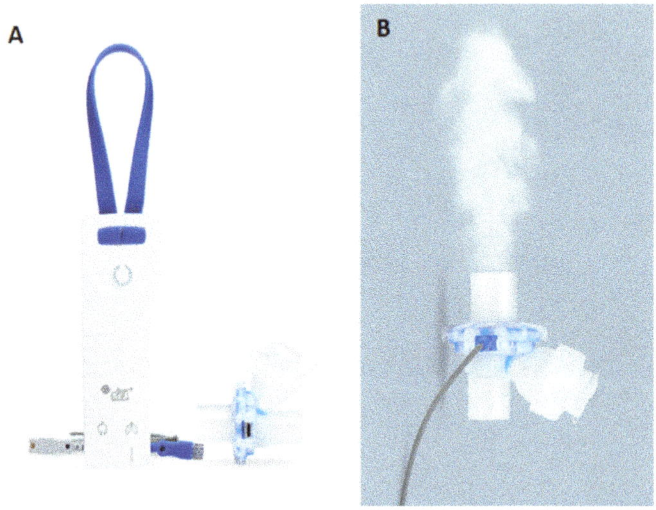

Figure 7.27. Photograph of eFlow® Inline Nebulizer (A) and delivery of drug substance from eFlow® Inline Nebulizer (B) (courtesy of PARI Pharma GmbH).

provided during the remaining 25% of the cycle to further push the aerosol bolus into the lungs. The PDDS delivered about 50% of the nominal dose to the lungs [91, 92], in contrast to a dose of about 10% that is typically achieved using a jet nebulizer. The PDDS system was also configured to nebulize continuously as a hand-held device to patients who are extubated before completing their course of therapy. During the exhalation period, the aerosolized drug is stored in a chamber and is then delivered to the patient during the subsequent inhalation. In this way, the PDDS can operate in both breath-actuated and continuous modes for when a patient is mechanically ventilated and extubated, respectively. The estimated lung doses achieved for the two configurations were similar, which ensured that comparable doses were delivered before and after patient extubation [91].

7.4.3 Future nebulizer trends

7.4.3.1 Nebulizer: surface acoustic wave nebulizer (SAWN)

A recent advance in atomization methodology is the Surface Acoustic Wave Nebulizer (SAWN). This approach, which was introduced in 1995 [93] has since been applied in many areas including drug solution nebulization. This technique operates by applying an electric current to a piezoelectric material in contact with a dilute solution. A high-frequency acoustic wave (on the order of 10–30 MHz) is generated to about 3–4 wavelengths depth along the piezoelectric material, propagates into the liquid, and causes low-frequency Rayleigh instability on the liquid surface. In turn, this instability results in droplet formation using as little as 1 W of power (figure 7.28(a)). This process contrasts with that of a conventional ultrasonic nebulizer, which typically requires up to 10 W of power. Because the SAWN drives nebulization at a much higher frequency (10 MHz) but lower power (~1 W), no

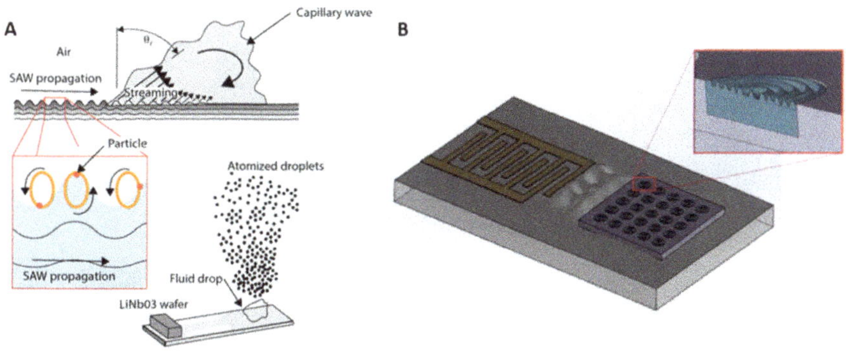

Figure 7.28. Surface acoustic wave (SAW) technology (A) (Reproduced from [5], with permission from Inhalation Magazine 2018) and a schematic representation of a low pass filter coupled to the surface of a Nebu~Flow device (B) (Reproduced with permission from *Respiratory Drug Delivery* 2022, RDD Online).

cavitation and minimal heat generation in the liquid are observed and therefore negligible degradation of dissolved drug would be expected. *In vitro* assessment indicated that SAW process has potential use in biomedical applications based on pre- and post-atomization results showing minimal protein degradation after the SAW extraction process [94, 95]. Further, plasmid DNA was shown to retain its biological activity when atomized using SAWN approach [96]. SAWN has also been shown to generate droplets with MMAD of <3 μm when nebulizing a low surface tension (~30 mN m^{-1}) liquid [97]. Due to its mechanism of droplet formation which eliminates the requirement for a mesh, clogging issue does not exist. Should SAWN be considered a next-generation nebulizer for delivery of inhaled biologics? It remains to be seen as successful adoption of the technology will rely heavily on device simplicity. Nebu-Flow (figure 7.28(b)) has adopted the SAW generator in a nebulizer that is currently in development and has reported promising data [98].

7.4.3.2 Nebulizer: personalized aerosol loading management (PALM)

The PALM nebulizer uses a high frequency piezoelectric element to draw drug solution through microfluidic hydrophilic channels using capillary action to generate high respirable fraction aerosols. The device is intended to fit in the user's palm and provides personalized, rapid feedback regarding patient use. Comparison of the PALM nebulizer to pMDI and Philips InnoSpire Go demonstrated superior aerosol performance [99]. PALM has not yet been evaluated in human clinical trials.

7.5 Soft mist inhalers

Soft mist inhalers are the most recent device type to reach the market, first introduced in 2003. As described by Wachtel [4], their design is intended to address many of the known limitations of pMDIs, DPIs, and nebulizers, including breath coordination, propellant use, and dry powder humidity sensitivity. SMIs are multi-dose devices that require no propellants, electronics, or external power source such as compressed air and rely solely on mechanical energy to generate small respirable

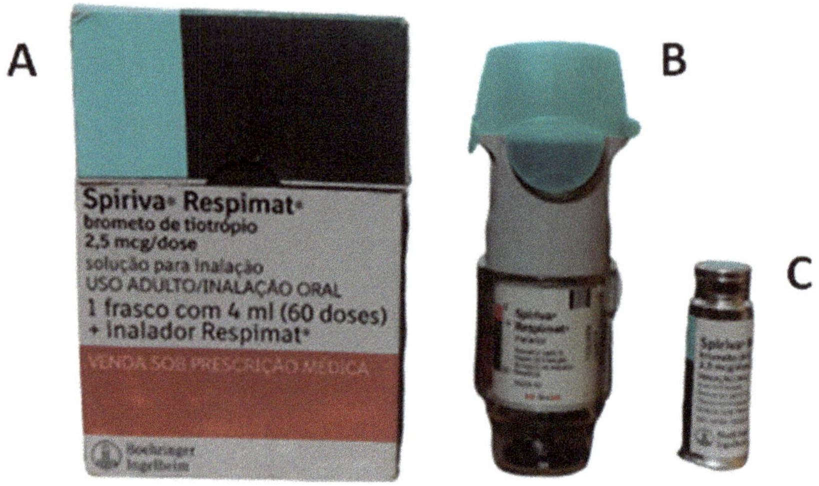

Figure 7.29. Spiriva® Respimat® Soft Mist Inhalers—Outer carton of Spiriva® Respimat® (A), Respimat® inhaler device (B) and Respimat® inhaler cartridge (C).

droplets. SMIs are intended to deliver small, metered doses of aqueous liquids for use in treating asthma and COPD.

The first SMI to be commercialized was the Respimat® Soft Mist™ Inhaler [100], shown in figure 7.29. The Respimat device is actuated by twisting its base, which causes a single dose of liquid to be drawn from a reservoir into a metering chamber through a capillary tube. The tube extends into a collapsible plastic bag that serves as the liquid reservoir and typically holds multiple doses of medication. Twisting the base of the device also tensions a spring. Next, pressing a button on the side of the device releases the preload on the spring, which forces the liquid in the holding chamber through a set of precision nozzles. Convergence of the liquid streams emitted from the nozzles results in atomization and formation of the soft mist with an FPF <5.0μm of approximately 60%–80% [4]. The patient is instructed to breathe through the device mouthpiece at the same time the button is pressed to release the dose and to ensure the complete dose is inhaled. Unlike a pMDI, which atomizes the entire dose volume essentially in 50–100 ms, a SMI atomizes the dose over a period exceeding one second and generates an aerosol bolus with a low forward velocity for optimal for drug delivery. The relatively slow atomization process is also intended to improve the patient's breath coordination. The high FPF that can be achieved with an SMI allows for greater lung deposition and greater overall efficiency compared to other inhaler designs. A limitation of the SMI is its ability to only handle low doses of medication, though this makes the SMI an attractive inhaler for delivery of potent drugs.

A new reusable Respimat for use with up to six disposable cartridges has been designed to reduce the inhaler's carbon footprint [101]. The standard Respimat® requires a patient to replace the inhaler once a month, but the new reusable Respimat can be used for up to six months. The reusable Respimat is a CE-marked inhaler and is available for use ex-US.

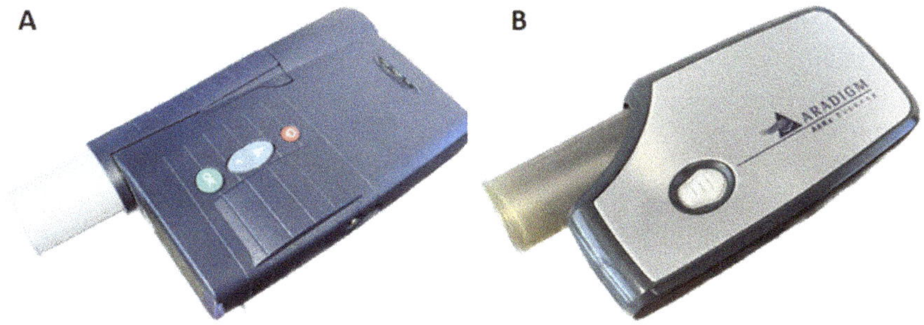

Figure 7.30. Picture of original electronic AERx™ device (A) and mechanical AERx Essence (B) device.

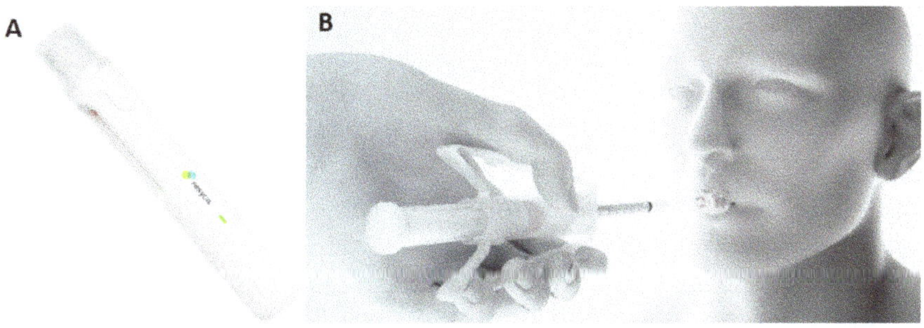

Figure 7.31. Representation of mechanical inhalation device i.e., pre-filled syringe inhaler (PFSI™) [A) and Pulmospray™ soft mist inhaler with Respi Lever Drive (B) (courtesy of Resyca).

The AERx™ device developed by the Aradigm Corporation is another small volume battery-powered inhaler that, similar to the SMI, was designed to aerosolize approximately 45 μl of liquid (figure 7.30). The AERx is considered a 'smart' inhaler as it has the capability to control aerosol generation as well as patient breathing parameters, including breath-hold. It also can record and download patient use information, and security is provided to block any unauthorized use. Liquid drug to be aerosolized using the AERx is provided in a strip containing multi-unit dose small blisters and a channel through which the drug solution flows, when the device is actuated, to a nozzle array comprised of multiple micron-sized holes. The liquid is then forced through the nozzle array to produce the aerosol. The blister strip is single use. Insulin was one of the drug solutions shown to be successfully aerosolized using the AERx [102]. To reduce cost, the AERx device was later simplified to include a mechanical version, AERx Essence, with no electronic feedback or heating conditioning features, however it generated larger droplet than the original AERx device.

Resyca, a joint venture between Recipharm and Medspray, has developed a mechanical drive inhaler integrating a single-use pre-filled syringe inhaler (PFSI®) that is capable of delivering up to 50 μl of drug solution per actuation with a gentle spray module. The drug is contained in a 1 ml glass syringe with integrated spray module that is attached to a base for administration (figure 7.31(A)). The syringe and spray module can be disposed of after dosing and the base can be re-used. This approach is intended to remove the need for cleaning and to reduce waste. A disposable nebulizer, the Pulmospray™ Soft Mist Inhaler used with a cartridge to deliver unit dose between 20 and 50 μl per actuation (figure 7.31(B)) [103]. A disposable version of the Respimat inhaler is the PulmoSpray™ (Resyca) which uses a Lever that can be tailored to the patient's breathing. It is a CE-marked disposable nebulizer system currently being evaluated in clinical trials for COVID-19 [104].

7.6 Patient adherence

Part of what makes a good inhalation product is its ability to promote patient adherence. Achieving this goal requires forward-looking approaches to inhaler design that consider why patients cannot follow their treatment regimens correctly or why they sometimes stop them entirely, and moreover how healthcare practitioners (HCPs) can obtain necessary feedback to properly train or intervene when self-care falls through. If 'successful asthma management is 10% medication and 90% education' [105], it was unfortunately observed that only 10% of HCPs were competent in providing the correct education to patients on the use of their pMDIs [106]. Thus, considerable motivation exists to provide other means of promoting adherence and to support the ability of HCPs to properly instruct patients on inhaler use.

The properties of an inhaler that can influence adherence, such as ease-of-use, convenience, and perception of benefit, have already been touched on for the different inhaler types covered in this chapter. More recent approaches to improving patient adherence include the concept of a 'smart' inhaler, which generally describes the inclusion of functionality into an inhaler design that will provide valuable information on inhaler use or misuse that can help the patient adhere to his or her treatment regimen. Such functionality can include electronic features that can monitor inhaler performance and patient inhalation parameters during dosing and record these data for use by the patient and/or HCP. Data obtained by the device are considered to be more reliable than information that may be related by the patient, who may provide an inaccurate assessment of their experience or even mislead the HCP about their inhaler use. These smart capabilities can provide invaluable feedback to assist the patient with proper inhaler technique and ultimately help develop a positive opinion about using the device and adhering to their regimen.

Mehta (2020) describes several electronic devices that have been introduced to monitor and evaluate adherence [57]. For example, Respiro® (Amiko, London, UK) is a device that can be coupled with any inhaler to record patient use. The device also provides software and communication capabilities to analyze and share use profiles. Electronic feedback functionality has also been adapted for use with some commonly marketed inhalers including Turbuhaler (SmartTurbo device), Diskus (SmartDisk device), and Breezhaler (EnerzAir device). Another inhaler, the ProAir Digihaler (Teva), is similar to a standard pMDI but is designed to simplify breath coordination and provide electronic monitoring and recording of patient inhalation and regimen adherence. Biocorp has developed Inspair [107], which is a stand-alone device that can be attached to the mouthpiece of any pMDI for recording of inhalation data. The information can be transmitted via Bluetooth to a smartphone to assist with patient education. These add-on approaches to obtaining data on patient inhaler use and inhalation parameters such as flow rate and inhaler resistance have been observed to accurately record real-world information pertaining to patient compliance. Digitalized DPIs have been developed as integrated or add-on connectivity for devices. A comprehensive list of marketed and under-development digitalized DPIs has been provided by Xiroudaki [108].

How to motivate patients to use their inhalers correctly is in focus due to the public health risks associated with poor compliance. Murphy *et al* (2012) document the negative impact of poor adherence on clinical outcomes (specifically, lung function) for difficult-to-treat asthma patients [109]. In addition to simplifying inhaler functionality through fewer and more intuitive user steps, addressing patient education and training by providing clear instructions for use and other ancillary aids such as online videos, chats, and telehealth feedback would be expected to improve patient comfort with their inhaler [110, 111]. Additionally, all inhalers are not created equal when it comes to patient understanding; for example, Chrystyn *et al* (2018) note that critical error frequencies tend to be higher for pMDIs than DPIs due to the need for breath coordination [112]. Lavorini *et al* (2014) also reported that 50%–60% of patients with asthma and COPD are unable to use their inhalers properly [113]. High error frequency leads to poor adherence, which is a weakness of pulmonary drug administration in general.

Chan *et al* (2022) conducted a review and meta-analysis of controlled clinical trials that evaluated the impact of electronic monitoring and intervention on patient outcomes. Their review was agnostic to the dosage form and route of administration but included 12 asthma and COPD studies. The authors observed through their analysis that, in general, electronic monitoring that provided feedback leading to some sort of intervention by an HCP or other instructor resulted in better clinical outcomes while no monitoring or monitoring with no follow up had no or less consistent impact [114]. Poor compliance has also been linked to poor outcomes in patients with severe asthma [115]. Furthermore, improving compliance was observed to result in lower incidence of exacerbation in asthmatic patients [116].

Some therapeutic regimens for respiratory diseases such as COPD and CF require the use of multiple inhalers to administer single drugs. For example, a bronchodilator may be prescribed for rescue therapy along with a corticosteroid for long-term control of exacerbations and/or an antibiotic to treat opportunistic lung infections. Requiring a patient to use multiple inhalers can result in even greater compliance and adherence issues than are seen for patients using just one inhaler. Banat *et al* (2023) describe advances in formulation and inhaler design that are enabling the development of combination therapies wherein two or more drugs may be simultaneously administered using one inhaler to improve the patient experience. The challenges and limitations in combination product design involve both the formulation, especially drug–drug compatibility, and dosing regimen, when the different active ingredients require very different therapeutic doses (e.g., a potent, low-dose β_2 agonist and a high-dose antibiotic). Nonetheless, many combination products have been successfully marketed, including Breztri Aerosphere® pMDI (budesonide/glycopyrronium/

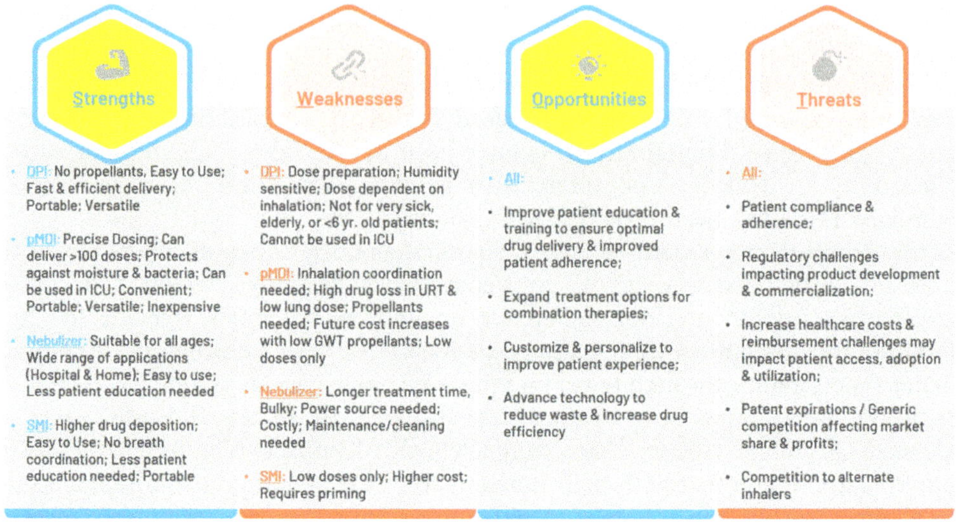

Figure 7.32. SWOT (strengths, weaknesses, opportunities, and threats) analysis for medical inhalers.

formoterol, AstraZeneca), Advair Diskus DPI (fluticasone/salmeterol, GSK), and Stiolto Respimat SMI (tiotropium/olodaterol, BI). It is noted that marketed combination products to date have focused on short- and long-acting asthma and COPD therapies. A more extensive list of these products is provided [110].

7.7 SWOT analysis

An overall SWOT (strengths, weaknesses, opportunities, and threats) analysis for medical inhalers is provided below to help the reader understand the SWOT for each inhaler. This analysis can be used to help plan for the development of inhalers for the products in mind (figure 7.32).

7.8 Conclusions

Oral inhalation is an established means of delivering therapeutic agents to the lungs. It can offer targeted local relief of respiratory issues using doses that would be toxic when delivered orally or parenterally and it can also be applied to administer drugs for systemic therapy. As drug/device combination products, inhaled therapies provide a much higher barrier to entry for competitors than oral dosage forms due to their complex development and registration pathways. Effective drug delivery to the lungs requires the use of an inhaler, of which four primary classes exist: pMDIs, DPIs, nebulizers, and SMIs. Advances in the design and function of these inhalers have contributed to an increasing market share for inhalation products; nonetheless, a review of the current state of inhaler technology recognized that further improvements to dosing efficiency and patient adherence/compliance are important for continuing and expanding this market.

The pMDIs are widely used to deliver asthma and COPD therapies. They employ a propellant to aerosolize microliter volumes of potent molecule solutions or suspensions for direct delivery to the local site of action. Rapid dose administration independent of the patient's respiratory ability has made pMDIs the product of choice for patients experiencing compromised breathing such as during an asthma attack. CFC propellants with ozone-depleting potential, such as Freon-11, initially used in pMDIs have been replaced with HFA-134a or similar non-ozone-depleting propellants. Active efforts are currently directed at replacing these propellants due to their global warming potential.

DPIs can be used to deliver a wide range of dose sizes from single- or multi-dose inhalers. There are many different DPI designs that have been developed and marketed. They are commonly associated with asthma, COPD, and CF therapies, but have also been used to administer systemic therapies such as insulin. Both active and passive DPIs are discussed, where it is clearly stated that flow rate independent drug delivery cannot be achieved via an active DPI. Various dispersion engines are available for powder dispersion in passive DPIs, and their designs are important in defining inhaler resistance. In addition, an impaction parameter, d_a^2Q, is an *in vitro* estimate of *in vivo* lung delivery and is therefore highly recommended for use rather than d_a or FPD/FPF alone because respiratory deposition relies on both d_a and Q. This parameter should also be considered when designing a DPI since it accounts for particle velocity at the exit of the inhaler mouthpiece. Turbulence and high particle velocities are generated during powder dispersion and should be dissipated before they reach the patient. Lower d_a^2Q is favored to minimize URT deposition and maximize TLD. Dispersion and impaction serve as competing parameters and play an important role in achieving flow-rate independent performance in most passive DPIs. Powder dispersion is a complex phenomenon, and one cannot assume that high resistance and low resistance inhalers disperse powder in the same manner. The choice of formulation also plays an important role as larger particles in lactose blends are likely to have greater URT deposition than formulation without large carrier particles such as engineered powders. Furthermore, with engineered particle formulations, high TLD can be achieved even from low resistance devices without requiring high deagglomeration velocities since the dispersion and impaction effects are more balanced. A cutoff of 1 kPa has been proposed as a metric to gauge patient ability to use a DPI, which would eliminate the need for patients to inhale forcefully when using a DPI. Open-inhale-close DPIs have been developed to reduce dose preparation and inhalation errors; for example, NEXThaler and Aspire demonstrated significant reductions in dose preparation errors to less than 1%. Device design should be accompanied by well-tested IFUs to improve user experience and usability. With Aspire, two common errors (i.e., exhalation prior to inhalation and breath-hold) are avoided and can be removed from the IFU.

Nebulizers are available primarily as jet or vibrating mesh-type devices that use compressed air sources or piezoelectric elements, respectively, to aerosolize and deliver liquid medication for up to several minutes. They can administer dose volumes up to several milliliters and can be used in both home and hospital/critical care settings. Nebulizers are available in different configurations that vary in delivery efficiency based on their operating mode, i.e., continuous, breath-enhanced, or breath-actuated. All nebulizers are powered inhalers that do not rely on the patient's breathing ability to aerosolize or present the dose for inhalation. New nebulizers (SAWN) have also been developed to remove clogging issues that can occur with vibrating mesh nebulizers. SMIs deliver small bolus doses of liquid medication gently without using propellants. They are currently used to deliver small, metered doses of aqueous liquids to treat asthma and COPD and have become an attractive inhaler for delivery of potent molecules. SMIs do not require as much breathing coordination with device actuation as pMDIs because of their slow generation of an aerosol bolus and long spray times. All inhaler classes continue to undergo advances in device and formulation design that will improve efficiency and patient convenience. Lastly, integrated and add-on monitoring devices for connectivity to inhalers are trending in order to reduce errors and positively affect patient adherence. These tools are becoming essential for improvement of patient outcomes and more data on their acceptability, cost effectiveness and clinical outcomes continue to be gathered.

About the author

Dr Nani Kadrichu is a pharmaceutical drug/device development professional with 25+ years of recognized expertise in the aerosol science field. She is currently owner and principal of Inspired - Pulmonary Solutions LLC, providing pulmonary drug delivery consulting services ranging from nonclinical evaluation through commercial readiness. Previously, Nani held positions of increasing responsibility within Inhale Therapeutic Systems, Nektar Therapeutics, and Novartis Pharmaceuticals, during which time she participated in development of small molecule and biologic combination products (including inhaled insulin) for pulmonary administration and developed/invented numerous complex pulmonary delivery platforms and novel aerosol characterization methods. Nani holds a BS in Chemistry and MS in Engineering from West Virginia University, and a PhD in Aerosol Science (minor in Chemical Engineering) from the University of California at Los Angeles (UCLA). Nani has authored/co-authored numerous publications and patents.

Acknowledgments

The author would like to acknowledge Andy Clark and Jeffry Weers for their insightful reviews and helpful comments.

References

[1] Stein S W and Thiel C G 2017 The history of therapeutic aerosols: a chronological review *J. Aerosol. Med. Pulm. Drug Deliv.* **30** 20–41

[2] https://fiercepharma.com/pharma/after-years-development-and-fda-rejection-novartis-calls-it-quits-advair-generic-and-takes

[3] Zhong H, Chan G, Hu Y, Hu H and Ouyang D 2018 A comprehensive map of FDA-approved pharmaceutical products *Pharmaceutics* **10** 263

[4] Wachtel H, Kattenbeck S and Dunne S 2017 The respimat® development story: patient-centered innovation *Pulm. Ther.* **3** 19–30
[5] Nebrink O 2018 Nebulizer technology past to present *Inhal. Mag.*
[6] Smith I J, Bell J, Bowman N, Everard M, Stein S and Weers J G 2010 Inhaler devices: what remains to be done? *J. Aerosol Med. Pulm. Drug Deliv.* **S2** 25–37
[7] Clark A R 2022 Half a century of technological advances in pulmonary drug delivery: a personal perspective *Front. Drug Deliv.* **2** 1
[8] Newman S P 2005 Principles of metered-dose inhaler design *Respiratory Care* **50** 1177–88
[9] Crompton G K 1982 Problems patients have using pressurized aerosol inhalers *Eur. J. Respir Dis.* **63** 57–65
[10] Clark A R 2021 Metered atomization for respiratory drug delivery *PhD Thesis* Loughborough University of Technology, Loughborough, UK
[11] Fletcher G E 1975 Factors affecting the atomization of saturated liquids *PhD Thesis* Loughborough University of Technology, Loughborough, UK
[12] Myatt B, Gavtash B, Hodges L and Cooper A 2022 The combined effect of valve and spray orifice diameters on pMDI plume force respiratory drug delivery *Respiratory Drug Delivery (RDD) Conference 2022 (Orlando, FL)*
[13] Djukanovic R, Wilson J W and Britten K M *et al* 1992 Effect of an inhaled corticosteroid on airway inflammation and symptoms in asthma *Am. Rev. Respir. Dis.* **145** 669–74
[14] Dekhuijzen P N R, Batsiou M and Bjermer L *et al* 2016 Incidence of oral thrush in patients with COPD prescribed inhaled corticosteroids: effect of drug, dose, and device *Respir. Med.* **120** 54–63
[15] ICF 2021 Market characterization of the U.S. metered dose inhaler industry(Stratospheric Protection Division Office of Air and Radiation U.S. Environmental Protection Agency Washington, D.C.)
[16] de Boer A H, Hagedoorn P and Grasmeijer F 2022 Dry powder inhalation, part 1: ancient history and precursors to modern dry powder inhalers *Expert Opin. Drug Deliv.* **19** 1033–44
[17] Newman S P, Weisz A W, Talaee N and Clarke S W 1991 Improvement of drug delivery with a breath actuated pressurised aerosol for patients with poor inhaler technique *Thorax* **10** 712–6
[18] Price D, Thomas M, Mitchell G, Niziol C and Featherstone R 2003 Improvement of asthma control with a breath-actuated pressurised metred dose inhaler (BAI): a prescribing claims study of 5556 patients using a traditional pressurised metred dose inhaler (MDI) or a breath-actuated device *Respir. Med.* **97** 12–9
[19] Mahmoud R A A, Tony A M, Boshra M S and Abdelrahman M A *et al* 2022 Addition of inhalation training devices and smartphone application to verbal counseling for asthmatic patients *J. Clin. Nurs. Res.* **6** 76–9
[20] Tony S M, Abdelrahman M A, Osama H, Elgendy M O and Abdelrahim M E A 2021 The effect of adding a training device and smartphone application to traditional verbal counseling in asthmatic children *Pulm. Ther.* **7** 549–62
[21] Kouri A and Gupta S 2023 Mobile health for asthma *Chest Pulmonary* **1** 100002
[22] Biddiscombe M F and Usmani O S 2018 Is there room for further innovation in inhaled therapy for airway disease? *Breathe* **14** 216–24
[23] Pritchard J and Usmani O 2022 The greenest inhaler: a patient-centric approach *Eur. Med. J. Respir.* **10** 2–7

[24] U.S. Food and Drug Administration (FDA) 2020b Drugs@FDA: FDA-Approved Drugs. https://accessdata.fda.gov/scripts/cder/daf/index.cfm
[25] Pritchard J 2020 The climate is changing for metered-dose inhalers and action is needed *Drug Design Dev. Ther.* **14** 3043–55
[26] Atkinson N 2022 Considerations for robust clinical and commercial manufacturing of next generation sustainable metered dose inhalers *Respiratory Drug Delivery 2022* 75–86
[27] Perry M 2023 Considerations when switching from current PMDI propellants to new lower gwp propellants *ONDrug Deliv.* **145** 6–9
[28] Ding B, Small M and Scheffel G 2018 Holmgren. maintenance of inhaler preference attribute importance and satisfaction in prescribing physicians and patients with asthma, COPD, or asthma-COPD overlap syndrome consulting for routine care *Int. J. Chron. Obstruct. Pulmon. Dis.* **13** 927–36
[29] Bar-Katz V, Woolley N J and Vitello E 2021 Economic analysis of NHS England's policy to reduce the carbon impact of inhalers by encouraging a rapid prescribing switch from pressurised metered dose inhalers (PMDIs) to dry powder inhalers (DPIs) *Value Health* **25** S65 POSA161
[30] Usmani O 2019 Choosing the right inhaler for your asthma or COPD patient *Therap. Clin. Risk Manag.* **15** 461–72
[31] Righton L 2021 Six inhaler sustainability myths and why they must be busted *On Drug Deliv.* **127** 30–4
[32] Kuehl P, Corr S and Leach C 2022 Safety, tolerance and pharmacokinetics of HFA-152a in healthy volunteers *Respiratory Drug Delivery 2022* 1–9
[33] Slowey A and Hayes A 2022 The use of accelerated stability storage to fast-track the development of a new metered dose inhaler incorporating the greener propellant HFA-152 *Respiratory Drug Delivery 2022* 263–6
[34] Berkenfeld K, Lamprecht A and McConville J T 2015 Devices for dry powder drug delivery to the lung *AAPS Pharm. Sci. Tech.* **16** 479–90
[35] Anderson A, Atkins O, Backman B, Cipolla D and Clark A *et al* 2022 Inhaled medicines: past, present, and future *Pharmacol. Rev.* **74** 48–118
[36] de Boer A H, Hagedoorn P and Grasmeijer F 2022 Dry powder inhalation, part 2: the present and future *Expert Opin. Drug Deliv.* **19** 1045–59
[37] Harper A and Sanders M J 2022 Dry powder inhalers—more than 170 years of development; where to next? *Inhal. Mag.*
[38] Weers J and Clark A 2017 The Impact of inspiratory flow rate on drug delivery to the lungs with dry powder inhalers *Pharm. Res.* **34** 507
[39] Weers J G *et al* 2019 Idealhalers versus realhalers: is it possible to bypass deposition in the upper respiratory tract? *J. Aerosol Med. Pulm. Drug Deliv.* **32** 55–69
[40] Begat P, Morton D A V, Shur J, Kippax P, Staniforth J N and Price R 2009 The role of force control agents in high-dose dry powder inhaler formulations *J. Pharm. Sci.* **98** 2770–83
[41] Mahar R, Chakraborty A and Nainwal N 2022 The influence of carrier type, physical characteristics, and blending techniques on the performance of dry powder inhalers *J. Drug Deliv. Sci. Technol.* **76** 760
[42] Stokes G G 1851 On the effect of the internal friction of fluids on the motion of pendulums *Trans. Cambridge Philosophical Soc.* **9** 8–106

[43] Finlay W H 2001 *The Mechanics of Inhaled Pharmaceutical Aerosols* (San Diego, CA: Academic)

[44] Weers J, Kadrichu N and Rao N 2019 Is aerodynamic diameter a good metric for understanding regional lung deposition? *Respiratory Drug Delivery Europe (Lisbon)* **2019** 59–66

[45] Stahlhofen S, Rudolf G and James A C 1989 Intercomparison of experimental regional aerosol deposition data *J. Aerosol Med.* **2** 285–308

[46] Borgström L, Olsson B and Thorsson L 2006 Degree of throat deposition can explain the variability in lung deposition of inhaled drugs *J. Aerosol Med.* **19** 473–83

[47] Hannon J, Donovan M, Gibbons A, Xu Z, Curtiw R, Smyth H and Clark A 2016 Novel high efficiency inhaler for PDE5i lung delivery *Respiratory Drug Delivery 2016* 519–22

[48] Weers J, Lyons S, Tarara T, Miller D P, Malloy L, Weers A, Saavedra K, Heller D and Curtis R 2020 The AOS™ DPI: A capsule-based dry powder inhaler with four distinct dispersion elements *Respiratory Drug Delivery 2020* 459–62

[49] Clark A R and Hollingworth A M 1993 The relationship between powder inhaler resistance and peak inspiratory conditions in healthy volunteers—implications for *In Vitro* testing *J. Aerosol Med.* **6** 99–110

[50] Clark A R, Weers J G and Dhand R 2020 The confusing world of dry powder inhalers: it is all about inspiratory pressures, not inspiratory flow rates *J. Aerosol Med. Pulm. Drug Deliv.* **33** 1–11

[51] Cardwell N D, Zee J, Kadrichu N, Rao N and Clark A R 2014 Flow field characterization of three dry powder inhalers *Respiratory Drug Delivery 2014* 501–6

[52] Harris D 2015 The advantages of designing high-resistance swirl chambers for use in dry-powder inhalers *ONDrug Deliv.* **57** 10–3

[53] Weers J G and Tarara T E 2014 The pulmosphereTM platform for pulmonary drug delivery *Therap. Deliv.* **5** 277–95

[54] Weers J G, Clark A R, Rao N, Ung K, Haynes A, Khindri S K, Perry S A, Machineni S and Colthorpe P 2015 *In vitro–in vivo* correlations observed with indacaterol-based formulations delivered with the breezhaler *J. Aerosol Med. Pulm. Drug Deliv.* **28** 268–80

[55] https://consumermedsafety.org/safety-articles/mix-ups-between-five-different-inhalers-that-all-include-ellipta-as-part-of

[56] Grant A C, Walker R, Hamilton M and Garrill K 2016 The ELLIPTA® dry powder inhaler: design, functionality, *in vitro* dosing performance and critical task compliance by patients and caregivers *J. Aerosol. Med. Pulm. Drug Deliv.* **28** 474–85
Erratum in *J. Aerosol Med. Pulm. Drug Deliv.* **29** 218

[57] Mehta P P 2021 Dry powder inhalers: a concise summary of the electronic monitoring devices *Ther. Deliv.* **12** 1–6

[58] Corradi M, Chrystyn H, Cosio B G, Pirozynski M, Loukides S, Louis R, Spinola M and Usmani O S 2014 NEXThaler, an innovative dry powder inhaler delivering an extrafine fixed combination of beclometasone and formoterol to treat large and small airways in asthma *Expert Opin. Drug Deliv* **11** 1497–506

[59] Serafin C, Maltz D, Glusker M, Lin J and Weers J 2016 Aspirations for usability: successfully including human factors in the design of the USSC-03 inhaler *Respiratory Drug Delivery 2016* 477–80

[60] Glusker M, Axford G, Le J, Lin J, Maltz D and Paterson D *et al* 2016 USSC-03: a modular breath-actuated multi-dose dry powder inhaler system with telehealth capability *Respiratory Drug Delivery 2016* 449–53
[61] Glusker M, Chiao A, Axford G, Serafin C, Summers J P and Downing J 2017 Multidose inhaler. WO 2017/12583 A1
[62] Akkerman-Nijland A M, Grasmeijer F, Kerstjens H A M, Frijlink H W, van der Vaart H, Vonk J M, Hagedoorn P, Rottier B L, Koppelman G H and Akkerman O W 2020 Colistin dry powder inhalation with the Twincer™: an effective and more patient friendly alternative to nebulization *PLoS One* **15** e0239658
[63] Westerman E M, de Boer A H, Le Brun P P H, Touw D J, Roldaan A C, Frijlink H W and Heijerman H G M 2007 Dry powder inhalation of colistin in cystic fibrosis patients: a single dose pilot study *J. Cyst. Fibrosis* **6** 284–92
[64] Sibum I, Hagedoorn P, de Boer A H, Frijlink H W and Grasmeijer F 2018 Challenges for pulmonary delivery of high powder doses *Int. J. Pharmaceut.* **548** 325–36
[65] Schwarz C 2015 Colobreathe® for the treatment of cystic fibrosis-associated pulmonary infections *Pulm. Therap.* **1** 19–30
[66] NCT01764841 2017 Ciprofloxacin Dry Powder for Inhalation in Non-Cystic Fibrosis Bronchiectasis (Non-CF BE) (RESPIRE 1)
[67] Moraga-Espinoza D, Hefnawy A, Brunaugh A D, Li Y, Smyth H D C and Atkins P 2022 Design and aerosol performance of a novel dry powder nebulizer for high dose delivery *Respiratory Drug Delivery 2022*
[68] Beller K D 2022 CLIPhaler—inhalation device design reduced to the maximum *ONDrug Deliv.* **140** 60–3
[69] Personal communication with K D Beller
[70] O'Neil J A and Villasmil-Urdaneta L A 2023 A path forward in the development of new aerosol drug delivery devices for pediatrics *Respiratory Med.* **211** 107210
[71] Everard M L, Clark A R and Milner A D 1992 Drug delivery from jet nebulisers *Arch. Dis. Child.* **67** 586–91
[72] O'Callaghan C and Barry P W 1997 The science of nebulized drug delivery *Thorax* **52** S31–44
[73] McCallion O N M, Taylor K M G, Thomas M and Taylor A J 1995 Nebulization of fluids of different physicochemical properties with air-jet and ultrasonic nebulizers *Pharm. Res.* **2** 1682–8
[74] Ari A and Fink J B 2020 Recent advances in aerosol devices for the delivery of inhaled medications *Expert Opin. Drug Deliv.* **17** 133–44
[75] Martin A R and Finlay W H 2015 Nebulizers for drug delivery to the lungs *Expert Opin. Drug Deliv.* **12** 889–900
[76] Scherer T, Geller D E, Owyang L, Tservistas M, Keller M, Boden N, Kesser K C and Shire S J 2011 A technical feasibility study of dornase alfa delivery with eFlow® vibrating membrane nebulizers: aerosol characteristics and physicochemical stability *J. Pharm. Sci.* **100** 98–109
[77] Hertel S P, Winter G and Friess W 2015 Protein stability in pulmonary drug delivery via nebulization *Adv. Drug Deliv. Rev.* **93** 79–94
[78] Hadaker L E A and Hatley H M 2010 *In vitro* characterization of the I-neb adaptive aerosol delivery (AAD) system *J. Aerosol Med. Pulm. Drug Deliv.* **23** S11–20

[79] Nikander K, Taylor G and Warren S 2010 Mode of breathing—tidal or slow and deep—through the I-neb adaptive aerosol delivery (AAD) system affects lung deposition of 99m Tc-DTPA *J. Aerosol Med. Pulm. Drug Deliv.* **23** S37–43
[80] Moody G B, Luckett P M, Shockley C M, Huang R and Ari A 2020 Clinical efficacy of vibrating mesh and jet nebulizers with different interfaces in pediatric subjects with asthma *Respir. Care* **65** 1451–63
[81] Moustafa I O F, ElHansy M H E and Al Hallag M *et al* 2017 Clinical outcome associated with the use of different inhalation method with and without humidification in asthmatic mechanically ventilated patients *Pulm. Pharmacol. Ther.* **45** 40–6
[82] Abdalln M *et al* 2022 A comparison of the aerogen vibrating mesh nebuliser versus a standard jet nebuliser to deliver bronchodilators in moderate to severe asthma in the emergency department *Emerg. Med.* **39** 243–68
[83] Edge R and Butcher R 2019 Vibrating mesh nebulizers for patients with respiratory conditions: clinical effectiveness, cost-effectiveness, and guidelines *CADTH Rapid Response Report* https://pubmed.ncbi.nlm.nih.gov/31553547/
[84] Ari A 2015 Aerosol therapy in pulmonary critical care *Respir. Care* **60** 858–79
[85] Ari A, Fink J B and Dhand R 2012 Inhalation therapy in patients receiving mechanical ventilation: an update *J. Aerosol Med. Pulm. Drug Deliv.* **25** 319–32
[86] MacLoughlin R and Martin-Loeches I 2023 Not all nebulizers are created equal: considerations in choosing a nebulizer for aerosol delivery during mechanical ventilation *Expert Rev. Respir. Med.* **17** 131–42
[87] Pritchard J N, Hatley R H M, Denyer J and von Hollen D 2018 Mesh nebulizers have become the first choice for new nebulized pharmaceutical drug developments *Therap. Deliv.* **9** 121–36
[88] Sweeney L, McCloskey A P, Higgins G, Ramsey J M, Cryan S A and MacLoughlin R 2019 Effective nebulization of interferon-γ using a novel vibrating mesh *Respir. Res.* **20** 66
[89] NCT01969799 2013 Aerosolized Amikacin and Fosfomycin in Mechanically Ventilated Patients with Gram-negative Pneumonia (IASIS)
[90] NCT01799993 2013 Inhaled Amikacin Solution BAY41–6551 as Adjunctive Therapy in the Treatment of Gram-Negative Pneumonia (INHALE 1)
[91] Kadrichu N, Boc S, Corkery K and Challoner P 2013 *In vitro* efficiency of amikacin inhale, a novel drug-device delivery system *Crit. Care* **17** 81
[92] Kadrichu N and Daniher D 2018 Improvement of an *in vitro* model to assess delivered dose and particle size for a vibrating mesh nebulizer during mechanical ventilation *J. Aerosol. Med. Pulm. Drug Deliv.* **31** 94–102
[93] Kurosawa M, Watanabe T, Futami A and Higuchi T 1995 Surface acoustic wave atomizer *Sens. Actuators Appl. Phys.* **50** 69–74
[94] Cortez-Jugo C, Masoumi S, Chan P P Y, Friend J and Yeo L 2022 Nebulization of siRNA for inhalation therapy based on a microfluidic surface acoustic wave platform *Ultrason. Sonochem.* **88** 106088
[95] Qi A, Friend J and Yeo L 2011 A miniaturized surface acoustic wave atomizer with a disposable pump-free liquid supply system for continuous atomization *Proc. of the 2011 6th IEEE Int. Conf. on Nano/Micro Engineered and Molecular Systems (Kaohsiung, Taiwan, February 20–23)*
[96] Rajapaksa A, Qi A, Yeo L Y, Coppel R and Friend J R 2014 Enabling practical surface acoustic wave nebulizer drug delivery via amplitude modulation *Lab Chip* **14** 1858–65

[97] Witte C, Nazarzadeh E, Pritchard J, Reboud J and Cooper J M 2021 Surface acoustic wave nebulisation for targeted inhalation drug delivery to central and peripheral airways *Drug Delivery to the Lungs 2021*

[98] Pritchard J N and Nazarzadeh E 2022 Next generation nebulized therapy: opportunities for new treatments and devices *Respiratory Drug Delivery 2022*

[99] Brenker J, Al-mazi J G, Le A, Pal S, Ong H X, Traini D and Alan T 2022 Microfluidic aerosol generation: development of a next generation hand-held device for aerosol drug delivery *Respiratory Drug Delivery 2022*

[100] Dalby R, Spallek M and Voshaar T 2004 A review of the development of respimat soft mist inhaler *Int. J. Pharm.* **283** 1–9

[101] Wachtel H, Bambach T, Kattenbeck S, Meisenheimer M, Jost I and Weiland F 2020 The Re-usable respimat® soft mist™ inhaler: an effective propellant-free inhaler platform *Respiratory Drug Delivery 2020*

[102] NCT00331604 2006 Safety and efficacy of inhaled insulin in type 2 diabetes

[103] de K 2022 What happened to nebuliser innovation? *Drug Delivery to the Lungs*

[104] NCT04990830 2021 Effects of low molecular weight heparin therapy with soft-mist inhaler for COVID-19 induced hypoxemia

[105] Fink J B 2005 Inhalers in asthma management: is demonstration the key to compliance? *Respir. Care* **50** 598–600

[106] Baverstock M *et al* 2010 Do healthcare professional have sufficient knowledge of inhaler techniques in order to educate their patients effectively in their use? *Thorax* **65** A117–8

[107] Vuillecard J 2016 Leverage technology to overcome pulmonary drug delivery challenges *Ondrug Deliv.* **72** 18–21

[108] Xiroudaki S, Schoubben A, Giovagnoli S and Rekkas D 2021 DPI in the digitalization era current status and future perspectives in pharmaceutics *Pharmaceutics* **13** 1455

[109] Murphy A C, Proeschal A and Brightling C E *et al* 2012 The relationship between clinical outcomes and medication adherence in difficult to control asthma *Chest Clinic* **67** 751–53

[110] Banat H, Ambrus R and Csoka I 2023 Drug combinations for inhalation: current products and future development addressing disease control and patient compliance *Int. J. Pharm.* **643** 123070

[111] Sanders M 2022 Dry powder inhalers: a new look at what may be next *Inhal. Mag.* October 2022

[112] Chrystyn H, van der Palen J and Sharma R *et al* 2017 Device errors in asthma and COPD: systematic literature review and meta-analysis *Prim. Care Respir. Med.* **27** 22

[113] Lavorini F, G, Fontana A and Usmani O S 2014 New inhaler devices—the good, the bad and the ugly *Respiration* **88** 3–15

[114] Chan A H Y, Foot H and Pearce C J *et al* 2022 Effect of electronic adherence monitoring on adherence and outcomes in chronic conditions: a systematic review and meta-analysis *PLoS One* **17** e0265715

[115] Smith J R, Mildenhall S, Noble M, Mugford M, Shepstone L and Harrison B D 2005 Clinician-assessed poor compliance identifies adults with severe asthma who are at risk of adverse outcomes *J. Asthma* **42** 437–45

[116] Stern L, Berman J, Lumry W, Katz L, Wang L, Rosenblatt L and Doyle J J 2006 Medication compliance and disease exacerbation in patients with asthma: a retrospective study of managed care data *Ann. Allergy Asthma Immunol.* **97** 402–8

[117] Mason F, Tweedie A and Lewis D A 2015 Effect of the breath-actuated mechanism on the dispersion performance of the NEXThaler® *Drug Delivery to the Lungs 26*

[118] de Boer A H, Hagedoorn P, Woolhouse R and Wynn E 2012 Computational fluid dynamics (CFD) assisted performance evaluation of the Twincer™ disposable high-dose dry powder inhaler *J. Pharm. Pharmacol.* **64** 1316–25

[119] Beck-Broichsitter M, Knuedeler M-C, Seeger W and Schmehl T 2014 Controlling the droplet size of formulations nebulized by vibrating-membrane technology *Eur. J. Pharmaceut. Biopharmaceut.* **87** 524–9

IOP Publishing

Advances in Drug Delivery Systems for Healthcare
From concept to clinic
Piyush Pradeep Mehta and Arpana Parihar

Chapter 8

The usage of artificial intelligence in drug delivery—current trends and future outlook

Pintu K Rathod[1], Sumedh D Bahadure[1], Shahid I Mir[1], Shital Kolhe[1] and Sachin S Surwase

The usage of artificial intelligence (AI) in drug delivery has emerged as a promising field that has the potential to revolutionize the pharmaceutical industry. AI techniques, such as machine learning and deep learning, are being increasingly employed to enhance various aspects of drug delivery, including drug formulation, targeting, release mechanisms, and personalized medicine. Over the last decade, increasing interest has been attracted towards the application of AI technology for analysing and interpreting the biological or genetic information, accelerated drug discovery, and identification of the selective small-molecule modulators or rare molecules and prediction of their behaviour. Application of the automated workflows and databases for rapid analysis of the huge amounts of data and artificial neural networks (ANN models) for development of the novel hypotheses and treatment strategies, prediction of disease progression, and evaluation of the pharmacological profiles of drug candidates may significantly improve treatment outcomes. The utilization of AI in drug delivery is poised to transform the pharmaceutical industry and improve patient care. By leveraging AI's capabilities in data analysis, prediction, and optimization, drug discovery, personalized medicine, and drug delivery systems can be revolutionized. However, careful consideration of ethical, legal, and regulatory aspects is necessary to harness the full potential of AI while ensuring patient safety and privacy. The future of AI in drug delivery holds immense potential. Advancements in machine learning, deep learning, and natural language processing will enable more sophisticated analysis of complex biological data. Integration of AI with other technologies, such as nanotechnology and robotics, will pave the way for innovative drug delivery platforms.

[1] All authors contributed equally.

doi:10.1088/978-0-7503-5613-8ch8

Additionally, the application of AI in clinical decision-support systems and real-world evidence analysis will further optimize drug delivery strategies.

8.1 Introduction

In the field of drug discovery, artificial intelligence (AI) has proven potential by improving drug development and delivery accuracy, efficiency, and speed. AI is a broad term that refers to software that simulates human cognition to accomplish and learn from complicated tasks. It includes a subfield known as machine learning, which includes algorithms trained with data to produce models for performing challenging tasks. Deep learning is a machine learning technique that employs layers of neural networks to perform the most intricate functions without the assistance of humans. These artificial intelligence techniques can be used to design and develop pharmaceutical formulations that can target and release drugs at specific sites in the body. ANN models, information technology along with the wireless communication technology, can be used to create advanced drug delivery techniques to overcome the drawbacks of conventional drug delivery systems. This approach has the potential to improve treatment efficacy, reduce side effects, and improve patient outcomes [1]. AI-powered drug delivery systems are also being used to optimize drug dosages, predict drug interactions, and identify potential drug candidates [2]. The incorporation of AI into drug delivery systems is a significant step toward personalized medicine, and it is expected to play a critical role in the future of healthcare [3]. The incorporation of AI in drug delivery systems has demonstrated enormous potential for improving drug efficacy, reducing toxicity, and improving patient outcomes [4]. AI has transformed drug delivery by providing sophisticated tools for predicting drug absorption, distribution, metabolism, and excretion [5]. It has also enabled the development of novel drug delivery systems that can target specific cells, tissues, and organs [6]. AI can aid in the design and optimization of drug delivery methods, as well as the identification of new drug targets, by utilizing machine learning algorithms [7, 8].

Current trends of using AI for drug delivery include the development of smart drug delivery systems, personalized medicine, and nanotechnology-based drug delivery [9]. AI algorithms are used in smart drug delivery systems to control the release of drugs at specific times and locations in the body, allowing for precise drug delivery and reducing the risk of side effects [10]. Personalized medicine, on the other hand, employs AI to tailor drug delivery to a person's specific genetic makeup, medical history, and lifestyle [3]. Nanotechnology-based drug delivery uses nanoparticles to deliver drugs to specific cells and tissues, increasing drug efficacy while decreasing toxicity [11]. AI in drug delivery has a bright future, with the potential to significantly improve drug delivery efficiency and patient outcomes. However, there are still issues to be addressed, such as the regulatory framework for AI-based drug delivery systems and the ethical implications of using AI in healthcare. Nonetheless, the potential benefits of AI in drug delivery make it an exciting area for pharmaceutical research and development (figure 8.1).

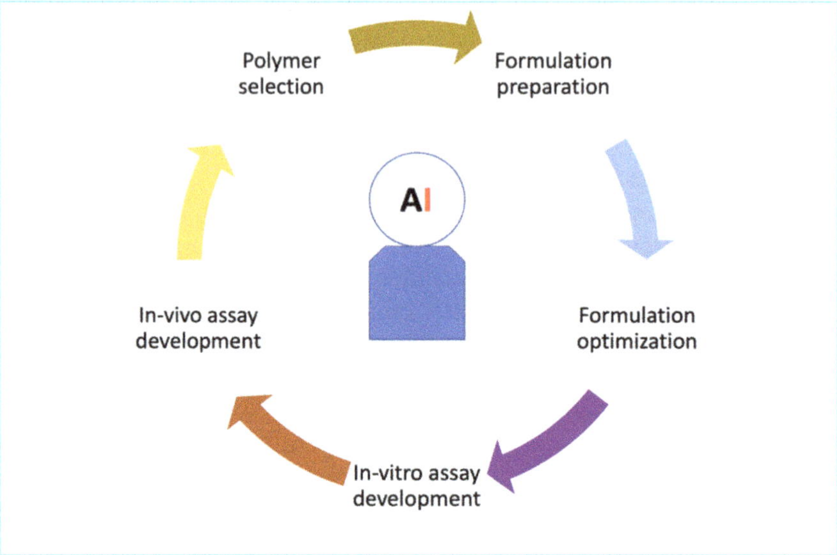

Figure 8.1. Areas where artificial intelligence can play an important role.

8.2 Why AI in drug delivery

To improve the effectiveness and safety of pharmaceuticals, AI has become more and more prevalent in drug delivery. The capacity of AI to analyse massive quantities of data to find patterns and forecast results is one of the technology's primary benefits in the medication delivery industry. This capability can assist to enhance drug formulations and distribution strategies. AI may also be used to customise medicine delivery by adjusting the dosage for every patient depending on their genetic profile and medical background.

8.3 Various tools and software in drug delivery

In the health sector, AI plays a crucial role in data management, drug design and suggesting the best treatment for patients. AI has historically reduced material waste and improved time efficiency in the development of pharmaceutical products. The quantitative structure property relationship (QSPR) aids in resolving issues with formulation dissolving, stability, porosity, etc. A model expert system (MES) typically determines the input parameters, whereas the ANN model links the desired outcomes to the formulation's parameters to simplify the formulation's development. Mathematical tools are being used for product development, for example, in order to understand more about the relationship between tablet shape and dissolution pattern, and computational fluid dynamics were investigated for application in tablet filling and compression [12]. The ANN model has proved its importance for the optimization, and forecasting of release patterns related to delivery systems like solid dispersions, beads, pellets, liposomes, and transdermal patches [2]. Quality by design (QBD) plays a crucial role in research by helping in choosing appropriate excipients. QBD also helps in life cycle management of products. Terbinafine nanoparticles that had been prepared showed improved skin penetrability and quadrupled skin absorption. By incorporating sorafenib into nanoparticles, its anti-cancer effectiveness was examined, and the anti-cancer activity of these nanoparticles was improved [13]. Numerous researchers are investigating the use of AI in the treatment of colorectal cancer with various applications, including predicting the efficacy of oxaliplatin and bevacizumab and the toxicity profile of irinotecan, as well as employing magnetotactic bacteria as an anti-cancer therapy [14].

8.4 The significance of AI in formulation development

The design of the novel medicinal compound necessitates its subsequent inclusion in an appropriate pharmaceutical formulation with the required delivery properties. In this discipline, AI has the potential to substitute for the conventional randomized process [14] By utilizing QSPR, many computational methods may tackle challenges faced in formulation development, such as porosity, stability, dissolution concern and so on [15]. Decision-support technologies employ regulation algorithms to determine the nature, type and proportion of additives based on the physicochemical parameters of the medicine, and they function through a feedback system to track and intermittently adjust the entire procedure on an ongoing basis [16]. MES provides formulation design options as well as suggestions based on the input parameters, whereas the ANN model uses backpropagation learning to connect formulation variables to the intended consequent action, concurrently controlled by the control module, ensuring development of formulations devoid of errors [16]. Various mathematical techniques, such as discrete element modelling (DEM), the finite element method, and computational fluid dynamics (CFD), have been used to examine the effects of powder flow properties on the die-filling and tablet compression processes [17, 18]. CFD could be employed to investigate how tablet geometry affects the dissolving profile. AI and these mathematical models working together could greatly speed up the production of medicinal products [19]. Designing drug delivery systems generally comes with some limitations, such as the inability to forecast the correlation between formulation parameter and actions [20]. This is connected to unforeseen circumstances and therapeutic results. Several different types of intelligent drug releasing systems must incorporate, rates of drug release, on-demand dose adjustment, drug stability and targeted release. Appropriate strategies are helpful for managing both the amount of drugs and the duration of drug release in self-monitoring systems. In order to forecast the efficacy of therapeutic dosing and the capability of drug delivery dosage forms, AI techniques can be helpful [21].

8.5 Using AI techniques for designing new medicines and delivery systems

AI techniques can also be used to design predictive models, find biomarkers, establish links between gene expression profiles and clinical characteristics, and encourage tailored treatments [21, 22]. Outside the initial stages of finding drugs or development, AI approaches have been used to quickly recognize bioactive compounds among millions of chemicals, evaluate kinetic curves, and assess data variables in chemical reactions, and direct conventional research. These methods can reduce the amount of time and money spent [23]. Furthermore, machine learning methods aid drug metabolism modeling, including associations with metabolic enzymes, links throughout drug molecules and biological results, and metabolic outcomes, which could result in better predictions of metabolic pathways and possible adverse effects of novel drugs candidates [24]. An ANN model was used to construct an automated system for evaluating compound metabolic changes in order to categorize medication candidates as cytochrome P450 substrates [25].

8.5.1 Synthesis of peptides

Several peptides have been developed under this situation and tested using screening methods and QSAR model analysis of biological data. For assessing organ-targeting peptides produced from a random phage-peptide library employing the phage display technique, an ANN model has been suggested. A multilayer system of completely interconnected neurons that had been trained to map input datasets to associated output datasets was known as a trained neural network. Statistics from training and test sets showed that ANN models were effective in identifying peptides that target specific organs from huge peptide libraries. ANN models were additionally utilized to forecast peptide binding to immune response targets and human leukocyte antigens [26].

8.5.2 Discovering new antimycobacterial medications

An ANN model for integrating significant descriptors for medication layout has been developed in an effort to minimize the potential hazard of being resistant to multiple drugs of tuberculosis while developing more effective antimycobacterial therapies. Virtual screening strategies for discovering novel antimycobacterial medicines have grabbed attention in recent years. In order to build the model, A feedforward system was programmed up for carrying out nonlinear regression within clustered descriptors and minimal inhibitory concentrations. Numerous structural databases were evaluated utilizing cheminformatics methods capable of identifying compounds as potential experimental assay options [27].

8.5.3 Predicting the efficacy of medication dosage and delivery techniques

Employing a machine learning framework, researchers created a data-driven predictive system designed for simulating pathogen–drug dynamics and forecasting the efficacy of dosage regimens and medicine delivery systems [28].

8.5.4 Quick bioactive agent identification and medication release monitoring

To prevent sexually transmitted diseases, an ANN model was developed to investigate the empirical correlations that exist between physiological factors and the releasing pattern of a targeted medication delivery system using an intravaginal gel-type formulation. ANN models were used to assess the impact of extrinsic/intrinsic and dosage parameter factors on the diffusivity of sodium dodecyl sulfate. The ANN model assisted in accurately predicting the influence of intrinsic factors on drug release profiles [29]. An adaptive modelling and control approach for automated drug distribution and post-surgical blood pressure regulation has been presented based on generalized fuzzy neural network, an intelligent modelling tool [30]. After training, the model's suitability for controlling an online adaptive system was evaluated. As the adaptive controller, a real-time feedforward generalized fuzzy neural network with a linear feedback loop was used. In simulation testing, it was shown that the adaptive fuzzy neural technique is capable of modeling system nonlinearities and uncertainties as well as assessing how the medicine affects blood pressure. The method's potential for gaining additional knowledge about the specifics of each drug's reaction was proven by an assessment of the fuzzy logic's capability to change the configuration of a controller for pancuronium distribution that is based on pharmacodynamic and pharmacokinetic models [31, 32]. We employed a trained ANN model and pharmacokinetic simulations to design controlled-release dosage forms. The inputs and outputs were determined by the formulation parameters and the total amount of medicine release over time, respectively. ANN models can also be used during the pre-formulation phase of controlled-release formulations for oral administration [31, 33]. In order to foresee the physicochemical characteristics of the controlled-release matrix tablets, an ANN model was created using computer aided design (CAD)/chem software [31].

8.5.5 Making connections between release patterns and formulation factors

ANN models are efficient at optimizing modified-release formulations that use solid dosage forms, as well as for predicting dissolution and release characteristics. Prediction of release profile and drug stability is aided by generalized regression neural network (GRNN) and connectionist models [31, 32]. GRNN has been used to create extended-release aspirin pills [33]. To create optimal aspirin tablets, in order to forecast formulation characteristics and process variables, an optimized GRNN model was implemented. The results showed no disparity that exists between the drug release patterns predicted by GRNN and those empirically observed according to the difference and similarity factors (f1 and f2). This demonstrates GRNN's applicability for modeling extended-release pills [34].

8.6 AI applications in the design of drug dosage forms

There are numerous examples of drug delivery systems that utilize AI. ANN models are helpful for optimizing modified-release products, including the solid dosage forms, in addition to the prediction of dissolution and release profiles [35, 36].

ANN models have also been applied to formulate the most potent dosage forms and predict the features of sustained release dosage forms' disintegration [37]. GRNN was used in the design of the extended-release aspirin pills. In order to create the best aspirin tablets, an enhanced GRNN model has been used to forecast formulation attributes and process parameters. Diclofenac sodium extended-release pills have been optimized through the multilayer perceptron (MLP) neural network and backpropagation algorithm. For the controlled administration of diclofenac sodium, GRNN has been used to develop multi-unit particle systems, model the impacts of causative factors on the release profile of the medication from compressed matrix pellets, and provide the best formulation.

The formulation of isradipine-containing osmotic tablets has been optimized using a combination of response surface methodology (RSM) and ANN approaches [34]. For the manufacture of glipizide push–pull osmotic pump pills, an ANN model and design expert system have been used. In addition to conducting dissolving testing, the ANN model optimized the process and a variety of formulation parameters. Additionally, ANN models have been used to forecast theophylline tablet response factors, release parameters, and plasma concentrations [38]. Polymers were chosen using a screening procedure and a feedforward backpropagation ANN model in order to increase mucoadhesion. The most important input factors and appropriate polymers for optimizing multi-polymeric propranolol buccal tablets were precisely determined using the MLP network [39]. NeuralShell2 has been proven to provide the best overall prediction when predicting the dissolving characteristics of controlled-release tablets using a variety of ANN model software programmes [40]. Table 8.1 shows various examples of drug delivery systems that utilize AI.

8.7 Application of AI in the design of drug delivery systems

Current developments in multimodal nanomedicine have already provided appropriate opportunities for AI-based optimization. To improve the targeting and effectiveness of tumor treatment, for instance, various classes of nanoparticles were delivered simultaneously. In particular, gold nanoparticles were first employed for target to tumor locations. By employing infrared light to photothermally heat the particles, the clotting cascade was initiated. To enhance tumor penetration, irinotecan-loaded multifunctional mesoporous silica nanoparticles (MSNPs) were administered in combination with iRGD, a tumor-penetrating peptide, and irinotecan. Nanoparticles have proven to be excellent at stabilization and delivering synergistic combinations such as PLGA-PEG nanoparticles for encapsulating and co-localizing siRNA and cisplatin-prodrug, two distinct classes of therapeutics. Nanoparticles can be used to deliver medications that work in synergy with other therapeutic techniques. The center of the multifunctional up-conversion of core/porous silica shell (UCSNs), which have an outer covering of porous silica for precise targeting using magnetic imaging, is the dual-functional up-conversion nanoparticles (UCNPs) embedded with cisplatin and demonstrated to enhance radiotherapy. According to accounts, UCSNs could successfully deliver cisplatin to

Table 8.1. AI application in drug delivery systems.

Drug delivery systems	Drug	AI methodologies used	Purpose	References
Matrix tablet	Metformin HCl	Elman dynamic neural networks, decision trees, and ANN model (GA optimizer tool or Monte Carlo simulations)	Dissolution characteristics correctly described from hydrophobic and aqueous matrix tablets exhibiting controlled-release profiles	[41]
Beads	Verapamil	ANN Model CAD/ Chem	The influence of formulation factors and method on the drug release profile from multi-articulate beads	[42]
Pellets	Theophylline	ANN Model	Give meaningful information on pellet qualities and establish the linkages between formulation parameters, pelletization processes, and important process variables	[43]
	Theophylline	Neuro-fuzzy systems	Pellet aspect ratio prediction and characterization	[44]
	Theophylline	MLP neural network	Estimation of the dissolving pattern of matrix-controlled-release theophylline pellets	[44]
Microspheres	Aspirin-loaded calcium alginate	ANN Model RSM	Prediction of *in vitro* drug release profile	[45]
Solid dispersion	Carbamazepine-Soluplus®-poloxamer	MLP network with three layers of feedforward and a mixture experimental design	The influence of solid dispersion composition on drug dissolving rate was investigated	[46]
	Nimodipine-PEG	ANN Model	Forecast for the optimization process	[47]
Implants	Dexamethasone	ANN model	Determining the formulation properties and medication release profiles from the coatings on cochlear implants	[48]

Liposomes	Leuprolide acetate	ANN model (nonlinear differential transfer functions); feedforward backpropagation network and MLR	Estimating drug entrapment percentages in liposomal formulations; forecasting the best composition for a certain reaction and learning more about the impact of the development steps and formulation variables on product attributes	[49, 50]
Transdermal formulation	Ketoprofen hydrogel	ANN model and RSM GMM and face-centered central composite (CCD)	For optimizing the vehicle composition; drug release rate estimation	[51]
Hydrodynamically balanced systems, suppositories, pulmonary delivery	Paracetamol	ANN model	Aided in properly predicting drug release characteristics and identifying critical elements influencing drug release	[52]
Controlled-release formulations	Clopidogrel	Fuzzy logic algorithms and ANN model	Investigating the impacts of formulation components on release characteristics and refining drug formulations helps with the creation of sustained-release formulations.	[53]
Emulsions	Rifampicin	ANN model	For the development of stable emulsions, optimization, and modelling of the complicated interactions between formulation factors and their impacts on final product quality have been used	[54]
Microparticles	Benznidazole chitosan	ANN model	Optimizing the formulation of benznidazole chitosan microparticles	[55]

(Continued)

Table 8.1. (*Continued*)

Drug delivery systems	Drug	AI methodologies used	Purpose	References
Nanomaterials	Tri-block poly(lactide)–poly (ethylene glycol)–poly (lactide) (PLA–PEG–PLA) c	ANN model	Determine the physicochemical characteristics of nanoparticles with theragnostic against a wide range of diseases	[56]
	Verapamil hydrochloride	Spherical central composite design	Effects of formulation parameters, optimization, and modelling are evaluated	[57]
		DL neural network model based on PBPK	Based on NP physicochemical properties, the tumour model, and the kind of cancer, estimate the effectiveness of NP delivery to tumours in mice	[13]
	Cell penetrating peptide	Random forest machine learning model	Prioritize suitable excipients for a novel drug	[58]
		Convolutional neural network (CNN)	Examine holographic images of single particles while precisely distinguishing and quantifying the particle's size, including its reflective index, utilising the information obtained	[59]
		Fuzzy logic	Effective in determining dose of the drug for intracellular administration	[59]
Long-acting polymeric injectable	Olaparib-PLGA and salicylic acid-PLGA MP (SA-PLGA)	Light gradient boosting machine (LGBM)	Forecasting fractional drug release with high accuracy	[48]

tumors for efficient radio/chemotherapy and luminescence/magnetic dual-mode imaging for tumor targeting [60]. Porous scaffolds that can instantly release the target drug are a promising approach for controlled release and dosing. When placed under an external magnetic field, a microporous ferrogel made of alginate and patterned with Fe_3O_4 nanoparticles, for instance, showed reversible deformation. This allowed for the stepwise release of many molecules, such as mitoxantrone (a type II topoisomerase inhibitor), plasmid DNA, and even whole cells. Gene therapy is the pinnacle of precision medicine since it allows for the correction, eradication, or prevention of patient-specific mutations. Nanocarriers are crucial for the efficient delivery of oligonucleotides for gene therapy and for enabling their action at the target region. Different kinds of nanoparticles for siRNA delivery have been assessed via animal models. According to studies, siRNA can be transported *in vivo* using self-assembled nucleic acid nanoparticles, poly(ethylene imine) polymeric nanoparticles, lipid nanoparticles, and polysaccharide-based nanoparticles composed of chitosan or cyclodextrin. The recent clinical acceptance of the first siRNA-based nanomedicine, patisiran, a lipid nanoparticle enclosing siRNA for alleviating hereditary transthyretin amyloidosis was a major development. Nanothermodynamics was also used to increase the precision of nanoparticle-based photothermal and radiation therapies by directing nanoparticles into the tumour region before therapy in animal models. For instance, PEGylated WS2 nanosheets with high near-infrared absorbance for photothermal therapy were first located by computed tomography imaging in a mouse breast cancer model before being photoactivated. These nanosheets showed excellent biocompatibility and successfully photo ablated the tumors when injected intravenously and intra-tumoral. When administered intravenously and into the tumor, these nanosheets demonstrated great biocompatibility and effective photoablation of the tumors [60]. Machine learning, a combination of data-analytical techniques for creating predictive models from a multidimensional dataset, is being used more and more in drug discovery and delivery. The complicated interrelationship between nanogels and biological systems can be studied using machine learning, which enables users to create models that learn from huge datasets and forecast expected consequences. Figure 8.2 shows that there are four main parts to machine learning (ML): input variables, feature approaches, model or algorithm training, and output: delivery solutions.

Given that administering an incorrect dose might have negative side effects, lead to the discovery of new drugs, and result in medication combinations, ML can be used to precisely predict the best drug dosage from a complicated dataset. Predicting the drug release profile of both the system as a whole and of individual components is employed in the design of drug delivery systems. ML can also forecast medication toxicity, including ototoxicity, hepatotoxicity, nephrotoxicity, neurotoxicity, and cardiotoxicity, as well as the stability of formulation [59]. Furthermore, the ANN model has been developed to predict the entrapment efficiency and particle size of noscapine-loaded PEG–PLA nanoparticles utilizing a variety of variables such as the number of blocks, polymer molecular weight, and polymer-to-drug ratio. The polymer molecular weight and polymer weight-to-drug ratio had the most

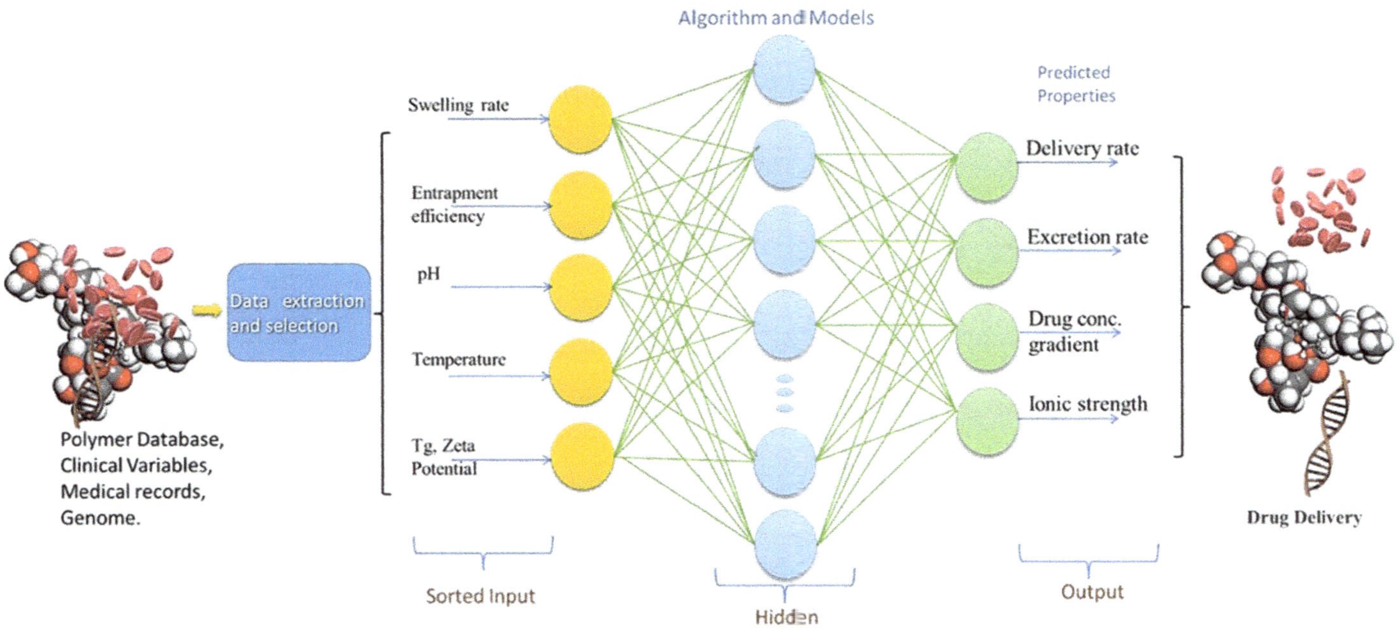

Figure 8.2. Key elements of neural networks used for drug delivery in nanogels. Reprinted from [59], copyright (2022), with permission from Elsevier.

significant impacts on particle size, and entrapment efficiency, respectively. Carbon nanotubes with adequate stability, mechanical properties, and thermoelectrical conductivity were widely utilized in theragnostic applications. CNTs can identify organic components with the help of an ANN model. The physical characteristics of quantum dot semiconductor optical amplifiers have been estimated with greater precision thanks to the usage of ANN models with powerful computational capabilities over conventional numerical models. In order to determine the correlations between the input factors and the output result, an ANN model was utilized in the construction of nano systems [61]. DOPC (1,2 Dioleoyl-snglycero-3-phosphocholine) and DSPE-PEG 2000 (1,2 Distearoyl-snglycero-3-phosphoethanolamine-N [amino (polyethylene glycol) 2000] are the examples of lipids used for the synthesis of liposome, used as a drug delivery vehicle for targeted therapy [61]. Using microfluidic technology, liposome formulations were made by combining the lipid solution and aqueous phase in a particular proportion. To create the lipid solution, ethanol was used to dissolve the components of DSPE-PEG 2000, DOPC and cholesterol in varied proportion. The aqueous phase comprises varying amounts of a solution of sodium chloride in Milli-Q water depending on the experiment. The two solutions have been loaded into 10 ml polypropylene injection, with the lipid solution going into pump 2 and the aqueous phase continuing into pumps 1 and 3. Mixing took place in a microfluidic tank linked to the earlier complete needles. Prior to combining, two requirements had to be satisfied: the total flow rate (TFR) and the flow rate ratio (FRR). One method was created to handle every TFR and FRR combination the machine could perform. 2 ml of liposome suspension was intended to be produced during the entire run duration (in seconds). Finally, using the temperature control device that had been managed by the Dolomite Flow Control Center Software, the temperature was changed. Because of the trapped air and dead space in the tubes, each experiment needed a cleaning run. After discarding the cleaning solution, a fresh run was started to gather the 2 ml of suspension in an Eppendorf tube. The samples' ethanol was then evaporated in a rotary evaporator after liposome synthesis. The samples were taken after 2 h of vaporization at 30 mbar, and Milli-Q water was added to make up the ethanol volume [61] (figure 8.3).

8.8 ML for *in vitro* optimization

In vitro testing refers to experiments that are conducted outside of a living organism, typically in a laboratory setting. In drug development, *in vitro* testing is used to evaluate the effects of a drug on cells, tissues, and organs outside of the body. *In vitro* testing is often used as an initial screening step to identify promising drug candidates before moving to *in vivo* testing. While *in vitro* testing has many advantages, such as cost-effectiveness, ease of use, and the ability to control experimental conditions, it also has several limitations. One of the primary limitations is that it does not fully capture the complexity of the human body, which can lead to discrepancies between *in vitro* and *in vivo* results. Additionally, *in vitro* testing may not accurately predict the toxicity or efficacy of a drug *in vivo*, as it does not take into account factors such as metabolism and pharmacokinetics [61]. ML models can be trained on a variety of

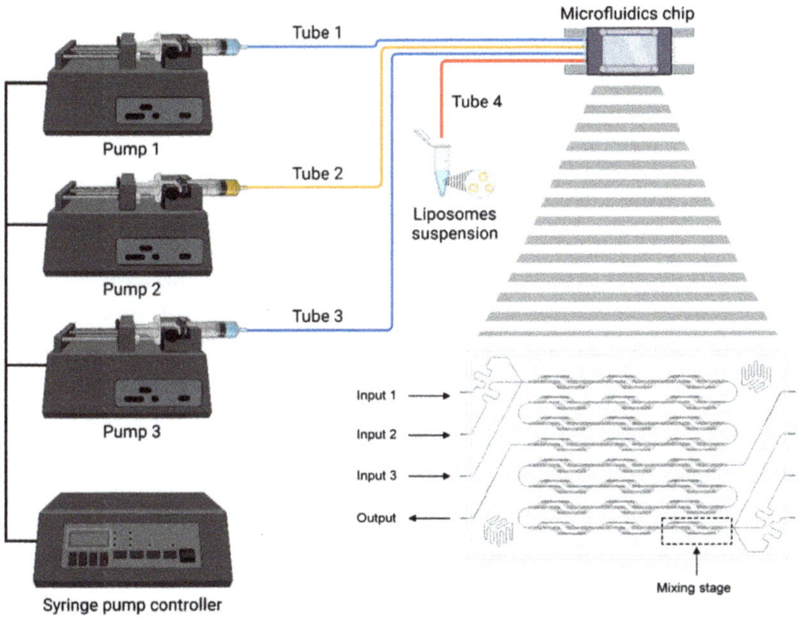

Figure 8.3. Microfluidic system scheme showing the preparation of liposome suspension. Reprinted with permission from [61], copyright (2022) American Chemical Society.

data sources to optimize the *in vitro* effects of drugs. These data sources can include chemical and structural properties of the drug, genomic and proteomic data from the target cells or tissues, and gene expression profiles from the host cells. By analyzing these data sources, machine learning models can identify patterns and relationships that can be used to optimize the dosages, timing, and delivery methods of drugs [62]. One example of *in vitro* optimization of drug effects using ML is the identification of novel drug candidates for cancer treatment. ML models can be trained on large datasets of chemical and structural data to predict the potency and selectivity of a drug candidate against cancer cells. These models can then be used to optimize the dosages and delivery methods of the drug *in vitro* to maximize its efficacy and minimize toxicity. Another example is the optimization of antiviral drugs for treating viral infections such as COVID-19. Machine learning models can be trained on genomic and proteomic data from the virus, as well as gene expression profiles from the host cells, to predict the optimal dosages, timing, and delivery methods of the drug to inhibit viral replication and minimize host cell toxicity [63]. ML models have several advantages in optimizing the *in vitro* effects of drugs. They can analyze large and complex datasets, identify patterns and relationships that may be difficult for humans to detect, and make predictions based on this analysis. Additionally, these models can be used to optimize drug dosages and delivery methods in a cost-effective and time-efficient manner. However, there are also limitations to the use of ML in *in vitro* optimization. One limitation is that the accuracy of the models is dependent on the quality and completeness of the data used for training. Additionally, ML models may be limited by the lack of diversity in the training data, which can lead to overfitting or bias in the predictions. Finally, ML models may not capture the full complexity of the biological systems involved, which can limit their predictive power in some cases [64].

8.9 ML for *in vivo* optimization

In vivo testing refers to experiments that are conducted in living organisms, typically animals, to evaluate the effects of a drug on the whole body. *In vivo* testing is a critical step in drug development, as it provides important information on the pharmacokinetics, toxicity, and efficacy of a drug in a complex biological system. ML models can be trained on a variety of data sources to optimize the *in vivo* effects of drugs. These data sources can include pharmacokinetic and pharmacodynamics data, imaging data, and biomarker data. By analyzing these data sources, machine learning models can identify patterns and relationships that can be used to optimize the dosages, timing, and delivery methods of drugs [65]. One example of *in vivo* optimization of drug effects using machine learning is the optimization of chemotherapy for cancer treatment. ML models can be trained on pharmacokinetic and pharmacodynamics data, as well as imaging data, to predict the optimal dosages, timing, and delivery methods of chemotherapy drugs to maximize their efficacy and minimize toxicity. Additionally, machine learning models can be used to identify biomarkers that can be used to predict patient response to chemotherapy and personalize treatment plans. Another example is the optimization of insulin therapy for diabetes management. ML models can be trained on continuous glucose monitoring data and insulin dosing data to predict the optimal insulin dosages and delivery methods to maintain stable blood glucose levels. Additionally, ML models can be used to identify patient-specific factors that may affect insulin sensitivity and adjust treatment plans accordingly [66]. ML models have several advantages in optimizing the *in vivo* effects of drugs. They can analyze large and complex datasets, identify patterns and relationships that may be difficult for humans to detect, and make predictions based on this analysis. Additionally, ML models can be used to personalized treatment plans based on patient-specific factors, such as biomarkers or genetic data [67]. However, there are also limitations to the use of ML in *in vivo* optimization. One limitation is that the accuracy of the models is dependent on the quality and completeness of the data used for training. Additionally, ML models may be limited by the lack of diversity in the training data, which can lead to overfitting or bias in the predictions. Finally, these models may not capture the full complexity of the biological systems involved, which can limit their predictive power in some cases [68].

ML has the potential to revolutionize drug development and treatment optimization in a variety of ways beyond those discussed above. One promising area is the development of ML models for predicting drug toxicity. By analyzing large datasets of patient data and drug interactions, ML models can help identify potential safety concerns before drugs are released to the market [69]. Another potential application is the use of ML models for drug repurposing. By analyzing the chemical properties of existing drugs and the genomic data of different diseases, these models can identify existing drugs that could be repurposed for new indications. This approach could potentially save time and money in drug development by using existing drugs with known safety profiles [70]. Finally, the development of personalized medicine is a key area where ML can make a significant impact. By analyzing large datasets of patient data, including genomic data, ML models can identify patient-specific factors that may affect drug efficacy or toxicity. This approach could enable more personalized treatment plans, tailored to the specific needs and characteristics of individual patients [71].

In the future, we can expect to see continued advancements in the use of ML in drug development and treatment optimization. As larger and more diverse datasets become available, ML models will become increasingly accurate and powerful. Furthermore, the integration of ML with other emerging technologies, such as CRISPR and gene editing, could lead to even more exciting breakthroughs in personalized medicine and drug development [72].

The development of new drugs is a complex and time-consuming process that requires the evaluation of the drug's efficacy and safety in both *in vitro* and *in vivo* settings. Traditional trial-and-error approaches to drug development can be costly and inefficient, leading to high failure rates and long development timelines. Machine learning models provide a powerful tool for optimizing the effects of drugs in both *in vitro* and *in vivo* settings, potentially leading to more effective and efficient drug development and treatment. In this chapter, we discuss the use of trained machine learning models to optimize the *in vitro* and *in vivo* effects of drugs, with a focus on examples and applications in drug development [63].

8.10 Future directions: how will it aid in better targeted drug formulations and future resources savings

The framework in the present formulation development may change with the use of AI and multiscale modeling methods. Computational approach can provide pharmaceutical scientists with multiscale optics that reveals chemical, mathematical, physical, and data-driven details in areas such as polymorphism, precision medicine, formulation screening, and chemical stability. Machine learning and AI algorithms can produce data-driven predictions from enormous amounts of accumulated experimental data in order to build the quantitative prediction model. The development process can be greatly accelerated by a well-designed AI system, which can also optimize formulations, reduce costs, gather and conserve formulation-specific information and experience, and maintain consistency in the products [73]. In addition to this, implantable devices and closed-loop medicine delivery are the future through AI-based regulated procedures. The full scope of 3D printing for automated drug delivery, such as 3D tablets, is still not realized. Future researchers will benefit greatly from the integration of AI and machine learning into this since with the help of these technologies, interactive, intelligent, real-time surveillance systems for the individualized care of the elderly and disabled, even at home, could be created. The future goal and success of the growing closed-loop therapeutic system can thus be realized through the combined efforts of healthcare professionals, engineers, researchers, businesses, and users [74]. Many senior citizens live in the community but could receive little assistance from close relatives or carers, posing health risks. Robotic assistants have been noticed to plug some of the current gaps in elderly patients such as reminding of regular activities and directing them through unfamiliar situations.

8.11 Startups and companies working on AI dependent drug delivery

Many industries are utilizing AI in their approach to increase patient's health by using their database, machine or both. Patient data will help the patient and their health consultant to understand the core of the patient's regime and its response, ultimately this will assist health professionals to update their prescription according to the patient. Startups not only working for treatment but they are also working in diagnostics to provide fast and accurate alerts to patient and their care givers, which will decrease the chances of emergency resulting in depletion of mortality rate.

Insilico Medicine is a company that works in drug discovery as well as drug development. It provides its facilities from chemistry of a molecule to its biological effect till its clinical trial. Using AI in its working helps to decrease cost of treatment with enhancement in rate of success (https://insilico.com/) [75]. Compound ISM3091 was developed for treatment of solid tumors. They also had received a letter of approval for its initial investigational new drug (IND) application from United States Food and Drug Administration (USFDA) (https://www.eurekalert.org/news-releases/990417) [76].

Nanopin (https://www.nanopintech.com/) [77] is a company aimed to developing a fast and accurate diagnosis of infectious diseases. It is integrating AI with its diagnostic assays for fast detection of infectious diseases like COVID-19, HIV, TB, etc., to reduce mortality caused by these diseases. Biosymetrics is company that primarily looks into drug discovery. They utilize machine learning to connect experimental and clinical data to find new effective drug targets. They launched software named Augusta (https://www.biosymetrics.com/blog/biosymetrics-launches-augusta-architect) [78], a machine learning platform which is very user-friendly and helps its user with fast data processing in various fields like drug discovery, drug development, precision medicine and diagnostics. Augusta not only made the process faster, but has also economically viable. Lumee™ is a Conformité Européenne (CE) mark approved oxygen detecting biosensor device made by Profusa which helps in monitoring oxygen level in patients suffering from peripheral artery disease and critical limb ischemia (https://profusa.com/profusa-receives-cemark/) [79, 80]. Profusa works on biosensors that work on chemistry happening inside the body to monitor a person's health and disease conditions. Profusa are working on an injectable device that can predict the influenza infection in its very early state (https://profusa.com/profusa-and-partners-announce/) [81]. Profusa also received a grant from Defense Advanced Research Project Agency and United States Army for making implantable biosensors which will help keep a check on soldiers to understand their body chemistry for better performance (https://www.snapmunk.com/conspiracy-fact-or-fiction-darpa-invests-in-implantable-chips/) [82].

In chronic diseases patients generally forget to adhere to their treatments, which can lead to serious consequences. Propeller Health (https://propellerhealth.com/) [83] is aiming to take care of chronic patients by keeping check on their daily activities and uptake of medicines to give them personalized medication. This platform also provides connections to all individuals in the healthcare system to increase effectiveness of their platform and treatment. They have made biosensors for users to analyse their breathing pattern and this trains them to improve their health with the help of their associated clinicians. London based company Amiko provides digital machines related to respiratory diseases in accordance with improving health of patients. Amiko has developed Respiro® to assist doctors and patients in maintaining constant dose. Its AI works by analyzing data related to dose volume, orientation of inhaler, resistance of inhaler, duration of inhalation, peak inspiratory flow to get maximum precision of dose. The 'Respiro Mobile' app transfers this data to a smartphone or computer paired with it and helps patients and healthcare professionals to interpret its results [84, 85].

8.12 SWOT analysis

As depicted in figure 8.4, AI is a very powerful technique that enables fast and accurate diagnosis with the appropriate medicine regime. Due to Its capacity of data collection and economically efficient operations many industries are opting for AI over present-day technology. AI is a totally data- and machine-driven technique, hence it is avoids the human approach. AI is an emerging field; its limited data and novelty are the main reason it is in not in the mainstream yet. AI in healthcare can play a crucial role with its ability to be available at any time for

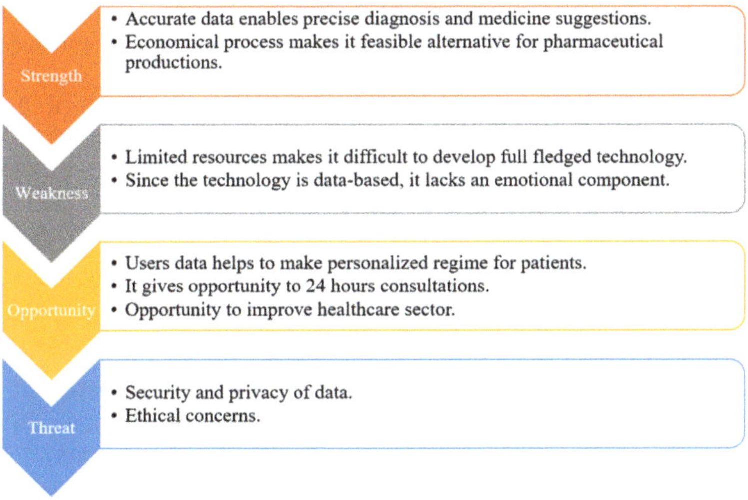

Figure 8.4. SWOT analysis for AI in drug delivery.

patient-specific responses. With every advancement in technology, there is raised the question of ethical concerns for the security of consumers, as this information can be misused, so there needs to be protected privacy and security of patients and their health data.

8.13 Conclusion

In conclusion, AI has significant potential to revolutionize drug delivery by enabling the development of more efficient, precise, and personalized treatments. AI-based drug delivery systems can help in identifying the optimal drug dosage, delivery route, and timing, as well as predicting potential side effects and adverse reactions. AI can significantly reduce the time and cost involved in the drug development process, ultimately leading to faster and more effective treatments. However, there are still a number of issues that need to be resolved, such as the need for high-quality data, regulatory barriers, and ethical concerns related to privacy and data ownership. Nevertheless, with continued research and development, In the coming years, AI has the potential to revolutionize drug delivery and enhance patient outcomes.

References

[1] Das K P and Chandra J 2022 Nanoparticles and convergence of artificial intelligence for targeted drug delivery for cancer therapy: current progress and challenges *Front Med. Technol.* **4** 1067144

[2] Hassanzadeh P, Atyabi F and Dinarvand R 2019 The significance of artificial intelligence in drug delivery system design *Adv. Drug Deliv. Rev.* **151** 169–90

[3] Schork N J 2019 Artificial intelligence and personalized medicine *Precision Med. Cancer Therapy* **178** 265–83

[4] Gao J, Karp J M, Langer R and Joshi N 2023 The future of drug delivery *Chem. Mater.* (ACS Publications) Vol 35 pp 359–63

[5] Singh A V, Ansari M H D, Rosenkranz D, Maharjan R S, Kriegel F L and Gandhi K *et al* 2020 Artificial intelligence and machine learning in computational nanotoxicology: unlocking and empowering nanomedicine *Adv. Healthc. Mater.* **9** 1901862

[6] Paul D, Sanap G, Shenoy S, Kalyane D, Kalia K and Tekade R K 2021 Artificial intelligence in drug discovery and development *Drug Discov. Today* **26** 80

[7] Bannigan P, Aldeghi M, Bao Z, Häse F, Aspuru-Guzik A and Allen C 2021 Machine learning directed drug formulation development *Adv. Drug Deliv. Rev.* **175** 113806

[8] Selvaraj C, Chandra I and Singh S K 2021 Artificial intelligence and machine learning approaches for drug design: challenges and opportunities for the pharmaceutical industries *Mol. Divers.* **26** 1893–913

[9] Egorov E, Pieters C, Korach-Rechtman H, Shklover J and Schroeder A 2021 Robotics, microfluidics, nanotechnology and AI in the synthesis and evaluation of liposomes and polymeric drug delivery systems *Drug Deliv. Transl. Res.* **11** 345–52

[10] Raijada D, Wac K, Greisen E, Rantanen J and Genina N 2021 Integration of personalized drug delivery systems into digital health *Adv. Drug Deliv. Rev.* **176** 113857

[11] Patra J K, Das G, Fraceto L F, Campos E V R, Rodriguez-Torres M, del P and Acosta-Torres L S *et al* 2018 Nano based drug delivery systems: recent developments and future prospects *J. Nanobiotechnol.* **16** 1–33

[12] Blasiak A, Khong J and Kee T 2020 CURATE. AI: optimizing personalized medicine with artificial intelligence *SLAS Technol* **25** 95–105
[13] Reker D, Rybakova Y, Kirtane A R, Cao R, Yang J W and Navamajiti N *et al* 2021 Computationally guided high-throughput design of self-assembling drug nanoparticles *Nat. Nanotechnol.* **16** 725–33
[14] Mitsala A, Tsalikidis C, Pitiakoudis M, Simopoulos C and Tsaroucha A K 2021 Artificial intelligence in colorectal cancer screening, diagnosis and treatment. A new era *Curr. Oncol.* **28** 1581–607
[15] Mehta C H, Narayan R and Nayak U Y 2019 Computational modeling for formulation design *Drug Discov. Today* **24** 781–8
[16] Schneider G and Clark D E 2019 Automated de novo drug design: are we nearly there yet? *Angew. Chem. Int. Ed.* **58** 10792–803
[17] Rantanen J and Khinast J 2015 The future of pharmaceutical manufacturing sciences *J. Pharm. Sci.* **104** 3612–38
[18] Ketterhagen W R, am Ende M T and Hancock B C 2009 Process modeling in the pharmaceutical industry using the discrete element method *J. Pharm. Sci.* **98** 442–70
[19] Chen W, Desai D, Good D, Crison J, Timmins P and Paruchuri S *et al* 2016 Mathematical model-based accelerated development of extended-release metformin hydrochloride tablet formulation *AAPS Pharm. Sci. Tech.* **17** 1007–13
[20] Yildirim O, Gottwald M, Schüler P and Michel M C 2016 Opportunities and challenges for drug development: public–private partnerships, adaptive designs and big data *Front. Pharmacol.* **7** 461
[21] Rost B and Sander C 1993 Prediction of protein secondary structure at better than 70% accuracy *J. Mol. Biol.* **232** 584–99
[22] Mjolsness E and DeCoste D 2001 Machine learning for science: state of the art and future prospects *Science* **293** 2051–5
[23] Fox T and Kriegl J M 2006 Machine learning techniques for in silico modeling of drug metabolism *Curr. Top. Med. Chem.* **6** 1579–91
[24] Korolev D, Balakin K V, Nikolsky Y, Kirillov E, Ivanenkov Y A and Savchuk N P *et al* 2003 Modeling of human cytochrome P450-mediated drug metabolism using unsupervised machine learning approach *J. Med. Chem.* **46** 3631–43
[25] Jung E, Kim J, Choi S H, Kim M, Rhee H and Shin J M *et al* 2010 Artificial neural network study on organ-targeting peptides *J. Comput. Aided Mol. Des.* **24** 49–56
[26] Zhang G L, Khan A M, Srinivasan K N, August J T and Brusic V 2005 Neural models for predicting viral vaccine targets *J. Bioinform. Comput. Biol.* **3** 1207–25
[27] Sardari S, Kohanzad H and Ghavami G 2014 Artificial neural network modeling of antimycobacterial chemical space to introduce efficient descriptors employed for drug design *Chemometr. Intell. Lab. Syst.* **130** 151–8
[28] Li Y, Lenaghan S C and Zhang M 2012 A data-driven predictive approach for drug delivery using machine learning techniques *PLoS One* **7** e31724
[29] Lee Y, Khemka A, Yoo J W and Lee C H 2008 Assessment of diffusion coefficient from mucoadhesive barrier devices using artificial neural networks *Int. J. Pharm.* **351** 119–26
[30] Fatouros D G, Nielsen F S, Douroumis D, Hadjileontiadis L J and Mullertz A 2008 In vitro–*in vivo* correlations of self-emulsifying drug delivery systems combining the dynamic lipolysis model and neuro-fuzzy networks *Eur. J. Pharm. Biopharm.* **69** 887–98

[31] Peppas N A 1985 Analysis of Fickian and non-Fickian drug release from polymers *Pharm. Acta Helv.* **60** 110–1

[32] Ibrić S, Jovanović M, Djurić Z, Parojčić J and Solomun L 2002 The application of generalized regression neural network in the modeling and optimization of aspirin extended release tablets with Eudragit® RS PO as matrix substance *J. Control. Release* **82** 213–22

[33] Ho D, Wang P and Kee T 2019 Artificial intelligence in nanomedicine *Nanoscale Horiz.* **4** 365–77

[34] Ivić B, Ibrić S, Cvetković N, Petrović A, Trajković S and Djurić Z 2010 Application of design of experiments and multilayer perceptrons neural network in the optimization of diclofenac sodium extended release tablets with Carbopol® 71G *Chem. Pharm. Bull. (Tokyo)* **58** 947–9

[35] Ibrić S, Djuriš J, Parojčić J and Djurić Z 2012 Artificial neural networks in evaluation and optimization of modified release solid dosage forms *Pharmaceutics* **4** 531–50

[36] Khan A M, Hanif M, Bukhar N I, Shamim R, Rasool F and Rasul S *et al* 2020 Artificial neural network (ANN) approach to predict an optimized pH-dependent mesalamine matrix tablet *Drug Des. Devel. Ther.* **14** 2435–48

[37] Chaibva F, Burton M and Walker R B 2010 Optimization of salbutamol sulfate dissolution from sustained release matrix formulations using an artificial neural *Pharmaceutics* **2** 182–98

[38] Takayama K, Morva A, Fujikawa M, Hattori Y, Obata Y and Nagai T 2000 Formula optimization of theophylline controlled-release tablet based on artificial neural networks *J. Control. Release* **68** 175–86

[39] Munasur A P, Pillay V, Choonara Y E, Mackraj I and Govender T 2008 Comparing the mucoadhesivity and drug release mechanisms of various polymer-containing propranolol buccal tablets *Drug Dev. Ind. Pharm.* **34** 189–98

[40] Bozič D Z, Vrečer F and Kozjek F 1997 Optimization of diclofenac sodium dissolution from sustained release formulations using an artificial neural network *Eur. J. Pharm. Sci.* **5** 163–9

[41] Petrović J, Ibrić S, Betz G and Urić Z 2012 Optimization of matrix tablets controlled drug release using Elman dynamic neural networks and decision trees *Int. J. Pharm.* **428** 57–67

[42] Vaithiyalingam S and Khan M A 2002 Optimization and characterization of controlled release multi-particulate beads formulated with a customized cellulose acetate butyrate dispersion *Int. J. Pharm.* **234** 179–93

[43] Peh K K, Lim C P, Quek S S and Khoh K H 2000 Use of artificial neural networks to predict drug dissolution profiles and evaluation of network performance using similarity factor *Pharm. Res.* **17** 1384–8

[44] Huang Y, Yao Q, Zhu C, Zhang X, Qin L and Wang Q *et al* 2015 Comparison of novel granulated pellet-containing tablets and traditional pellet-containing tablets by artificial neural networks *Pharm. Dev. Technol.* **20** 670–5

[45] Yuksel N, Turkoglu M and Baykara T 2000 Modelling of the solvent evaporation method for the preparation of controlled release acrylic microspheres using neural networks *J. Microencapsul.* **17** 541–51

[46] Medarević D P, Kleinebudde P, Djuriš J, Djurić Z and Ibrić S 2016 Combined application of mixture experimental design and artificial neural networks in the solid dispersion development *Drug Dev. Ind. Pharm.* **42** 389–402

[47] Barmpalexis P, Kachrimanis K and Georgarakis E 2011 Solid dispersions in the development of a nimodipine floating tablet formulation and optimization by artificial neural networks and genetic programming *Eur. J. Pharm. Biopharm.* **77** 122–31

[48] Bannigan P, Bao Z, Hickman R J, Aldeghi M, Häse F and Aspuru-Guzik A *et al* 2023 Machine learning models to accelerate the design of polymeric long-acting injectables *Nat. Commun.* **14** 1–12
[49] Moussa H G, Husseini G A, Abel-Jabbar N and Ahmad S E 2017 Use of model predictive control and artificial neural networks to optimize the ultrasonic release of a model drug from liposomes *IEEE Trans. Nanobiosci.* **16** 149–56
[50] Husseini G A, Mjalli F S, Pitt W G and Abdel-Jabbar N M 2009 Using artificial neural networks and model predictive control to optimize acoustically assisted doxorubicin release from polymeric micelles *Technol. Cancer Res. Treat.* **8** 479–88
[51] Takayama K, Takahara J, Fujikawa M, Ichikawa H and Nagai T 1999 Formula optimization based on artificial neural networks in transdermal drug delivery *J. Control. Release* **62** 161–70
[52] Belič A, Grabnar I, Karba R and Mrhar A 2003 Pathways of paracetamol absorption from layered excipient suppositories: artificial intelligence approach *Eur. J. Drug Metab. Pharmacokinet* **28** 31–40
[53] Tan C and Degim I T 2012 Development of sustained release formulation of an antithrombotic drug and application of fuzzy logic *Pharm. Dev. Technol.* **17** 242–50
[54] Miwa A, Yajima T, Ikuta H and Makado K 2008 Prediction of suitable amounts of water in fluidized bed granulation of pharmaceutical formulations using corresponding values of components *Int. J. Pharm.* **352** 202–8
[55] Leonardi D, Salomón C J, Lamas M C and Olivieri A C 2009 Development of novel formulations for Chagas' disease: optimization of benznidazole chitosan microparticles based on artificial neural networks *Int. J. Pharm.* **367** 140–7
[56] Asadi H, Rostamizadeh K, Salari D and Hamidi M 2011 Preparation of biodegradable nanoparticles of tri-block PLA-PEG-PLA copolymer and determination of factors controlling the particle size using artificial neural network *J. Microencapsul.* **28** 406–16
[57] Li Y, Abbaspour M R, Grootendorst P V, Rauth A M and Wu X Y 2015 Optimization of controlled release nanoparticle formulation of verapamil hydrochloride using artificial neural networks with genetic algorithm and response surface methodology *Eur. J. Pharm. Biopharm.* **94** 170–9
[58] Feger G, Angelov B and Angelova A 2020 prediction of amphiphilic cell-penetrating peptide building blocks from protein-derived amino acid sequences for engineering of drug delivery nanoassemblies *J. Phys. Chem.* B **124** 4069–78
[59] Adekoya O C, Yibowei M E, Adekoya G J, Sadiku E R, Hamam Y and Ray S S 2022 A mini-review on the application of machine learning in polymer nanogels for drug delivery *Mater. Today Proc.* **62** S141–4
[60] Sansare S, Duran T, Mohammadiarani H, Goyal M, Yenduri G and Costa A *et al* 2021 Artificial neural networks in tandem with molecular descriptors as predictive tools for continuous liposome manufacturing *Int. J. Pharm.* **603** 120713
[61] Rebollo R, Oyoun F, Corvis Y, El-Hammadi M M, Saubamea B and Andrieux K *et al* 2022 Microfluidic manufacturing of liposomes: development and optimization by design of experiment and machine learning *ACS Appl. Mater. Interfaces* **14** 39736–45
[62] Hartl D, de Luca V, Kostikova A, Laramie J, Kennedy S and Ferrero E *et al* 2021 Translational precision medicine: an industry perspective *J. Transl. Med.* **19** 1–14

[63] Vamathevan J, Clark D, Czodrowski P, Dunham I, Ferran E and Lee G *et al* 2019 Applications of machine learning in drug discovery and development *Nat. Rev. Drug Discov.* **18** 463–77

[64] Yang F, Zhang Q, Ji X, Zhang Y, Li W and Peng S *et al* 2022 Machine learning applications in drug repurposing *Interdiscip. Sci.* **14** 15–21

[65] Zhang L, Zhang H, Ai H, Hu H, Li S and Zhao J *et al* 2018 Applications of machine learning methods in drug toxicity prediction *Curr. Top. Med. Chem.* **18** 987–97

[66] Keutzer L, You H, Farnoud A, Nyberg J, Wicha S G and Maher-Edwards G *et al* 2022 Machine learning and pharmacometrics for prediction of pharmacokinetic data: differences, similarities and challenges illustrated with rifampicin *Pharmaceutics* **14** 1530

[67] Kim H, Kim E, Lee I, Bae B, Park M and Nam H 2020 Artificial intelligence in drug discovery: a comprehensive review of data-driven and machine learning approaches *Biotechnol. Bioprocess Eng.* **25** 895–930

[68] Yeh Y C, Huang T H, Yang S C, Chen C C and Fang J Y 2020 Nano-based drug delivery or targeting to eradicate bacteria for infection mitigation: a review of recent advances *Front. Chem.* **8** 286

[69] Réda C, Kaufmann E and Delahaye-Duriez A 2020 Machine learning applications in drug development *Comput. Struct. Biotechnol. J.* **18** 241–52

[70] Guengerich F P 2011 Mechanisms of drug toxicity and relevance to pharmaceutical development *Drug Metab. Pharmacokinet.* **26** 3–14

[71] M Fu L 2014 Machine learning and tubercular drug target recognition *Curr. Pharm. Des.* **20** 4307–18

[72] Haiyan B, Shuxun Y, Ying W and Xin Y 2013 Application of computer aided medicine design in development of medicine *2013 Fourth Int. Conf. on Intelligent Systems Design and Engineering Applications* (Piscataway, NJ: IEEE) 129–34

[73] Wang W, Ye Z, Gao H and Ouyang D 2021 Computational pharmaceutics-A new paradigm of drug delivery *J. Control. Release* **338** 119–36

[74] Sharma R, Singh D, Gaur P and Joshi D 2021 Intelligent automated drug administration and therapy: future of healthcare *Drug Deliv. Transl. Res.* 1–25

[75] https://insilico.com/ (accessed 29 June 2023)

[76] EurekAlert! Insilico medicine receives IND approval for novel AI-designed USP1 inhibitor for cancer https://eurekalert.org/news-releases/990417 (accessed 29 June 2023)

[77] Nanopin Technologies A novel approach to infectious disease detection https://nanopintech.com/ (accessed 29 June 2023)

[78] BioSymetrics Launches Augusta™ architect—biosymetrics https://biosymetrics.com/blog/biosymetrics-launches-augusta-architect (accessed 29 June 2023)

[79] Profusa, Inc. Join the conversation …with your body https://profusa.com/ (accessed 29 June 2023)

[80] Profusa, Inc. Profusa receives CE mark approval to market the wireless lumee® oxygen platform for continuous, real-time monitoring of tissue oxygen https://profusa.com/profusa-receives-cemark/ (accessed 29 June 2023)

[81] Profusa, Inc. Profusa and partners announce initiation of study to measure early signs of influenza through biosensor technology https://profusa.com/profusa-and-partners-announce/ (accessed 29 June 2023)

[82] A Biotracker implantable in the skin just got $7.5 million in government grant money https://snapmunk.com/conspiracy-fact-or-fiction-darpa-invests-in-implantable-chips/ (accessed 29 June 2023)
[83] Propeller health: a precision digital health company https://propellerhealth.com/ (accessed 29 June 2023)
[84] Amiko Upgrading respiratory care https://amiko.io/ (accessed 29 June 2023)
[85] Mehta P P 2020 Dry powder inhalers: a concise summary of the electronic monitoring devices *Therapeut. Delivery* **12** 1–6

Chapter 9

ML in drug delivery—current scenario and future trends

Prakash Muthudoss, Hussain Ali, Gobi Ramasamy, Ravikiran Allada, Elisabeth Fink, Vivekanandan Kalaiselvan, Balaji Jayakrishnan, Saurabh Shahane, Manikandan Ramalingam, Lakshmi Kanakaraj, Ilango Kaliappan and Amrit Paudel

Machine learning (ML) has enabled transformative applications and emerged as a domain-agnostic decision-making tool as a virtue of its rapid democratization. The authors believe that a systematic assortment of important publications on this issue is indispensable in this context. In terms of data ingestion, data curation, data pre-processing, data handling, and model cross-validation, this review gathers together several studies that have demonstrated a minimum ML framework approach. In general, ML models are described as black-box models, with limited information supplied about their transparency. The authors propose techniques based on the US Food and Drug Administration (FDA)'s current good ML practice (GMLP) in order to improve the ML framework and minimize the aforementioned gap, especially for data. Considering this, the conversation around a model's logic and interpretability are additionally provided. Explicitly, the authors explore the challenges and constraints that ML execution confronts throughout the development of pharmaceuticals. In this context, a structural approach in statistics is presented to allow the scientist to assess the quality of data and incorporate important ideas and techniques that would be implemented in modern ML. The data analytics tetrahedron proposed here can be applied to data of any size. To further contextualize, selected case studies capturing good practices are highlighted to provide pharmaceutical scientists, pharmaceutical ML enthusiasts, readers, reviewers, and regulatory authorities an exposure to fundamental and cutting-edge techniques of ML and data science with respect to chemistry, manufacture, and control (CMC) of drug products. In addition, the authors believe that leveraging ML within CMC procedures can assist in improving decision-making, increasing quality, and enhancing the speed of pharmaceutical product development.

doi:10.1088/978-0-7503-5613-8ch9

9.1 Digital pharmaceutical development

9.1.1 Introduction

One of the most important steps in the pharmaceutical development of new medicines is drug formulation. 'Product development is more of an art than a science' and 'development relies on iterative trial-and-error approach' are, two of the most commonly heard phrases. Recently, the utilization of advanced innovation in the pharmaceutical industry (hereinafter termed 'digital pharmaceutical development') has been investigated in order to overcome such experience-based product development and unravel important information. That is, data learning platforms such as ML, artificial neural networks (ANN), and deep learning (DL) are one of the most fascinating as well as active areas of research and application.

Alan Turing in 1950 asked 'Can machines think?' Artificial intelligence (AI) enables the machine to think, that is, without any human intervention, the machine will be able to make decisions [1]. AI is a multidisciplinary field that coordinates ideas from computer science, statistics, ML, and data analysis to understand as well as extract insights from the ever-increasing amounts of data. In the author's purview, AI can be considered as individual assistance in making decisions, however, AI just achieves the tasks set for it; ML applies statistical learning algorithms to build smart systems; and the next machine advancement featured is ANN, which imitates neuron cells in human brains to process information [2]. Precisely, ML and ANN learn from provided data and then teach the machines/computers. However, DL represents the technology at its best, resembling multi-connected biological neurons' functionality in the brain [3]. In summary, AI is considered as an umbrella discipline that makes machines extract various hidden information which is otherwise uninterpretable by humans (figure 9.1) that aids in enhancing the intelligence of machines as part of the industry 4.0 revolution. These approaches help in incubating a predictive approach which reduces the innovation

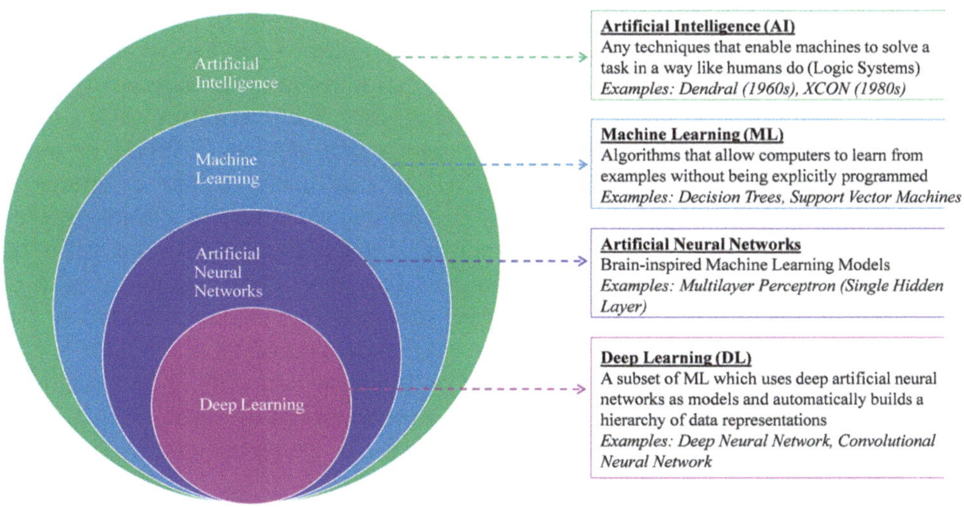

Figure 9.1. Data learning approaches.

phase that shortens launch time, as well as strengthening quality and safety while meeting budgeted costs [4].

9.1.2 Motivation and objectives of this review

For prediction modelling, methods from the ML domain and its broader field of AI have seen a rapid increase in popularity. ML has emerged as a domain-agnostic decision-making tool, and the authors anticipate that a systematic aggregation of pertinent papers on this theme would be of paramount significance to pharmaceutical communities. This review article is dedicated to the pioneering groups who, between 1990 and 2000, pioneered the use of AI/ML in pharma, including researchers like Rowe [5], Burbidge, York [6–9], Leuenberger [2, 10–12], Takayama [13, 14], Peck [15], Agatonovic-Kustrin [16–24], Bozic [25], and Yliruusi [26–29].

While the benefits of ML and AI are exciting, the development of complex data-driven prediction models necessitates careful quality and appropriateness assessment to ensure their performance, safety, and usability before they are applied and disseminated in practice. Previous reviews summed up ML applications regarding drug discovery [30], metabolomic biomarkers [31], polymorphism screening, drug product development [32–36], drug discovery and development [37], manufacturing and scale-up [38]. Similarly, many of the currently available ML review papers emphasize decision-making, particularly when leveraging big data analytics. Despite the fact that the number of existing reviews on this topic is exponentially increasing, none of them appear to be focused on the context of good practice. The beginning stage for this review is to focus on providing systematic procedures in applying ML algorithms for data analytics (a neglected area).

FDA's long-standing commitment to developing and implementing innovative methods to the regulation of digital technologies exemplifies the aforementioned embracement. The FDA delivers an activity plan that fills in as a guide for building up a framework for AI/ML-based products [39–41]. One of the action plans emphasises the need of building GMLP, which is similar to good software engineering or good quality system practice as well as including data management, feature extraction, training, interpretability, assessment, and documentation. The authors believe that the new framework for software as medical devices (SaMD), as well as guidelines and quality standards for AI/ML in healthcare, might be integrated across disciplines [40–44]. The purpose of this review is to present a brief, intuitive introduction to the data analytics tetrahedron (DAT), constraints, and good ML practice so that researchers may use ML in their everyday operations to improve and foster smarter decisions. In this perspective, this review will be structured in four sections, with the following details:

Part 1: Establishes the DAT background on the basic concepts of data, statistics, ML and first principles required for digital pharmaceutical development.

Part 2: Emphasizes the difficulties in applying ML on data (specific barriers in data analytics).

Part 3: Compilation of case studies of ML in pharmaceutical product development (CMC) with a special focus on data.

Part 4: Challenges and outlook.

9.2 Part 1: data analytics tetrahedron

In the era of data-driven decision making, it is deemed pivotal in clearly understanding the cross-disciplinary concepts, core principles, methods, assumptions and domain knowledge. This is crucial since datasets in the pharmaceutical industry are frequently small and sparse. To overcome such limitations and fully comprehend the benefits in the realm of digital pharmaceutical development, for the first time, the data analytics tetrahedron (figure 9.2) as pyramid is proposed where the base corresponds to data analytics formalism. Secondly, the four triangular facets rest on this formalism and relate to the following: (i) data, (ii) statistics, (iii) ML, as well as (iv) first principles. It is proposed that a systematic implementation of the data analytics tetrahedron (DAT) can boost the digitalization of pharmaceutical development by converting it from a trial-and-error approach to a rationale methodology, thereby, facilitating accelerated, interdisciplinary, and integrative research.

9.2.1 DAT-data

Data (as measurements) is usually collected in the form of 'variables' that can take any value based on concept or characteristic [45]. Stevens proposed four different types of scales (figure 9.3) which are 'nominal', 'ordinal', 'interval', and 'ratio', unifying both qualitative and quantitative variables [45]. In experimentation, variables are either defined as independent or dependent. The independent variables are considered as 'explanatory or predictor or precedent or antecedent or causal or feature' terms while the dependent variables are termed 'consequent or effect or response or outcome or target'. Every measured outcome can be a random variable having a specific pattern called 'distribution'. Depending on the data type, the probability distribution can be discrete or continuous. The most common continuous distribution is the Gaussian or normal distribution [46]. Probability distribution is essential in analytics as mostly the

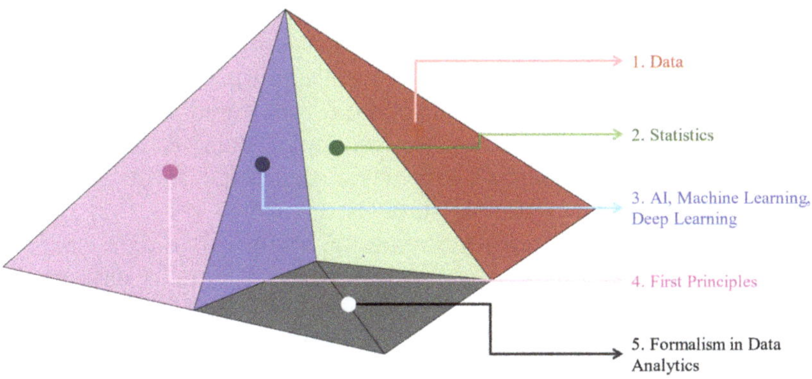

Figure 9.2. Data analytics tetrahedron (DAT).

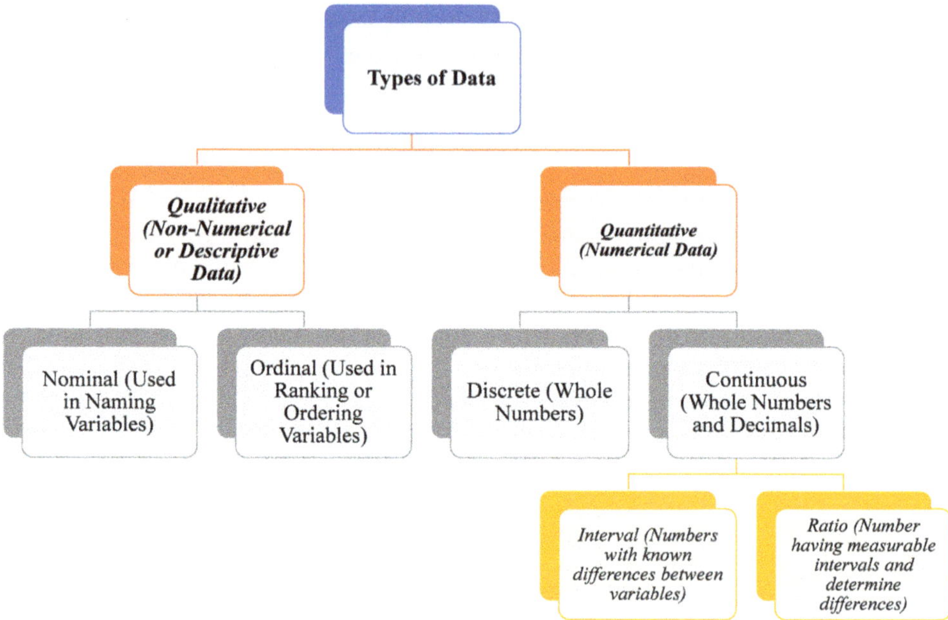

Figure 9.3. Types of data.

decision is made based on sample data to make an inference about the population. In order to infer the population from the sample, quality of input data or data quality is considered a major challenge [47]. Understanding the variable types will determine how they are described, the level of complexity involved, as well as the type of statistical test that can be applied. The data types are provided in below.

9.2.1.1 Small data versus big data

Data naming standards as either 'small' or 'big' have a long-standing history dating back to the early nineteenth century [48]. We have slipped into a 'data-istic' society as a result of the industry 4.0 revolution, which has resulted from a rise in huge volumes of data and very sophisticated technologies. According to Ozkose *et al* (2015) [49], further classification of data can be based on '5Vs', volume (quantity or size of data, in gigabytes/GB, terabytes/TB, petabytes/PB, exabytes/EB, zettabytes/ZB, yottabytes/YB), velocity (speed of data collection), value (data should enrich process under study), variety (format of data, structured or unstructured), and veracity (quality of data) the format. For example, 'data' is defined as data that takes less storage space, arrives slowly, has a structured format, and is of high quality or ready-to-use, whereas 'big data' is defined as data that requires more storage space, appears at a faster rate/streaming, and involves data cleaning as well as data preparation as additional steps. In summary, data is data that is easily accessible, organizable, explainable, and usable that enables rapidly correlated, informative, and actionable meaningful insights. Mining big data without having *a priori* hypothesis, on the other hand, is considered statistical theatrics, however, such analysis can also help in generation of unknown information. Apart from the 5Vs, the other information that differentiates data from big data is variability, visualization, location (local PC versus cloud or multiple servers), longevity (specific duration versus infinite time), reproducibility in case of loss (easy with data while difficult with big data), stakeholder risk (higher with big data than data) [50]. Big data must be derived from high-quality data in order to produce meaningful insights. The authors believe that there is no such thing as big data without data. Typical pharmaceutical product design phase generating data and big data are shown in figure 9.4.

The case studies (section 9.4 and part 3) surveyed that have been recently published demonstrate that the amount of data that were employed in digital pharmaceutical development employing ML is from ~few tens to few thousands, which is to be considered 'data' based on the '5Vs' definition.

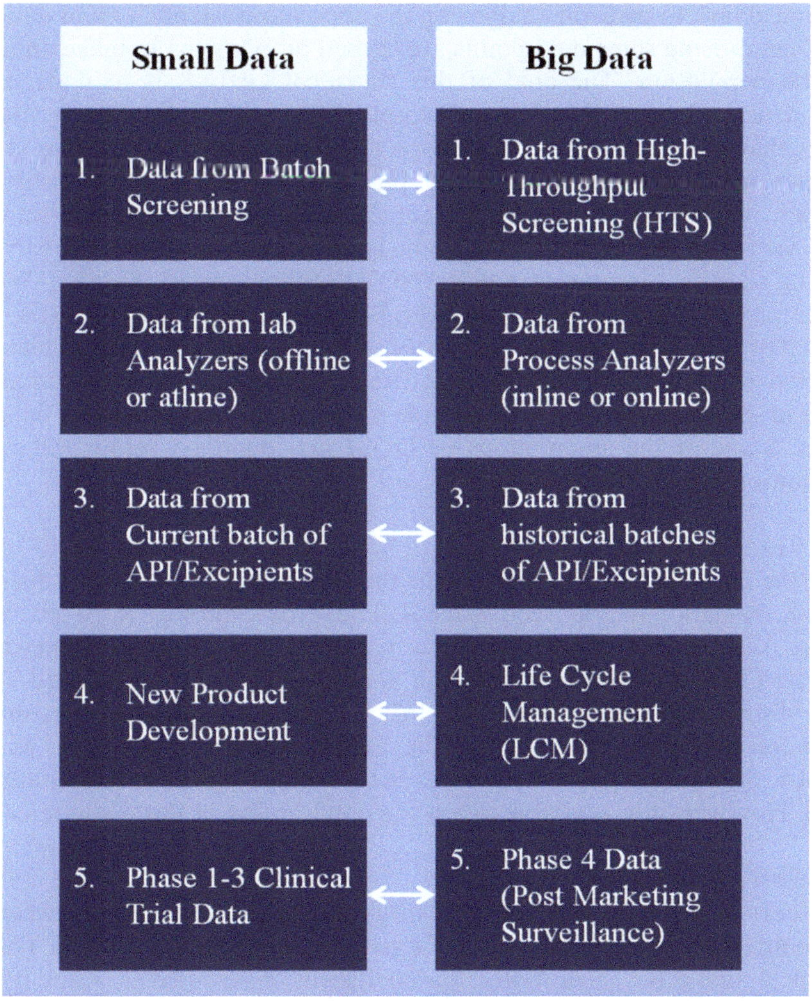

Figure 9.4. Typical pharmaceutical CMC sources and scenarios that generate small data and big data.

9.2.2 DAT: statistics

Statistics, in general, are at the heart of data analytics, and there are two types: descriptive and inferential [51]. Briefly, descriptive statistics provide numerical measures summarizing the data with respect to location (quartiles, percentiles), central tendency (mean, median, mode), dispersion (standard deviation, inter quartile range), shape or symmetry of a dataset's distribution (skewness), and tailedness of distribution (kurtosis) [52]. Graphical descriptive measures involve histogram, scatter plot, QQ plot, boxplot, treemap, violin plot that help in extracting patterns pertaining to the data under investigation [53]. Descriptive statistics do not benefit either decision-making or providing conclusions about the data. While conducting statistical analysis, the two essential notions that are worthwhile mentioning are population and sample [54]. Population can be a complete set of data points from a set of related items that exist. Sometimes it would be an astronomical task to perform analysis on the population. Hence a set of data termed 'sample' comprising some data points are chosen or extracted to make an inference about the population. The goal of this statistical analysis is to understand the characteristics of both population and sample [54]. In a broader context, descriptive numbers that summarize data with respect to population and sample are called 'parameter' and 'statistic', respectively [52, 53]. To infer characteristics of the population, inferential statistics is sought. It compares the available sample and predicts the future outcomes. The outcome is presented as scores of probabilities by employing statistical testing tools like ANOVA, Student *t*-test, Kruskal–Wallis test etc are employed [51, 53, 55–61]. However, before deciding on any analysis, whether inferential or ML, it is a good idea to verify some assumptions which will hereinafter be referred to as data qualification metrics (DQM) [52, 53]. To summarize, the 'garbage in–garbage out' (GIGO) principle is frequently used to address data quality concerns. Some of the assumptions or DQM are identified below and a concise representation is provided in table 9.1.

9.2.2.1 Test for normality

Most of the linear ML algorithms assume that the data follows normal distribution. That said, evaluation metrics such as the Kolmogorov–Smirnov (K–S) test, Shapiro–Wilk test, Anderson–Darling test, Cramer–von Mises test, D'Agostino skewness test, Anscombe–Glynn kurtosis test, and the Jarque–Bera test were utilized to assess whether distribution follows normality [62, 63]. Of these, the most recommended measure for normality assessment is the Shapiro–Wilk test [46, 64]. As already mentioned, the normality assumption has been found to work for larger sample sizes ($n > 30$). However, it is advisable to test the applicability of this assumption.

9.2.2.2 Test for linearity

Pearson correlation test is utilized to quantify the linear association between two or more continuous variables and is part of a parametric statistical test [65]. The output of the calculation is the generation of the coefficient represented as 'r' and it takes on the values between -1 (negative correlation) and $+1$ (positive correlation), that is, 'r'

Table 9.1. Data quality metrics [46, 53].

Test	What for?	Decision rule
Kolmogorov–Smirnov (K–S) test, Shapiro–Wilk test, Anderson–Darling test, Cramer–von Mises test, D'Agostino skewness test, Anscombe–Glynn kurtosis test, and the Jarque–Bera test	Test for normality	Null hypothesis: $p > 0.05$, data follow normal or Gaussian distribution Alternate Hypothesis: p-value < 0.05 indicates data does not follow normal distribution
Hartley's Fmax, Cochran's test, Levene's test, and Bartlett's test	Test for homogeneity of variance (Homoscedasticity)	Null hypothesis: $p > 0.05$, data demonstrates homogeneity of variance or equal variance; Alternate hypothesis: p-value < 0.05 indicates data does not demonstrate equal variance
Scatter plot matrix (SPLOM)	Test for linearity	Pairwise groupings of continuous variables
Variance inflation factor (VIF)	Test for multicollinearity	Values <5 indicate less or no, Values 5–10 indicate moderate; Values >10 indicate severe multicollinearity
Graphical, univariate or multivariate (parametric or non-parametric)	Test for outliers	A data point that has extreme values (either large or small) than nearest value
Prediction power score (PPS)	Test for prediction	PPS lies between '0' (no predictive power) and '1' (perfect predictive power)
Hopkin's test, elbow method, Silhoutte method, hierarchial cluster analysis (HCA)	Test for clustering (dimensionality reduction in *x*-direction)	To identify the presence of clusters in data; To identify the number of clusters
Vapnik–Chervonen–Kis dimension, curve-fitting SSDMs, MSE loss versus training/test split	Sample size determination methodologies (SSDMs)	Minimum generalizability error; Sample sufficiency

is best represented as numericals with values ranging from −1 to 0 to +1. Values closer to +1 represent absolute positive correlation while values closer to −1 represent absolute negative or opposite correlation [66]. Values closer to 0 mean no correlation among variables.

9.2.2.3 Test for multicollinearity

Before we start applying ML models, we need to understand the correlation between independent variables. This is considered crucial because it will become impossible to disentangle the effect of individual predictor variables on model's classification accuracy or regression metrics error. In other words, the multicollinearity induces high variance in the performance of the model, thereby making it susceptible to minor changes in unseen futuristic data. Also, in cases of feature selection, such high correlations could cause uncertainties. Variance inflation factor (VIF) is one of the most commonly employed tests to assess the multicollinearity [46]. VIF is determined by calculating the correlation strength of individual variables. The resulting VIF values would be high if an explanatory variable had a strong correlation with at least one other independent variable. In general, the presence of multicollinearity is justified if the VIF values are >5. Consequently, choosing the right explanatory variables may be occasionally difficult.

9.2.2.4 Test for homogeneity of variance

The homogeneity of variance or homoscedasticity is one of the data qualifying criteria that is regarded a necessity when executing any ML for data analytics. Hartley's Fmax, Cochran's test, Levene's test, and Bartlett's test are examples of statistical tests used to assess homoscedasticity in datasets [67]. The majority of these assessments have been demonstrated to be sensitive to non-normality. Levene's test is the evaluation that is less prone to departures from normality. Because heteroscedasticity leads to overfitting of ML models, inhomogeneity in variances must be assessed on each dataset.

9.2.2.5 Test for outliers

Outliers are data points that differ significantly from other values and can reveal information about a domain as well as the data gathering method [68]. Discrimination and identification of outliers, on the other hand, is regarded as a critical task. An outlier may be termed as a global outlier if its value is significantly different from the rest of the data. If it solely deviates from the data point that originated from a certain context, it is referred to as a contextual outlier. If a set of data points differs greatly from the rest, they can also be labelled as outliers [69]. Outliers exist for a variety of causes, including the following: (i) incorrect data entry; (ii) identification and failure to code missing values; (iii) noise; (iv) extreme data distribution for some specific variables [69]. The outlier detection methods [70–72] can be broadly classified into: (i) graphical visualization (boxplot, histogram, scatter plot); (ii) Univariate parametric Z-scores (dataset size $n > 30$ and normal distribution), extreme Studentized deviate (identifies outlier in normally distributed data), Grubb's test (identifies only one outlier in normally distributed data), Tietjen–Moore test (user to specify number of outliers), Dixon's test (dataset size <10); (iii) univariate non-parametric (Hampel's test, Quartile test), and multivariate detection (robust PCA, k-nearest neighbors, Mahalanobis distance). Application, number of observations in the dataset, dataset type (continuous or categorical), dataset distribution (parametric or non-parametric), and/or analysis level (univariate or multivariate) all influence which outlier detection algorithms are used [70–74]. For non-parametric unsupervised and other approaches to outlier detection please refer to articles [75, 76].

9.2.2.6 Test for prediction

The concept of 'correlation is not causation' is widely acknowledged in the data science and statistics profession. That is, there might be a linear positive or linear negative correlation between two variables, but no causality. In real-world data analytics, the relationships between two variables can be either symmetric or asymmetric, and linear or nonlinear. In such scenarios, tools like predictive power score (PPS) are beneficial. The PPS score is calculated by considering each variable as both feature and target [77]. The estimated PPS values are asymmetric around the matrix, which means that if the variable as a feature effects the goal, the vice versa does not have to hold true. The learning algorithm currently deployed to calculate PPS is decision trees (DTs) and is a part of non-parametric statistical test [77]. The employed algorithm helps in identifying linear or nonlinear relationships, requires less feature pre-processing, is robust in handling outliers (does not overfit), can be employed for both classification and regression, handles both categorical and continuous variables, and is much faster in calculation. The value spectrum of PPS lies between 0 (no predictive power) and 1 (perfect predictive power). Through PPS we can figure out how useful a variable would be in predicting the values of another variable in each dataset and since it normalizes the data (as default) it is much more reliable. More recently, PPS is used as an alternative to correlation matrix, especially to predict the feature importance as well as to help in feature selection [77].

9.2.2.7 Test for clustering

In exploratory data analysis, pattern identification and dataset bias reduction, determining the structure of multi-dimensional data is a major challenge [78]. Clustering algorithms have been widely utilized for this purpose, and it is now regarded as a ubiquitous data analysis tool [78]. Clustering algorithms, on the other hand, will search for and identify clusters in data even if they do not exist. It is a good idea to analyze a dataset's clustering propensity or randomness before applying a clustering algorithm to it. The Hopkins statistic, which analyses the distances between a sample of data points and their nearest neighbor, is recognized to be a reasonable estimate of randomness in a data collection [78]. If the data is not clustered, the average distances between the two sets of distances should be similar. Hopkins' statistic distribution may be studied using a threshold scale (0–1) to determine data clusterability. The data is regularly/uniformly spaced if the value is between 0.01 and 0.3, randomly spaced if the value is 0.5, and highly clusterable if the value is >0.7 [79]. Also, inference using statistical hypothesis testing is possible wherein the null hypothesis (HO, $p > 0.05$) states that the data is unclusterable or uniform while the alternate hypothesis (HA, $p < 0.05$) states that the data can be grouped or clustered. Understanding the clustering tendency is critical since it aids in the reduction of bias as well as in the selection of more explainable ML models [78].

9.2.2.8 Sample size determination methodologies (SSDMs)

For high performance, a specific cut-off, or minimum generalizability error, appropriate sample size determination methodologies (SSDMs) are required [80]. Sample size is always an issue in the pharmaceutical sector, due to cost, raw material availability, and uncommon disorders. One of the requirements of DAT is to assist in calculating the sample sufficiency. Traditional statistical sample size (n) calculations may not provide a strategy for estimating sample size that reduces error or improves the accuracy of predictive ML models [81]. A more rigorous method employing the Vapnik–Chervonenkis dimension may be used to compute the sample size for qualitative ML models [82]. According to Balki *et al* (2019) [81], curve-fitting SSDMs depended on experimentally evaluating model performance at certain sample sizes (wherein performance testing procedures (PTPs) for classification and regression are employed). Recently, model mean squared error loss function in relation to training-test split was carried out [83].

9.2.3 DAT-ML

With the advent of the high-performance computing and sophisticated algorithms, the art of learning to solve a problem from available data is approached. The data consist of a known set of independent variables called 'features' and the machine learns the unknown function on feature variables as well as constructing a good approximation that is called learning '*f*' which is represented as

$$y = f(x) + E(\text{model error}) \tag{9.1}$$

where, '*y*' is dependent variable, '*x*' is the independent features, '*f*' is the function learnt while developing the model and '*E*' is the error associated in the approximation.

In general, two paradigms of digital pharmaceutical development exist: (i) statistics or hypothesis-driven, (ii) data or ML driven. Usually, the former approach is based on 'if given a problem', what kind of data are required in solving the problem? [56, 84]. With statistical approaches, there is a mathematically proven theory behind the applied model, but data must also meet certain strong assumptions [85] (cf section 9.2.2 and subsections describing DQM). Moreover, when we know the function to describe the data, we can utilize traditional statistical methods [86]. The latter approach, ML, is based on the idea of automating as well as building analytical models so that algorithms can learn continually with the help of available data [87, 88] as well as extract the mathematical function behind the data, especially without applying any theory [87]. That said, both paradigms (statistical learning or ML) drive each other complementarily. In other words, theu use a systemic approach to solve a problem, while using data-driven approaches to gain additional insights from already completed experiments [89].

9.2.3.1 Supervised versus unsupervised learning

ML includes a substantial number of algorithmic approaches that can be broadly categorized as supervised or unsupervised approaches. Supervised learning endeavors to predict the target or dependent variable based on the provided input labelled or independent variables. On the other hand, when no target is provided, the strategy is termed unsupervised learning and the employed algorithms find patterns or create clusters of data points. This article provided the labels of various algorithms that are classified under the supervised and unsupervised learning

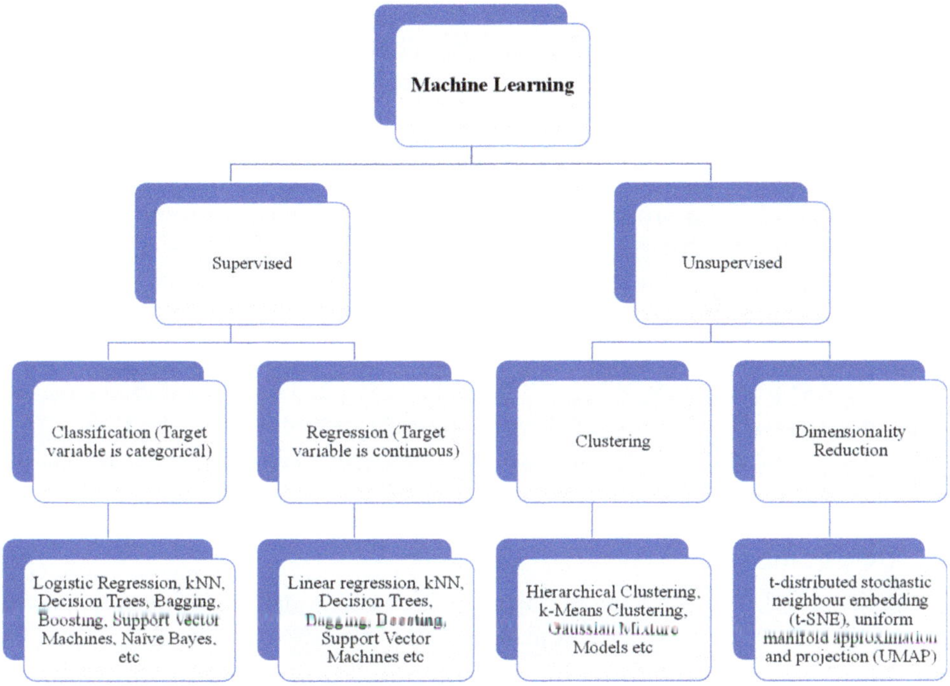

Figure 9.5. Pedigree of ML approaches.

(figure 9.5). However, there are excellent review articles that provide an in-depth understanding on the working mechanism of the ML algorithms [32, 33, 35–38, 90, 91]. When the dependent variable is continuous, we employ regression or quantitative analysis while if the dependent variable is categorical, classification or qualitative analysis is employed. Consequently, data being inspected, determine the available ML methods in predicting the 'target variable'.

9.2.4 DAT: first-principles modelling

One of the major drawbacks of ML is explainability of the derived solutions. To overcome this, in recent years, several researchers have demonstrated that combining a first-principles approach with ML can solve real-world data of practical importance. The above-mentioned hybrid approach is, in fact, a viable avenue. Historically, inventions come first, followed by theories that describe the governing functions and limitations. That is, solutions to complex science and engineering problems require novel methodologies that are able to integrate traditional modelling approaches with state-of-the-art ML techniques [92]. Another avenue where ML techniques have come in handy to overcome the limitations of a multi-model is first-principles-informed ML [42, 93–95], where integration is growing in consensus and helps in combining the existing knowledge with data science [95]. A physics-based or chemistry-based model as substitute to one or more of the ML-based modules helps in achieving good generalization and explainability that helps in predicting previously unseen data as well as providing insights to otherwise black-box models [96, 97]. This integration is unaffected by the data volume or veracity [98]. The noisy data cannot be incorporated with the multiphysics models. This practice of setting the domain-based constraint for ML framework that is referred to as first-principles-informed ML tries to get the better of both universes which could integrate noisy data and mathematical models involving partial differential equations [42]. Finally, we suggest here that extensive use of first-principles-based ML approaches accelerates solving pharmaceutical development problems and thus incentivizes the digitized drug product and process design.

9.3 Part 2: specific barriers in data analytics

Despite the high potential of ML applications in pharmaceutical development, the benefits appear a long way off due to the following cited significant challenges and specific barriers: (i) lack of data, (ii) the availability of high-quality data, (iii) sample representativeness and sample randomness (inherent training data bias), (iv) data leakage, and (v) the lack of ML frameworks [99].

9.3.1 Data quality

The quality of the database used to train the ML model can have a substantial influence on the outcomes of an automated or fully data-driven technology [100]. That is, one of the most serious issues in ML is a lack of high-quality data (for both small and big), which may be ascribed to inauthentic data collection, incompleteness, unrepresentativeness, inconsistency, and unreliability [101–103]. There is currently a lack of comprehensive research of quality standards and quality assessment tools for data science. That said, the DQMs provided in section 9.2.2 can be considered as a good starting point for generating an informed assessment related to data quality [52, 53].

9.3.2 Data quantity

Unless the data meets the 5V's criterion, the amount of the data to be examined is deemed small. In such circumstances, merely increasing the dataset size may not be beneficial. Li and Chao (2021) have demonstrated that the combination of good quality and smaller quantity of data can reach the optimum performance [83]. However, the data quantity, on the other hand, may be regarded essential for determining the uncertainty of the investigated parameters [104, 105]. Furthermore, because statistics and ML models are extensively adopted for inference and decision-making, in this context, uncertainty quantification (UQ) is used to evaluate the reliability and efficiency of ML-based predictions [104, 105]. The confidence interval or prediction interval can be used to estimate UQ [104, 106]. That is, the data quality and quantity do share a connection and are not mutually exclusive [83, 101–103]. On the other hand, working with less data accentuates the virtues of reduced data collection costs, cheaper annotation costs, shallow training models, lower hardware costs, and shorter training durations [83]. To summarize, in order to accomplish sustainable ML, it is vital to strike a balance between data quality and quantity, which may be aided by analyzing as well as recognizing the bias coupled with variance associated with the data (see section 9.3.3).

9.3.3 Bias and variance (B–V)

Understanding the errors associated with prediction, whether in hypothesis-driven or machine-driven statistical data analysis, is vital. The errors in prediction are ordinarily portrayed as either bias or variance [107]. Bias is referred to as the difference in values between the original data and the predicted data; on the other hand, for any slight change in the training dataset, the expected values will contrast drastically and this change in sum is referred to as the variance [108]. Navigating between different sources of error that cause bias and variance aids in accentuating data quality, data quantity, and the ML framework, resulting in more precise and accurate ML models. In supervised ML, we assume a definitive link between independent variables/feature(s) and dependent variables/target. To estimate this unknown relationship, a model function called '*f*' is used, which accurately depicts the relationship between features and target (refer to equation (9.1)). Bias or variance are two potential reasons why the ML model may not perform adequately.

Conceptually, in practice, model function '*f*' is almost always unknown and must be determined using a model with a specified training set [108]. A wide variety of ML methods are employed, like linear regression (LR), support vector machines (SVMs), DTs, random forest (RF). If the employed model oversimplifies the underlying function and lacks attention to the training data a 'bias' error is generated [105, 108]. It is defined as the difference between the model's average prediction and the true value. The algorithm's ability to establish relevant relationships between features ('*x*') and the outputs of the target ('*y*') variables is lost, resulting in a high level of error on both training and test data (leading to underfitting) [109]. On the other hand, the predicted value for a particular training data is indicated as '*f1*^'. A different '*f2*^' is obtained using a new set of training data, and so on. The degree by which '*fn*^' changes across various training sets is called variance [109]. The variance characterizes the dispersion in the data and describes the uncertainty of model prediction for a given dataset. A high variance model pays close attention to training data and does not generalize the test or real-world data and the obtained error is termed as 'variance' error [105, 108, 109]. As a result, while these models perform well on training data, their error rates on test data are high (leading to overfitting). Specific indicators called DQM that help assess ML data readiness as part of digital pharmaceutical development to address data bias and variance, have been mentioned in section 9.2.2 [52, 53, 110, 111].

Mathematically, model error or mean square error (MSE) is defined as the difference in prediction between the test and training sets, and it is necessary to keep it as low as possible. Two major sources of error are (i) reducible (bias as well as variance), and (ii) irreducible [112], as depicted in equations (9.2) and (9.3).

$$\text{Mean squared error (model)} = \text{reducible error} + \text{irreducible error}. \tag{9.2}$$

$$\text{Mean squared error (model)} = \text{bias}^2 + \text{variance} + \text{irreducible error}. \tag{9.3}$$

The bias and variance both contribute to the reducible error and, reducing these two would allow us to create more accurate as well as precise models [113].

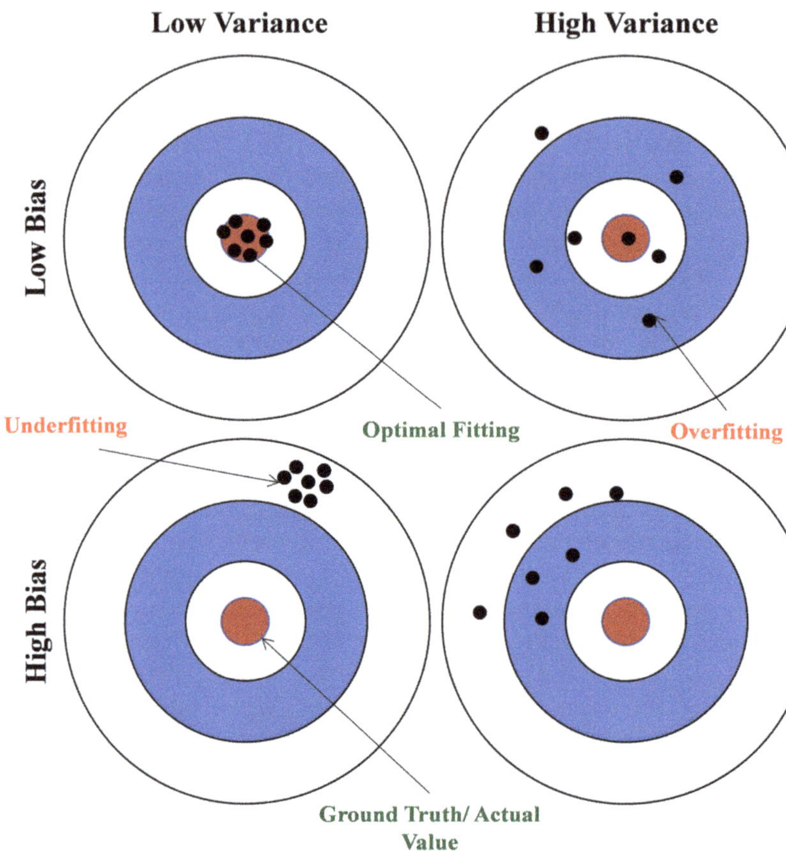

Figure 9.6. Understanding bias and variance impact on fitting the predicted versus actual data values.

The irreducible error, on the other hand, is caused by instrument, sample, or sampling-related reasons. Using a bulls-eye diagram, the bias and variance can be graphically illustrated, figure 9.6, and four alternative scenarios can be plotted, each exhibiting a mix of high and low bias and variance (low bias/variance, low bias/high variance, high bias/low variance, high bias/high variance) [114, 115]. Given the random heterogeneity in the training data we collect, each hit represents an individual realization of ML model. When the data quality and quantity are good, the prediction is optimal, hitting the bulls-eye, but when training data fails any attributes of DQM, the model makes weaker predictions. The outcome of these various realizations is a dispersion of strikes on the target.

9.3 4 Data leakage

Target or dependent-variable leakage and training-test dataset contamination are the two major categories of leakage. In the first scenario, training data contains information about the target, but similar data is not available when the model is used for real-world prediction [116, 117]. In the second case, there is mismatch between training and test records (data-driven model) or sample and population data (hypothesis-driven model), especially with respect to data [109, 118–120]. That is, the data employed results in excellent performance on the training set (and possibly even the validation data), but poor performance in production or real-world data.

9.3.5 Lack of ML frameworks

Even though several studies look into the pharmaceutical applications of various AI models, the authors believe that methodical ML frameworks are lacking with respect to open-standard processes like cross-industry standard data mining processes (CRISP-DM) [121–124]. This is also demonstrated by the FDA's recent draft guidance on software as medical device [41]. Our main contribution in this review paper is a CRISP-DM-style framework that focuses more on good practice that benefits students, academics, regulators, and researchers in order to advance research in this domain.

9.4 Part 3: case studies

9.4.1 Chemistry, manufacturing, and control (CMC)

Combinatorial chemistry, molecular simulations, and high throughput screening have complemented and expanded in size for the characterization of active pharmaceutical ingredients (APIs) or drug substances [3, 125–129]. Numerous experiments on the prediction of API properties such as melting point, solubility, and so on have been reported. This review focusses on all stages of the life cycle of drug product development, usually after early discovery phase, where the activities are known as CMC. CMC entails manufacturing a pharmaceutical or biopharmaceutical using similar raw materials, comparable procedures, well-defined drug product specifications, and end-product testing which ensures that the developed product is safe, effective, and consistent between batches. The flow of CMC activities is shown in figure 9.7. These ensure the following batches are produced and submitted to FDA, including clinical or pilot or engineering or process validation batches, details of which are provided below.

Clinical batches are made to produce drugs used in clinical studies, whereas the pilot batches are required to demonstrate quality, stability as well as the consistency [130].

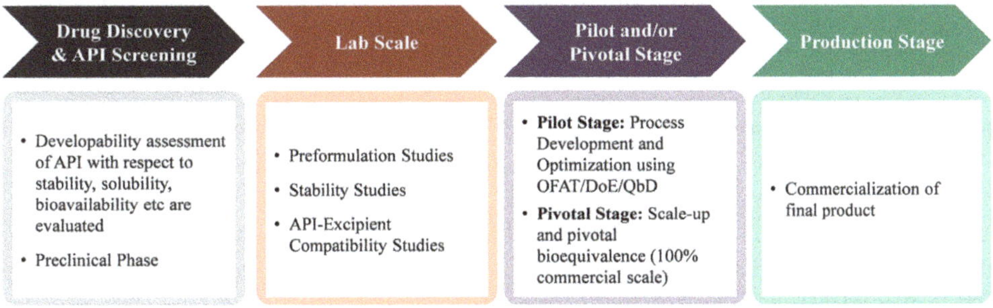

Figure 9.7. Key components in the stages of CMC of product development, starting from API screening to preformulation (lab scale) to pilot or pivotal clinical stage to commercialization (production scale).

Data collected from both clinical and pilot batches are submitted to the FDA in the CMC technical section for review. After the drug is approved, the manufacturer needs to increase the size of the batch (usually termed as commercial batch) [130]. While doing so, the manufacturer needs to meet the specifications as described in CMC [131]. To do the scale-up, the sponsor may need to make manufacturing batches and process validation batches. That said, clinical batches can be the same as pilot batches, and process validation batches can be the same as commercial batches [130]. As mentioned already, at each of these stages, both qualitatively similar composition and equivalent manufacturing processes are to be adopted [132]. Despite the high-level advancements (whether at the quantum or classical level that happens in drug discovery), the speed for decision-making as well as extrapolation to CMC stages are a serious setback, especially when moving from pilot scale to commercial drug product development stages [130–132], ML models are being adopted as an interface to overcome such setbacks.

This review is not intended to suggest what is correct or incorrect, but rather to extensively examine those publications that have adhered to the basic minimum of GMLP.

9.4.2 ML approach in material property investigation

9.4.2.1 API screening

Ghosh *et al* [133], demonstrated that adopting data-driven digitization approaches such as ML, especially in the prediction of crystallization tendency, may be regarded as a considerable advancement in the field of pharmaceutical sciences. Authors catalogued the 'Pfizer dataset' on API crystallization experiments based on investigation types, solvent system employed, nature of solid forms which were carried out between 2005 and 2017. The ML models employed were random forest regression (RFR), support vector machine regression (SVMR) and neural networks (NN). The authors concluded that the RFR approach outperformed the other two ML methods in terms of size of training dataset, feature extraction from models involving API and solvents. The other parameter that was included in the models was the molecular property of the API. The study's highlight is that, despite the fact that it only employed a dataset (88 organic molecules), the rigorous production measures used for ML model design helped to achieve a high precision with a low error of 20% to predict the crystallization propensity with desired API properties. The overview of this paper is provided in figure 9.8.

9.4.2.2 Nanocrystals

The prediction of formation propensity of nanocrystals has been considered next to an impossible task. The reasons sighted are the complex interplay between material properties, experimental conditions, and manufacturing procedures. He *et al* [134] thoroughly collated API nanocrystals which were manufactured using three different preparation methods involving ball wet milling (BWM), high-pressure homogenization (HPH) and antisolvent precipitation (ASP). Through this extensive literature survey, the authors have compiled 910 nanocrystal datasets along with polydispersity index data from 341 datasets. Once trained, newly prepared

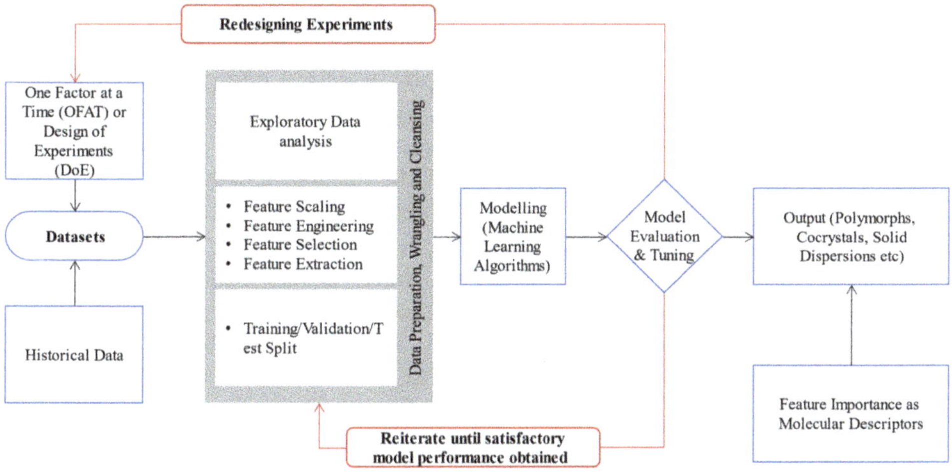

Figure 9.8. Generic data-driven digitization flowchart towards the prediction of the propensity of formation of diverse solid-state forms and formulationsof drug molecules (modified based on Ghosh *et al* [134]).

nanocrystals were validated in order to understand the model's robustness, generalization ability as well as prediction accuracies. Highlights of the paper include the following: (a) three split strategies 80% train, (b) 10% validation, and 10% test dataset, as well as (c) 10-fold cross-validation.

9.4.2.3 Solid form screening

Pereira (2020) [135] employed trained ML models on molecules derived from the Elsevier database (Reaxys©) that contains 40 462 molecules (belonging to crystalline as class A: 37 790 structures; polymorphic as class B: 2167 structures; and amorphous as class C: 503 structures). The author employed the following GMLP-like different models (reduced error pruning tree (REPTree), RF, SVMs, deep learning multilayer perceptron networks (dMLP)), feature selection (RF based feature importance and correlation-based feature subset selection (CFS)), handling class imbalance (base-classifier, CostSensitiveClassifier, class weight parameters). Even without crystallisability data, the proposed model can accurately predict crystallization propensity, enabling for the discovery of suitable crystalline compounds of new or existing small organic molecules.

ML offers numerous benefits over traditional statistical approaches in drug design, making it highly important in the development and optimization of preformulation. The vast majority of frequently used ML models are nonlinear, and therefore potentially capable of mimicking interactions that linear quantitative structure-activity relationship models may not effectively describe. The reported use of ML models in the prediction of solubility enhancements, as well as their efficient use in final dosage formulations, stimulates additional study into their potential usage in pharmaceutical preformulation research. Recent studies on the ML approaches for the prediction of the solubility of drug like molecules in aqueous media as published by Lovrićh *et al* [136] and by Francoeur and Koes [137] reflect a strong potential in streamlining preformulation phase. Also, the solvent selection for various formulation designs could be assisted by ML models [134].

Understanding and formulating the drug-phospholipid complex is considered a daunting task. Gao *et al* [138] developed ML as well as simulation involving molecular dynamics in combination with design of experiments. In order to achieve this objective, the authors, web-scraped the data on drug-phospholipid complexes published between 1999 and 2019. The inclusion of articles was based on complexation rate of $\geqslant 80\%$. Various molecular descriptors for both API and phospholipids were also incorporated. ML models employed were RF, SVM, k-nearest neighbour (kNN), DT, naïve Bayes (NB) classifier and boosting algorithms (LightGBM). A five-fold cross-validation technique was used to model and tune hyperparameters, as well as optimize and validate the training datasets. An unseen or test dataset was utilized as an external validation strategy. The performance of the model was studied using the following metrics like accuracy, recall, F1-score, precision, and area under the curve. By simply amalgamating the ML and molecular dynamics domains, drug screening as well as formulation development efficiency may be accomplished. In this study, amalgamation yielded a successful prediction with respect to the features accountable for drug-phospholipid complexation.

9.4.3 ML in formulation development

9.4.3.1 Drug product design and optimization

Despite the fact that ML has been effectively incorporated in several different facets of the pharmaceutical sector, drug product development is still primarily directed by expert knowledge [139]. Generally acceptable, however, the availability of difficult to synthesize or expensive molecules in the initial phases of formulation research might limit drug product development even when expert knowledge is available. To overcome such scenarios, Zhao *et al* [140] devised prediction models that can enable us in identifying critical formulation components and process parameters, thereby, minimizing the number of trials required. The prediction approach, on the other hand, was very accurate and generalizable without collapsing to variances/overfitting. The major highlight of this study was that the authors implemented dataset selection (historical dataset between 1990 and 2018), train-validation-test split (80%/10%/10%), feature selection, algorithm selection (Bagging models/RF, boosting models/LightGBM, DL model), and regression model metrics (R2, MAE, RMSE). In conclusion, a quick and reliable prediction model capable of forecasting the solubilizing capabilities of cyclodextrin (CD) systems was established. In another attempt, Thomas *et al* [141] utilized the power of ML approaches to derive the compacted powders' mechanical property merely using components' material properties. The highlights of the model include inclusion of linear regression and nonlinear regression (using second-order polynomial function) models, data qualification metrics (feature transformation like normalization, testing for multicollinearity like VIF), three different k-fold cross-validation on the best model like Stratify-By-Batch (SBB), Leave-One-Batch-Out (LOBO), Leave-One-API-Out (LOAO) were approached. Although, it has been long assumed that Young's modulus is proportional to tensile strength, the authors demonstrated that this assumption is critically dependent on API as well as excipient mechanical properties and recommend that nonlinear models be progressively employed instead of linear models. Gao *et al* [142] recently advanced ML- and AI-based models for predicting formulation factors for poorly soluble drugs such as composition prediction of self-emulsifying drug delivery systems (SEDDS) [142] and physical stability prediction of amorphous solid dispersion (ASD) [143].

9.4.3.2 Pharmaceutical process design and optimization

To date, there has been a disparity in correlating the extensively studied material attributes with respect to manufacturability and processability. Experiment correlation is currently achieved by a trial-and-error approach that alternates between end-product testing and process parameter tweaking. However, these are random trials, and where to restart in the event of a failure is a million-dollar question. Hayashi *et al* [144] employed a boosted tree (BT) ML model to correlate the drug substance (81 model API utilized in this study) critical material attributes with the tensile strength of directly compressed API/excipient compacts. This research focused on eliminating multicollinearity, adding four-fold cross-validation, utilized sensitivity analysis to increase the BT model's accuracy. The authors concluded that the BT model was successful in extracting quantitative causal relationship between the API properties and desired tensile strength. The feature of importance was d10 particle size, modal diameter, elastic recovery, moisture content.

One other significant barrier that fraternities come across is cost-effective as well as successful technology transfer. Millen *et al* [145], successfully applied ML model for the wet granulation scale-up. The particle size distribution (PSD) of dry granulate was calculated using sieve analysis and laser diffraction methods, yielding novel parameters such as the coefficient of determination (R2) and slope of the PSD line. The determined novel parameters were utilized in correlating the wet granulated tablets' tensile strength of laboratory batches (21 training sets) and commercial batches (21 test batches). The scale-up decision-making process was assisted by ML algorithms, with the gradient boosted regression trees (GBRT) algorithm achieving the lowest error rates. Good practice of this study was as follows: the authors addressed multicollinearity, developed stepwise regression for feature selection, and performed hyperparameter tuning and cross-validation on the best method.

9.4.3.3 Pharmaceutical quality by design (QbD)

One other area in the pharmaceutical development that generates lot of datasets is quality by design (QbD). QbD and statistics have been in existence for a long time. Nevertheless, they model only the linear explorative/regressive data. Likewise, there has been a lot of understanding that the QbD data might involve nonlinearity as well as time-dependency. Klemenčič and Mihelič [38] have reviewed the current practices in the pharmaceutical QbD arena. Despite the fact that chemometrics has been widely used, nonlinear data mining techniques have yet to find a place in small-molecule process-related data. ML implementation to process data has been successfully executed in biopharmaceutical manufacturing [146–150]. ML in the small-molecule pharmaceutical development can be considered as an attractive area of research with subsequent articles where there is an attempt to unravel the nitty-gritty underpinning the manufacturing process.

Until now, it has been of common misconception that data analytics or ML for small size data is near to impossible which is naturally true with respect to the QbD or analytical QbD (AQbD) or design of experiments where the size is ~5 to ~50 or similar. According to International Conference on Harmonization guidelines (ICH Q8R), QbD is 'a systematic approach to development that begins with predefined objectives and emphasizes understanding and control, based on sound science and quality risk management'. With respect to datasets, recently, the authors of [150] proposed self-validated ensemble methods (SVEMs) that utilize a modified version of commonly known fractionally-weighted bootstrapping. When compared to typical statistical models like degrees of freedom (dof), SVEM's predicted accuracy is greater by an order of magnitude. On the other hand, because SVEM works well with smaller datasets, the following benefits are realized: (i) decreased experimentation time, resulting in (ii) lower costs for innovation while (iii) boosting the speed to market. In most circumstances, it is always good practice to thoroughly understand both raw material attributes and process parameters in advance in order to ensure the quality and performance of the finished product. Moreover, this understanding will facilitate better communication between those involved in R&D and technology transfer at the manufacturing units. Gams *et al* [149] introduced hybrid feature selection (ML-based and expert-driven) of both material attributes and process parameters, as well as innovative algorithm selection (from ML-based, human-based as well as metalearning approaches which involves DT along with human interaction), of which, metalearning models outperformed other approaches. One of the study's key conclusions is that the suggested model is particularly well-suited for assessing manufacturing processes with limited datasets. This was attributed to the innovation approach that blends the human-computer interaction which also provides improved performance and quality.

9.4.4 ML approach in end-product testing

Historically, and also today, the formulation of oral solid dosage forms of any active pharmaceutical ingredients was regarded as more of an art than a science [151]. In order to understand the quality and performance of both drug substances and drug product, compendial monograph (pharmacopeial) procedures have been drafted by agencies around the globe like US Pharmacopoeia-National Formulary (USP/NF), the European Pharmacopoeia (EP), the Japanese Pharmacopoeia (JP), the Indian Pharmacopoeia (IP), and the British Pharmacopoeia (BP) that provide standardized methods and specifications tests [152]. A blend of historical approach and regulatory philosophy, which asserts 'show me it works and then do not change process, material, or release testing procedures' was demonstrated to be very congruent [153]. The identification, purity, and microbiological tests of pharmaceutical ingredients and excipients are few of the compendial tests for oral solid dosage forms [154]. The quality as well as performance of finished dosage forms are categorized based on the following: (i) test for assay, which is availability of declared drug's strength; (ii) test for content uniformity which denotes that each dosage unit has a consistent amount of drug within an acceptable level of uncertainty; (iii) test for related substances that necessitates the finished dosage form should not generate hazardous compounds as well as; (iv) test for dissolution studies that simulates the release profile of a dosage form at predefined rates [155–157]. Both compendial (high pressure liquid chromatography/HPLC, gas chromatography (GC), Fourier transform infrared spectroscopy (FTIR), Karl Fisher titration, microbiological tests) and non-compendial analytical techniques (x-ray diffraction, particle size analyzer, dissolution apparatus) are used to measure these tests [158].

The end-product testing of drug substance or solid dispersions or finished dosage forms for poorly water-soluble drugs are considered as a daunting task, especially with respect to the physical stability of high energy amorphous phase. In this context, Han *et al* [159] have used ML modelling to predict the physical stability of amorphous solid dispersion (ASD) as one of the potential ways towards strategic formulation development. Mendyk *et al* [160], utilized in-house data which turned out to be more homogeneous, and extensively characterized than literature-based data. The models performed better with the in-house datasets. The models were selected from rule-based systems, RF, artificial neural networks, fuzzy logic, and genetic programming. The train–test split was 90%:10% and the uncertainty in prediction (as RMSE) was addressed using 10-fold cross-validation. The structure or features of in-house data included composition of excipient 1 and 2 (molecular weight, molecular descriptors), particle size, surface, pore volume, differential scanning calorimeter (DSC) and FTIR features of powder system, formulation method, time dissolved amount of API in particular time. The contributing features were selected using a variance–covariance matrix. Interestingly, the interaction between powder systems of bicalutamide-polyvinyl pyrrolidone (PVP) and bicalutamide-poly ethylene glycol (PEG) was detected using the FTIR peak at 1260 cm^{-1} as evidenced by Ab Initio modelling. Among a relatively large number of attributes (out of ~3600), the ML model discovered the FTIR feature at 1260 cm^{-1} as the most important contributor, which was also found to surrogate the amorphous solid dispersions' final product performance.

Understanding the effects of environmental factors (such as pH, temperature, and humidity) is perceived as critical. There have been fewer studies that have systematically investigated such factors. However, in one of the studies, King *et al* [161] utilized a range of experimental and supplemented findings using ML approaches. Often the performance of complex/biological molecules like antibodies is assumed based on thermal stability. In order to investigate this assumption, firstly, the protein sequences were unfolded using clustering algorithms for meaningful amino acid residues. Next, the algorithm SVMRs with radial basis kernel (SVR-RBF) were selected. In order to reduce the overfitting procedures nested cross-validation loop and iterative selection of features within this loop were employed. The authors demonstrated that the pH was more influential than thermal stability. As predictable, ML has aided the researchers in their decision-making.

9.4.5 ML approach in *in vitro* drug release and *in vivo* pharmacokinetic predictions

The content of drug and its uniformity in and the release of drug molecule from formulated products at the desired rate and to the desired extent are the prerequisites for obtaining optimal efficacy. There has been abundant research towards implementing in-line process analytical technology (PAT) solutions such as near infrared (NIR) spectroscopy for content uniformity monitoring during drug product manufacturing. The statistical models built from such process monitoring data builds the basis for predicting content and uniformity of the drug in the product, serving as the basic framework to achieve a real-time release of the drug product [162]. The disintegration and drug dissolution are the other key quality attributes for solid oral dosage forms and are tested *in vitro* as a surrogate of *in vivo* behaviour, during product development. While in-line PAT as real-time release testing (RTRT) for content uniformity is well established within academic research and is in industrial practice, similar approaches for dissolution/disintegration performance have emerged only in recent years. Several attributes related to raw material, formulation, underlying drug product process and interaction among them can influence the microstructure of the final product that governs drug dissolution and release. So comprehensive statistical modelling solutions considering process dynamics and material variation are evolving as a tool to predict the *in vitro* drug release behavior [163]. The *in vitro* drug release data are often empirically fitted using models like Nernst–Brunner, Higuchi, Krosmeyer–Peppas to obtain model parameters and use for further prediction [164]. However, a sufficiently large amount of data would be required to develop a robust statistical model and to validate correlation per product/process. Galata *et al* [165] recently reported the application of ML approach using the PSD, NIR spectra and compression force as input for developing surrogate models for a real-time drug dissolution testing of a sustained-release tablet [165]. The ANN model performed best to demonstrate the influence of matrix polymer PSD and was thus identified as the critical material attribute (CMA) for the drug release. Likewise, Nagy *et al* found that an ANN model, developed based on NIR PAT data of extended release tablet formulation manufacturing, outperformed the prediction powder of *in vitro* drug dissolution profile compared to the linear partial least regression (PLS) model [166]. Antonio Susto *et al* [167] used historical manufacturing data including raw material parameters, coating data, loss on drying and pellet size statistics in an ML algorithm (LASSO) to develop predictive models for the drug dissolution variability. Akseli and co-workers from Boehringer-Ingelheim Pharmaceuticals Inc. developed a predictive framework for the disintegration and breaking force of a tablet using an ML tool [168]. Benomar *et al* [169] employed hierarchical Bayesian approach for modelling the dissolution profiles of sustained-release suppositories formulations. The use of ANN and genetic programming (GP) has been successfully demonstrated for dissolution modelling of solid lipid extrudate [170]. GP enabled direction modelling of drug dissolution versus extrudate dimension reduction over time as well as indirect modelling through Weibull fitting. Salazar-Jiménez *et al* [171] addressed the problem of dimensionality reduction for the dissolution prediction using ML. The authors used various feature selection algorithms to identify the most relevant variables subset. The emerging approach of applying ML in the context of continuous manufacturing of solid oral dosage forms towards the prediction of *in vitro* drug release is depicted in figure 9.9.

The ultimate task of drug product performance evaluation is to examine the correlation between *in vitro* drug release data with *in vivo* performance (IVIVC) of the

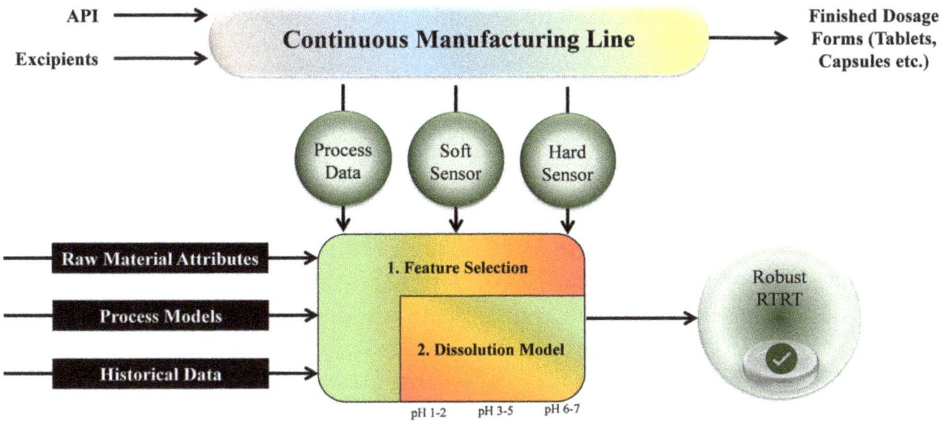

Figure 9.9. Schematic representation the ML enabled RTRT for the *in vitro* dissolution/drug release modeling of solid oral dosage forms. Hard sensors could be various PAT tools (e.g. NIR, Raman, FTIR, Terahertz (THz)) and soft sensors could include real-time recording of temperature, pressure, humidity, shear forces, compression/compaction forces, torque.

developed formulation. An application of advanced modelling and simulation beyond current numerical deconvolution practice of IVIVC is highly desirable to reduce drug formulation and process optimization effort. Such models could be either PBPK ones or statistical data-driven models such as ML that can help setting virtual bioequivalence study using the framework of *in vitro–in silico–in vivo* correlation (IV–IS–IVC). Yamashita *et al* have shown the use of a genetic algorithm called gene expression programming (GEP) for the search of nonlinear function in the IVIVC of the sustained-release oral formulation of diltiazem [172]. The authors presented a powerful yet simpler empirical modelling approach for describing a complex input–output relationship in the context of modelling IVIC data. Population pharmacokinetic (popPK) modelling is an area where various types of nonlinear models are popularly used with the goal towards building a covariate model for each PK parameter. Also, for popPK modelling, GEP approach has been shown to be useful for automatic extrapolation [173]. Ogami *et al* [174] recently developed an ANN-PK model using patients PK data as input for predicting the drug clearance (CL). By further employing the ANN predicted CL to a one-compartment absorption model and thereby calculating the drug concentration, the parameter of ANN was further updated via back propagation methodology. The RMSE of prediction and the model convergence of ANN-PK model were found to be superior to that of the classical popPK model, evidencing the better prediction accuracy. The readers are referred to an excellent recent review published by McComb *et al* for further details and the potential of ML application to the field of pharmacokinetics and the whole of pharmacometrics [175].

9.4.6 ML in translational development of drug product and device

There are two basic types of software being used in healthcare; the first type is used for medical purposes (software products used to make clinical decisions) such as ‘software as a medical device’ and ‘software in a medical device’ (intended as an accessory to a medical device). The second type of software, that used for non-medical purposes (e.g., administrative, financial), is not considered as medical devices. SaMD is standalone software products intended to be used for one or more medical purposes that perform these purposes without being part of a hardware medical device. For example: treatment planning software, and automated radiological image processing software. Software in a medical device (SiMD) is embedded software programs, firmware, or micro-codes essential for the functioning of a medical device, for example: software used to drive or control the motors and the pumping of a medication infusion pump. As the applications of software products as medical devices have increased in disease diagnosis therapy and surgeries, they have been regulated in many countries [176, 177].

In the US, the FDA was granted the authority to regulate the manufacturing and marketing of medical devices in 1976. The Centre for Devices and Radiological Health with the FDA is responsible for ensuring the safety, effectiveness, quality of medical devices and communicate the risk and other science-based information to the public [178, 179]. Although the medical devices regulation in EU controls to ensure that devices are safe and effective, it has now been further extended to post-market clinical follow-up data for all medical devices including software used in healthcare [180]. In India, the ministry of health & Family Welfare, government of India, notified the Medical Devices Rule in 2017 for regulating devices including software.

Tremendous volumes of healthcare data and rapid growth of health technology methods have opened a new window for use of AI and ML in healthcare, including in regulatory sciences. There are many pharmaceutical and other technology industries and governmental projects that have invested in developing AI/ML-based tools for clinical practice where patients or end users are beneficiaries. However, those study outcomes are yet to be published. After the review of available literature, the applications of AI/ML in clinical practice, can be considered as medical devices as per the regulation. The Ideal AI/ML must be composed of tools for monitoring and remote management of chronic diseases, imaging applications for diagnostic support and clinical decision support tools to facilitate the choice of treatment [181]. The AI/ML implementation for better patient care and its regulatory pathway also must be clear; implementation is completely dependent on the trained clinical or biomedical engineers or technicians. In the case of regulatory requirements, dependence is on the assessment of level of risk associated with the use of AI/ML in clinical practice. Generally, its risk can be classified into administrative or procedural errors, quality related issues, software design, patient's co-morbid conditions or biocompatibility. The number of approved AI/ML as medical devices has increased substantially in US and Europe mainly for use in radiology. However, there is no specific regulatory pathway for AI/ML-based medical devices in the USA or Europe [182].

Reiterating, the case studies (table 9.2) surveyed that have recently been published show that the quantity of data used in digital pharmaceutical development using ML was on average between 10 and 3000, which is deemed 'data' according to the '5Vs' criterion.

Table 9.2. Synopsis of case studies demonstrating size of data (data analytics) and GMLP.

Data size	Objective	Inputs/variables	GMLP	Output(s)	Reference
28	Prediction of powder compactability of tablets using core/shell technique	Four input variables: concentration of shell material, concentration of core material, type of shell material, type of core material	28-run DoE, 6 ML and deep learning, algorithms, model generalizability	Tensile strength; brittleness index	[183]
88	Prediction of crystallization propensity (from 11 000 experiments)	Experiments conducted between 2005 and 2017 at Pfizer Inc. with 88 organic API molecules 1000 descriptors of API and solvent physicochemical properties	GMLP followed were train–test–split, ~4 different algorithms and understanding the feature importance	API crystallisation	[133]
646	Prediction of the physical stability of solid dispersions	24 variables related to: formulation (including molecular weight, melting point, hydrogen bonding for both drug and polymer); experimental conditions (including temperature, relative humidity, and storage time)	GMLPs followed were train–test–split using improved maximum dissimilarity algorithm, eight different ML algorithms, hyperparameter tuning, understanding the feature importance, orthogonal approaches using molecular modelling	Stability results	[159]
910	Prediction of nanocrystal formation from three manufacturing methods (three different preparation methods involving BWM, high-pressure homogenization (HPH) and antisolvent precipitation (ASP))	API and stabilizer descriptors	Highlights include (a) three split strategy 80%:10%:10% train: validation:test dataset, (b) models: deep neural networks (DNN), SVM, DT, LightGBM, RF, PLS, kNN (c) 10-fold cross-validation	Nanocrystal size and PDI	[134]
3000	Forecast the complexation ability of various cyclodextrins	Diverse set of organic molecules collected from published literature from the year 1990 to 2018. The final dataset with 3000 formulations for the predictive model building contained 1320 guest molecules and eight CDs	GMLP followed were train–test–split, ~4 different algorithms, regression metrics	API-cyclodextrin inclusion complexation	[140]

9.4.7 Advanced concepts

In the following we briefly introduce three advanced concepts in ML, transfer learning, generative models, and sequential learning. All are to date comparably new but promising first results indicate that a broader use will be beneficial.

9.4.7.1 ML for vaccinology

At least 650 000 fatalities per year are recorded worldwide because of the influenza virus. Vaccination development has been one of the most significant medical and pharmaceutical discoveries in history, and vaccine strategies are now used to manage virus epidemics. However, present procedures may not always give protection, and understanding why current vaccinations work in some people but not in others is critical in developing better vaccines. Over the last two decades, ML has also revolutionized the area of vaccine development. Using ML algorithms, in combination with existing advancements in computational biology, allows for the unbiased extraction of information to identify immune cell types and genes that stimulate stronger antibody responses to influenza vaccinations. VaxiJen was the first reverse vaccinology technique to use ML, and it has demonstrated good antigen prediction results. Ong *et al* [184] employed VaxiJen-ML in conjunction with VaxiJen to predict COVID-19 vaccine candidates. On the other hand, the Oxford Vaccine Group is utilizing ML on biological data to study human responses to vaccine dosages and has released SIMON (Sequential Iterative Modelling OverNight), an open-source programme. According to Tomic *et al* [185] (Oxford Vaccine Group), time-consuming work to comprehend with the goal of improving the vaccine's effectiveness was the need of the hour, 'the major aims of SIMON project are to understand why some individuals who receive the vaccine are protected against flu while others get infected and to predict if an individual will respond appropriately to the vaccine.' This project also identified the important cellular biomarkers through data mining approach FluPRINT [186]. A new ML technique is used to forecast an individual's mortality risk to COVID-19 based on electronic health records, vitals, and lab findings obtained during hospitalization [186]. The developed model presents a more broadly applicable and generalized technique for predicting the group of people most vulnerable to COVID-19 as well as who need immediate medical attention. The COVID-19 pandemic has inspired researchers all over the world to work at breakneck speed, integrating diverse types of data and submitting them to an advanced analytical model to extract effective clinical development programmes. The unprecedented collaboration between Janssen and MIT researchers resulted in the deployment of advanced ML approaches that aid in tracking pandemics, forecasting hotspots, harnessing data to understand riskier populations, and leveraging data to provide informed decisions about freedom to travel to the workplace, among other things. In summary, ML and DL were applied to identify biomarkers, vulnerable groups of patients, and forecasting the spread. It was reported that using ML saved a significant amount of investment as well as time to comprehend data that would otherwise have been unachievable within the existing time scale, and it is also predicted that ML might prevent new disease outbreaks.

9.4.7.2 Hyphenation of multiphysics models

Within the context of digital pharmaceutical development, elucidating the structure–process–properties relationship across the molecular level to nano-, meso-, micro-level hierarchy of pharmaceutical materials and formulated systems and underlying processes enables developing the desired functionality in crystals, particles and formulated products, thereby improving the process and product performance as well as the therapeutic outcome. The scientific principles and rational methods that enable us to predict *a priori* the performance of pharmaceutical materials, formulations and processes need to encompass wider time- and length-scales. To understand mechanistically the crucial physics and chemistry involved in a certain formulation and/or process, advanced simulation approaches such as MD simulation [187], computational fluid dynamics (CFD) [188], discrete element modelling (DEM) [189, 190], finite elemental method (FEM) [191], population balance model (PBM) [192], PBPK modelling [193, 194] either in isolation, or in combination [195]. Routine use of such elaborate and high-resolution models to address CMC cases is often hindered by the prohibitively computational expenses and lengthy run times. In this context, bridging such mechanistic modelling approaches with ML approaches can help unravelling various unanswered issues within pharmaceutical development. Some of the recently published exciting use cases are presented below.

One of the most successful approaches that helps in connecting the data from material properties (API and excipients) to formulation has been multiscale modelling. However, the authors have observed that multiscale modelers who create large datasets from a variety of sources and resolutions are frequently constrained in their capacity to integrate them successfully so as to derive a more logical design and development. Homogeneous mixing of solid particles is one of the most basic determinants for attaining content homogeneity as well as reproducible batch manufacturing processes such as drying, blending, and granulation. Mixing of solid particles is a critical yet least-understood technique. DEM is a first-principles modelling approach that provides a basic mechanistic knowledge of particle mixing, but is practically limited by availability of computational resources and power. ML embedded with multiscale modelling can be used to probe whether patterns or trends or correlations in data are causal, and similarly interrogate physics-based mechanistic models with uncertainty. Kumar *et al* [98] used an innovative approach integrating ML and time-series forecasting via auto regressive integrated moving average (ARIMA) models to simulate a complex pharmaceutical problem that involved developing an agitation protocol to ensure uniform solid mixing. Instead of simulating for the entire physical operation time, which is prohibitively large, the authors chose to simulate for one minute (65 simulations and typical timeframe were ~1 month) of operation using a high-fidelity modelling technique like DEM. The ARIMA model was then used to anticipate the mixing behavior and the point of homogeneity. The developed ML model shows good predictability and agreement between the ARIMA, and DEM predictions and the error between these models was

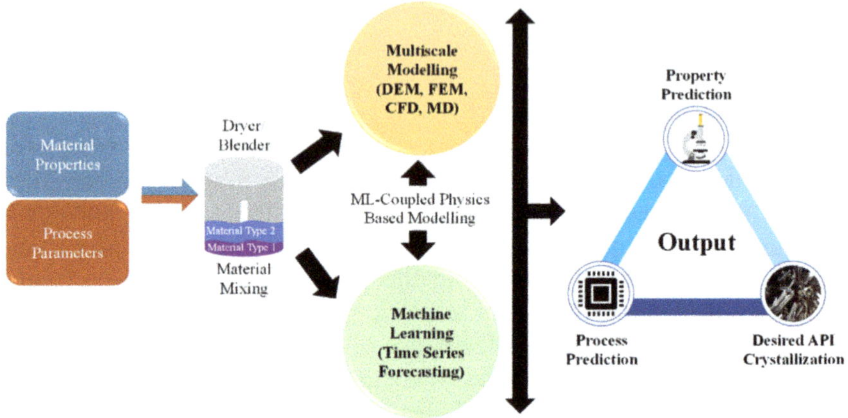

Figure 9.10. Integration of multiphysics models like DEM with ML (ARIMA) for the modelling of pharmaceutical dry powder mixing.

~2.5%, which is considered negligible. A snapshot of this paper is provided in figure 9.10. In summary, combining fundamental tools with revolutionary ML models reduces computational time while also providing promising insights and guiding the creation of a mechanistic framework that identifies key characteristics that most substantially affect the drying process.

It is anticipated that these models would have infinite possibilities from an industrial standpoint in terms of PAT, predictive control, automation, and so on. We anticipate that bridging first-principles simulations with ML models, as well as forecasting approaches such as ARIMA, will aid in overcoming lengthy computational constraints, and we hope that more researchers will be interested in this ingenious approach.

9.4.7.3 Hyphenation of physiological models with ML

ML has been exploited by a community of scholars to predict interactions and the miscibility of poorly soluble APIs in water-soluble polymers, both of which are considered paramount factors in pragmatic product development and formulation decisions. In one such study, Gao *et al* [196] integrated multidisciplinary computational tools (ML, solid-state simulation using molecular dynamics and bioavailability prediction using PBPK modelling). Around 674 dissolution curves were web-scraped from the 'Web of Science' database. Explanatory variables (like formulation composition, dissolution method parameters, *in vitro* release testing timepoints, and molecular descriptors) were 374 and one target variable (percent drug dissolved). Feature selection involves recursive feature elimination (RFE) method in order to prune the non-contribution explanatory variables. Two dissolution types involved target variables like 'spring and parachute' (11%) and 'maintain supersaturation' (89%). The class imbalance was addressed using random undersampling approach, and stratified sampling. All the datasets (674) were split into train–test at 80%:20% ratio. The target variable was considered both as qualitative (classification model) and as quantitative (regression model). To achieve high ML model generalizability, five-fold cross-validation was employed, along with several performance metrics for both classification-based and regression-based models. Once the historical data was extensively researched the next step involved application of molecular dynamics (solid-state property investigation) to extract the mechanism behind dissolution followed by application of PBPK models to predict bioperformance. The authors subsequently applied the established model to the poorly water-soluble drug Vemurafenib (VEM) and reported that the Vem-HPMCAS solid dispersion had a higher bioavailability and dissolving rate. While dealing with complex problems of pharmaceutical development, one needs to consider that having mechanistic understanding and data obtained from high fidelity models like that mentioned above would improve the predictive power of even simpler ML methods.

9.4.7.4 Transfer learning

Until now, the idea of memory, generalizability as well as the extrapolation of inferences learnt from training data are some of the missing components in traditional ML systems. Transfer learning has been demonstrated to be an effective approach for successfully bridging this gap as well as effectively dealing with small amounts of data [197]. Moreover, it is well-accepted that the properties of materials are interconnected, hence, this trait facilitates application of transfer learning [198]. Multiple disciplines have articulated ML-based transfer learning principles, although widespread adoption of this promising technology in pharmaceutical science (especially CMC-related) has yet to occur. Conversely, there have been a few publications that have embraced this essential transfer learning strategy. Yamada *et al* [199] developed a Python package termed XenonPy. MDL consists of pretrained models that were obtained by feeding structure-property relationships data of diverse materials onto neural networks and other supervised ML models. The authors further present successful applications in prediction of polymeric heat capacity, thermal conductivity of organic polymers, thermal conductivity of inorganic crystals as well as transferability across organic and inorganic materials. Grisoni *et al* [200] show the successful experimental application of deep ML to membranolytic anti-cancer peptides (ACPs). In the first step, the model was trained on 10 000 presumably α-helical cationic amphipathic peptides that represented amino acid sequences in one-letter code. In the second step, this model was then fine-tuned on only 26 known ACPs. This resulting model was then used to generate unique and novel amino acid sequences and it was shown that this method can successfully accelerate the search for peptides which are active against cancer cells. Similarly, Lee and Asahi [201] developed a transfer learning application employing crystal graph convolutional neural networks (TL-CGCNN) using 118 286 computed data samples from the Materials Project Database (MPD) to construct crystal graphs. The authors showed that a pretrained CGCNN could predict numerous output parameters on a smaller dataset with better prediction accuracy. DeepPharm (amalgamated transfer and multitask learning model) was recently proposed by [159]. A large collection of publicly available datasets consisting of 500 000 molecules with ~157 targets were employed to create the DeepPharm pre-training model. The pretrained model was then applied to datasets consisting of FDA approved drugs (~1104). Marginal improvement in accuracy over the classical ML approaches was demonstrated.

9.4.7.5 Generative models

Material characterization properties are often only tediously and expensively obtained. Material databases are hence incomplete, difficult to obtain and generally not widely shared or publicly accessible. Especially when combining results from the literature, comparability of values is not always given. Generative models aim to fill those gaps in the resulting datasets but anticipating missing values. These are successful in cases when the original, complete dataset is too small to apply transfer learning as NNs generally need more data. Hatakeyama-Sato and Oyaizu [202] describe a generative model for extrapolating prediction in material informatics. They demonstrate their proposed approach on a database covering 12 000 compounds and over 25 types of experimental properties. Since the original data sources for this database focused on different properties, there were many missing values. Richardson *et al* [203] introduced a flow-based model called Monte Carlo flow, which was used as imputer to estimate missing values. This method was also compared to established imputers such as generative adversarial network, autoencoders and variational autoencoders.

9.4.7.6 Sequential learning

Because of the time intensity and associated cost of experiments it is often not possible to explore an entire parameter space systematically. A choice of limited experiments must be made, often resulting in a design of experiment. When conducting material investigations aimed at generating a dataset for predictive modeling, not all experiments are equally supportive. Sequential learning (SL) provides a systematic approach to iteratively identify the most beneficial next step to reduce the number of essential experiments and hence speed up material discovery. Ling *et al* [204] present an algorithm (FUEL) which suggests the next candidate to test based on maximizing some selection function over the unmeasured candidates. Based on a random initial dataset, an RF model is trained paired with an uncertainty function leading to a next suggested experiment. In four test cases the performance of FUEL SL was compared to random guessing and Bayesian SL. In these test cases an optimal candidate for a maximal response function had to be found with as few experiments as possible. Rohr *et al* [205] compare SL methods for oxygen evolution reaction (OER) catalyst discovery in high-dimensional composition spaces, where they define discovery of a good catalyst to identification of a composition whose activity is in the top percentile of all compositions in the search space. Their results show that not all SL methods are equally suited for a given problem. This indicates that more research in this already very promising strategy for experimental will be beneficial.

9.5 Challenges and outlook

Even though the industry 4.0 revolution has resulted in improved performance and scientific breakthroughs in how we operate, the pharmaceutical industries' adoption of digitalization may pose a number of significant challenges that need to be addressed first with respect to regulatory agencies, academia, private and government sectors [204]. While ensuring the quality, safety, and efficacy of AI/ML as medical devices by regulatory agencies, barriers such as a quality management system, data exchange and privacy, standardization of data, lack of guidance, intellectual property challenges, risk-based systematic inspection etc are expected [206]. Other areas to be addressed such as monitoring real-world use, and exchange of information (benefit, risk, alert, recall) with key users such as clinicians and patients. The FDA has made significant progress in creating digital health regulations, with intentions to develop AI/ML-based SaMD and construct a total product life cycle (TPLC) regulatory framework that allows for research and development while ensuring product quality. Because AI/ML devices learn from real-world data, appropriate regulatory considerations are necessitated. FDA recently released a GMLP and plans to integrate with quality management systems.

Some of the building blocks of rational product design, included in the published case studies that we have cited above, comprise molecular dynamics, PBPK, DEM/CFD simulations, and other multiphysics modeling. Such high fidelity modeling and simulations often consume massive time and resources that when combined with AI/ML can be reduced dramatically. Thus the speed of model-based prediction can speed up so that entire digital pharmaceutical development becomes a reality. Moreover, there is an emerging stride of using advanced experimental methodologies such as synchrotron x-ray scattering, high speed and high-resolution imaging, and various forms of non-ambient experiments, wide diversity of advanced modular and continuous manufacturing including process analytics, QbD etc. These experiments will generate a massive data storm that is quite difficult to be analyzed in the traditional way, which has impeded their implementation in past. However, with the emergence of advanced data analytics (AI, ML, DL, computer vision) the application of such advanced methodologies is being realized in drug development settings. In parallel, quantum computing is in emergence and can benefit the massive computational requirements. The other unexplored areas in the traditional analytics phase are unstructured data which is an inevitable in the AI/ML/DL arena.

There is huge scope for capacity building in both private and government sector laboratories (like drugs and pharmaceuticals) in AI/ML testing. An accreditation system of such testing laboratories by independent authority should be put in place. On the other hand, allocating sufficient and appropriate resources to data science teams should be regarded as mandated, and establishing data science as a separate function can also be viewed as a viable investment. Biotech investors (like Xtalpi, Insitro, Tempus), pharma majors (like Abbvie, Johnson and Johnson, Pfizer, Boehringer-Ingelheim, AstraZeneca, Novartis, Sanofi, Roche, Bristol Myers Squibb, Merck and Co) invest abundantly in AI-based data-driven drug discovery. On the other hand, the FDA invested $83 million in digitalization to encourage scientific breakthroughs in genomics, blockchain, and real-time analytics concerning pharmaceutical, food safety and medical device programmes. However, this will be an acute challenge for developing, low- and middle-income countries or start-up pharmaceutical companies. Nevertheless, adoption of digitalization and the return on investment in such cutting-edge technologies are both rapid and favorable.

Briefly, the SWOT analysis (figure 9.11) of AI reveals its strengths in automation, pattern recognition, decision making, scalability, and personalization. However, challenges arise due to data dependency, lack of transparency, and limited contextual understanding. Opportunities lie in innovation, new applications, enhanced customer experience, research advancements, and cost reduction. Threats include ethical concerns, job displacement, and security risks. By leveraging strengths, addressing weaknesses, and capitalizing on opportunities, AI can revolutionize industries and improve society. It is crucial to navigate the challenges responsibly and strategically, ensuring ethical guidelines, investment in education, and prioritizing cybersecurity. Overall, AI's potential for positive impact remains promising.

9.6 Conclusion

ML and deep learning, when democratized, have undeniably modernized the potential to improve efficiency in the pharmaceutical product development process. This review serves as an update to the applications of ML in pharmaceutical development with the emphasis on six domains: (i) a brief introduction to statistics and ML, as well as the significance of combining statistics with ML; (ii) the first review to describe the integration of AI and ML for effective decision making in the context of CMC; (iii) our chapter highlights the value of ML in analytical development and stability prediction; (iv) similarly, as advocated by FDA on GMLP for software as medical devices, we are also providing a systematic framework and best practice in the essence of ML applications in pharmaceutical development; (v) we establishe the tone for the digitalization trend in pharmaceutical product design, development, and manufacturing. This is deemed critical because, in the near future, continuous manufacturing will indeed be required, with advanced data analytics involving AI/ML/DL playing a significant role; (iv) moreover, examples incorporating advanced principles linking multiscale modelling with ML to efficiently extract the physics behind pharmaceutical operations are presented.

In summary, we have highlighted several examples of how ML tools might be harnessed to address inherent challenges encountered during drug formulation development, and to aid in the development and characterization of both conventional and non-conventional drug formulations. In order to extend the application of ML in the pharmaceutical sciences in the future years, close multidisciplinary collaboration between industry, academia, AI and ML enthusiasts, and regulatory authorities will be essential. Similarly, combining digitalization with pharmaceutical development can help pharmaceutical scientists move away from trial-and-error based pharmaceutical product development, resulting in more accurate, quick, accessible, and cost-effective solutions. Importantly, the ML space allows for the

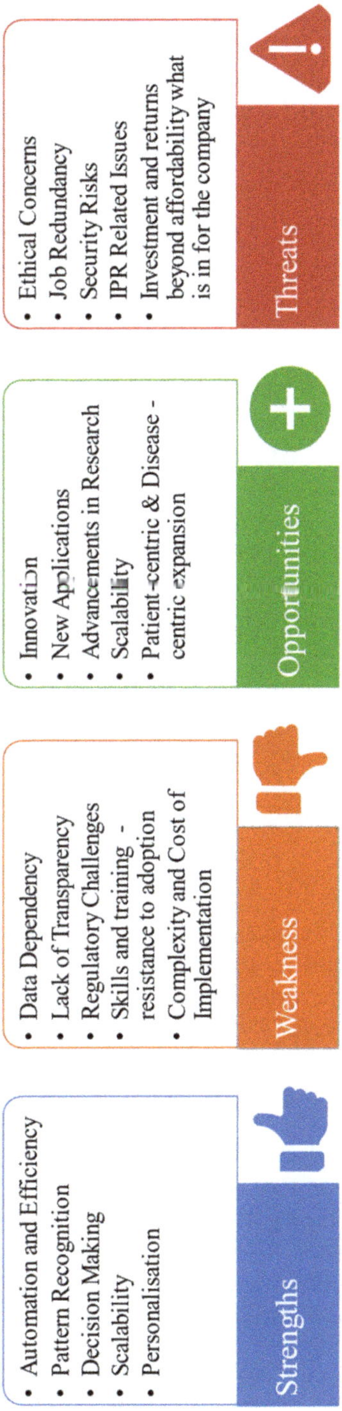

Figure 9.11. SWOT analysis of AI in pharmaceutical set-up.

development of novel materials, the discovery of advanced drug delivery systems, as well as the incorporation of new knowledge. According to the authors, the use of ML to harness the industry 4.0 revolution is uniquely positioned and ML application at various phases of pharmaceutical product development will increase the number of applications in the forthcoming years.

Author contributions

All authors have contributed equally. All authors have read and agreed to the published version of the manuscript.

Acknowledgments

PM acknowledges the Greatlakes Institute of Management Mr Raman (PGP-BABI), Ms Sneha Gorle (PGP-BABI/Accenture), Mr Shyam Muralidharan (PGP-AIML/Lead Consultant, Infosys, Chennai), Ms Shruti Karki (PGP-BABI), Mr Pratesh Kalyani (PGP-AIML), Mr Sampath (Ford Chennai), Mr Kamal (Hyundai, Chennai), Mr Ram (EY, Bangalore), Mr Nishant Bhaskar (PGP-AIML), Ms Savitha Puttaswamy (Sabre Technologies, Bangalore) who helped on structured learning of statistics, ML, deep learning; SS and PM acknowledge the Hack-Weekly group for AI/ML enthusiasts involving Mr Vetrivel, Mr Atif Hassan, Mr Sayantan Basu, Ms Ankita Chatterjee, Ms Manpreet Kaur, Ms Antaripa Saha, Mr Manish Sharma, Mr Ishan Dutta and; SS acknowledges images created using Canva.com.

Conflicts of interest

The authors declare no conflict of interest.

References

[1] Turing A M 1950 Computing machinery and intelligence *Parsing the Turing Test: Philosophical and Methodological Issues in the Quest for the Thinking Computer* ed R Epstein, G Roberts and G Beber (Dordrecht: Springer) pp 23–65

[2] Bourquin J, Schmidli H, van Hoogevest P and Leuenberger H 1998 Advantages of artificial neural networks (ANNs) as alternative modelling technique for data sets showing non-linear relationships using data from a galenical study on a solid dosage form *Eur. J. Pharm. Sci.* **7** 5–16

[3] Göller A H *et al* 2020 Bayer's in silico ADMET platform: a journey of ML over the past two decades *Drug Discov. Today* **25** 1702–9

[4] Wang W, Ye Z, Gao H and Ouyang D 2021 Computational pharmaceutics—A new paradigm of drug delivery *J. Control. Release* **338** 119–36

[5] Rowe R C and Roberts R J 1998 Artificial intelligence in pharmaceutical product formulation: neural computing and emerging technologies *Pharm. Sci. Technol. Today* **1** 200–5

[6] Plumb A P, Rowe R C, York P and Doherty C 2002 The effect of experimental design on the modeling of a tablet coating formulation using artificial neural networks *Eur. J. Pharm. Sci.* **16** 281–8

[7] Plumb A P, Rowe R C, York P and Brown M 2005 Optimisation of the predictive ability of artificial neural network (ANN) models: a comparison of three ANN programs and four classes of training algorithm *Eur. J. Pharm. Sci.* **25** 395–405

[8] Shao Q, Rowe R C and York P 2007 Investigation of an artificial intelligence technology—Model trees *Eur. J. Pharm. Sci.* **31** 137–44

[9] Aksu B, Paradkar A, de Matas M, Özer Ö, Güneri T and York P 2013 A quality by design approach using artificial intelligence techniques to control the critical quality attributes of ramipril tablets manufactured by wet granulation *Pharm. Dev. Technol.* **18** 236–45

[10] Bourquin J, Schmidli H, van Hoogevest P and Leuenberger H 1997 Application of artificial neural networks (ANN) in the development of solid dosage forms *Pharm. Dev. Technol.* **2** 111–21

[11] Bourquin J, Schmidli H, van Hoogevest P and Leuenberger H 1998 Pitfalls of artificial neural networks (ANN) modelling technique for data sets containing outlier measurements using a study on mixture properties of a direct compressed dosage form *Eur. J. Pharm. Sci.* **7** 17–28

[12] Bourquin J, Schmidli H, van Hoogevest P and Leuenberger H 1998 Comparison of artificial neural networks (ANN) with classical modelling techniques using different experimental designs and data from a galenical study on a solid dosage form *Eur. J. Pharm. Sci.* **6** 287–300

[13] Takahara J, Takayama K and Nagai T 1997 Multi-objective simultaneous optimization technique based on an artificial neural network in sustained release formulations *J. Control. Release* **49** 11–20

[14] Takayama K, Fujikawa M and Nagai T 1999 Artificial neural network as a novel method to optimize pharmaceutical formulations *Pharm. Res.* **16** 1–6

[15] Kesavan J G and Peck G E 1996 Pharmaceutical granulation and tablet formulation using neural networks *Pharm. Dev. Technol.* **1** 391–404

[16] Agatonovic-Kustrin S, Zecevic M, Zivanovic L J and Tucker I G 1998 Application of artificial neural networks in HPLC method development *J. Pharm. Biomed. Anal.* **17** 69–76

[17] Agatonovic-Kustrin S, Zecevic M, Zivanovic L and Tucker I G 1998 Application of neural networks for response surface modeling in HPLC optimization *Anal. Chim. Acta* **364** 265–73

[18] Agatonovic-Kustrin S, Wu V, Rades T, Saville D and Tucker I G 1999 Powder diffractometric assay of two polymorphic forms of ranitidine hydrochloride *Int. J. Pharm.* **184** 107–14

[19] Agatonovic-Kustrin S, Tucker I G and Schmierer D 1999 Solid state assay of ranitidine HCl as a bulk drug and as active ingredient in tablets using DRIFT spectroscopy with artificial neural networks *Pharm. Res.* **16** 1477–82

[20] Agatonovic-Kustrin S, Zecevic M and Zivanovic L 1999 Use of ANN modelling in structure–retention relationships of diuretics in RP-HPLC *J. Pharm. Biomed. Anal.* **21** 95–103

[21] Alany R G, Agatonovic-Kustrin S, Rades T and Tucker I G 1999 Use of artificial neural networks to predict quaternery phase systems from limited experimental data *J. Pharm. Biomed. Anal.* **19** 443–52

[22] Agatonovic-Kustrin S, Wu V, Rades T, Saville D and Tucker I G 2000 Ranitidine hydrochloride x-ray assay using a neural network *J. Pharm. Biomed. Anal.* **22** 985–92

[23] Agatonovic-Kustrin S, Tucker I G, Zecevic M and Zivanovic L J 2000 Prediction of drug transfer into human milk from theoretically derived descriptors *Anal. Chim. Acta* **418** 181–95

[24] Agatonovic-Kustrin S, Beresford R and Razzak M 2000 Determination of enantiomeric composition of ibuprofen in solid state mixtures of the two by DRIFT spectroscopy *Anal. Chim. Acta* **417** 31–9

[25] Zupančič Bozič D, Vrečer F and Kozjek F 1997 Optimization of diclofenac sodium dissolution from sustained release formulations using an artificial neural network *Eur. J. Pharm. Sci.* **5** 163–9

[26] Murtoniemi E, Merkku P, Kinnunen P, Leiviskä K and Yliruusi J 1994 Effect of neural network topology and training end point in modelling the fluidized bed granulation process *Int. J. Pharm.* **110** 101–8

[27] Murtoniemi E, Yliruusi J, Kinnunen P, Merkku P and Leiviskä K 1994 The advantages by the use of neural networks in modelling the fluidized bed granulation process *Int. J. Pharm.* **108** 155–64

[28] Taskinen J and Yliruusi J 2003 Prediction of physicochemical properties based on neural network modelling *Adv. Drug Deliv. Rev.* **55** 1163–83

[29] Rantanen J T, Laine S J, Antikainen O K, Mannermaa J-P, Simula O E and Yliruusi J K 2001 Visualization of fluid-bed granulation with self-organizing maps *J. Pharm. Biomed. Anal.* **24** 343–52

[30] Lavecchia A 2015 Machine-learning approaches in drug discovery: methods and applications *Drug Discov. Today* **20** 318–31

[31] McComb M and Ramanathan M 2020 Generalized pharmacometric modeling, a novel paradigm for integrating ML algorithms: a case study of metabolomic biomarkers *Clin. Pharmacol. Ther.* **107** 1343–51

[32] Bannigan P, Aldeghi M, Bao Z, Häse F, Aspuru-Guzik A and Allen C 2021 ML directed drug formulation development *Adv. Drug Deliv. Rev.* **175** 113806

[33] Damiati S A 2020 Digital pharmaceutical sciences *AAPS PharmSciTech.* **21** 206

[34] Sutariya V, Groshev A, Sadana P, Bhatia D and Pathak Y 2013 Artificial neural network in drug delivery and pharmaceutical research *Open Bioinforma.* J **7** 49–62

[35] Réda C, Kaufmann E and Delahaye-Duriez A 2020 ML applications in drug development *Comput. Struct. Biotechnol.* J **18** 241–52

[36] Kapoor Y *et al* 2021 Flexibility in drug product development: a perspective *Mol. Pharm.* **18** 2455–69

[37] Talevi A *et al* 2020 ML in drug discovery and development Part 1: a primer *CPT Pharmacometr. Syst. Pharmacol* **9** 129–42

[38] Klemenčič J and Mihelič J 2019 Application of algorithms and ML methods in pharmaceutical manufacture http://ipsitransactions.org/journals/papers/tir/2019jan/p4.pdf

[39] USFDA 2021 Good machine learning practice for medical device development: guiding principles https://fda.gov/media/153486/download

[40] USFDA 2021 Proposed regulatory framework for modifications to artificial intelligence/ML (AI/ML)-based software as a medical device (SaMD)-discussion paper and request for feedback https://fda.gov/media/145022/download

[41] USFDA 2021 Artificial intelligence/ML (AI/ML)-based software as a medical device (SaMD) action plan *USFDA* 4023–4 https://www.fda.gov/medical-devices/software-medical-device-samd/artificial-intelligence-and-machine-learning-software-medical-device

[42] Karniadakis G E, Kevrekidis I G, Lu L, Perdikaris P, Wang S and Yang L 2021 Physics-informed ML *Nat. Rev. Phys.* **3** 422–40
[43] de Hond A A H *et al* 2022 Guidelines and quality criteria for artificial intelligence-based prediction models in healthcare: a scoping review *npj Digit. Med.* **5**
[44] USFDA 2021 Good ML practice for medical device development: guiding principles
[45] Stevens S S 1946 On the theory of scales of measurement *Science* **103** 677–80
[46] Saravanan D, Muthudoss P, Khullar P and Rose Venis A 2021 Quantitative microscopy: particle size/shape characterization, addressing common errors using 'analytics continuum' approach *J. Pharm. Sci.* **110** 833–49
[47] Cleophas T J and Zwinderman A H 2011 *Statistical Analysis of Clinical Data on a Pocket Calculator* (Dordrecht: Springer) 1st edn
[48] Jifa G and Lingling Z 2014 Data, DIKW, big data and data science *Procedia Comput. Sci.* **31** 814–21
[49] Özköse H, Arı E S and Gencer C 2015 Yesterday, today and tomorrow of big data *Procedia —Soc. Behav. Sci.* **195** 1042–50
[50] Baldassarre M 2016 Think big: learning contexts, algorithms and data science *Res. Educ. Media* **8** 69–83
[51] Sutanapong C and Louangrath P I 2015 Descriptive and inferential statistics *Int. J. Res. Methodol. Soc. Sci.* **1** 22–35
[52] Saravanan D, Muthudoss P, Khullar P and Rose Venis A 2021 quantitative microscopy: particle size/shape characterization, addressing common errors using 'analytics continuum' approach *J. Pharm. Sci.* **110** 833–49
[53] Muthudoss P *et al* 2022 Topologically directed confocal Raman imaging (TD-CRI): advanced Raman imaging towards compositional and micromeritic profiling of a commercial tablet components *J. Pharm. Biomed. Anal.* **210** 114581
[54] Vickers A J 2005 Parametric versus non-parametric statistics in the analysis of randomized trials with non-normally distributed data *BMC Med. Res. Methodol.* **5** 35
[55] Halsey L G 2019 The reign of the p-value is over: what alternative analyses could we employ to fill the power vacuum? *Biol. Lett.* **15** 20190174
[56] Kim J and Bang H 2016 Three common misuses of P values *Dent. Hypotheses* **7** 73
[57] Marshall G and Jonker L 2011 An introduction to inferential statistics: a review and practical guide *Radiography* **17** e1–6
[58] Allua S and Thompson C B 2009 Inferential statistics *Air Med. J.* **28** 168–71
[59] Ragni M, Kola I and Johnson-Laird P N 2018 On selecting evidence to test hypotheses: a theory of selection tasks *Psychol. Bull.* **144** 779
[60] Byrne G 2007 A statistical primer: understanding descriptive and inferential statistics *Evid. Based Libr. Inf. Pract.* **2** 32–47
[61] Trafimow D and MacDonald J A 2017 Performing inferential statistics prior to data collection *Educ. Psychol. Meas.* **77** 204–19
[62] Ghasemi A and Zahediasl S 2012 Normality tests for statistical analysis: a guide for non-statisticians *Int. J. Endocrinol. Metab.* **10** 2
[63] Shapiro S S, Wilk M B and Chen H J 1968 A comparative study of various tests for normality *J. Am. Stat. Assoc.* **63** 1343–72
[64] Mohd N and Bee Y 2011 Power comparisons of Shapiro-Wilk, Kolmogorov-Smirnov, Lilliefors and Anderson-Darling tests *J. Stat. Model. Anal.* **2** 13–4

[65] Mukaka M M 2012 Statistics corner: a guide to appropriate use of correlation coefficient in medical research *Malawi Med. J.* **24** 69–71
[66] Onwuegbuzie A J and Daniel L G 1999 Uses and misuses of the correlation coefficient https://eric.ed.gov/?id=ED437399%0Ahttp://eric.ed.gov/?id=ED437399
[67] Conover W J, Guerrero-Serrano A J and Tercero-Gómez V G 2018 An update on 'a comparative study of tests for homogeneity of variance' *J. Stat. Comput. Simul.* **88** 1454–69
[68] Aggarwal C C 2017 An introduction to outlier analysis *Outlier Analysis* (Berlin: Springer) pp 1–34
[69] Filzmoser P and Gregorich M 2020 Multivariate outlier detection in applied data analysis: global, local, compositional and cellwise outliers *Math. Geosci.* **52** 1049–66
[70] Walfish S 2007 A review of statistical outlier methods *Pharm. Technol.* 1–5 http://statisticaloutsourcingservices.com/Outlier2.pdf
[71] Chromiński K and Tkacz M 2010 Comparison of outlier detection methods in biomedical data *J. Med. Informatics Technol.* **16** 89–94
[72] Leys C, Klein O, Dominicy Y and Ley C 2018 Detecting multivariate outliers: use a robust variant of the Mahalanobis distance *J. Exp. Soc. Psychol.* **74** 150–6
[73] Zimek A and Filzmoser P 2018 There and back again: outlier detection between statistical reasoning and data mining algorithms *WIREs Data Min. Knowl. Discov.* **8** 6
[74] Goldstein M and Uchida S 2016 A Comparative evaluation of unsupervised anomaly detection algorithms for multivariate data *PLoS One* **11** p e0152173
[75] Domingues R, Filippone M, Michiardi P and Zouaoui J 2018 A comparative evaluation of outlier detection algorithms: experiments and analyses *Pattern Recognit.* **74** 406–21
[76] Ilango V, Subramanian R and Vasudevan V 2012 A five step procedure for outlier analysis in data mining *Eur. J. Sci. Res.* **75** 327–39
[77] GitHub—8080labs/ppscore: Predictive Power Score (PPS) in Python *Bamboolib—a GUI for Pandas DataFrames* 2021 (https://github.com/8080labs/ppscore) (accessed 19 November 2021)
[78] Cross G R and Jain A K 1982 Measurement of clustering tendency *Theory Appl. Digit. Control* (Amsterdam: Elsevier) pp 315–20
[79] Banerjee A and Dave R N 2004 Validating clusters using the Hopkins statistic *2004 IEEE Int. Conf. Fuzzy Syst. (IEEE Cat. No.04CH37542)* Vol 1 pp 149–53
[80] Figueroa R L, Zeng-Treitler Q, Kandula S and Ngo L H 2012 Predicting sample size required for classification performance *BMC Med. Inform. Decis. Mak.* **12** p 8
[81] Balki I *et al* 2019 Sample-Size determination methodologies for ML in medical imaging research: a systematic review *Can. Assoc. Radiol. J.* **70** 344–53
[82] Mpoudeu M and Clarke B 2019 Model selection via the VC dimension *J. Mach. Learn. Res.* **20** 1–26
[83] Li Y and Chao X 2021 Toward sustainability: trade-off between data quality and quantity in crop pest recognition *Front. Plant Sci.* **12** 811241
[84] Allison D B, Brown A W, George B J and Kaiser K A 2016 Reproducibility: a tragedy of errors *Nature* **530** 27–9
[85] SAS Institute Inc. 2020 *ML with SAS Viya* (SAS Institute)
[86] Gupta S, Mateu J, Degbelo A and Pebesma E 2018 Quality of life, big data and the power of statistics *Stat. Probab. Lett.* **136** 101–4
[87] van der Aalst W 2016 Data science in action *Process Min* (Berlin, Heidelberg: Springer) pp 3–23

[88] Harpaz R, DuMouchel W, Shah N H, Madigan D, Ryan P and Friedman C 2012 Novel data-mining methodologies for adverse drug event discovery and analysis *Clin. Pharmacol. Ther.* **91** 1010–21

[89] Sivarajah U, Kamal M M, Irani Z and Weerakkody V 2017 Critical analysis of big data challenges and analytical methods *J. Bus. Res.* **70** 263–86

[90] Ray S 2019 A quick review of ML algorithms *2019 Int. Conf. Mach. Learn. Big Data, Cloud Parallel Comput* 35–9

[91] Greener J G, Kandathil S M, Moffat L and Jones D T 2021 A guide to ML for biologists *Nat. Rev. Mol. Cell Biol.* **23** 40–55

[92] Willard J, Jia X, Xu S, Steinbach M and Kumar V 2020 Integrating scientific knowledge with ML for engineering and environmental systems *arXiv* **1** 1–35 2003.04919

[93] Kaiser E *et al* 2014 Cluster-based reduced-order modelling of a mixing layer *J. Fluid Mech.* **754** 365–414

[94] Champion K, Lusch B, Kutz J N and Brunton S L 2019 Data-driven discovery of coordinates and governing equations *Proc. Natl Acad. Sci.* **116** 22445–51

[95] Hong R S *et al* 2021 Novel physics-based ensemble modeling approach that utilizes 3D molecular conformation and packing to access aqueous thermodynamic solubility: a case study of orally available bromodomain and extraterminal domain inhibitor lead optimization series *J. Chem. Inf. Model.* **61** 1412–26

[96] Liao Z *et al* 2021 Image-based prediction of granular flow behaviors in a wedge-shaped hopper by combing DEM and deep learning methods *Powder Technol.* **383** 159–66

[97] Rangarajan S 2022 Towards a chemistry-informed paradigm for designing molecules *Curr. Opin. Chem. Eng.* **35** 100717

[98] Kumar P *et al* 2020 A ML framework for computationally expensive transient models *Sci. Rep.* **10** 11492

[99] Chua I S *et al* 2021 Artificial intelligence in oncology: path to implementation *Cancer Med.* **10** 4138–49

[100] Barragán-Montero A M *et al* 2021 Deep learning dose prediction for IMRT of esophageal cancer: the effect of data quality and quantity on model performance *Phys. Medica* **83** 52–63

[101] Liu J, Li J, Li W and Wu J 2016 Rethinking big data: a review on the data quality and usage issues *ISPRS J. Photogramm. Remote Sens.* **115** 134–42

[102] Sadiq S and Indulska M 2017 Open data: quality over quantity *Int. J. Inf. Manage.* **37** 150–4

[103] Cai L and Zhu Y 2015 The challenges of data quality and data quality assessment in the big data era *Data Sci. J.* **14** 2

[104] Tavazza F, DeCost B and Choudhary K 2021 Uncertainty prediction for ML models of material properties *ACS Omega* **6** 32431–40

[105] Abdar M *et al* 2021 A review of uncertainty quantification in deep learning: techniques, applications and challenges *Inf. Fusion* **76** 243–97

[106] Cai C, Poor H V and Chen Y 2020 Uncertainty quantification for nonconvex tensor completion: confidence intervals, heteroscedasticity and optimality *IEEE Trans. Inform. Theory* **69** 407–52

[107] Rodriguez J D, Perez A and Lozano J A 2010 Sensitivity analysis of k-fold cross validation in prediction error estimation *IEEE Trans. Pattern Anal. Mach. Intell.* **32** 569–75

[108] Mehta P *et al* 2019 A high-bias, low-variance introduction to ML for physicists *Phys. Rep.* **810** 1–124

[109] Chen J M, Zovko M, Šimurina N and Zovko V 2021 Fear in a handful of dust: the epidemiological, environmental and economic drivers of death by PM2. 5 pollution *Int. J. Environ. Res. Public Health* **18** 8688
[110] Beleites C, Neugebauer U, Bocklitz T, Krafft C and Popp J 2013 Sample size planning for classification models *Anal. Chim. Acta* **760** 25–33
[111] Dietterich T G 1998 Approximate statistical tests for comparing supervised classification learning algorithms *Neural Comput.* **10** 1895–923
[112] Hastie T, Tibshirani R, Friedman J H and Friedman J H 2009 *The Elements of Statistical Learning: Data Mining, Inference, and Prediction* **2** (Berlin: Springer)
[113] James G M 2003 Variance and bias for general loss functions *Mach. Learn.* **51** 115–35
[114] Room C 2020 Bias-variance trade-off *Statistics (Ber)* **8** 1
[115] Gudivada V, Apon A and Ding J 2017 Data quality considerations for big data and machine learning: going beyond data cleaning and transformations *Int. J. Adv. Softw.* **10** 1–20
[116] Picek S, Heuser A, Jovic A, Bhasin S and Regazzoni F 2019 The curse of class imbalance and conflicting metrics with ML for side-channel evaluations *IACR Trans. Cryptogr. Hardw. Embed. Syst.* **2019** 1–29
[117] Kaufman S, Rosset S, Perlich C and Stitelman O 2012 Leakage in data mining: formulation, detection, and avoidance *ACM Trans. Knowl. Discov. from Data* **6** pp 1–21
[118] Nayak S K and Ojha A C 2020 Data leakage detection and prevention: review and research directions *Machine Learning and Information Processing* ed D Swain, P Pattnaik and P Gupta (Singapore: Springer) Advances in Intelligent Systems and Computing vol 1101
[119] Alneyadi S, Sithirasenan E and Muthukkumarasamy V 2016 A survey on data leakage prevention systems *J. Netw. Comput. Appl.* **62** 137–52
[120] Greenland S, Schlesselman J J and Criqui M H 1986 The fallacy of employing standardized regression coefficients and correlations as measures of effect *Am. J. Epidemiol.* **123** 203–8
[121] Silva A J, Cortez P and Pilastri A 2020 Chemical laboratories 4.0: a two-stage ML system for predicting the arrival of samples *IFIP Int. Conf. on Artificial Intelligence Applications and Innovations* pp 232–43
[122] Wirth R and Hipp J 2000 CRISP-DM: towards a standard process model for data mining *Proc. of the 4th Int. Conf. on the Practical Applications of Knowledge Discovery and Data Mining* Vol 1 pp 29–40
[123] Martínez-Plumed F P, Contreras-Ochando F, Ferri L, Orallo C, Kull C, Lachiche M and Quintana M J 2019 CRISP-DM twenty years later: from data mining processes to data science trajectories *IEEE Trans. Knowl. Data Eng.* **33** 3048–61
[124] Nguyen G *et al* 2019 ML and deep learning frameworks and libraries for large-scale data mining: a survey *Artif. Intell. Rev.* **52** 77–124
[125] Lobell M *et al* 2006 In silico ADMET traffic lights as a tool for the prioritization of HTS hits *ChemMedChem.* **1** 1229–36
[126] Fraczkiewicz R *et al* 2015 Best of both worlds: combining pharma data and state of the art modeling technology to improve in silico pKa prediction *J. Chem. Inf. Model.* **55** 389–97
[127] Hillisch A, Heinrich N and Wild H 2015 Computational chemistry in the pharmaceutical industry: from childhood to adolescence *Chem. Med. Chem.* **10** 12
[128] Schuffenhauer A *et al* 2020 'Evolution of novartis' small molecule screening deck design *J. Med. Chem.* **63**

[129] Fogg M J *et al* 2006 Application of the use of high-throughput technologies to the determination of protein structures of bacterial and viral pathogens *Acta Crystallogr., Sect. D: Biol. Crystallogr.* **62** 1196–207

[130] DiFeo T J 2003 Drug product development: a technical review of chemistry, manufacturing, and controls information for the support of pharmaceutical compound licensing activities *Drug Dev. Ind. Pharm.* **29** 939–58

[131] Wahid R, Holt R, Hjorth R and Berlanda Scorza F 2016 Chemistry, manufacturing and control (CMC) and clinical trial technical support for influenza vaccine manufacturers *Vaccine* **34** 5430–5

[132] Cauchon N S, Oghamian S, Hassanpour S and Abernathy M 2019 Innovation in chemistry, manufacturing, and controls—a regulatory perspective from industry *J. Pharm. Sci.* **108** 2207–37

[133] Ghosh A *et al* 2019 Assessment of ML approaches for predicting the crystallization propensity of active pharmaceutical ingredients *Cryst. Eng. Comm.* **21** 1215–23

[134] He Y *et al* 2020 Can ML predict drug nanocrystals *J. Control. Release* **322** 274–85

[135] Pereira F 2020 ML methods to predict the crystallization propensity of small organic molecules *Cryst. Eng. Comm.* **22** 2817–26

[136] Lovrić M *et al* 2021 ML in prediction of intrinsic aqueous solubility of drug-like compounds: generalization, complexity, or predictive ability *J. Chemom.* **35** 7–8

[137] Francoeur P G and Koes D R 2021 SolTranNet–a ML tool for fast aqueous solubility prediction *J. Chem. Inf. Model.* **61** 2530–6

[138] Gao H *et al* 2020 Predicting drug/phospholipid complexation by the lightGBM method *Chem. Phys. Lett.* **747** 137354

[139] Boyd B J *et al* 2019 Successful oral delivery of poorly water-soluble drugs both depends on the intraluminal behavior of drugs and of appropriate advanced drug delivery systems *Eur. J. Pharm. Sci.* **137** 104967

[140] Zhao Q, Ye Z, Su Y and Ouyang D 2019 Predicting complexation performance between cyclodextrins and guest molecules by integrated ML and molecular modeling techniques *Acta Pharm. Sin.* B **9** 1241–52

[141] Thomas S, Palahnuk H, Amini H and Akseli I 2021 Data-smart ML methods for predicting composition-dependent Young's modulus of pharmaceutical compacts *Int. J. Pharm.* **592** 120049

[142] Gao H, Jia H, Dong J, Yang X, Li H and Ouyang D 2021 Integrated in silico formulation design of self-emulsifying drug delivery systems *Acta Pharm. Sin.* B **11** 3585–94

[143] Dong J, Gao H and Ouyang D 2021 PharmSD: a novel AI-based computational platform for solid dispersion formulation design *Int. J. Pharm.* **604** 120705

[144] Hayashi Y *et al* 2018 Modeling of quantitative relationships between physicochemical properties of active pharmaceutical ingredients and tensile strength of tablets using a boosted tree *Drug Dev. Ind. Pharm.* **44** 1090–8

[145] Millen N, Kovačević A, Djuriš J and Ibrić S 2020 ML modeling of wet granulation scale-up using particle size distribution characterization parameters *J. Pharm. Innov.* **15** 535–46

[146] Severson K, VanAntwerp J G, Natarajan V, Antoniou C, Thömmes J and Braatz R D 2015 Elastic net with Monte Carlo sampling for data-based modeling in biopharmaceutical manufacturing facilities *Comput. Chem. Eng.* **80** 30–6

[147] Severson K A, VanAntwerp J G, Natarajan V, Antoniou C, Thömmes J and Braatz R D 2018 A systematic approach to process data analytics in pharmaceutical manufacturing *Multivariate Analysis in the Pharmaceutical Industry* (Amsterdam: Elsevier) pp 295–312

[148] Hong M S, Sun W, Lu A E and Braatz R D 2020 Process analytical technology and digital biomanufacturing of monoclonal antibodies *Am. Pharm. Rev.* https://americanpharmaceuticalreview.com/Featured-Articles/569427-Process-Analytical-Technology-and-Digital-Biomanufacturing-of-Monoclonal-Antibodies/
[149] Gams M, Horvat M, Ožek M, Luštrek M and Gradišek A 2014 Integrating artificial and human intelligence into tablet production process *AAPS Pharm. Sci. Tech.* **15** 6
[150] Lemkus T, Ramsey P, Gotwalt C and Weese M 2021 Self-validated ensemble models for design of experiments *Chemom. Intell. Lab. Syst.* **219** 104439
[151] Allen L V 1998 The art, science, and technology of pharmaceutical compounding *Washington, USA Am. Pharm. Assoc.* **2** https://ebusiness.pharmacist.com/PRODUCTFILES/84999507/Sample
[152] Koch W F, Hauck W W, de Mars S S and Williams R L 2010 Measurement science for food and drug monographs: toward a global system *Pharm. Res.* **27** 1203–7
[153] Sivaraman A and Banga A 2015 Quality by design approaches for topical dermatological dosage forms *Res. Rep. Transdermal Drug Deliv.* **4** 9–21
[154] Shabir G A 2004 A practical approach to validation of HPLC methods under current good manufacturing practices *J. Valid. Technol.* **0** 210–8
[155] Andreas C J *et al* 2018 Introduction to the OrBiTo decision tree to select the most appropriate *in vitro* methodology for release testing of solid oral dosage forms during development *Eur. J. Pharm. Biopharm.* **130** 207–13
[156] Yuwono M and Indrayanto G 2005 Validation of chromatographic methods of analysis *Profiles of Drug Substances, Excipients and Related Methodology* (Elsevier) pp 243–59
[157] Hubert C, Lebrun P, Houari S, Ziemons E, Rozet E and Hubert P 2014 Improvement of a stability-indicating method by quality-by-design versus quality-by-testing: a case of a learning process *J. Pharm. Biomed. Anal.* **88** 401–9
[158] Woodcock J 2004 The concept of pharmaceutical quality *Am. Pharm. Rev.* **7** 10–5
[159] Han R *et al* 2019 Predicting physical stability of solid dispersions by ML techniques *J. Control. Release* **311–312** 16–25
[160] Mendyk A *et al* 2020 Data-driven modeling of the bicalutamide dissolution from powder systems *AAPS Pharm. Sci. Tech.* **21** 111
[161] King A C, Woods M, Liu W, Lu Z, Gill D and Krebs M R H 2011 High-throughput measurement, correlation analysis, and machine-learning predictions for pH and thermal stabilities of Pfizer-generated antibodies *Protein Sci.* **20** 1546–57
[162] European Medicines Agency 2012 Guideline on real time release testing (formerly guideline on parametric release) *EMA/CHMP/QWP/811210/2009-Rev1* p 10 https://ema.europa.eu/en/documents/scientific-guideline/guideline-real-time-release-testing-formerly-guideline-parametric-release-revision-1%7B%5C_%7Den.pdf
[163] Pawar P, Wang Y, Keyvan G, Callegari G, Cuitino A and Muzzio F 2016 Enabling real time release testing by NIR prediction of dissolution of tablets made by continuous direct compression (CDC) *Int. J. Pharm.* **512** 96–107
[164] Costa P and Lobo J M S 2001 Modeling and comparison of dissolution profiles *Eur. J. Pharm. Sci.* **13** 123–33
[165] Galata D L *et al* 2021 Real-time release testing of dissolution based on surrogate models developed by ML algorithms using NIR spectra, compression force and particle size distribution as input data *Int. J. Pharm.* **597** 120338
[166] Nagy B *et al* 2019 Application of artificial neural networks for process analytical technology-based dissolution testing *Int. J. Pharm.* **567** p 118464

[167] Susto G A and McLoone S 2015 Slow release drug dissolution profile prediction in pharmaceutical manufacturing: a multivariate and ML approach *2015 IEEE Int. Conf. Autom. Sci. Eng* 1218–23

[168] Akseli I *et al* 2017 A practical framework toward prediction of breaking force and disintegration of tablet formulations using ML tools *J. Pharm. Sci.* **106** 234–47

[169] Abdelhafid B *et al* 2020 Hierarchical Bayesian approach applied to the formulation of sustained-release suppositories and dissolution profile modeling *J. Appl. Pharm. Sci.* **11** 55–62

[170] Mendyk A *et al* 2015 From heuristic to mathematical modeling of drugs dissolution profiles: application of artificial neural networks and genetic programming *Comput. Math. Methods Med.* **2015** 863874

[171] Salazar-Jiménez J E, Sánchez-Carvajal J D, Quiros-Gómez B and Arias-Londoño J D 2017 Automatic feature selection in the SOPFs dissolution profiles prediction problem *Bioinforma. 2017—8th Int. Conf. Bioinforma. Model. Methods Algorithms, Proceedings; Part 10th Int. Jt. Conf. Biomed. Eng. Syst. Technol. BIOSTEC 2017* **3** 52–8

[172] Yamashita F, Fujita A, Zhang X, Sasa Y, Mihara K and Hashida M 2012 Computer-based evolutionary search for a nonlinear conversion function for establishing *in vitro–in vivo* correlation (IVIVC) of oral drug formulations *Drug Metab. Pharmacokinet.* **27** 280–5

[173] Yamashita F, Fujita A, Sasa Y, Higuchi Y, Tsuda M and Hashida M 2017 An evolutionary search algorithm for covariate models in population pharmacokinetic analysis *J. Pharm. Sci.* **106** 2407–11

[174] Ogami C *et al* 2021 An artificial neural network−pharmacokinetic model and its interpretation using Shapley additive explanations *CPT Pharmacometr. Syst. Pharmacol* **10** 760–8

[175] McComb M, Bies R and Ramanathan M 2021 ML in pharmacometrics: opportunities and challenges *Br. J. Clin. Pharmacol.* **88** 1482–99

[176] Luzi D and Pecoraro F 2012 Medical device software: a new challenge *Stud. Health Technol. Inform.* **180** 885–90

[177] McCarthy A D and Lawford P V 2015 Standalone medical device software: the evolving regulatory framework *J. Med. Eng. Technol.* **39** 7

[178] Razavi S *et al* 2021 The future of sensitivity analysis: an essential discipline for systems modeling and policy support *Environ. Model. Softw* **137** 104954

[179] Zhang P 2019 A novel feature selection method based on global sensitivity analysis with application in ML-based prediction model *Appl. Soft Comput.* J **85** 105859

[180] Martelli N *et al* 2019 New European regulation for medical devices: what is changing? *Cardiovasc. Interv. Radiol* **42** 1272–8

[181] Angehrn Z *et al* 2020 Artificial intelligence and ML applied at the point of care *Front. Pharmacol* **11** 759

[182] Muehlematter U J, Daniore P and Vokinger K N 2021 Approval of artificial intelligence and ML-based medical devices in the USA and Europe (2015–20): a comparative analysis *Lancet Digital Health* (Elsevier Ltd) Vol 3 pp e195–203

[183] Lou H, Chung J I, Kiang Y H, Xiao L Y and Hageman M J 2019 The application of ML algorithms in understanding the effect of core/shell technique on improving powder compactability *Int. J. Pharm.* **555** 368–79

[184] Ong E, Wong M U, Huffman A and He Y 2020 COVID-19 coronavirus vaccine design using reverse vaccinology and ML *Front. Immunol* **11** 1581

[185] Tomic A, Tomic I, Rosenberg-Hasson Y, Dekker C L, Maecker H T and Davis M M 2019 SIMON, an automated ML system, reveals immune signatures of influenza vaccine responses *J. Immunol.* **203** 749–59

[186] Estiri H, Strasser Z H, Klann J G, Naseri P, Wagholikar K B and Murphy S N 2021 Predicting COVID-19 mortality with electronic medical records *npj Digit. Med.* **4** 15

[187] Müller P, Bonthuis D J, Miller R and Schneck E 2021 Ionic surfactants at air/water and oil/water interfaces: a comparison based on molecular dynamics simulations *J. Phys. Chem.* B **125** 406–15

[188] Boehling P *et al* 2021 Validating a numerical simulation of the consigma(R) coater *AAPS PharmSciTech.* **22** 10

[189] Lin Q, Cao P, Meng J, Cao R and Zhao Z 2020 Strength and failure characteristics of jointed rock mass with double circular holes under uniaxial compression: insights from discrete element method modelling *Theor. Appl. Fract. Mech.* **109** 102692

[190] Kumar A, Radl S, Gernaey K V, De Beer T and Nopens I 2021 Particle-scale modeling to understand liquid distribution in twin-screw wet granulation *Pharmaceutics* **13** 928

[191] Meynard J, Amado-Becker F, Tchoreloff P and Mazel V 2021 Use of impulse excitation technique for the characterization of the elastic anisotropy of pharmaceutical tablets *Int. J. Pharm.* **605** 120797

[192] Muthancheri I, Chaturbedi A, Bétard A and Ramachandran R 2021 A compartment based population balance model for the prediction of steady and induction granule growth behavior in high shear wet granulation *Adv. Powder Technol.* **32** 2085–96

[193] Kushwah V, Arora S, Tamás Katona M, Modhave D, Fröhlich E and Paudel A 2021 On absorption modeling and food effect prediction of rivaroxaban, a BCS II drug orally administered as an immediate-release tablet *Pharmaceutics* **13** 283

[194] Pinto J T, Cachola I, Pinto J F and Paudel A 2021 Understanding carrier performance in low-dose dry powder inhalation: an *in vitro*–in silico approach *Pharmaceutics* **13** 297

[195] Benque B and Khinast J G 2021 Estimating inter-patient variability of dispersion in dry powder inhalers using CFD-DEM simulations *Eur. J. Pharm. Sci.* **156** 105574

[196] Gao H, Wang W, Dong J, Ye Z and Ouyang D 2021 An integrated computational methodology with data-driven ML, molecular modeling and PBPK modeling to accelerate solid dispersion formulation design *Eur. J. Pharm. Biopharm.* **158** 336–46

[197] Yosinski J, Clune J, Bengio Y and Lipson H 2014 How transferable are features in deep neural networks? ArXiv:1411.1792

[198] Jain A *et al* 2013 Commentary: the materials project: a materials genome approach to accelerating materials innovation *APL Mater.* **1** 011002

[199] Yamada H *et al* 2019 Predicting materials properties with little data using shotgun transfer learning *ACS Cent. Sci.* **5** 1717–30

[200] Grisoni F, Neuhaus C S, Gabernet G, Müller A T, Hiss J A and Schneider G 2018 Designing anticancer peptides by constructive ML *ChemMedChem.* **13**

[201] Lee J and Asahi R 2021 Transfer learning for materials informatics using crystal graph convolutional neural network *Comput. Mater. Sci.* **190** 110314

[202] Hatakeyama-Sato K and Oyaizu K 2021 Generative models for extrapolation prediction in materials informatics *ACS Omega* **6** 14566–74

[203] Richardson T W, Wu W, Lin L, Xu B and Bernal E A 2020 McFlow: monte carlo flow models for data imputation *2020 IEEE/CVF Conf. on Computer Vision and Pattern Recognition (CVPR) (Seattle, WA)* 14193–202

[204] Ling J, Hutchinson M, Antono E, Paradiso S and Meredig B 2017 High-dimensional materials and process optimization using data-driven experimental design with well-calibrated uncertainty estimates *Integr. Mater. Manuf. Innov.* **6** 207–17

[205] Rohr B *et al* 2020 Benchmarking the acceleration of materials discovery by sequential learning *Chem. Sci.* **11** 2696–706

[206] Pasas-Farmer S and Jain R 2021 Artificial intelligence in drug discovery and development: challenges and recommendations *AAPS Newsmazagine* https://aapsnewsmagazine.org/aapsnewsmagazine/articles/2021/jul21/cover-story-jul21

Chapter 10

Soft mist inhaler delivery of biologics

Diana A Fernandes

When treating local or systemic conditions, pulmonary drug delivery offers direct access to the lung, yielding a faster onset of the drug action, while avoiding the stomach and liver's metabolic activity. Soft mist inhalers (SMIs) have been gradually found to be more effective and convenient than other devices due to their slower aerosol plume and ease of handling. This not only results in a higher deposition profile but also in increased patient adherence. Additionally, SMIs' underlying mechanism seems to expose the sprayed drug to a lower risk of shear-stress induced degradation, which is encouraging in those for which conformational structure might be more sensitive, as in the case of biologics. Developing a biologic/SMI combination product has however its own challenges, and therefore patient-, technical (device, formulation)- and regulatory-driven considerations should be regarded for its safe and effective administration. In this chapter, these aspects are further explored. Research and current clinical outlook of SMI delivery of biologics is also reviewed and a SWOT analysis presented.

10.1 Introduction

The pulmonary route of drug administration remains the gold standard for the treatment of local respiratory diseases. Its use is also gradually being extended to the treatment of systemic disorders [1–3]. The lungs offer a unique and direct channel for drugs to be delivered straight to their target(s), or alternatively, enter the blood stream and reach systemic circulation. This results in a faster drug onset while circumventing proteolytic activity in the stomach and the first-pass metabolism in the liver, when compared to the oral route of administration [2, 4]. Therefore, the delivered dose can be reduced, and potential adverse side effects mitigated [3, 5]. Moreover, when compared to the injectable route of administration, despite all the advancement witnessed in understanding patient fear of needles [5] or rendering micro-needles less painful and/or easy-to-use [6], portable inhalation devices do not

doi:10.1088/978-0-7503-5613-8ch10

pose the same pain perception concerns whilst allowing for a more convenient treatment routine, more likely to be adopted by the patient.

Nebulizers, pressurized metered dose inhalers (pMDIs), dry powder inhalers (DPIs) and SMIs are different types of devices currently available on the market to attain pulmonary drug delivery [1, 3]. Each presents advantages and disadvantages according to the target disease, patient condition and adherence, type of dosage form (liquid- or dry powder-based) and type of active pharmaceutical ingredient (API) i.e., biologic or small molecule. However, for SMIs, increasing data showcases not only a greater patient adherence due to the ease of handling but also a higher deposition profile in the lungs attributed to the slower aerosol plume with a larger duration, when compared with other portable devices [2].

In addition, the underlying mechanism yielding the soft mist upon SMI actuation, exposes the sprayed API to a lower risk of degradation induced by shear stress [7]. This feature is particularly relevant in the case of biologics with a 3D conformational structure, that when compromised, might trigger immunogenic reactions, sometimes dangerous and/or fatal for the patient [4, 8, 9]. The European Medicines Agency (EMA) and US Food and Drug Administration (FDA) define biologics or biological (medicinal) products as any pharmaceutical drug product manufactured, extracted, or semi synthesized from a biological source (human, animal, plant, fungal or microbial) [10, 11] aiming to prevent, treat and/or cure injuries and/or diseases. These usually comprise nucleic acid derivatives (antisense oligonucleotides—ASO, microRNAs, Anti-micro-RNAs, messenger RNA, aptamers, RNA interference—RNAi, genes), peptides, recombinant proteins (interferons, interleukins, lung surfactant proteins, hormones, therapeutic enzymes, antibodies, and others), lung surfactants, virus, living cells or even tissues. When compared to small molecules, biologics therapeutic action can be more specific and potent towards its target, allowing for a lower dose to be employed and a narrower range of adverse side effects to take place [12].

Despite being promising, enabling a biologic-based therapy using an SMI has its own challenges. The patient, SMI features, dosage form, formulation, molecule, and regulatory requirements must be considered when designing such a combination product. Patient's adherence, lung's anatomy, physiology, and clearance mechanisms will ultimately determine drug deposition profile, absorption, and overall efficiency. Despite favouring absorption, the liquid nature of the SMI dosage form also makes the biologic more vulnerable to conformational changes and the formulation to microbial burden, shortening its long-term stability and safety [4] when compared to dry powder-based dosage forms. As a result, preservatives must often be added to the formulation, complexifying this process as well as the regulatory approval, considering that the relevant guidance documents discourage their use, while requiring extra documentation to ascertain its safety in the concentration range included [2, 13]. High-dose biologic formulations may display high viscosity and/or surface tension that, in turn, hamper device performance, requiring again formulation adjustments/add-ons.

Nowadays, there is only one reported biologic, a low molecular weight heparin, undergoing clinical development with an SMI—Pulmospray™ (https://resyca.com/) by Recipharm (Sweden) [14]. However, the first SMI device—Respimat® (https://

www.respimat.com/), by Boeringher Inghelheim (Germany)—was approved for the first time almost 20 years ago. In the present chapter, some background for the development of SMI delivery will be provided followed by an overview of patient, technical (device, formulation) and regulatory considerations when conceptualizing and designing an SMI combination product. A review of the research and current clinical outlook of soft mist inhaler delivery of biologics is also presented.

10.2 Towards soft mist inhalation delivery

Nebulizers, pMDIs, DPIs and SMIs are the main types of devices currently available to manage inhalation therapy. Nebulizers feature a sterile liquid that is atomized into an aerosol. Most of the commercially available nebulizers rely on jet (or pneumatic), ultrasonic, or mesh technology, ranging from bulky to portable set-ups. For a thorough understanding of the underlying mechanisms inherent to each, the author recommends the reading of cited articles [15–17]. Nebulizers only require tidal breathing allowing patients, from children to seniors, with or without cognitive and/or physical impairment to use them in the absence of agency or any specific training. Nonetheless, the non-metered dosing regimen results in long administration periods, inaccurate, low delivered dose, and drug waste, which requires a larger amount of drug to be included at the start in the product. Moreover, in the case of ultrasonic nebulizers, poor aerosolization and biologic degradation of concentrated, viscous solutions or suspensions has been previously reported in the literature [17, 18].

The pMDIs deliver a metered multi-dose of single or combined drugs in solution or suspension together with a liquefied gas propellant under pressure, through a portable metal canister. To actuate the device, the patient presses down the top of the canister that aerosolizes its content, while coordinating with inhalation. Upon actuation, the gas propellant evaporates [2, 3]. Chlorofluorocarbons (CFC) were the first gas propellants to be employed. However, the cold Fréon effect exerted in the back of the patient's throat culminating in temperature drops to −20°C would interrupt the inhalation manoeuvre. Besides this, the depleting effect of CFCs on the ozone layer triggered the research for alternative propellants [3, 19, 20]. Hydrofluoroalkanes (HFAs), such as HFA-134a, HFA-227 and HFA152a have been the most regularly used as replacements despite still contributing, albeit to a lower extent, to the greenhouse effect. HFA propellants' impact on the aerodynamic performance differs from that of CFCs. Furthermore, the drug also tends to be swallowed by the patient [1]. To address this, auxiliary systems, such as spacers and facemasks, have been developed and coupled to pMDIs, favoring evaporation of the propellant, the deceleration of the spray and the collection of larger droplets so that oropharyngeal deposition is reduced, and lung's drug intake increased [1, 16]. From a biologic standpoint, the formulation process is hindered due to the poor solubility and stability of these molecules in the commonly used propellants, requiring a carrier-based strategy to be implemented.

DPIs deliver single- or multi-dose solid dosage forms through the patient's inspiratory flow effort and the turbulence induced inside the device upon actuation, resulting from its intrinsic resistance to aerosolization [21]. The solid nature of a DPI formulation renders it less prone to undergo liquid-mediated degradation mechanisms that compromise stability of the API, especially if this is a biologic. From a supply chain perspective, this could even represent a lighter resource and financial load as cold transport might not be required. On the other hand, it can also aggravate treatment emergent adverse events (TEAEs) such as a cough. TEAEs, cough included, might be caused by the type of molecule, dose, formulation, age group and even sex. However, cough seems to be predominant in solid dosage forms, as depicted in figure 10.1 [22, 23]. Contrary to pMDIs, DPIs do not require propellants. However, the formulation exercise can be halted by other factors. An additional drying and particle engineering (D&PE) step is required, entailing a combination of excipients simultaneously showcasing patient adherence, inhalation precedence, API stabilization potential and D&PE compatibility, to be determined [4]. Freeze drying followed by a milling-based technology, spray drying or most recently spray freeze drying [24, 25] are some examples of D&PE technologies that have been investigated within the inhalation framework. The increasing availability of high-throughput analytical tools, such as differential scanning fluorimetry, and even artificial intelligence and machine learning algorithms [26] to support formulation screening methodologies is allowing this challenge to be addressed in reduced time with microgram (μg) range or no sample requirement [4]. SMIs deliver a single- or multi-metered dose, propellant-free drug solution using one of (at least) two underlying mechanisms—the colliding jets or the Rayleigh jets principle. In the colliding jets principle, two liquid jets, from the same source, are forced through a uniblock nozzle that makes them collide while yielding a liquid sheet that breaks up into fine droples. On the other hand, Rayleigh jets are extruded from micro-nozzles of well-defined geometry that break into monodisperse droplets, twice their pore size [48]. These mechanisms result in a slower aerosol plume that facilitates coordination between inhalation and device actuation, yielding a higher deposition profile ranging from 65%–80%, when compared

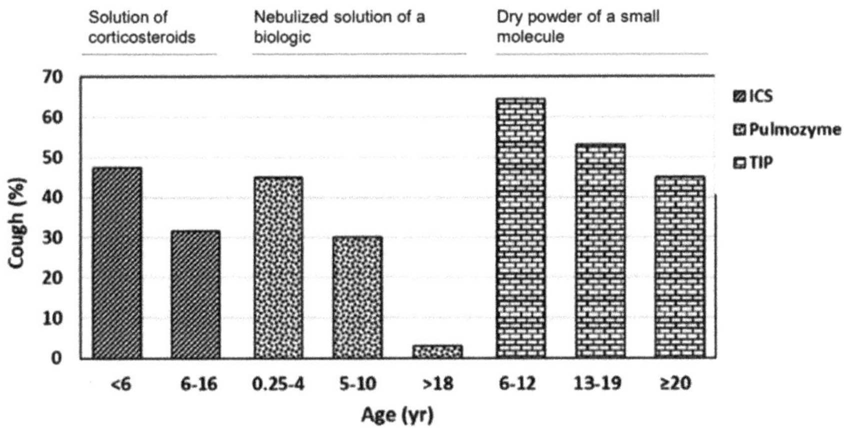

Figure 10.1. Cough incidence percentage as a function of age group for an inhaled solution of corticosteroids (ICS), for a nebulized solution of a biologic (rHDNase, Pulmozyme) and for a dry powder of a small molecule, Tobramycin, (TIP). Reprinted from [22], copyright (2020) with permission from Elsevier.

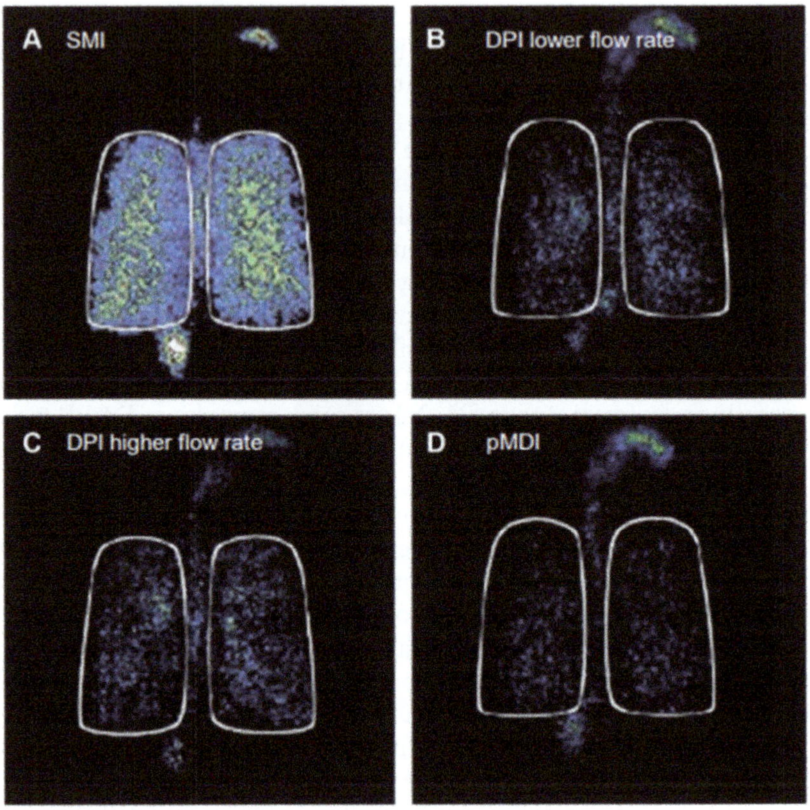

Figure 10.2. Scintigraphy images for an SMI—Respimat® (A), a DPI actuated at a lower flow rate—Turbuhaler® (B), a DPI actuated at a higher flow rate—Turbuhaler® (C) and a pMDI—(D). Reproduced from [19] originally published by and used with permission from Dove Medical Press Ltd.

with nebulizers, pMDIs and DPIs (figure 10.2) [7]. The milder aerosolization could also be beneficial for shear-stress sensitive molecules, as is the case of some biologics.

The first SMI to be developed was Respimat® by Boehringer Ingelheim and was made commercially available in 2004 to support asthma and chronic obstructive pulmonary disease (COPD) small molecule therapy, in Europe [7].

The Respimat® inhaler design has undergone several key evolution steps, as depicted in figure 10.3.

Respimat® turned out to be a cylindrical-shaped, handheld, pocket-sized oral inhalation device with a cap, a gray-colored body and a clear base. The cartridge storing the liquid formulation consists of an aluminum cylinder with a collapsible and double-walled plastic bag. To use the device, the patient removes the clear base, inserts the cartridge in the gray-colored body, assembles the clear base and turns this until it clicks. The patient is then expected to open the cap and press the dose-release button. The clear base should then be turned and the dose-release button pressed until a fully developed spray has been generated—priming. Once primed, the device is prepared for use. To provide convenience and ensure proper usage, the inhaler incorporates a dose

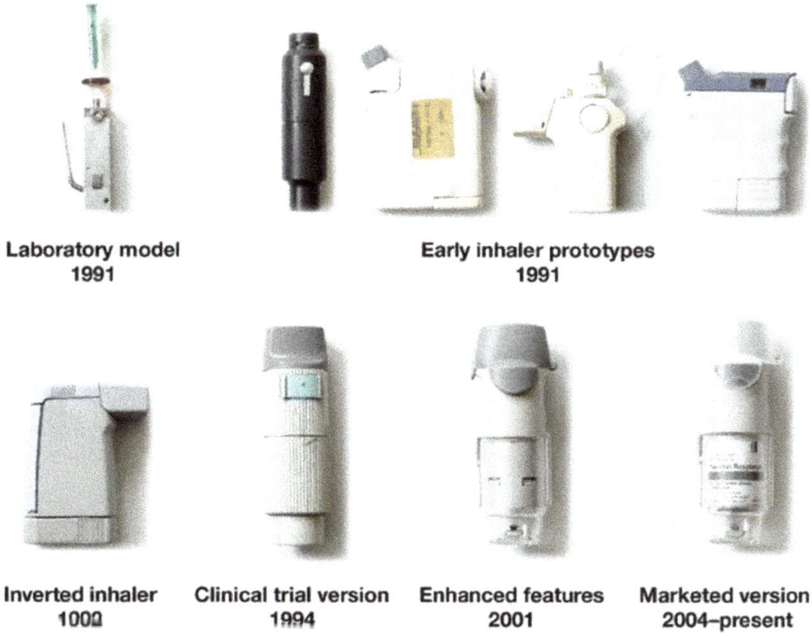

Figure 10.3. Evolution of Respimat® Inhaler Devic. Reproduced from [47] CC BY 4.0.

indicator that shows the remaining number of actuations in the device. Furthermore, the mouthpiece cap is designed in distinct colors. For instance, the Spiriva® Respimat® (tiotropium bromide) inhaler features an aqua or blue cap, the Striverdi® Respimat® (olodaterol) inhaler has a yellow cap, and the Spiolto® Respimat® (tiotropium/olodaterol) inhaler is identified by its light green cap. These color-coded caps aid users in identifying the mouthpiece cover and assist in product identification. The Respimat® inhaler design, with its compact size, precise dosing mechanism, and user-friendly features, aims to enhance the delivery of medication for respiratory conditions.

From a patient standpoint, relative feedback on Respimat® against other devices was quite positive. According to a review of Respimat® preference studies carried out by Hodder and Price [27], patients seem to accept well the use of an SMI based treatment when compared to other alternatives (figure 10.4). Nearly 75 % of patients with COPD and asthma preferred Respimat® over a pMDI (figure 10.4(A)) or Turbuhaler® DPI (figure 10.4(B0) and almost 65 % over Diskus® DPI (figure 10.4(C)). This was mainly attributed to ease of handling and carrying, despite Respimat® scoring significantly worse on size, than pMDI and Turbuhaler®. SMI delivery has since gained followers and other players have been joining this arena with their own SMI devices to support combination product development. In the next section, an overview of patient, technical and regulatory considerations for the development of SMI combination products is presented.

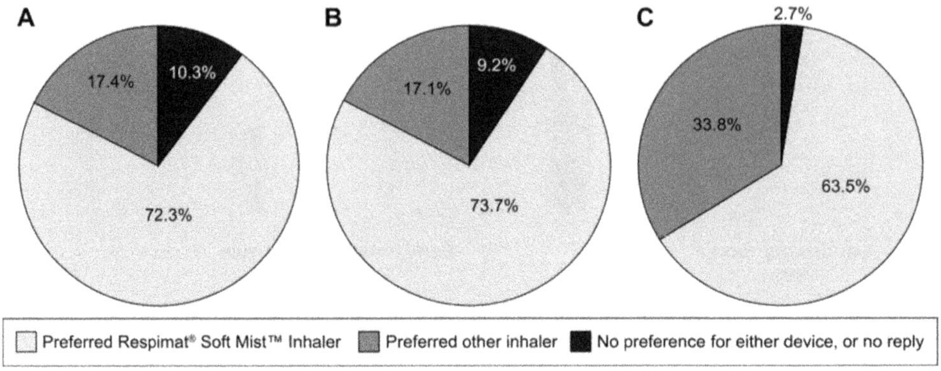

Figure 10.4. Proportions of patients indicating preference for Respimat® SMI versus alternative inhaler devices in three studies, using the Patient Satisfaction and Preference survey. Reproduced from [19] originally published by and used with permission from Dove Medical Press Ltd.

10.3 Developing a soft mist inhaled combination product: considerations

Combination products pertain to the sets composed of drug/device, biologic/device, drug/biologic, or drug/device/biologic, that are physically, chemically, or otherwise combined or mixed and produced as a single entity [28]. These may also include products packaged together and products that are separately packaged but need to be used together [29]. When conceptualizing and designing an SMI combination product, patient-, technical- and regulatory-driven considerations should be jointly weighted to enable a safe and effective delivery platform. Considering the scope of the present chapter, the author will focus on biologic/device (SMI) combination product.

10.3.1 Patient

The patient's adherence, lungs anatomy and physiology may condition the conceptualization and design of an SMI combination product.

10.3.1.1 Adherence

Patient adherence can be defined as '(...) an active, cooperative and voluntary participation of the patient in following recommendations from a healthcare provider'. It encompasses three steps over time [30]:

- Initiation, corresponding to the first dose the patient takes.
- Implementation, defined as the extent to which a patient's actual dosing corresponds to the prescribed dose, from initiation until the last one.
- Persistence, which is the length of time between initiation and the last dose.

Non-adherence determinants can be multiple. Based on World Health Organization (WHO), the causes of non-adherence can be grouped in socioeconomic-, healthcare provider and system-, patient-, therapy- and condition-related factors [31] that naturally overlap with each other. From a socioeconomic standpoint, medication adherence rates in respiratory conditions, such asthma and COPD, are lower among patients with low income or limited insurance/social coverage [32]. To circumvent this, these patients might look for complimentary or alternative medication (CAM) like herbal remedies, massage, acupuncture, yoga, spirituality/religion [32, 33].

The healthcare provider–patient relationship, also affected by the healthcare system in play, is one of the leading causes for non-adherence. Miscommunication between parties (healthcare provider and patient) and absence of medication controller strategies are the main contributors for non-adherence stemming from access to healthcare (how easy it is to schedule an appointment with a specialist), language barriers, (if the patient's native language is not the same as the healthcare provider), misinformation on treatment options by both that limits discussion, inability of the healthcare provider to clearly convey the prescribed treatment procedure, unavailability of helpful training content and insufficient consultation time [30, 32–34]. Healthcare provider cultural competence, i.e., her/his/their ability to grasp the likelihood for the cultural background of the patient to impact adherence, has also been identified as an important aspect. Patient medication beliefs towards a self-management approach, namely the necessity for a medication and the level of concern to administer it according to the respective posology, differs among cultural backgrounds and may be influenced by family experiences and historical facts rooted in medical abuse of racial and ethnic minority populations. Culture and background also influence a patient's positioning on CAM. Many patients with asthma use CAM for managing their condition and some studies have reported that certain racial and ethnic groups, including African Americans and Latinos, are more likely to use CAM for managing their asthma [32, 33]. Another patient-related factor believed to have a toll in adherence is mental health. Research suggests that depression symptoms can contribute to a higher risk of poor medication adherence in patients with asthma. Among young inner-city children with asthma, maternal depressive symptoms have been linked to adherence difficulties. Diverse samples of adolescents, young adults and seniors with asthma have also been found to have poor medication adherence when experiencing depressive symptoms [32].

The type of therapy, specifically the treatment regimen, type of API (small molecule or biologic) and dosage form also influence adherence. The patient's preference lies in the possibility of easy and independent self-management, reduced number of products in a combination therapy scenario for the lowest number of dosing times. From a type of molecule perspective, diverse patient experience has been reported and there is an overall lack of qualitative data to assess patients' response to biologic-based treatments: corticosteroids are perceived for some as more beneficial, familiar and less dreadful than biologics; adult patients described a positive response in terms of reduced burden of disease and treatment and others, a reduced benefit from biologic-based therapies over time. Cost, onset of efficacy and long-term side effects have weight on the patient decision making for a biologic-based therapy [35]. From a dosage form stance, there is again a lack of qualitative data to assess patients' preference on inhaled solid versus liquid dosage forms as adherence in this context seems to be driven by device-related factors like ease of handling and carrying [19]. However, cough and dry throat are more incident for solid dosage forms, as previously mentioned.

10.3.1.2 Lung's anatomy and physiology

Understanding the structure and function of the airways is critical to develop safe and effective drug delivery platforms targeting the lungs. The lung airways can be divided into two main regions: the conducting airway and the respiratory airway [36, 37]. The Weibel-A mathematical model provides a widely accepted description of their layout, dividing the lung into 24 stages [38]. The respiratory airway differs from the conducting airway in terms of physical characteristics as it facilitates gas exchange, with a surface area of approximately 100 m^2 compared to the 2–3 m^2 of the conducting airway. Both types of airways are lined with mucus gel that contains water, glycoproteins, inorganic salts, lipids, proteins, and DNA [39]. Aerosol particles deposit in this mucus and dissolve to release the active drug. The volume of fluid in the lung for particles to dissolve is limited and the thickness of the lung lining fluid layer varies between central and peripheral lungs. The alveoli are lined with pulmonary surfactant, which plays a dual role of reducing surface tension and defending against inhaled pathogens and particles. This surfactant also extends the residence time of drugs within the lung, but can cause aggregation of large molecules, such as biologics, leading to their elimination or immunogenic events. However, it can enhance absorption of lower molecular weight biologics such as peptides [40].

The mechanisms involved in particle deposition in the lungs include inertial impaction, gravitational sedimentation, Brownian diffusion, interception, and electrostatic precipitation [41]. Inertial impaction occurs in the conducting airways, while gravitational sedimentation and Brownian diffusion occur in the respiratory airways. Interception and electrostatic precipitation can occur in both the conducting and respiratory airways. Particle size, shape, breathing rate, inhalation volume, and patient health condition all affect particle deposition. Understanding the specific pattern of deposition is important for determining local doses, redistribution, and clearance of deposited particles. After particle deposition in the lungs, the drug may be subjected to various *in vivo* mechanisms such as mucociliary clearance, clearance by macrophages, and protease degradation, both extra- and intracellularly [36]. Mucociliary clearance involves ciliated cells driving trapped particles in the mucus from the lower airways to the pharynx, where they can be swallowed and degraded in the gastrointestinal tract or ejected. Macrophages migrate to the particles and phagocytize them via chemotaxis involving opsonization and disintegrate them once they are internalized. As to protease degradation, there is low activity in the lung. However, the higher the biologic molecular weight, the more vulnerable it becomes.

10.3.2 Technical considerations: device and formulation

From a technical stance, when developing a biologic/SMI combination product, the following criteria must be attained:

- The aerodynamic particle size distribution (aPSD) should be in accordance with the target deposition site in the lungs (PSD typically ranges from 1–5 μm or below 10 μm);
- The biologic structure must be maintained so no immunogenic response mechanism is triggered while posing a safety risk for the patient.

- The process through which a biologic/SMI combination product is obtained must be simple, scalable, with a low manufacturing capacity burden and cost-effective.

Device and formulation development are thus intertwined and should occur, ideally, in parallel.

10.3.2.1 Device considerations

One of the critical aspects of any inhalation therapy device, is its ability to deliver a precise and constant respirable fraction of particles effectively and reproducibly, for optimal deposition in its target [7]. Droplet size distribution consistency is particularly relevant to achieve this. Jin *et al* (2022) [42] have recently used a computational fluid dynamic approach to further understand the atomization process generating the droplets in an impingement system commonly used in SMI. The results of their numerical analysis indicated that the angle of impingement and the velocity distribution of the jet are significantly influenced by the flow conditions inside the nozzle, and these factors have a significant impact on the atomization characteristics. An increase in the impingement angle and pressure at the nozzle inlet results in a greater X-direction velocity component of the liquid jet, leading to a more forceful impact at the impingement point, which directly affects the fluctuation and breakup pattern of the liquid sheet, resulting in smaller droplets. Furthermore, the Y-direction velocity component of the liquid jet affects the velocity and diffusion of the liquid sheet, so the X- and Y-direction velocities of the liquid jet have a critical impact on the breakup length of the liquid sheet. As to the materials used in the device and/or the device components (cartridge), these should shield the biologic solution from any source of contamination, whether this a leachable, or of microbial nature. Also, these materials should be robust enough to prevent the liquid formulation from evaporation while avoiding the biologic adherence to the inner wall of the cartridge. These materials should also be environmentally sustainable and light to favour patient adherence [27, 28].

10.3.2.2 Formulation considerations

SMI formulations must be sterile [13]. Moreover, biologics must endure their respective manufacturing process, device actuation and, following administration, evade mucociliary clearance, clearance by macrophages and protease degradation. In addition, their high molecular weight and strong negative charge, hinders their passive diffusion across the cellular membrane. Formulation compounds beside the biologic should be kept to a minimum to avoid compatibility issues while expediting development and regulatory process. However, the liquid nature of SMI formulations might entail the use of buffers (e.g. sodium citrate), salts (e.g. sodium chloride, calcium chloride) and preservatives (e.g. quaternary ammonias like benzalkonium chloride) [1, 43] to help maintaining the biologic conformational structure in the long run, whether by pH control, functional activity enhancement and microbial burden management. An alternative to preservatives, as the most used are sometimes associated with hypersensitive reactions [43] and discouraged by the relevant guidance's for biologic/SMI combination products [13], are self-preserving excipients (e.g. propylene glycol, glycerin, sodium chloride) that render the same effect. Surfactants can also be added in the case of highly concentrated biologic solutions to decrease surface tension and maintain droplet size distribution within target, while having a stabilizing effect on the biologic. Respaud *et al* (2014) [44] have reported that the addition of surfactants to antibody formulations at concentrations appropriate for lung administration markedly reduced the formation of medium or large aggregates enabling a safer delivery.

10.3.3 Regulatory considerations

Despite being discussed last, regulatory strategy should precede, ideally, device and formulation development. Selecting in advance the regulatory approval pathway allows one to identify the type and burden of analytical testing required to prove safety and efficacy of the biologic/SMI combination product. Several guidance documents for the development and testing of biological products and devices are available in regulatory agencies webpages, but frequently as standalone constituents, instead of combined. This might hamper the determination of the regulatory center that should supervise its approval [45].

EMA defines an SMI as a metered dose inhaler. The safety and effectiveness of medicines used in combination with a medical device is part of a centralised procedure application for the medicinal product. Biologics should fall under Advanced therapies category, although this should be confirmed on a case-by-case basis as currently it seems to only include gene, cell or tissue-based therapies [49].

FDA, on the other hand, defines an SMI as an inhalation spray. Accroding to the 'Early Development Considerations for Innovative Combination Products' guidance for industry and FDA staff [28], the developers should consult with the FDA's Office of Combination Products (OCP), which, based on section 503(g) of the Act, is responsible for assigning a lead agency center with primary jurisdiction over the review and regulation of the respective biologic/SMI combination product. This lead agency should be defined based on the biologic/SMI combination product primary mode of action (PMOA). PMOA is defined as 'the single mode of action of a combination product that provides the most important therapeutic action of the combination product.' For instance, if the PMOA of a device-biologic combination product could be attributed to its biological product constituent, the agency component responsible for premarket review of that biological product would have primary jurisdiction for the combination product. In the case of a biologic/SMI combination product, the Center for Biologics Evaluation and Research (CBER) could be designated as the lead agency, considering the PMOA definition mentioned above. CBER is, however, expected to collaborate with OCP and other agency components, such as the Center for Devices and Radiological Health (CDRH), as necessary, to identify and evaluate the information required for a regulatory submission. FDA advises the submission of a single application for a combination product but there might be cases where it may determine that an application for each constituent part is warranted. The marketing application type submitted should coincide with the PMOA of the biologic/SMI combination product. If PMOA is biologic-driven, then a 351(a) BLA for a biologic, or a 351(k) BLA for a biosimilar or interchangeable biological product is to be followed. There are previously launched biologic/inhalation device combination products that might help pave the way for a biologic/SMI combination product: Survanta (beractant, surfactant) by AbbVie (1991), Pulmozyme (dornase alfa, enzyme) by Roche (1993), Afrezza (insulin, peptide) by MannKind Corporation (2014) and Exubera (insuline, peptide) by Pfizer (2017) [50]. In addition, there are also a few biologic/SMI clinical programs currently ongoing that might shed light on possible regulatory pathways.

10.4 Current research and clinical outlook

Despite the approval of Respimat® in 2004, very few studies coupling this SMI with biologics have been led. Carrigy *et al* (2017) [18] conducted a comparative study on titer reduction and delivery rate of active anti-tuberculosis bacteriophage (phage) D29 with three inhalation devices—a vibrating mesh- (Aerogen Solo with Pro-X Controller), a jet nebulizer (Pari LC Sprint with Pari Boy SX Compressor) and a SMI (Respimat®). They have found that the jet nebulizer was not a good option for aerosolizing phage D29, as it caused a significant reduction in titer during droplet generation. For animal inhalation studies requiring large amounts of D29 aerosol, the vibrating mesh nebulizer could be more suitable. Interestingly, the SMI was considered a promising option for self-administration of D29 aerosol as it allowed a high titer delivery of phage D29 in a fast and convenient manner. A US patent was filed claiming that the Respimat® inhaler can deliver over 75% of biologically active IFN-ω and manganese superoxide dismutase for the treatment of diabetes [46]. Other SMI-like devices were tested as was the case of the AERx® aerosol system. In a study comparing it to a jet nebulizer, the AERx® was found to be more efficient in delivering IFNα2b, DNase, and rh-IL-4 receptor. However, this system is no longer available.

Nowadays, there is only one reported biologic, a low molecular weight heparin (LMWH), undergoing clinical development (NCT04990830) with an SMI—Pulmospray™ [14]. The COVID-19-induced acute respiratory distress syndrome can cause severe hypoxemia and high mortality in hospitalized patients. A clinical trial was conducted with Pulmospray™ to deliver low-molecular-weight heparin to these patients. The Device Group (40 patients) received low-molecular-weight heparin via the SMI twice a day, while the Control Group (40 patients) received standard therapy. The study found that low-molecular-weight heparin significantly improved breathing capability, particularly in cases of severe hypoxemia, when delivered via a SMI. The treatment was well-tolerated and decreased the need for oxygen treatment. A larger follow-up trial is currently being conducted to determine the extent to which soft-mist LMWH attenuates lung injury and hypoxemia in COVID-19.

10.5 Concluding remarks

In the present chapter, SMI delivery of biologics was further explored. SMIs address some of the limitations showcased by other available devices: conversely to nebulizers, these allow for a metered dose to be delivered; contrary to pMDIs, these do not require propellants to mediate aerosolization; and when opposed to DPIs, these do not require an extra D&PE step, do not rely on patient respiratory capacity and are less likely to induce cough and dry throat. SMIs' deposition profile is also higher when compared with the other devices. From a biologic standpoint, SMIs' underlying mechanism responsible for the generation of a soft mist seems to expose the biologic to a lower shear-stress-based degradation. On top of this, data showed an increased patient adherence towards SMI when compared to other treatment options. Despite the positive features, developing a biologic/SMI combination product has its own challenges for which patient-, technical- and regulatory-driven considerations must be regarded. Patient's adherence might be affected by socioeconomic-, healthcare provider and system-, patient-, therapy- and condition-related factors that naturally overlap with each other. Adherence is lower for patients with low income, poor insurance/ social coverage that limits access to healthcare and who have a poor relationship with the healthcare provider due to miscommunication between parties. Patients that are open to CAM or whose healthcare provider lacks culture competence also show low adherence. On the other hand, patient's lung anatomy and physiology will determine particle deposition and absorption. These should be taken into account when setting the technical approach for the combination product. Device and formulation aspects should be weighted so the aerodynamic particle size distribution (aPSD) corresponds to the target deposition site in the lungs (PSD typically ranges from 1–5 μm or below 10 μm); the biologic conformational structure is maintained (if that is the case) and no immunogenic response mechanism is triggered posing a safety risk for the patient; the process through which a biologic/SMI combination product is obtained is simple, scalable, with a low manufacturing capacity burden and cost-effective while supported by a robust supply chain strategy. Defining the regulatory strategy is pivotal, even before beginning technical development. This will help anticipate which type and burden of analytical testing is required to prove safety and efficacy of the biologic/SMI combination product. In the case of a biologic/SMI combination product, in which the PMOA is biologic-driven the regulatory center will be the Center for Biologics Evaluation and Research (CBER). If the API is a biologic, then a 351(a) BLA should be filed; if the API is a biosimilar or interchangeable biological product, then a 351(k) BLA should be pursued. Despite the approval of Respimat® in 2004, very few studies have been led, coupling this SMI or a similar type of device with biologics, and only one biologic product, an LMWH, is currently under clinical development with a different SMI device—Pulmospray™, by Resica. However, both research and clinical results demonstrate the suitability of SMIs for biologic therapy, encouraging their future adoption for the treatment of local and systemic conditions. To conclude, a strengths, weaknesses, opportunities, and threats (SWOT) analysis is proposed to overview these for SMI delivery of biologics previously explored in this chapter (figure 10.5).

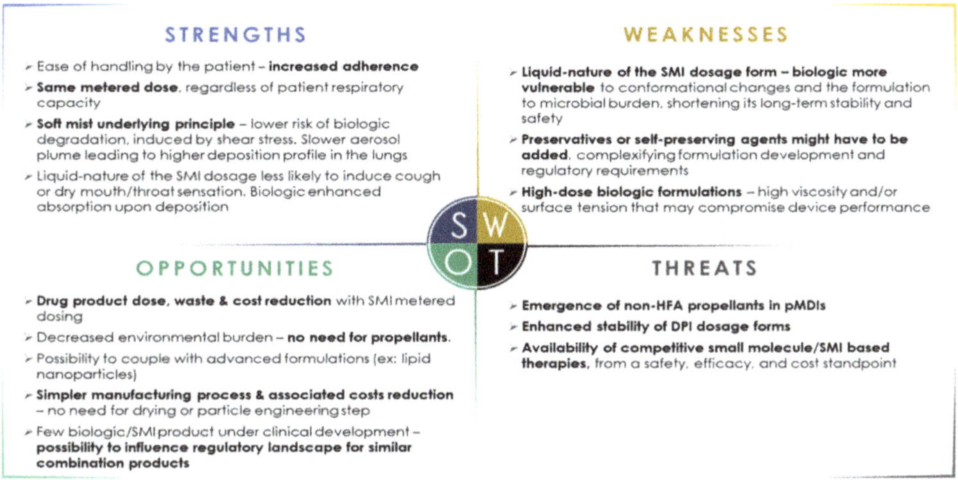

Figure 10.5. Strengths, weaknesses, opportunities, and threats (SWOT) analysis of SMI delivery of biologics.

About the author

Diana Fernandes is a Consultant and Founder at OnResp, Denmark. OnResp is a strategic partner for Pharma, Biotech, Medical device companies, and research institutes, expediting dry powder and soft mist inhalation solutions for the delivery of biologics and small molecules via the pulmonary and nasal routes. OnResp offers three distinct consulting services, including: (i) CMC technical project leadership; (ii) advisory from concept to lab and production; and (iii) on-demand training focusing on respiratory drug product development. For further information and inquiries, interested individuals and organizations can reach out to OnResp by sending an email to info@onresp.com.

References

[1] Dalby R and Suman J 2003 Inhalation therapy: technological milestones in asthma treatment *Adv. Drug Deliv. Rev.* **55** 779–91

[2] Dalby R, Spallek M and Voshaar T 2004 A review of the development of respimat® soft mist TM inhaler *Int. J. Pharm.* **283** 1–9

[3] Sorino C, Negri S, Spanevello A, Visca D and Scichilone N 2020 Inhalation therapy devices for the treatment of obstructive lung diseases: the history of inhalers towards the ideal inhaler *Eur. J. Intern. Med.* **75** P15–8

[4] Fernandes D A, Costa E, Leandro P and Corvo M L 2022 Formulation of spray dried enzymes for dry powder inhalers : an integrated methodology *Int. J. Pharm.* **615** 121492

[5] Weers J G *et al* 2010 Pulmonary formulations: what remains to be done? *J. Aerosol Med. Pulm. Drug Deliv.* **23** S5–23

[6] Mitragotri S, Burke P A and Langer R 2014 Overcoming the challenges in administering biopharmaceuticals: formulation and delivery strategies *Nat. Rev. Drug Discovery* **13** 655–72

[7] DalbyR V and Spallek M 2004 A review of the development of Respimat® Soft Mist™ Inhaler *Int. J. Pharm.* **283** 1–9

[8] Fernandes D A, Leandro P, Costa E and Corvo M L 2021 Dry powder inhaler formulation of Cu,Zn-superoxide dismutase by spray drying: a proof-of-concept *Powder Technol.* **389** 131–7

[9] Ibrahim M, Wallace I, Ghazvini S, Manetz S, Cordoba-rodriguez R and Patel S M 2023 Protein aggregates in inhaled biologics: challenges and considerations *J. Pharm. Sci.* **112** P1341–4

[10] FDA, What are 'biologics' questions and answers (https://www.fda.gov/about-fda/center-biologics-evaluation-and-research-cber/what-are-biologics-questions-and-answers)

[11] European Medicines Agency, Biological medicine (https://www.ema.europa.eu/en/glossary/biological-medicine)

[12] Skalko-Basnet N and Press D 2014 Biologics : the role of delivery systems in improved therapy *Biologics* **8** 107–14

[13] FDA 2002 Nasal spray and inhalation solution, suspension, and spray drug products — chemistry, manufacturing, and controls *Final* 10–15 (https://www.fda.gov/media/70857/download)

[14] Erelel M *et al* 2021 Early effects of low molecular weight heparin therapy with soft-mist inhaler for covid-19-induced hypoxemia: a phase IIb trial *Pharmaceutics* **13** 1–13

[15] Dessanges J 2001 A history of nebulization *J. Aerosol Med.* **14** 65–71

[16] Stein S W and Thiel C G 2017 The history of therapeutic aerosols : a chronological review *J. Aerosol Med. Pulm. Drug Deliv.* **30** 20–41

[17] Labiris N R and Dolovich M B 2003 Pulmonary drug delivery. Part II: the role of inhalant delivery devices and drug formulations in therapeutic effectiveness of aerosolized medications *Br. J. Clin. Pharmacol.* **56** 600–12

[18] Carrigy N B *et al* 2017 Anti-tuberculosis bacteriophage D29 delivery with a vibrating mesh nebulizer, jet nebulizer, and soft mist inhaler *Pharma. Res.* **34** 2084–96

[19] Dekhuijzen P N, Lavorini F and Usmani S 2016 Patients ' perspectives and preferences in the choice of inhalers : the case for Respimat® or Handihaler® *Patient Prefer. Adher.* **10** 1561–72

[20] Newman S P 2017 Drug delivery to the lungs: challenges and opportunities *Ther. Deliv.* **8** 647–61

[21] Negro R W D 2015 Dry powder inhalers and the right things to remember: a concept review *Multidiscip. Respir. Med.* **10** 13

[22] Sahakijpijarn S, Smyth H D C, Miller D P and Weers J G 2020 Post-inhalation cough with therapeutic aerosols: formulation considerations *Adv. Drug Deliv. Rev.* **165–166** 127–41

[23] Depreter F, Pilcer G and Amighi K 2013 Inhaled proteins: challenges and perspectives *Int. J. Pharm.* **447** 251–80

[24] Sebastião I B *et al* 2019 Bulk dynamic spray freeze-drying. Part 1 : modeling of droplet cooling and phase change *J. Pharm. Sci.* **108** 2063–74

[25] Yuh-Fun Maa C C H, Nguyen P A, Sweeney T and Shire S J 1999 Protein inhalation powders: spray drying vs spray freeze drying *Pharm. Res.* **16** 249–54

[26] Narayanan H, Dingfelder F, Butté A, Lorenzen N, Sokolov M and Arosio P 2021 Machine learning for biologics : opportunities for protein engineering, developability, and formulation *Trends Pharmacol. Sci.* **42** 151–65

[27] Nicolaas P and Dekhuijzen F L 2016 PPA-82857-patients—perspectives-and-preferences-in-switching-inhalers *Dovepress* **12** 1561–72 https://www.ncbi.nlm.nih.gov/pmc/articles/PMC4993394/pdf/ppa-10-1561.pdf

[28] FDA 2006 Early Development Considerations for Innovative Combination ProductsFDA-2020-D-1455 Office of the Commissioner, Office of Clinical Policy and Programs, Office of Combination Products https://www.fda.gov/regulatory-information/search-fda-guidance-documents/early-development-considerations-innovative-combination-products
[29] Tian J *et al* 2022 Bioactive materials regulatory perspectives of combination products *Bioact. Mater.* **10** 492–503
[30] Menditto E *et al* 2020 Patient centric pharmaceutical drug product design—the impact on medication adherence *Pharmaceutics* **12** 1–23
[31] Chaudri N A 2004 Adherence to long-term therapies—evidence for action *Ann. Saudi Med.* **24** 221–2
[32] Mcquaid E L 2018 Barriers to medication adherence in asthma: the importance of culture and context *Ann. Allergy, Asthma Immunol.* **121** 37–42
[33] McQuaid E L and Landier W 2018 Cultural issues in medication adherence: disparities and directions *J. Gen. Intern. Med.* **33** 200–6
[34] Stegemann S, Ternik R L, Onder G, Khan M A and van Riet-Nales D A 2016 Defining patient centric pharmaceutical drug product design *AAPS* J. **18** 1047–55
[35] Felice K M D 2020 Patients perception of risks and benefits of biologic therapy *Inflamm. Bowel Dis.* **26** 147–9
[36] Labiris N R and Dolovich M B 2003 Pulmonary drug delivery. Part I: physiological factors affecting therapeutic effectiveness of aerosolized medications *Br. J. Clin. Pharmacol.* **56** 588–99
[37] Smyth H D C and Hickey A J 2011 *Controlled Pulmonary Drug Delivery* (New York: Springer) 1st edn
[38] 2015 *Pulmonary Drug Delivery Advances and Challenges* ed A Nokhodchi and G P Martin (New York: Wiley)
[39] Huck B C *et al* 2022 Models using native tracheobronchial mucus in the context of pulmonary drug delivery research: composition, structure and barrier properties *Adv. Drug Deliv. Rev.* **183** 114141
[40] Liang W, Pan H W, Vllasaliu D and Lam J K W 2020 Pulmonary delivery of biological drugs *Pharmaceutics* **12** 1–28
[41] Darquenne C 2006 Particle deposition in the lung *Encyclopedia of Respiratory Medicine* (Elsevier) pp 300–4
[42] Jin W, Xiao J, Ren H, Li C, Zheng Q and Tong Z 2022 Three-dimensional simulation of impinging jet atomization of soft mist inhalers using the hybrid VOF-DPM model *Powder Technol.* **407** 117622
[43] Johnson N F 2018 Pulmonary toxicity of benzalkonium chloride *J. Aerosol Med. Pulm. Drug Deliv.* **31** 1–17
[44] Respaud R *et al* 2014 Effect of formulation on the stability and aerosol performance of a nebulized antibody *MAbs* **6** 1347–55
[45] Couto D S, Perez-breva L, Saraiva P and Cooney C L 2012 Lessons from innovation in drug-device combination products *Adv. Drug Deliv. Rev.* **64** 69–77
[46] Fröhlich E and Salar-Behzadi S 2021 Oral inhalation for delivery of proteins and peptides to the lungs *Eur. J. Pharm. Biopharm.* **163** 198–211
[47] Wachtel H, Kattenbeck S, Dunne S and Disse B 2017 The Respimat® Development Story: Patient-Centered Innovation *Pulmon. Therapy* **3** 19–30
[48] Komalla V *et al* 2023 Advances in soft mist inhalers *Exp. Opin. Drug Del.* **20** 1055–70

[49] https://www.ema.europa.eu/en/human-regulatory-overview/medical-devices#medicinal-products-used-in-combination-with-a-medicaldevice-section (accessed October 2023)
[50] https://www.ondrugdelivery.com/delivering-biologics-with-soft-mist-inhalers-a-market-poised-to-expand/ (accessed October 2023)

IOP Publishing

Advances in Drug Delivery Systems for Healthcare
From concept to clinic
Piyush Pradeep Mehta and Arpana Parihar

Chapter 11

Computational approaches for antibody-based drug design

Sude Gunes[1], Ipek Arkca[1], Seref Berk Atik[1], Fulden Ulucan-Karnak Humeyra Taskent Sezgin[2] and Arzu Uyar[2]

This chapter includes various aspects of antibodies with a major emphasis on computational tools in antibody design. In this scope, current antibody databases, computational tools, and approaches for modelling antibodies and nanobodies, the structure, and interface prediction are analyzed. On the other hand, various antibody design techniques such as grafting, the significance of antibody–drug conjugates, and how computational methods contribute to the development of therapeutic antibodies are discussed with relevant strategies in the literature. Lastly, the production cost and the rising market value of antibodies are emphasized.

11.1 Introduction

The emergence of the hybridoma technique in 1975 as well as the established approaches in science and technology improved the prevalence of antibodies in research and clinics. In 2022, 138 monoclonal antibodies (mAbs) were reported to be in late-stage clinical trials. 104 mAbs were reported to be approved by the United States Food and Drug Administration (US FDA). Currently, the significance of antibodies was considered to demonstrate a remarkable increase since the reported antibodies were being used in the treatment of various diseases including cancer, multiple sclerosis, asthma, and rheumatoid arthritis [1]. In addition, the role of antibodies in vaccine development was also pointed out. In this scope, several antibodies were expressed to have a potential for their usage in the presence of SARS-CoV-2 infection. Moreover, the usage of antibodies in other infectious diseases including respiratory syncytial virus, anthrax, and *Clostridioides difficile*

[1] These authors contributed equally.

[2] Corresponding authors.

doi:10.1088/978-0-7503-5613-8ch11

was specified, and these antibodies were known to be approved by FDA [2]. Currently, antibody and antibody-based pharmaceuticals are also among the 10 most valuable research & development projects, which are ranked by the net present value, as highlighted in the EvaluatePharma 2022 report [3], which provides a global view of the pharmaceutical market. The top-ranked drug molecule with a 12.1 billion dollars net present value is a monoclonal antibody for the treatment of Alzheimer's Disease, named Gantenerumab developed by Roche and MorphoSys companies.

Research that yields successful solutions to both antibody- and other biomolecules-related questions requires laborious experimentation, which is time- and cost-intensive, and is intrinsically tied to technology. Thanks to rapid developments in technology, computational power has a much wider place in the health care industry, specifically and importantly, it plays a vital role in developing new drug molecules and therapeutics for the treatment of diseases. In this respect, computational tools are both complementary and strong, fast alternatives. Computational tools demonstrated significant impact in various fields such as drug discovery with the progress in science and computational power. Recently, the prevalence of computational tools has led pharmaceutical companies to include these tools for drug discovery research; we all have witnessed how fast computational tools were applied in the race to find a drug molecule against COVID-19. With the help of artificial intelligence (AI) tools, Pfizer developed Paxlovid against COVID-19 and obtained emergency use authorization in less than 12 months [4].

Moreover, Cox and Gupta (2022) reported more than 150 computational tools with various applications in the scope of cheminformatics and structure-based drug design [5]. In addition, the application of machine learning and deep learning in drug discovery was also indicated. The computational tools were indicated to provide the evaluation of desired properties in the drug such as potency and stability in the scope of multiple-parameter optimization (MPO). Recently, machine learning and deep learning have had enormous potential to speed up, improve and optimize protein properties, which improve performance and safety as well as shortening times and costs for the development and production processes. Computational design and discovery of new antibody or antibody-based therapeutics would make immunotherapy more affordable.

This chapter focuses on the structure-function-dynamics of antibodies and their importance in the pharmaceutical sector and summarizes how recent computational tools play a vital role in the development and production of antibody and antibody-based therapeutics. We present here general protocols for how to use current computational tools efficiently. In the last part of this chapter, we focus on the great market value of these antibody-based targeted therapies, growing investment of pharmaceutical industry into mAb therapies as the personalized medicine field is expanding.

11.2 Antibody structure and function

Monoclonal antibodies, also called immunoglobulins (Igs), have five isotypes: IgA, IgD, IgE, IgG, and IgM. IgGs are the most relevant immunoglobulins for

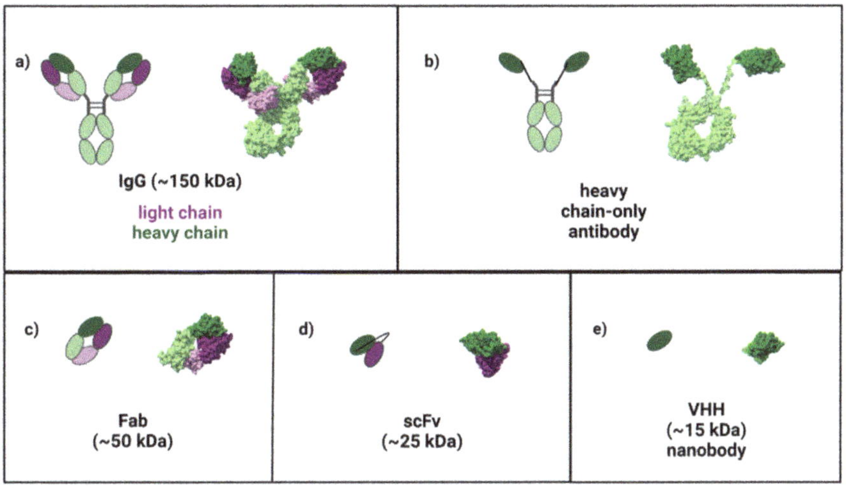

Figure 11.1. Schematic representations and structures of different antibody formats. (a) full IgG, (b) heavy chain-only antibody, (c) Fab (fragment antigen binding) region which is composed of one constant and one variable domain of each of the heavy and the light chains. (d) scFv, single-chain variable fragment which is an engineered antibody fusing heavy (VH) and light chains (VL) of immunoglobulins by a short polypeptide linker. (e) VHH antibody (or nanobody) is the antigen binding fragment of heavy chain-only camelid antibodies. UCSF Chimera was used to prepare 3D protein images in all figures of this chapter [11].

therapeutic purposes with a molecular weight of around 150 kDa. IgGs can bind to their specific target with nanomolar to picomolar affinities. IgGs are Y-shaped molecules, made up of four chains; two heavy (H) and two light (L) chains (figure 11.1). The N-terminal part of heavy and light chains have variable domains, which are together responsible for binding to the target antigen. Specifically, the complementarity determining regions (CDRs) on the variable domains of heavy and (VH and VL) recognize and bind to the target antigen. There are two copies of identical VH and VL domains binding identical sites on two antigen molecules (figure 11.1). Other parts of an IgG molecule are called constant domains (CH or CL); three CHs in heavy chain (CH1, CH2 and CH3) and one CL in light chain. The four chains in IgGs are held together with highly conserved disulfide bonds and non-covalent interactions such as electrostatic interactions, hydrogen bonds, van der Waals interactions and hydrophobic effect [6, 7].

In addition to full-length monoclonal antibodies, there are antibody fragments which are smaller in size. Each of the two arms of the Y-shaped IgG, which is composed of VH and CH1 of heavy chain, and whole light chain, is called Fab (antigen binding fragment) (figure 11.1(c)). When the two variable domains from the heavy and light chains are joined together through a linker peptide, this molecule is called the single-chain variable fragment (scFv) (figure 11.1(d)). These antibody fragments carry the specificity of an antibody to its corresponding antigen in a much smaller size and become very useful when size is important in such cases as quick clearance from blood or deep tissue penetration. The dimerized constant domains of heavy chains are called constant or crystallizable fragment (Fc) in antibodies.

In addition to conventional antibodies, there are heavy chain-only antibodies discovered in camelids and sharks in the 1990s. Unlike standard IgGs, these antibodies are missing the light chain and CH1 domain from the heavy chain [8, 9]. N-terminal domain of a heavy chain-only antibody, a single domain, is enough to bind to its antigen with nanomolar to picomolar affinity (figure 11.1(b)). This single domain when isolated from the whole antibody is called a nanobody or VHH. Small size, thermal and chemical stability, and ease of production of nanobodies makes them attractive new antibody fragments in the field of antibody engineering. We would like to direct the reader's attention to the section called nanobodies for more details on these molecules. There are also various other forms of engineered antibody fragment. They are not in the scope of this book chapter. Goulet and Atkins wrote an excellent review on these molecules [10].

11.2.1 Antigen recognition and binding

Overall, the amino acid sequences of antibodies are relatively conserved. This is reflected in antibody structures. Each variable and constant domain folds into a globular-like immunoglobulin fold. The highest variation in amino acid sequence is observed in the complementarity determining regions (CDRs) of the variable domains (VH and VL). These variable regions are close in 3D structure, and all together form the paratope and are responsible for antigen recognition. The paratope's complementary region on the antigen is called the epitope. How these CDR regions are positioned depends on the targeted antigen. Antibodies targeting a small antigen can have their CDRs close and create an opening just enough for the antigen to bind. On the other hand, antibodies targeting larger antigens have wide CDRs surfaces, thus creating an area appropriate for the antigen binding [12]. An antibody's CDRs and its antigen interact through reversible non-covalent interactions. These interactions are electrostatic interactions, hydrogen bonds, Van der Waals forces, and hydrophobic forces. Which of these forces are dominant when binding depends on the antigen type. For example, antibodies that target protein antigens can have many aromatic amino acids at the binding interface and these amino acids generally take part in van der Waals and hydrophobic interactions [13].

11.2.2 Fragment crystallizable (Fc)

In the early days, when intact IgGs were treated with papain large fragments one third of the size of the whole IgG was produced. Later, it was understood that one fragment was able to bind the antigen which is called Fab today. Another similar-sized fragment was not binding to the antigen, and it was easily crystallized, which is called the crystallizable fragment or Fc. In IgGs, the dimer of heavy chain constant domains forms the Fc region. Fc region of an IgG can bind to Fc receptors on immune cells and initiate various immune activation mechanisms for destruction of the foreign body such as antibody-dependent cellular cytotoxicity (ADCC), antibody-dependent cell-mediated phagocytosis (ADCP) and complement-dependent cytotoxicity (CDC) [14].

11.2.3 Antibody function

Antibodies can be examined under five different classes: IgA, IgD, IgE, IgG, and IgM. These classes are separated by their function in the body and their targets. After binding their target antigen, antibodies either directly neutralize the target or they recruit immune cells and assist in elimination of the target. In antibody structure, both the variable and constant domains have certain functions for a properly functioning immune system [15]. The variable region of the antibody is responsible for recognizing the targeted antigen. This recognition is mostly mediated through the CDRs from both the light and heavy chain. The constant region of the antibody is responsible for mediating the interaction with immune cells and activating the immune system for destruction of a foreign body.

An antibody can trigger many processes in the body through molecular interactions. There are four responses to the antibody–antigen interaction: neutralization, antibody-mediated cytotoxicity, CDC and using an antibody as a cargo for drug delivery [18]. Neutralization occurs when a designed antibody blocks the interaction of the target. For example, when an antibody and a viral antigen on a virus' surface form a complex, the antibody inhibits virus' entry into the cell. In another case, an antibody binding to a cell surface protein or receptor inhibits cellular signalling progress. Several ligand-blocking antibodies are on the market such as Bevacizumab, which is used for treatment of colorectal cancer via blocking vascular epidermal growth factor (VEGF) [16] Antibody–receptor interaction can prevent a ligand binding to that receptor. For example, trastuzumab is used for blocking HER2 receptor in breast cancer [16]. Blocking of receptor–ligand interaction causes disruption in signaling pathway leading to loss of cellular activity or activation of apoptotic pathways.

Antibodies could be used as targeting agents because of the specificity of antibodies for their antigen. Abs can carry toxins, drugs, cytokines, or radioisotopes to the target site. These molecules are called antibody–drug conjugates. It is advantageous to use antibodies for drug delivery because the drug can be used in higher doses due to antibody–antigen specificity and despite higher doses it can be less toxic for healthy cells because of targeted delivery. The reader is advised to check out the section on antibody–drug conjugates below. Both are ways that the host immune system interacts with therapeutic antibodies. While ADCC uses the effector cell of the host, CDC uses C1 complex of the host. Antibody binds its specific antigen from variable domains on the surface of a target cell, then the Fc region of the antibody interacts with effector cells such as natural killer cells or macrophages initiating ADCC. The targeted cell is destroyed by an immune effector cell [16]. On the other hand, CDC is a complex that is composed of plasma and cell surface protein and has a role in cell lysis [17]. CDC occurs when the C1 complex binds to the antibody–antigen complex, starts a series of complement protein reactions, and creates a complex that damages the target cell's membrane [18].

Depending on the type of response expected such as blocking or immune cell-mediated destruction of target, there are various kinds of engineered antibodies. All are developed through costly, laborious experimental techniques like phage display or animal immunization. Developing computational methods can reduce the number of possible candidate antibodies or antibody fragments tested in these costly experimental screening processes. In addition, molecular level details of the binding interface can be acquired.

11.3 Computational tools for antibody design

Servers and tools that are currently not accessible are omitted in this chapter. Computational methods have great potential to design and generate novel, successful and developable biologics such as enzymes, peptides, and antibodies. The development process of an antibody might take up to ~12 years. The process would include target validation, discovery, early screening, lead candidate, and its optimization, preclinical and clinical trials and finally the production [19]. Therefore, early design and fast development of a potent candidate antibody is needed to meet the market demand, especially during unprecedented times such as a pandemic. Computational tools extensively help reduce the number of experiments and cost since they can suggest or accurately predict the optimum conditions, therefore reducing the wide design space. Several state-of-the-art methods are available that can be used in designing antibody and antibody-based structures. These methods are reviewed in recent review articles and books [20–22]. Also, there are a couple of excellent benchmark studies that compare structure modeling tools in terms of antibody modeling [23]. In this section, we present useful general protocols that show how to use antibody-specific computational tools and how to incorporate general others, which are used in the drug discovery, for antibody structure design, antibody–antigen interface prediction, antibody affinity maturation, prediction of developability and immunogenicity.

11.3.1 Antibody databases

The availability of larger and more accurate datasets is a prerequisite for computational tools to assess and create antibody structures. There are several databases either free or commercial that can be used for therapeutic antibody development. Some databases use sequence data, e.g., International Immunogenetics Information System (IMGT [24, 25], abYsis [26], iReceptor [27], Observed Antibody Space (OAS, [28]), AbDiver [29], and AntiBERTy [30]. Some of the sequence-based databases such as abYsis include artificially engineered sequence information. There are several databases that include structure information, e.g., IMGT/3D-Structure-DB [31], Structural Antibody Database (SabDAb [32], abYsis [26] and AbDb [33], Immune Epitope Database (IEDB [34]. The Protein Data Bank (RCSB [35]) is the main resource for 3D structure of any biomolecular system; therefore, it is always an option. There are also resources that combine sequence and structure data with available experimental data such as binding affinity (SAbDab [32] and PDBBind [36]), binding energy (SKEMPI [37], which is not an antibody-specific database), mutation (AB-Bind [38] or epitope-specific antibody sequence IEDB [34]).

11.3.2 Structure prediction

Even a human body might produce around 10^{12} different antibodies [39, 40], however, there are only ~3250 human antibody 3D structures available as of March 2023 in SAbDab [32]. At that point, computational structure modeling tools would be very helpful since antibodies are highly conserved in terms of both structure and sequence of their framework region. Therefore, classical methods like homology modeling using either available antibodies or proteins in general would yield promising antibody models. Besides classical methods, machine learning- and deep learning-based methods that use either sequence or structure datasets are recently hot tools in the field. Machine learning ones either learn inputs to generate outputs that describe the relationship in the system components, called supervised learning, or learn the hidden patterns (unsupervised learning) in the input and predict if new data has the same or similar pattern(s). Deep learning-based methods are a subclass of machine learning, and they mimic the human brain with the help of deep neural networks which the data is trained on.

Figure 11.2 shows a summary of general protocols to design an antibody. Starting from the known amino acid sequence information, an appropriate framework template selection is needed so that CDR loops can be incorporated easily. For this, databases such as SAbDab [32] can be used to find the closest sequence that is like the heavy (H) and light (L) chains. Then, the relative orientation of the VH and VL domains can be determined using tools such as Rosetta [41] to define the correct shape of the binding site of the antibody—*paratope*. The next step would be the modeling of functionally important CDR loops in an antibody. For this, ABlooper [42], RosettaAntibodyDesign [43], Parapred [44], proABC-2 [45, 46], FREAD [47] and AntBO [48] can be used. AntBO [48] tool outperforms other approaches and uses Absolut! [49] to obtain binding affinity calculation for each generated conformation in AntBO. In addition, general protein or Ab-specific structure prediction tools, which can provide complete modeling of a protein, can also be used such as AlphaFold [50], Chroma [51], LYRA [52], tFold [53], and NanoNet (optimized for VHH) [54].

The next step is the side-chain prediction and refinement using tools such as Rosetta [55, 56]. The full model having the CDRs and side-chains can be energetically optimized using Rosetta [57]. Besides these great tools, one can use free webservers/packages or commercial tools that are either physics- and/or machine-learning-based such as RosettaAntibodyDesign [43] and ABodyBuilder2 [58, 59]. The latter is currently the fastest free webserver. ABodyBuilder2 server is an antibody homology modeling pipeline that includes all the steps explained above. ABodyBuilder2 has a lower accuracy (< 3 Å) for the CDR-H3 loops compared to other methods such as ABlooper that uses graph neural network [42]. However, it is a faster (~30 sec) method compared to some others. Ruffolo *et al* (2022) developed DeepAB that can predict an antibody structure in 10 min, which is dependent on Rosetta [59]. DeepAB is a recurrent neural network encoder-decoder model that can learn features from amino acid sequence of the query antibody. Its CDR-H3 loop prediction accuracy is 2.33 Å. This algorithm is specifically designed for antibody

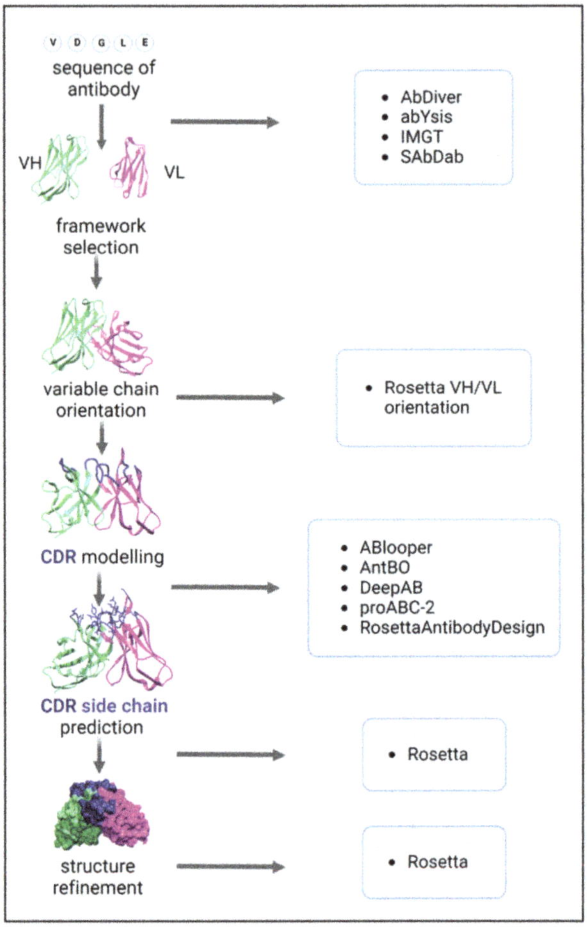

Figure 11.2. Antibody modeling involves creating a 3D representation of an antibody-based on its amino acid sequence. This is done by identifying the framework templates and positioning the VH/VL domains in relation to each other, in cases where they come from separate molecules. The CDRs are then added to the framework, and the final step is to improve the accuracy of the entire structure through energy optimization. Server/tool names are alphabetically ordered. The figure is adapted from [21] CC BY 4.0.

structure prediction, but not for nanobodies (please see section titled Nanobodies for more details). The same group developed another method called IgFold [60], which can predict a structure in less than one minute. IgFold provides accurate predictions for nanobody structures. In addition to these free servers and packages, there are commercial packages available such as BioLuminate (Schrödinger Inc., www.schrodinger.com), Biovia (Accelrys, https://www.3ds.com/products-services/biovia/), MOE (CCG, www.chemcomp.com) and SmrtMolAntibody (Macromoltek, www.makromoltek.com) tools, which also offer other useful modules in addition to structure modelling and interaction detection.

Current computational tools yield significant results, however, CDR-H3 loop prediction is still challenging since CDR-H3 loops with very similar sequences can adopt different conformations [61–63]. Kuroda and Tsumoto (2023) visually inspected CDR-H3 regions in 370 different VHH antibodies and identified three main structural classes in CDR regions as helical bending, kinked and extended conformation and eight subclasses (chapter 2 in reference [25]). A recent great tool, AlphaFold2 [50], which predicts 3D structures from the sequence by using the template structures and multiple sequence alignment data, is unfortunately not applicable to CDR-H3 loop modelling, yet, since 3D structures of antibodies are currently limited. However, AlphaFold-Multimer [64] can be used to predict antibody–antigen complex structures in an hour. EquiFold [65] performs better than AlphaFold-Multimer and IgFold and predicts 3D structures of antibodies in 1 sec with a similar or better accuracy compared to the others. A general protocol to model loop regions in antibodies can be found in the study of Marin and Marcatili (2023) where both advantages and disadvantages of loop modelling methods are discussed (chapter 3 in reference [25]).

11.3.3 Interface prediction

Experimentally determined 3D structures of antibody–antigen complexes provide crucial information about the critical interactions between them. However, these complexes are big, therefore experimental determination requires more time and money. Currently, there are rapid computational methods that can predict antibody–antigen interface, so called paratope–epitope contacts. In this part, we summarize these tools that are either paratope-, epitope-, or paratope–epitope-focused and provide a general protocol and suggested tools, shown in figure 11.3. Application of machine learning and deep learning in the epitope–paratope interface prediction is crucial for the rational design of antibodies as well as diagnostics and vaccine development. The most recent and free paratope prediction tools are proABC-2 (convolutional neural network) [45, 46], Parapred (deep learning) ([44], AntibodyInterface Prediction (support vector machine) [66], ABlooper (graph neural network) [59], and AntiBERTa [67]. The predicted paratope structures can be further optimized in terms of binding affinity using tools such as mmCSM-AB [68] or mCSM-AB2 [69]. CDR regions on the paratope comprise most of the directly interacting residues with the epitope. However, there are also residues in the framework region, which interact with the antigen. For this, Paratome [70] tool can be advantageous to identify these residues in the framework region that might have a role in the antigen recognition. AntibodyInterface Prediction, AG-Fast-Parapred and proABC-2 are the best performing tools for the paratope prediction.

Knowing antibody sequence/structure results in better epitope prediction and this is called antibody-specific epitope prediction. When the epitope is not known, the epitope prediction methods become very useful. Linear epitope prediction servers, which are currently available and active, are ABCpred [71], BepiPred-2.0 [72], iBCE-EL [73], and SVMTriP [74].

PEASE [75] is a free webserver to design and predict the epitope of a given antibody sequence. REBELOT repository (chapter 13 in reference [25]) uses an energy decomposition method called matrix of local coupling energies (MLCE) [76–78],

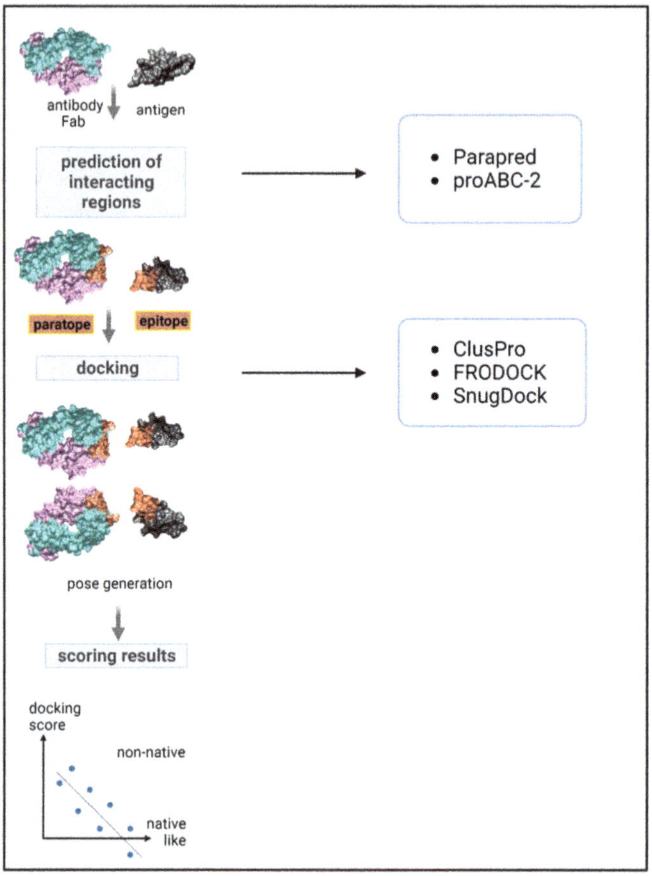

Figure 11.3. Antibody interface prediction is the process of determining the specific amino acid residues on an antibody that interact with an antigen. This can be thought of as a type of molecular docking, which aims to recreate the binding interaction between the antibody and antigen. Ideal binding poses are selected by scoring structures as native and non-native. Server/tool names are alphabetically ordered. The figure is adapted from [21] CC BY 4.0.

and PECAN [79] is a free repository that can be used for both epitope and paratope prediction. SEPPA 3.0 [80], Epitopia [81, 82] and Discotope 2.0 [83] are other free webservers. After finding the correct antibody–antigen complex, the specific interactions in these complexes need to be identified. For this, molecular docking tools are great resources to sample and analyze several possible complex conformations. Some tools can even perform and/or offer antibody-specific docking and scoring such as **ClusPro** [84, 85], **SnugDock** [41, 86] and FRODOCK 2.0 [87]. One can also use general protein docking tools such as ATTRACT [88], **HADDOCK** [89, 90], Hex [91], GRAMM-X [92], PatchDock [93, 94], pyDock [95], **Swarmdock** [96], and PIPER (Schrödinger, [97, 98] (The tools written in bold in the last two sentences are the ones that can also perform flexible docking, which considers conformational changes in the structures).

On the other hand, consideration of epitope information during antibody design is also crucial for more accurate structure prediction with better specificity and affinity. Recently, a monoclonal antibody that is the first computationally designed antibody, which entered clinical trials, called AU-007, is a promising therapeutic antibody that targets IL-2 for the treatment of cancer. The monoclonal antibody was designed by the company, Biolojic Design and presently by Aulos Bioscience Inc. According to the developer company's report [105], the epitope information was included during the design process of the AU-007 antibody. Currently, the details of the design process were not found to be available in any article. However, several posters and a video presentation were observed to be available on Aulos Bioscience Inc.'s website [99]. AU-007 was reported to be the first computationally designed human immunoglobulin G1 (IgG1) monoclonal antibody in clinical trials that inhibits tumor growth by binding to the CD25 interacting part of IL-2. In this scope, the binding of IL-2 to IL-2R dimer which contains CD122 and CD132 subunits was indicated to be maintained while the IL-2 binding to the IL-2R trimer which is composed of CD25, CD122, and CD132 subunits was blocked. This approach was pointed out to be significant since the decline in toxicity can be achieved by blocking the binding. On the other hand, the Fc domain of the antibody was indicated to contain LALA double mutations (Leu to Ala) as an effector silent [100]. The computational design of AU-007 is mainly composed of three steps including finding template antibody, determination of mutations for certain positions to obtain higher binding affinity, and analysis of binding as well as humanness. Machine learning was observed to be used in all these steps [99, 101].

Molecular dynamics (MD) simulations are also very effective in elucidating antibody–antigen interactions and different CDR conformations at all-atom level. One can perform an MD simulation for antibody-only, antigen-only and/or antibody–antigen complex in a wild-type or mutant form to investigate the dynamics of the system of interest in a range of changing environments such as pH, temperature, pressure. There are several examples of MD software such as AMBER [102], **CHARMM** [103], Desmond [104], **Gromacs** [105], and **NAMD** [106] etc (their names are alphabetically ordered, and freely available ones are written in bold).

Childers and Daggett (2023) summarized how to integrate MD simulations into the effort of understanding antibody–antigen systems (chapter 5 in reference [25]). Fine *et al* (1986) and Shenkin *et al* (1987) performed the first MD simulations of antibodies to predict antibody hypervariable loop conformations [107, 108]. A study by Yamashita (2023) suggests an umbrella sampling (US) method that follows a multistep targeted MD simulation (US/mTMD). They explained the application steps of this method to hen egg-white lysozyme and its antibody HyHEL-10 and analysis of MD simulation, however, the simulation results are not provided (chapter 4 in reference [25]).

Tucs *et al* (2023) applied constrained geometric all-atom simulation method called FRODAN to study the dynamics of IgG2a monoclonal antibody (chapter 6 in reference [25]). They also combined FRODAN with Monte Carlo Tree Search (MCTS) method (a type of reinforcement learning algorithm) [109, 110]. They analyzed the distribution of domain-domain distance values and noticed that their results overlapped with the experimental findings by Bongini *et al* [111, 112]. The FRODAN in combination with MCTS yielded all-atom conformation for the IgG2a with an RMSD value of 5.8 Å with respect to the target structure.

Bekker and Kamiya groups used MD to predict CDR-H3 structure [113] and antibody–antigen complex [114], also to refine/rank rigid-body antibody–antigen docking decoys [115]. Later, the same groups performed high-temperature MD simulations using Gromacs to estimate the thermal stability of seven different single-domain antibodies (chapter 8 in reference [25]). They showed a good correlation between the fraction of native contacts (Q-value, [116]) and experimental melting temperatures and identified potential stabilizing mutants.

Zhang and Dalby (2023) computationally characterized an anti-TNF-alpha antibody fragment called Fab A33 (chapter 9 in reference [25]). First, they modelled the structure using RosettaCM [117], then applied MD in Gromacs to identify the flexible regions in the Fab. They predicted the mutational ΔΔGvalues using Rosetta cartesian_ddg method [118] and suggested single point mutations that improve the stability of the Fab.

Jia and Sun (2023) studied the deamidation of asparagine residues on CDR regions from 25 different antibodies, which can affect binding potency of antibodies (chapter 10 in reference [25]). They developed a structure-based Asn deamidation predictive model by applying six different supervised machine learning methods partial least squares (PLS), K-nearest neighbor (KNN), (SVM, random forests (RF), naïve Bayes classifier (NBC), and artificial neural network (ANN). Their predictive model uses different types of descriptors such as pentapeptide deamidation half-life, Asn torsion angles and local secondary structure information, normalized B-factor values for key carbon atoms in the backbone and side-chains, percent solvent accessibility and percent side-chain solvent accessibility, and nucleophilic attack C–N distance. According to their cross-validation accuracy values, the RF algorithm outperformed the others. Also, they applied MD using Schrödinger Desmond to obtain insights on the deamidation in antibodies and calculated cumulative time occupancy for the nucleophilic attack C–N distance throughout the trajectories. Their analysis correctly predicted 12 out of 17 Asn residues that have deamidation tendency.

Qiao *et al* (2021) computationally analyzed 350 antigen–antibody complexes using molecular mechanics and MD simulations. They extracted antibody-interacting residues on the antigens and examined them according to secondary structure, residue population, binding affinity, and structural stability. For each complex, molecular mechanics calculations were applied to obtain energy-minimized structures. Then, they used DSSP program to define secondary structure information for each extracted region from antigens. 350 complexes were classified into four groups (helix, sheet, turn, and coil) according to the secondary structure information. Turn was the most popular one. They noticed that they are mostly charged polar residues with a small population of hydrophobic residues and hydrophilic interactions are dominant. Three complexes were selected from each group and a single MD run applied for each complex to observe if there is any change on the stability of secondary structure [119].

Bai *et al* (2021) computationally designed a single-chain, biparatopic bispecific antibody that targets *Staphylococcal enterotoxin* B (SEB) and blocks its interaction with the T-cell receptor (TCR) [120]. They mixed two anti-SEB antibodies, namely 14G8 and 6D3, which can block SEB–TCR interactions. They performed extensive MD simulations (18.9 microseconds) where almost all simulations have two replicates and found that the designed bispecific antibody MB102a allosterically affects SEB–TCR association. They observed that the SEB–TCR complex dissociated after 159 ns of the simulation in the presence of the antibody. A similar observation was obtained for the SEB–TCR-MHC II complex after the 460 ns of the simulation. They also tested the effect of different linkers that connect 14G8 and 6D3 antibodies and found that the linkers have subtle effects on the antibody–SEB interactions.

11.3.4 Antibody grafting and humanization

An alternative antibody design is possible by using a technique called grafting where the CDR regions of the known antibody–antigen complex are transferred onto the framework of the candidate antibody structure (figure 11.4). Recently, Rangel *et al* (2022) used this method to design single-domain antibodies for SARS-CoV-2 [121]. They divide possible epitope regions into small fragments (at least four residues) to be used as a query for a structural search in a database of antigen-like and CDR-like interacting fragments. This database is used to find possible CDR-like fragments. Then, they combine identified CDR-like fragments and optimize the designed CDR motifs in terms of paratope–epitope contacts. The optimized motifs are grafted onto antibody frameworks. They tested their method on six different single-domain antibodies that target three different epitope regions including receptor binding domain (RBD) of the SARS-CoV-2 spike protein. However, another recent method by Ruffolo *et al* (2022) outperformed compared to earlier grafting approaches. Their DeepAb method uses a deep residual convolutional network to predict the variable fragment region. In addition, the structure formation was achieved using Rosetta [59].

Antibodies against specific antigens are usually generated by animal immunization and murine species are preferred due to their genetic similarity to humans. These non-human antibodies which are developed against a human disease antigen for medical treatment purposes must be modified to prevent any adverse immune reaction known as anti-drug antibodies (ADAs). One method can be replacing the variable fragment of a human IgG antibody with the variable fragments of antigen specific antibody creating a chimeric antibody with around 70% human sequence (figure 11.5). Another method is called humanization which involves CDR grafting of antigen-specific animal-derived antibody to a human antibody framework or modifying the animal-derived antibody to resemble human antibody framework (figures 11.4 and 11.5) [122]. However, humanization is not a direct method, grafting CDR regions of animal-derived antibody onto human antibody framework might create a loss in affinity to the antigen or a loss in stability of the antibody.

It is possible to compare the sequences of both framework and CDRs of animal-derived antibody with human antibodies. This allows choosing the best candidate

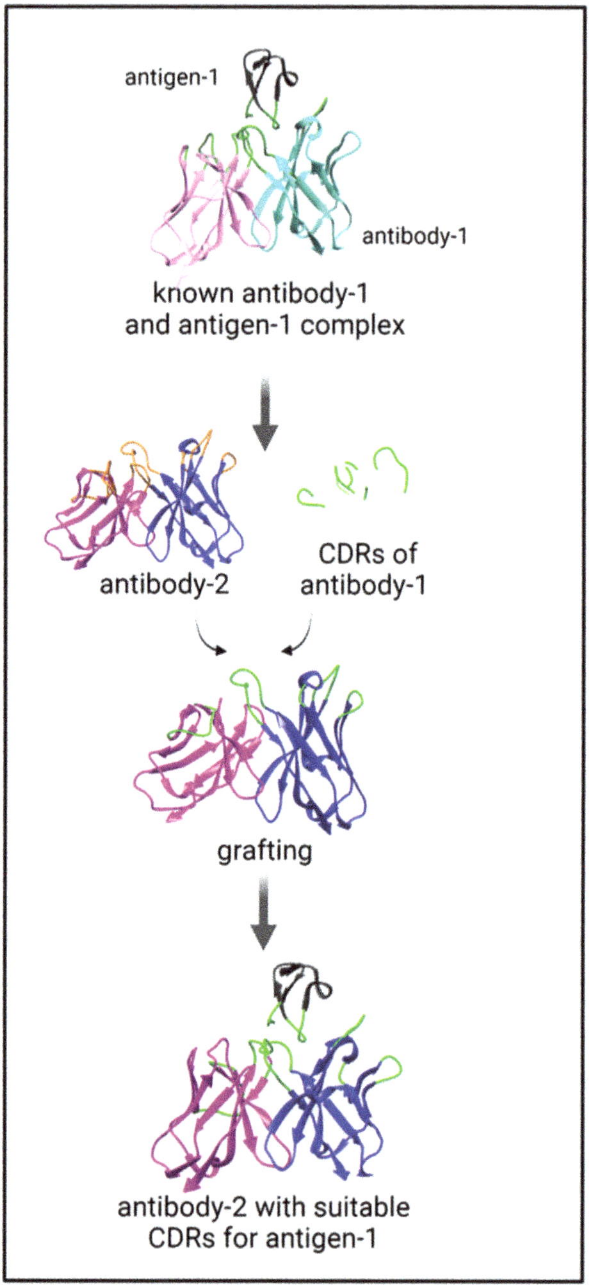

Figure 11.4. Antibody design aims to improve binding of an antibody to a desired antigen epitope. Model antibody–antigen complex can be generated with computational tools like docking and energy optimization. Well-known binding patterns (CDRs) of antibody from a model of antibody–antigen complex are taken and incorporated into another antibody template. The figure is adapted from [21] CC BY 4.0.

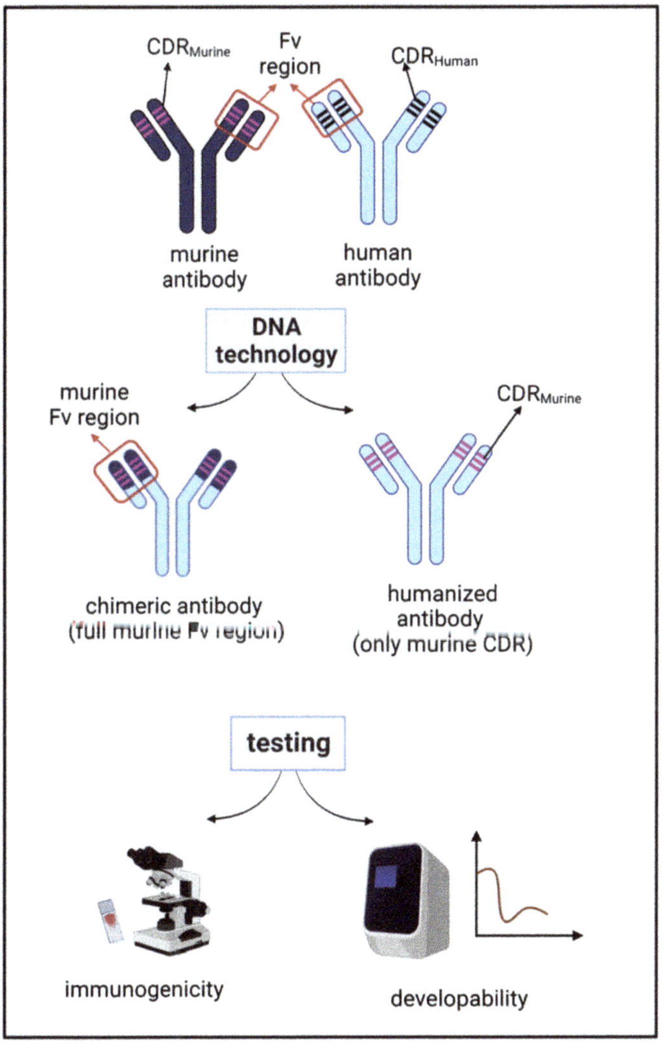

Figure 11.5. Method of creating chimeric or humanized antibodies. Raising antibodies against certain antigens in animals, such as murine species, is a common procedure. Humanization is required for antibody drug development to prevent undesired immune reaction and have desirable physical characteristics. The process of humanization involves changing the sequence of an animal-derived antibody to resemble a human antibody while maintaining its binding capacity and specificity. Following humanization, the engineered antibody is evaluated for developability and immunogenicity. Adapted from [21] CC BY 4.0.

human framework for the best binding CDR regions. This method is called super humanization [123]. Another method called resurfacing involves comparing the surfaces of variable regions of animal-derived antibody and the human antibody. There is high sequence similarity between murine and human antibody Fv regions but there are key surface residues that are different and these need to be humanized for therapeutic use [124]. Sequence comparison can be analyzed with statistical tools to give a humanness score to the sequence [125]. However, primary structure comparison is useful to a certain extent. Tools discussed below are taking the humanization process to the 3D structure level.

Recently, a couple of webservers and free tools have been developed by different groups to make the Ab humanization process easier and faster. CUMAb [126] Computational hUMan AntiBody design (enabled for academic use), is a free web-accessible method that uses an experimental or model antibody structure as input. Grafting of animal CDRs is systematically performed in CUMAb for thousands of human frameworks, then Rosetta atomistic simulations are used to rank the grafted designs by energy and structural integrity. Sang *et al* (2022) have developed an open-source computational pipeline called Llamanade, which offers a rational humanization of nanobodies with the help of big data [127]. CoDAH can predict humanizing mutations that either does not affect or affects minimally the folding stability of the structure. The source code for CoDAH is freely available for academic use [128].

Jayakody *et al* (2021) computationally humanized aldolase catalytic antibody 38C2 using homology modeling and generated a 3D atomistic model of humanized abzyme 38C2. Then, they investigated the stability of the structure, ligand binding and binding sites. They also performed quantum mechanical calculations to deeply investigate the catalytic residues at the binding site. The generated model was validated in terms of accuracy and reliability [129].

11.3.5 Developability

In addition to design and validation, the physicochemical properties of antibodies should be evaluated for developability. There are certain factors that affect the developability of an antibody such as aggregation, viscosity, poly-specificity and thermostability. Computational fast prediction of these factors could reduce late-stage risks and failures during the development and production processes and provide better optimized candidates. CamSol [130] can be used for solubility prediction and optimization of antibodies. Wolf Perez *et al* (2019) were able to engineer the developability of IgG4 monoclonal antibody by using CamSol [131].

Immunogenicity prediction is another very important step during antibody design and development to check the safety of an antibody. PITHA webserver is a machine-learning-based immunogenicity prediction algorithm for humanized and fully human therapeutics antibodies [132]. Their SVM algorithm uses sequence and structural properties of CDR regions such as hydrophobicity and cavity volume. The accuracy of the method is 83% for 29 different therapeutic antibodies.

Another tool, Therapeutic Antibody Profile (TAP) [133] is focused on the developability of antibodies. Developability here comprises immunogenicity, solubility, conformational stability, specificity, storability, and manufacturability. A high-affinity antibody might not have all good characteristics that are necessary for its developability [134]. TAP can offer a route to rapidly identifying drug-candidate antibodies that are likely to have poor developability. They build a homology model for each post-Phase-1 therapeutic antibody. Then, they measure the five TAP metrics, namely the total CDR length, surface hydrophobicity of the CDR patches, surface positive and negative charges, and structural Fv charge symmetry parameter. The total job time takes a couple of minutes if MODELLER is used for modeling, otherwise an hour since Sphinx H3 is used for CDR modeling [135].

11.4 Antibodies and antibody-based structures and their applications

11.4.1 Antibody drugs

Antibodies are immune system generated proteins highly specific to their target antigens. Antibodies can neutralize their target antigen by binding, or through effector function they can activate the host immune system after target binding, as explained in section 11.3. Table 11.1 gives a list of approved monoclonal antibody therapies against various disease targets.

11.4.2 Nanobodies

Single domain, antigen binding region of camelid heavy chain-only antibodies are known as nanobodies. It is possible to generate naïve, synthetic or antigen specific phage display libraries to screen for nanobodies (Nbs) against immunogenic proteins [136]. Nanobodies have specific features like small size (15 kDa), high affinity to their target antigen, ease of production, stability, better solubility, fast blood clearance, deep tissue penetration, multimerization or formatting possibility, and low immunogenicity. Nearly 90% sequence similarity exists between nanobodies and human antibodies. These advantages make nanobodies great tools for diagnosis and targeted therapeutics of cancer, infections, and autoimmune diseases [137–144]. Nanobodies can be in monovalent, bivalent, trivalent, pentavalent, bispecific, and biparatopic forms. Nanobodies specific for different antigens can be combined creating multivalent chimeric versions with high affinity or efficacy [145].

With the advances in recombinant DNA technology, numerous antibody fragments and chimeras have been created. Two of the most favorite versions are camelid heavy-chain variable domains (VHHs or nanobodies) and single-chain variable fragments (scFvs). The size and position of the CDR3 loop have significant differences between the human VH domain and the camelid VHH. The CDR3 loop length of nanobodies varies widely (3–28 amino acids). Generally, the antigen-binding surface of conventional mAbs is typically flat, however nanobodies can bind to concave, convex and hard to reach epitopes. Nanobodies can be utilized as an alternative to scFv because of their superior chemical and physical characteristics, such as higher solubility, stability, smaller size, and reduced production cost. Despite Nbs' superior qualities, scFvs continue to rule the clinic, with around ten treatments having received FDA approval and more than eighty in clinical trials. [146, 147].

To emphasize and highlight the trend of nanobody research, 'nanobody' term was searched from the PubMed database on 13 February 2023. There is an increasing trend in the total amount of research conducted on nanobodies. Between 1982–2003, there were only a few studies in this field, but after 2004 it accelerated. The number of articles doubled after 2019. Only 27 of them are the results of clinical trials. In table 11.2, 21 studies from clinical trials website are summarized with the nanobody

Table 11.1. List of approved antibody therapeutics in the market. Data extracted from http://clinicaltrials.gov/ct2/home.

Approval year	Brand name	Generic name	Target	Format	Disease type	Website
1986	OrthocloneOKT3	Muromonab-CD3	CD3	Murine IgG2a	Hybridoma/Janssen Biotech, Inc.	NA
1994	ReoPro®	Abciximab	GPIIb/IIIa	Chimeric IgG1Fab	Prevention of blood clots in angioplasty	NA
1997	MabThera, Rituxan®	Rituximab	CD20	Chimeric IgG	Non-Hodgkins lymphoma	https://www.rituxan-hcp.com
1998	Synagis®	Palivizumab	RSV	Humanized IgG	Prevention of respiratory syncytial virus infection	https://www.synagis.co.uk
1998	Remicade®	Infliximab	ITNFα	Chimeric IgG	Crohn's disease	https://www.remicade.com
1998	Herceptin®	Trastuzumab	HER2	Humanized IgG	Breast cancer	https://www.herceptin.com
2001	Campath®, Lemtrada®	Alemtuzumab	CD52	Humanized IgG	Chronic myeloid leukemia	https://www.lemtrada.com
2002	Humira®	Adalimumab	TNFα	Human IgG1	Rheumatoid arthritis	https://www.humira.com
2003	XOLAIR®	Omalizumab	IgE	Humanized IgG	Asthma	https://www.xolair.com
2004	Erbitux®	Cetuximab	EGFR	Chimeric IgG	Colorectal cancer	https://www.erbitux.com
2004	Avastin®	Bevacizumab	VEGF-A	Humanized IgG	Colorectal cancer	https://www.avastin.com
2004	Tysabri®	Natalizumab	ITGA4	Humanized IgG	Multiple sclerosis	https://www.tysabri.com
2006	Vectibix®	Panitumumab	EGFR	Human IgG2	Colorectal cancer	https://www.vectibix.com
2006	Lucentis®	Ranibizumab	VEGF-A	Humanized IgG1Fab	Macular degeneration	https://www.lucentis.com
2007	Soliris®	Eculizumab	C5	Humanized IgG2/4	Paroxysmal nocturnal hemoglobin uria	https://solirisgmg.com
2008	Cimzia®	Certolizumab pegol	TNFα	Humanized Fab, PEGylated	Crohn's disease	https://www.cimzia.com

2009	Stelara®	Ustekinumab	IL-12/23	Human IgG1	Psoriasis	https://www.stelarahcp.com
2009	Ilaris®	Canakinumab	IL-1β	Human IgG1	Muckle-Wells syndrome	https://www.ilaris.com
2009	Simponi®	Golimumab	TNFα	Human IgG1	Rheumatoid and psoriatic arthritis, ankylosing spondylitis	https://www.simponi.com
2009	Arzerra®	Ofatumumab	CD20	Human IgG1	Chronic lymphocytic leukemia	https://www.us.arzerra.com
2010	RoActemraActemra®	Tocilizumab	IL-6R	Humanized IgG	Rheumatoid arthritis	https://www.actemra.com
2010	Xgeva®, Prolia®	Denosumab	RANKL	Human IgG2	Bone loss	https://www.xgeva.com https://www.prolia.com
2011	Benlysta	Belimumab	BLyS	Human IgG1	Systemic lupus erythematosus	https://www.benlysta.com
2011	Yervoy®	Ipilimumab	CTLA-4	Human IgG1	Metastatic melanoma	https://www.yervoy.com
2012	Perjeta®	Pertuzumab	HER2	Humanized IgG1	Breast Cancer	https://www.perjeta.com
2012	ABthrax	Raxibacumab	B. anthrasis PA	Human IgG1	Anthrax infection	NA
2013	Gazyva®, Gazyvaro	Obinutuzumab	CD20	Humanized IgG1Glyco engineered	Chronic lymphocytic leukemia	https://www.gazyva.com
2014	Sylvant®	Siltuximab	IL-6	Chimeric IgG1	Castleman disease	https://www.sylvant.com
2014	Cyramza®	Ramucirumab	VEGFR2	Human IgG1	Gastric cancer	https://www.cyramza.com
2014	Entyvio®	Vedolizumab	α4β7integrin	Humanized IgG1	Ulcerative colitis, Crohn disease	https://www.entyvio.com
2014	Blincyto®	Blinatumomab	CD19, CD3	Murine bispecific tandem scFv	Acute lymphoblastic leukemia	https://www.blincyto.com

(*Continued*)

Table 11.1. (*Continued*)

Approval year	Brand name	Generic name	Target	Format	Disease type	Website
2014	Opdivo®	Nivolumab	PD-1	Human IgG4	Melanoma, non-small cell lung cancer	https://www.opdivo.com
2014	Keytruda®	Pembrolizumab	PD-1	Humanized IgG	Melanoma	https://www.keytruda.com
2015	Praxbind®	Idarucizumab	Dabigatran	Humanized Fab	Reversal of dabigatran-induced anticoagulation	https://pro.boehringer-ingelheim.com/us/products/praxbind/
2015	Portrazza	Necitumumab	EGFR	Human IgG1	Non-small cell lung cancer	https://www.lillymedical.com/en-us/medical-information/oncology/portrazza
2015	Unituxin®	Dinutuximab	GD2	Chimeric IgG	Neuroblastoma	https://www.unituxin.com
2015	Cosentyx®	Secukinumab	IL-17α	Human IgG1	Psoriasis	https://www.cosentyx.com
2015	Nucala	Mepolizumab	IL-5	Humanized IgG1	Severe eosinophilic asthma	https://www.nucala.com
2015	Praluent	Alirocumab	PCSK9	Human IgG1	High cholesterol	https://www.praluent.com
2015	Repatha®	Evolocumab	PCSK9	Human IgG2	High cholesterol	https://www.repatha.com
2015	Darzalex®	Daratumumab	CD38	Human IgG1	Multiple myeloma	https://www.darzalexhcp.com
2015	Empliciti®	Elotuzumab	SLAMF7	Humanized IgG	Multiple myeloma	https://www.empliciti.com
2016	Taltz®	Ixekizumab	IL-17α	Humanized IgG4	Psoriasis	https://www.taltz.com
2016	Cinqaero, Cinqair®	Reslizumab	IL-5	Humanized IgG	Asthma	https://www.cinqair.com
2016	Lartruvo	Olaratumab	PDGFRα	Human IgG1	Soft tissue sarcoma	NA

2016	Zinplava™	Bezlotoxuma	Clostridium difficile entero toxinB	Human IgG1	Prevention of Clostridium difficile infection recurrence	https://www.merckconnect.com/zinplava/coverage/
2016	Tecentriq®	Atezolizumab	PD-L1	Humanized IgG1	Bladder cancer	https://www.tecentriq.com
2016	Anthim®	Obiltoxaximab	B. anthrasis	Chimeric IgG1	Prevention of inhalational anthrax	https://anthim.com
2017	Siliq®, Lumicef®	Brodalumab	IL-17R	Human IgG2	Plaque psoriasis	https://www.siliq.com, https://www.kyowakirin.com/what_we_do/products/lumicef/index.html
2017	Tremfya®	Guselkumab	IL-23 p19	Human IgG1	Plaque psoriasis	https://www.tremfya.com
2017	Dupixent®	Dupilumab	IL-4Rα	Human IgG4	Atopic dermatitis	https://www.dupixent.com
2017	Kevzara®	Sarilumab	IL-6R	Human IgG1	Rheumatoid arthriti	https://www.kevzara.com
2017	Bavencio®	Avelumab	PD-L1	Human IgG1	Merkel cell carcinoma	https://www.bavencio.com/hcp
2017	Ocrevus®	Ocrelizumab	CD20	Humanized IgG1	Multiple sclerosis	https://www.ocrevus.com
2017	Hemlibra®	Emicizumab	Factor IXa, X	Humanized IgG4, bispecific	Hemophilia A	https://www.hemlibra.com
2017	Fasenra®	Benralizumab	IL-5Rα	Humanized IgG1	Asthma	https://www.fasenrahcp.com
2017	Imfinzi®	Durvalumab	PD-L1	Human IgG1	Bladder cancer	https://www.imfinzi.com
2018	Crysvita®	Burosumab	FGF23	Human IgG1	X-linked hypophosphatemia	https://www.crysvita.com

(*Continued*)

Table 11.1. (*Continued*)

Approval year	Brand name	Generic name	Target	Format	Disease type	Website
2018	Takhzyro®	Lanadelumab	Plasma kallikrein	Human IgG1	Hereditary angioedema attacks	https://www.takhzyro.com
2018	Poteligeo®	Mogamulizumab	CCR4	Humanized IgG1	Mycosis fungoides or Sézary syndrome	https://www.poteligeohcp.com
2018	Aimovig®	Erenumab	CGRPR	Human IgG2	Migraine prevention	https://www.aimovighcp.com
2018	Emgality®	Galcanezuma	CGRP	Humanized IgG4	Migraine prevention	https://www.emgality.com
2018	Ilumya®	Tildrakizumab	IL-23 p19	Humanized IgG1	Plaque psoriasis	https://www.ilumya.com
2018	Libtayo®	Cemiplimab	PD-1	Human mAb	Cutaneous squamous cell carcinoma	https://www.libtayo.com
2018	Gamifant®	Emapalumab	IFNγ	Human IgG1	Primary hemophagocytic lymphohistio cytosis	https://gamifant.com
2018	Ajovy®	Fremanezumab	CGRP	Humanized IgG2	Migraine prevention	https://www.ajovy.com
2018	Trogarzo®	Ibalizumab	CD4	Humanized IgG4	HIV infection	https://www.trogarzo.com
2018	Ultomiris®	Ravulizumab	C5	humanized IgG2/4	Paroxysmal nocturnal hemoglobin uria	https://ultomiris.com › ahus
2019	Cablivi®	Caplacizumab	vonWille brand factor	Humanized Nanobody	Acquired thrombotic thrombocytopenic purpura	https://www.cablivi.com
2019	Evenity®	Romosozumab	Sclerostin	Humanized IgG2	Osteoporosis in postmenopausal women at increased risk of fracture	https://www.evenity.com
2019	Skyrizi®	Risankizumab	IL-23 p19	Humanized IgG1	Plaque psoriasis	https://www.skyrizi.com
2019	Beovu®	Brolucizumab	VEGF-A	Humanized scFv	Macular degeneration	https://www.beovu.com

2019	Adakveo®	Crizanlizumab	P-selectin	Humanized IgG2	Sickle cell disease	https://www.hcp.novartis.com/products/adakveo/sickle-cell-disease/
2020	Vyepti®	Eptinezumab	CGRP	Humanized IgG1	Migraine prevention	https://www.vyepti.com
2020	Sarclisa®	Isatuximab	CD38	Chimeric IgG1	Multiple myeloma	https://www.sarclisa.com
2020	Tepezza	Teprotumumab	IGF-1R	Human IgG1	Thyroid eye disease	https://www.tepezza.com
2020	Uplizna®	Inebilizumab	CD19	Humanized IgG1	Neuromyelitis optica and neuromyelitis optica spectrum disorders	https://www.uplizna.com/eu/
2020	Enspryng®	Satralizumab	IL-6R	Humanized IgG2	Neuromyelitis optica and neuromyelitis optica spectrum disorders	https://www.enspryng.com
2020	Monjuvi®, Minjuvi	Tafasitamab	CD19	Humanized IgG1	Diffuse large B-cell lymphoma	https://www.monjuvi.com
2020	Inmazeb®	Atoltivimab, Maftivimab, and Odesivimab-ebgn	Ebola virus	mixture of 3 human IgG1	Ebola virus infection	https://www.inmazeb.com
2020	Danyelza®	Naxitamab	GD2	Humanized IgG1	High-risk neuroblastoma and refractory osteomedullary disease	https://danyelza.com
2020	Margenza®	Margetuximab	HER2	Chimeric IgG1	HER2+ breast cancer	https://www.margenzahcp.com
2021	Ebanga™	Ansuvimab	Ebola virus	Human IgG1	Ebola infection	https://www.ebanga.com
2021	Jemperli	Dostarlimab	PD-1	Humanized IgG4	Endometrial cancer	https://www.jemperlihcp.com

(Continued)

Table 11.1. (*Continued*)

Approval year	Brand name	Generic name	Target	Format	Disease type	Website
2021	Aduhelm®	Aducanumab	Amyloid-beta	Human IgG1	Alzheimer's disease	https://www.aduhelmhcp.com
2021	Evkeeza®	Evinacumab	Angiopoietin-like 3	Human IgG4	Homozygous familial hypercholesterolemia	https://www.evkeeza.com/s/
2021	Adtralza®	Tralokinumab	IL-13	Human IgG4	Atopic dermatitis	https://www.scottishmedicines.org.uk/medicines-advice/tralokinumab-adtralza-full-smc2403/
2021	Bimzelx®	Bimekizumab	IL-17A, F	Humanized IgG1	Psoriasis	https://www.ucb.com/our-products/Products/Bimzelx®
2021	Saphnelo	Anifrolumab	IFNAR1	Human IgG1	Systemic lupus erythematosus	https://www.saphnelo.com
2021	Rybrevant®	Amivantamab	EGFR, cMET	Human bispecific IgG1	NSCLC w/EGFR exon 20 insertion mutations	https://www.rybrevanthcp.com
2021	Tezspire®	Tezepelumab	Thymic stromal lymphopoietin	Human IgG2	Severe asthma	https://www.tezspirehcp.com
2022	Enjaymo®	Sutimlimab	C1s	Humanized IgG4	Cold agglutinin disease	https://www.enjaymo.com

2022	Vabysmo™	Faricimab	VEGF-A, Ang-2	Human/humanized IgG1 kappa/lambda, with domain crossover	wAMD, DME	https://www.vabysmo.com
2022	Kimmtrak®	Tebentafusp	gp100, CD3	Bispecific immunoconjugate (TCR-scFv)	Metastatic uveal melanoma	https://www.kimmtrak.com
2022	Opdualag™ (relatlimab + nivolumab combo)	Relatlimab	LAG-3	Human IgG4	Melanoma	https://www.opdualag.com
2022	Tecvayli™	Teclistamab	BCMA, CD3	Humanized bispecific IgG4	Multiple myeloma	https://www.tecvaylihcp.com
2022	Spevigo®	Spesolimab	IL-36 receptor	Humanized IgG1	Generalized pustular psoriasis	https://patient.boehringer-ingelheim.com/us/products/spevigo/
2022	Imjudo®	Tremelimumab	CTLA-4	Human IgG2A	Antineoplastic, liver cancer	NA
2022	Briumvi®	Ublituximab	CD20	Chimeric IgG1	Multiple sclerosis	https://www.briumvi.com
2022	Tzield™	Teplizumab	CD3	Humanized IgG1	Delay onset of type 1 diabetes	https://www.tzield.com
2023	Leqembi™	Lecanemab	Amyloid-beta proto fibrils	Humanized IgG1	Alzheimer's disease	https://www.leqembi.com

(*Continued*)

Table 11.1. (*Continued*)

Approval year	Brand name	Generic name	Target	Format	Disease type	Website
NA	Beyfortus	Nirsevimab	RSV	Human IgG1	RSV infection	NA
NA	NA	Narsoplimab	MASP-2	Human IgG4	Hematopoietic stem cell transplant-associated thrombotic microangiopathies	NA
NA	Zynyz™	Retifanlimab	PD-1	Humanized IgG4	Squamous cell carcinoma of the anal canal	https://www.zynyzhcp.com
NA	(Pending)	Omburtamab	B7-H3	Murine IgG1	CNS/leptomeningeal metastasis from neuroblastoma	NA
NA	Tuoyi	Toripalimab	PD-1	Humanized IgG4	esophageal squamous cell carcinoma	NA
NA	Tyvyt®	Sintilimab	PD-1	Human IgG4	Non-small cell lung cancer	NA
NA	NA	Penpulimab	PD-1	Humanized IgG1	Metastatic nasopharyngeal carcinoma	https://www.akesobio.com/en/rd-and-science/products-center/penpulimabinjection/
NA	NA	Tislelizumab	PD-1	Humanized IgG4	Esophageal squamous cell carcinoma	https://www.beigene.com/our-science-and-medicines/tislelizumab/

NA	Regen-Cov, Ronapreve	Casirivimab + imdevimab	SARS-CoV-2	Human IgG1	COVID-19	NA
NA	Regkirona®	Regdanvimab	SARS-CoV-2	Human IgG2	COVID-19	NA
NA	Xevudy	Sotrovimab	SARS-CoV-3	Human IgG3	COVID-19	—

Abbreviations in table 11.1: Angiopoietin 2 (Ang-2), B7 homolog 3 protein (B7-H3), B Lymphocyte Stimulator (BLyS), B-cell maturation antigen (BMCA). Complement protein 1s (C1s), Complement protein C5 (C5), Cluster of differentiation 3 (CD3), Cluster of differentiation 4 (CD4), Cluster of differentiation 19 (CD19), Cluster of differentiation 38 (CD38), Cluster of differentiation 52 (CD52), Calcitonin gene-related peptide (CGRP), Calcitonin gene-related peptide receptor (CGRPR), C-C chemokine receptor type (CCR4), Cytotoxic T-lymphocyte Antigen-4 (CTLA-4), Fibroblast growth factor 23 (FGF23), Epidermal growth factor receptor (EGFR), Glycoprotein (GP), Human epidermal growth factor 2 (HER2), Interleukin-1 beta (IL-1β), Interleukin-4 receptor alpha (IL-4Rα), Interleukin-5 (IL-5), Interleukin-5 receptor alpha (IL-5Rα), Interleukin-6 (IL-6), Interleukin-6 receptor (IL-6R), Interleukin 12/23 (IL-12/23), Interleukin 13 (IL-13), Interleukin-17 alpha (IL-17α), Interleukin-17 receptor (IL-17R), Interleukin-36 (IL-36), insulin-like growth factor 1 receptor (IGF-1R), Interferon gamma (IFNγ), Interferon-α/β receptor 1 (IFNAR1), Intracellular tumor necrosis factor alpha (ITNFα), Integrin alpha 4 (ITGA4), Lymphocyte activation gene-3 (LAG-3), Mannan-binding lectin-associated serine protease-2 (MASP-2), Mesenchymal–epithelial transition (MET), Protective antigen (PA), Programmed cell death protein 1 (PD-1), Programmed death-ligand 1 (PD-L1), Proprotein convertase subtilisin/kexin type 9 (PCSK9), Platelet-derived growth factor receptor alpha (PDGFRα), Respiratory syncytial virus (RSV), Receptor activator of nuclear factor kappa-B ligand (RANKL), Tumor necrosis factor α (TNFα), Severe acute respiratory syndrome coronavirus (SARS-CoV), Signaling lymphocytic activation molecule family member 7 (SLAMF7), Vascular endothelial growth factor A (VEGF-A), Vascular endothelial growth factor receptor 2 (VEGFR2), polyethylene glycol (PEG).

Table 11.2. List of nanobodies in clinical trials. Adapted from [178] and http://www.antibodysociety.org/resources/approved-antibodies/.

Nanobody	Condition or disease	Target	Features	Phase	Identifier	Sponsor
CD7 CAR-T cells infusion	Acute lymphocytic leukemiaNK/T-cell lymphomaT-lymphoblastic lymphoma	CD7	CAR-T	Phase I	NCT04004637	PersonGen BioTherapeutics (Suzhou) Co., Ltd
KN046	Advanced hepatocellular carcinoma	PD-L1/ CTLA4	Tetravalent bispecific	Phase I	NCT04601610	Jiangsu Alphamab Biopharmaceuticals Co., Ltd
CD22 CAR-T cells	B-cell lymphoma; Diffuse large B-cell lymphoma; Extranodal marginal zone lymphoma of mucosa-associated lymphoid tissue; Follicular lymphoma; Mantle cell lymphoma; Plasma cell neoplasm; Primary cutaneous follicle centre lymphoma	CD22	CAR-T	Phase I	NCT03999697	PersonGen BioTherapeutics (Suzhou) Co., Ltd
γδT-Cell infusion agent	B-cell leukemia		CAR-T	Early	Phase 1	NCT04439721
PersonGen	BioTherapeutics (Suzhou) Co., Ltd					
CD19/CD20 CAR-T cells	B-cell lymphoma	CD19/CD20	Bispecific CAR-T	Phase I	NCT03881761	Henan Cancer Hospital
αPD1-MSLN-CAR-T cells	Colorectal cancer	PD-1	CAR-T	Phase I	NCT05089266	Shanghai Cell Therapy Group Co.,Ltd
ALX-0651	Healthy volunteers	CXCR4	Bivalent bispecific	Phase I	NCT01374503	Ablynx, a Sanofi company
KN035	Hepatocellular carcinoma	PD-L1	Bivalent monospecific	Phase I	NCT03101488	3D Medicines (Sichuan) Co., Ltd.
		PD-L1		NA	NCT05156515	

68Ga-THP-APN09	Lung cancerMelanomaPD-L1PET/CT		PET/CT imaging agent			Peking University Cancer Hospital & Institute
αPD1-MSLN-CAR-T cells Non-small-cell lung cancer	Mesothelioma Wuhan Union Hospital, China	PD-1	CAR-T	Early	Phase I	NCT04489862
M1095	Psoriasis	IL17A/IL17F	Trivalent bispecific	Phase II	NCT03384745	Bond Avillion 2 Development LP
M1095	Psoriasis	IL17A/IL17F	Trivalent bispecific	Phase II	NCT05640245	MoonLake Immunotherapeutics AG
MSB0010841	Psoriasis	IL17A/IL17F	Trivalent	Phase I	NCT02156466	Merck KGaA, Darmstadt, Germany
BCMA nanobody CAR-T cells	Relapsed/refractory myeloma	CD8/4–1BB	CAR-T	Phase I	NCT03664661	Henan Cancer Hospital
ALX-0171	Respiratory syncytial virus lower respiratory tract infection	F-protein RSV	Trivalent monospecific	Phase II	NCT02979431	Ablynx, a Sanofi company
ALX-0061	Rheumatoid arthritis	IL6R	Bivalent albumin-conjugated	Phase II	NCT02518620	Ablynx, a Sanofi company
ATN-103	Rheumatoid arthritis	TNF	Trivalent albumin-conjugated	Phase II	NCT01063803	Ablynx, a Sanofi company
BI836880	Solid tumors	Angiopoietin/VEGF	Bivalent bispecific	Phase I	NCT02674152	Boehringer–Ingelheim
18F-FDG	Solid tumors			NA	NCT05436093	

(*Continued*)

Table 11.2. (*Continued*)

Nanobody	Condition or disease	Target	Features	Phase	Identifier	Sponsor
		CLDN18.2 expression	PET/CT imaging agent			Peking University Cancer Hospital & Institute
KN046	Squamous non-small-cell lung cancer	PD-L1/ CTLA4	Tetravalent bispecific	Phase III	NCT04474119	Jiangsu Alphamab Biopharmaceuticals Co., Ltd
M6495	Symptomatic knee osteoarthritis	ADAMTS-5	Bivalent bispecific	Phase I	NCT03583346	Merck KGaA, Darmstadt, Germany
ALX-0061	Systemic lupus erythematosus (SLE)	IL6R	Bivalent albumin-conjugated	Phase II	NCT02437890	Ablynx, a Sanofi company
Caplacizumab	Thrombotic thrombocytopenic purpura (TTP)	VWF	Bivalent monospecific	Phase III	NCT02878603	Sanofi

Abbreviations in table 11.2: Cluster of Differentiation 7 (CD7), Chimeric Antigen Receptor (CAR), Natural Killer/T (NK/T), Programmed Cell Death Protein 1 (PD-1), Programmed Death-Ligand 1 (PD-L1), Cytotoxic T-lymphocyte Antigen-4 (CTLA-4), Cluster of Differentiation-22 (CD22), Gamma delta (γδ), Cluster of Differentiation 19/Cluster of Differentiation 20 (CD19/CD20), C-X-C Motif Chemokine Receptor 4 (CXCR4), Gallium 68—Tris (Hydroxypyridinone)—Nanobody Targeting PD-L1 (68Ga-THP-APN09), Positron Emission Tomography/Computed Tomography (PET/CT), Mesothelin (MSLN), Interleukin-17A/Interleukin-17F (IL17A/IL17F), B-cell Maturation Antigen (BCMA), Cluster of Differentiation 8 (CD8), Tumor Necrosis Factor Receptor Superfamily 9 (4–1BB or TNFRSF9), Fusion protein (F-protein), Respiratory Syncytial Virus (RSV), Gontivimab (ALX-0171), Vobarilizumab (ALX-0061), Interleukin-6 Receptor (IL6R), Tumor Necrosis Factor (TNF), Ozoralizumab (ATN-103), Vascular Endothelial Growth Factor (VEGF), Fluorodeoxyglucose (FDG), Claudin18.2 (CLDN18.2), A Disintegrin and Metalloproteinase with Thrombospondin Motifs-5 (ADAMTS-5), Von Willebrand Factor (VWF).

name, condition or disease, target, features, phase, identifier, and sponsor information.

Nanobodies have main advantages in size, structure, affinity, stability, and ease of mass production. They are regarded as a viable therapeutic alternative to conventional mAbs, which frequently have limited efficacy and a high production cost. Indeed, several Nbs are already in phase I or II clinical trials, particularly for cardiovascular, neurodegenerative, or autoimmune diseases [148]. However, more than half of candidate drug molecules would fail in phase III trials [149]. Thus, it is better to fail earlier to reduce the cost and labor. More importantly, uncovering the reasons behind the failure in any phase is critical in developing better drug molecules. However, detailed reports on clinical trial failures mostly cover efficacy, safety, and toxicity results [149]. Immunogenicity risk could be one of the hidden reasons for Nb failure in the late stages of production as seen in the case of bococizumab by Pfizer [150]. At this point, computational methods would help designing nanobodies having better properties.

Computational modeling of nanobody 3D structure is much faster than antibody modeling. The technology for computer-aided nanobody design has made significant advancements in the previous few years and will become more and more dependable [151, 152]. Traditional lab based approaches to developing nanobody therapies still require many experiments before they reach the clinic. Computational approaches could speed up this process, allowing life-saving therapeutics to be designed and delivered much more quickly, or these methods detect poor candidates with high immunogenicity risk earlier.

Recent computational studies use MD simulations and/or machine learning methods to design and investigate nanobodies at molecular level. Liang *et al* (2022) compared five different deep learning-based protein structure prediction methods, namely AlphaFold2, RoseTTAFold, DeepAb, NanoNet, and tFold, in terms of RMSD and TM scores (topological similarity) on 60 known nanobody structures [23]. They concluded that the AlphaFold2 outperformed on the prediction of the framework region when both all-atom and C-alpha-only predictions were considered. AlphaFold2 was also good at predicting CDR1 and 2, however, its prediction quality was moderate in predicting the CDR3 region. tFold by Tencent AI lab was the best method in predicting all-atom structures with a good CDR3 region prediction that was better than the AlphaFold2 and RoseTTAFold predictions. DeepAb performed the worst since its algorithm is designed for antibody Fv regions. On the other hand, NanoNet performed best on the prediction of both framework and CDR regions although it is C-alpha-based prediction method. In terms of computational time, C-alpha-based NanoNet is the fastest method since it can process structures in parallel and provide results for 60 structures in 4.65 s while the others take minutes or hours.

Fernandez-Quintero *et al* (2023) performed MD simulations for anti-GFP binding nanobody and compared experimentally derived data from NMR to the MD-generated data to assess the quality of the simulations. Time-lagged independent component analysis tICA [153] was applied to MD data to identify slow modes of the CDR loops. Their results are in good agreement, especially for the CDR3 loop, which is critical for antigen recognition [62].

Baroroh *et al* (2022) computationally designed new mutants to improve binding affinity of the nanobody in complex with cortisol, which mostly interacts with the CDR1 region of the nanobody [154]. They used MODELLER to model mutant structures; BIOVIA Discovery Studio to prepare structures for docking process; AutoDockTools-1.5.6 for docking; Amber for MD simulations and analysis and MMPBSA.py for binding free energy calculations. Their calculations showed that substitution of hydrophobic residues in CDR2 and CDR3 regions increases the binding affinity of the nanobody. Therefore, their results might help in developing better diagnostic tools for cortisol. Hacisuleyman and Erman (2020) performed a benchmark testing on three different protein-nanobody complexes and proposed an algorithm to design better nanobodies [155]. They successively mutated each hypervariable residue on CDR regions and performed MD simulations for each mutated structure to find the optimum binding residues by calculating and updating the interaction energies with the antigen using evolutionary probability distributions. Their method revealed critical mutations that yield nanobodies with higher affinities, which are experimentally proven best binders.

Cheng *et al* (2019) studied Nb02, which is an anti-CD47 nanobody, to increase its binding affinity using computational methods [156]. They first modeled the Nb02 using homology modeling, then applied Rational Mutation Hotspots Design Protocol (RMHDP) to determine critical residues for mutation. RMHDP uses two criteria: residues on CDR that are within a specific distance with the antigen, and hot spots on CDR constant sequences. The overlapped residues from the two criteria are selected as potential mutations. ADAPT [157], which is a combination of computational and experimental protocols, was used to optimize the binding affinity.

Sang *et al* (2022) created an open-source computational pipeline called Llamanade by systematically analyzing nanobodies and human IgGs that revealed unique features of nanobodies. Their pipeline, which is guided by big data analysis, provides rational humanization of nanobodies. Llamanade is also experimentally validated for the humanization of the SARS-CoV-2 neutralizing nanobodies. They showed that the humanized nanobodies using Llamanade have a framework similar to human VH and excellent solubility and bioactivity values compared to non-humanized nanobodies [127].

11.4.3 Antibody–drug conjugates

Antibody–drug conjugates (ADCs) are molecules produced by covalent attachment of multiple copies of cytotoxic drug molecules to an antibody through synthetic linkers. The target antigen is present at higher levels in the target tissue than healthy tissue. ADC immunoconjugates join the cytotoxic small molecule drug with the specificity and longer half-life of antibodies together creating a tissue specific, targeted therapy with fewer side effects. Especially for the treatment of various cancers, antibodies in ADCs deliver the cytotoxic drug molecule to specific tissue or cell type. After Ab binding to its target on the cell surface, ADCs are taken inside the cell via lysosomal trafficking. Inside the lysosome, the antibody–drug conjugate is digested releasing the cytotoxic drug molecule into the cytosol and killing the cancer cell. This mechanism of action minimizes off-target effect of the cytotoxic drug compared to when the drug is administered solo [158]. Since 2010 there have been 13 ADCs approved and used in the clinic for targeted cancer therapy (table 11.3).

Computational approaches are implemented on ADC design to optimize these molecules, especially for cancer treatment. Finding the best ADCs against cancer is a highly difficult task that requires rational design. Antibody structures are computationally designed using either homology, fragment-based, or *ab initio* modeling in the development of ADCs [159]. The ideal target for ADCs can be chosen with the use of machine learning techniques. Also, to determine the most likely fit between antibodies and antigens and to comprehend the linker-drug interaction, homology modeling, molecular docking, and refinement can be used. The specificity of the molecules in the entire system is decided during this critical stage of ADC development. Another approach for elucidating issues that take antibodies and antigens into consideration is MD. By investigating potential antibody conformations that the antibody might acquire and providing crucial information on drug antibody complementarity, MD can be used in particular to assist in the selection of the optimum drug candidate [160].

Coumans *et al* (2020) developed an *in silico* screening platform to produce site-specific ADCs that can selectively reduce engineered cysteines [161]. Their hypothesis is based on introducing a linker-drug to the epitope–paratope region might reduce the new larger hydrophobic surface caused by the payload. They performed homology modeling for the Fab part of two antibodies using YASARA modeling program, then docked the linker-drug onto a specific position using AutoDock Vina. The linker-drug docking ended up around the cavity between the heavy and light chains. These results led the authors to choose suitable potential sites around the Fab cavity to engineer the antibody with cysteines. *In vivo* xenograft models showed that site-specific ADCs have better efficacy and exposure compared to randomly conjugated ADCs.

An interactive, all-in-one immunoinformatics platform called Drugena was developed by Papageorgiou *et al* [162]. Drugena suite is an antibody structural database and offers a command line-free and user-friendly platform to develop new potent molecules such as ADCs. The platform uses RCSB database to extract 3D structures and covers more than 5000 structures of all full-length antibodies (HFabFc and LFab) and antibody domain fragments from all species that are solved by either x-ray crystallography, NMR, or electron microscopy. Drugena also contains over 96 million entities (drugs or drugs derivatives) taken from the NCI database [163] of specialized antibodies for neurological disorders from RCSB by *in silico* ADC development. For each structure in the database at least one contains a complete variable or constant domain.

Lysine and cysteine residues are widely used for antibody–drug conjugation [164]. However, Gupta *et al* (2019) reported multivalent and affinity-guided antibody empowerment technology (MAGNET) as an alternative approach which does not

Table 11.3. A list of approved antibody drug conjugates (ADCs) in the market. Adapted from [178] and http://www.antibodysociety.org/resources/approved-antibodies/.

Approval year	Brand name	Generic name	Drug mechanism	Antigen target	Disease type	Website
2002	Zevalin®	Ibritumomab tiuxetan	ADCC, CDC, Apoptosis induction	CD20	Non-Hodgkin lymphoma	http://zevalin.com
2017	Mylotarg®	Gemtuzumab ozogamicin	DNA damage	CD33	Myeloid leukemia B-cell lymphoma	https://mylotarg.pfizerpro.com
2017	Besponsa®	Inotuzumab ozogamicin	DNA damage	CD22	Lymphoblastic B leukemia	https://www.besponsa.com/
2011	Adcetris®	Brentuximab vedotin	Microtubule disruptor	CD-30	Hodgkin's lymphoma	https://www.adcetris.com/
2013	Kadcyla®	Trastuzumab emtansine	Microtubule disruptor	HER-2	HER2+Breast cancer	https://www.kadcyla.com/
2019	Polivy®	Polatuzumab vedotin	Microtubule disruptor	CD79B	Large B-Cell lymphoma	https://www.polivy.com/
2018	Lumoxiti®	Moxetumomab pasudotox	Apoptosis induction	CD22	Refractory hairy cell leukemia	https://www.lumoxiti.com/
2019	Padcev®	Enfortumab vedotin	Microtubule disruptor	Nectin-4	Bladder cancer	https://www.padcev.com/
2019	Enhertu®	Trastuzumab deruxtecan	Topoisomerase inhibitor	HER2	HER2 positive breast cancer	https://www.enhertu.com/
2020	Trodelvy®	Sacituzumab govitecan	topoisomerase inhibitor	TROP2	Triple-negative breast cancer	https://www.trodelvyhcp.com/moa
2020	Blenrep®		Microtubule disruptor	BCMA	Myloma	

		Belantamab mafodotin				https://gskpro.com/en-gb/products/blenrep/home/
2021	Zynlonta®	Loncastuximab Tesirine-lpyl	Binds to the DNA minor groove and forms highly cytotoxic DNA interstrand crosslinks	CD19	B-cell lymphoma	https://www.zynlonta.com/
2022	Elahere®	Mirvetuximab soravtansine	Microtubule disruptor	folate receptor alpha (FRα)	Ovarian cancer	https://www.elahere.com/
2021	Tivdak®	Tisotumab vedotin	MMAE disrupts the microtubule network	TF-expressing cells	Cervical cancer	https://www.elahere.com/
NA	NA	Trastuzumab	duocarmazine	DNA damage	HER2	Breast cancer

Abbreviations in table 11.3: Antibody-dependent cellular cytotoxicity (ADCC), Complement-dependent cytotoxicity (CDC) monomethyl auristatin E (MMAE), cluster of differentiation 20 (CD20), cluster of differentiation 33 (CD33), cluster of differentiation-22 (CD22), human epidermal growth factor receptor 2 (HER2), Cluster of Differentiation 79B(CD79B), Trophoblast cell surface antigen 2 (TROP2), B-cell maturation antigen (BCMA), Cluster of differentiation 19 (CD19), Tissue factor (TF).

require pre-modification of the antibody [165]. In addition, MAGNET-based conjugation needs less process time for the incubation with linker-drug compared to lysine- and cysteine-based conjugation. On the other hand, computational approaches such as MD simulations and docking were used to design ADCs by including affinity linkers.

11.4.4 Antibody-based PROTACs

Proteolysis targeting chimeras (PROTACs) are heterobifunctional small molecules that function as targeted protein degraders. They consist of three main components: a ligand for the target protein, a ligand for the E3 ubiquitin ligase enzyme, and a linker that connects the two ligands. The target protein ligand binds to the protein of interest, while the E3 ubiquitin ligase ligand binds to the enzyme and brings it into proximity with the target protein. PROTACs work by recruiting an E3 ubiquitin ligase enzyme to a specific protein of interest leading to polyubiquitination and degradation of the protein by the proteasome. The linker is designed to keep the two ligands close in 3D space, allowing for efficient recruitment of the E3 ubiquitin ligase to the target protein. The main advantage of PROTACs is being able to target proteins considered 'undruggable' by other means and the potential for increased specificity and efficacy. PROTACs have shown promise in preclinical studies for the treatment of a variety of diseases, including cancer, neurodegenerative disorders, and viral infections [166].

Antibody-based PROTACs (AbTACs) or proteolysis-targeting antibodies (PROTABs) are inspired by PROTACs. AbTACs or PROTABs are designed to target proteins on the cell surface which are highly expressed, especially in cancer patients. These antibodies are bifunctional molecules with one binding site specific for one transmembrane E3 ubiquitin ligase and the other binding site is specific for target protein selected for degradation on the cell surface [167]. Wells and colleagues targeted immune checkpoint protein PD-L1 for degradation through AbTAC technology. They labeled PD-L1 with a bispecific antibody that can also bind to RNF43 which is an E3 ligase on the cell surface. PD-L1 was taken into the cell through endocytosis and degraded [168]. Tate and colleagues targeted bromodomain-containing protein 4 (BRD4) in HER-2 positive breast cancer cell lines with Trastuzumab-PROTAC conjugate. BRD4 was internalized through lysosomes and tissue specific BRD4 degradation was achieved [169]. The biotechnology company Genentech developed proteolysis-targeting antibodies (PROTABs) against the insulin growth factor 1 receptor (IGF1R), a receptor tyrosine kinase. IGF1R mediates growth factor signaling in various tissues and cancers and has been targeted with therapeutic antibodies before. The Genentech team demonstrated targeted degradation of cell surface proteins with bifunctional antibodies one site binding E3 ligase, the other site binding target protein IGF1R [170].

11.5 Production cost and market value of antibodies

Antibody therapeutics are one of the major focuses in the pharmaceutical market due to their advantageous properties such as specificity, potency, and metabolic stability compared to small-molecules [10]. As of August 2020, full-length naked mAbs (71.60%) and biosimilar full-length naked mAbs (23.19%) cover the bigger part of the approved and marketed mAbs in the United States or Europe [171]. Global antibody market size is around USD 162.17 billion in 2023 and is expected to be around USD 277.11 billion (2028) with approximately 11.31% of compound annual growth rate (CAGR), which is a good CAGR value for large biopharmaceutical companies [172].

11.5.1 Monoclonal antibodies

Monoclonal antibodies became attractive therapeutics since mAb production was streamlined in 1975, as shown in figure 11.6. Antibodies were defined as 'magic bullets' especially against cancer. There has been an exponential increase in estimated market value of mAbs since the discovery of rituximab in 1997 until now and the market is expected to grow. The fastest acceleration was shown after 2012. The top 10-selling monoclonal antibodies (blockbuster) drugs are shown in red in figure 11.6 below [173].

This trend remained the same according to the report of EvaluatePharma. In that report, four out of ten most valuable R&D projects are on monoclonal antibodies. The most valuable mAb projects are listed in terms of net present value as Gantenerumab (Roche and MorphoSys), intravitreal Pegcetacoplan (Apellis Pharmaceuticals), Epcoritamab (AbbVie and Genmab), Donanemab (Eli Lily), Tiragolumab (Roche), respectively [174]. In the last five years, the monoclonal antibody (mAb) market has more than doubled in size. Abbvie, Genentech, and Johnson & Johnson dominate the market. While mAbs target range is getting larger, medical applications in oncology and hematology remain the most prevalent. The mAb market has a strong pipeline and is expected to grow faster, reaching US$130–200 billion in value [175]. Since 1986 after the release of the first licensed mAb product, the procedures to manufacture therapeutic monoclonal antibodies (mAbs) have improved significantly. Due to the remarkable increase in demand for mAbs production, efforts were made to simultaneously enhance production capacity through building industrial manufacturing facilities and advancements in cell culture techniques to increase product titers. The cost of manufacturing the mAb product is estimated at $10 per vial, although actual costs will vary depending on configuration, batch size, and testing specifications. Fill/finish costs, which cover all processes for filling the vials and packaging, are highly dependent on dosage and product titer. However, in some circumstances, these costs cover a larger portion of the final product cost compared to the drug substance cost of goods (COG). The drug substance plant occupancy or utilization is the most significant potential cost driver since a high titer process would yield a product more than demand [176]. According to the report of Farid *et al* (2020), on a production level, the mAb industry's process innovations over the past 40 years have helped to drive down the published commercial COG/g numbers from over $10 000 per gram to $1000 or less per gram in the 1980s and 1990s to $10 or less per gram today [177]. Manufacturing costs include R&D costs and after those costs for clinical stages. A pharmaceutical company should consider almost ~$60M for

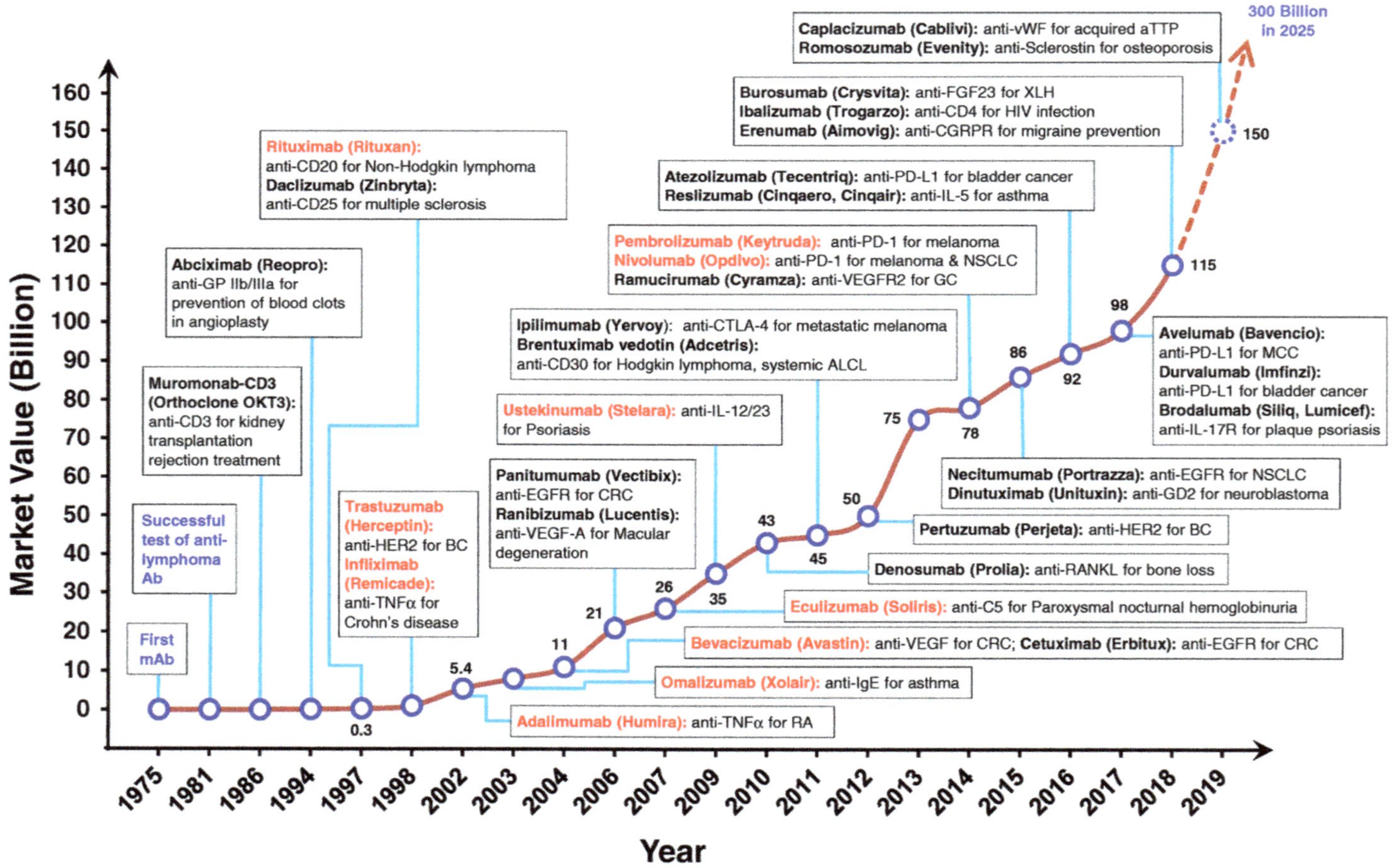

Figure 11.6. Timeline between 1975 and 2019 that depicts the successful development of therapeutic antibodies and their applications. The figure is taken from [173] under the license CC BY 4.0.

preclinical to Phase II trials, and ~\$70M for Phase III to the regulatory process for a potential biopharmaceutical drug candidate development process. And these numbers would be increased for low overall clinical success diseases like Alzheimer's almost 2.5-fold [177].

The COG can differ due to process modes. In a study by Klutz *et al* (2016), they compared different process modes in terms of production costs. The annual production capacity for fed-batch and continuous operation modes was set as 200 kg API. They calculated the production costs by using capital costs and operating costs which include many sub-costs. As a result of the study, while the fed-batch process has the total specific cost of goods as 59 euro $gram^{-1}$ mAb, the continuously operated process has 84 euro $gram^{-1}$ mAb. Upstream of the continuous process is expensive but downstream is about 8 euro $gram^{-1}$ mAb cheaper than the fed-batch process due to the use of chromatography resins. After these evaluations, the authors suggested a hybrid process that combines both processes' beneficial parts. Therefore, this hybrid process resulted in 50 euro $gram^{-1}$ mAb cost of goods, which means a 15% reduction in production costs [178]. Production costs can be arranged by using different processes for antibody production. The investigation of Mahal *et al* (2021) showed that continuous facilities offer COG reductions when there are only a few single upstream processes (USP) and downstream process (DSP) trains needed to meet smaller commercial demands. The cost-effectiveness of continuous manufacturing is decreased at bigger sizes when parallel continuous trains are used and the cost of media dominates the COG [179].

11.5.1.1 Selected monoclonal antibodies on the market or in clinical trials and leading companies

Lecanemab-BAN2401 (commercial name: LEQEMBI™) is a humanized IgG1 monoclonal antibody designed for the treatment of Alzheimer's Disease (AD) by affecting both aggregated soluble and insoluble forms of amyloid-beta. It was approved on January 6, 2023 by FDA using the Accelerated Approval Pathway for intravenous use in patients who are in the stages of AD such as mild cognitive impairment or mild dementia. LEQEMBI™ was designed and developed by Japanese pharmaceutical company Eisai Co., Ltd (www.eisai.com) in collaboration with Biogen Inc. (American multinational biotechnology company, www.biogen.com). Eisai also has had a strategic research agreement with the Swedish biopharma company BioArctic AB (www.bioarctica.se) since December 2007. However, Eisai has the final decision-making authority [180]. There have been eight clinical trials that include lecanemab (three completed and five active [181]). Phase 2 (NCT01767311 [182], estimated completion date February 2025 and sponsored by Eisai) aims to determine clinical efficacy and different dose response. Phase 2 results showed that the drug reduces amyloid-beta plaque formation in the brain in early AD patients. Phase 3 (NCT03887455, estimated completion date September 2027 and sponsored by Eisai [183]) to evaluate the efficacy of the drug, NCT04468659 (AHEAD 3–45 study, estimated completion date October 2027 [184]) aims to assess the effectiveness of the drug compared to a placebo. There are also two ongoing clinical trials (NCT05269394 [185] and NCT01760005 [186]: phase 2 and 3, both sponsored by Washington University School of Medicine) that aim to see if the treatment improves disease-related biomarkers.

Ozoralizumab (commercial name: Nanozora®) is a trimeric nanobody drug targeting pro-inflammatory cytokine tumor necrosis factor α (TNFα) for treatment of rheumatoid arthritis (RA). Ozoralizumab is developed by Taisho Pharmaceutical Co. Ltd under license from Ablynx, an affiliate of Sanofi, and was approved in Japan in September 2022 for treatment of rheumatoid arthritis in patients who did not respond well to conventional treatments (https://www.taisho.co.jp/global/news/2022/20220926001109.html). The medication is administered as a subcutaneous injection once every four weeks. The phase 2/3 OHZORA trial (TS152–3000-JA study, TS152–3001-JA study) was a randomized, placebo-controlled, double-blind study and was conducted from September 2018 to October 2020 at 78 different locations in Japan. Taisho Pharmaceuticals is evaluating the long-term safety and efficacy of ozoralizumab in another clinical trial (NCT04077567 [187]).

AU-007 Aulos Bioscience is a company with an interest in the computational design of antibody therapeutics [99]. AU-007, which was computationally designed by Biolojic Design and presently by Aulos Bioscience Inc., was indicated to be in Phase I for monotherapy for the patients with/having advanced solid tumor, and Phase II for a combined usage with aldesleukin for metastatic cancer (Phase I/II; NCT05267626). The clinical trial was indicated to continue till 2024 according to estimations and the safety, efficacy, tolerability, and pharmacokinetic profile of the AU-007 will be analyzed [188].

Genentech (acquired by Roche in 2009) is one of the leading companies in the field of antibody therapeutics. Genentech has 29 antibody or antibody–drug conjugate medicine in the market with bevacizumab (Avastin), rituximab (Rituxan), and trastuzumab (Herceptin) being the top selling drugs. Genentech currently has 71 molecules at different phases of clinical trials, mostly antibody drugs for treatment of various diseases in oncology, immunology, neuroscience, metabolism, infectious diseases, and ophthalmology (https://www.gene.com/medical-professionals/medicines). Genentech recently acquired Prescient Design to accelerate their protein therapeutic design with AI tools.

11.5.2 Bispecific antibodies

However, there have also been substantial limitations to traditional antibody treatment, despite the efficacy of several anti-tumor therapeutic antibody medicines. Low tumor penetration and retention rates are significant disadvantages of antibody treatment. Typically, only 20% of the administered dose of therapeutic mAbs targeting tumor-specific antigens interacts with the surface proteins of solid tumors, leaving the majority of these mAbs in circulation. This disparity illustrates the difficulties in effectively penetrating and being retained within solid tumor tissue [189]. In addition, even though most mAbs work to stop growth factors from interacting with their receptors, they seldom cause apoptosis of tumors since patients' immune systems are not strong enough to fight against tumors, particularly when T cells are not activated to do so. To get over the natural mAbs' restriction of only being able to bind one epitope, bispecific antibodies were postulated thirty years ago and have since undergone substantial research. Bispecific antibodies can concurrently bind to two distinct antigens, tumor cell receptors and cytotoxic immune cells [190]. This improved functionality may lead to fewer adverse effects and injections down the road. Additionally, from the viewpoint of a biopharmaceutical producer, producing a single molecule rather than two allows for fewer clinical studies and lower production costs. Vaccination, *in vitro*, and *in vivo* studies may increase the production costs, therefore using hosts like *Escherichia coli* and co-culturing methods are suggested for the bispecific antibody production [191].

11.6 Conclusions

We summarized the currently active and free computational tools to design therapeutic antibodies to understand their structure and dynamics better. Most of the tools take advantage of machine learning and deep learning and provide better results. Currently, it is possible to design an antibody 3D structure in seconds. The improvement in those computational tools would help develop better therapeutics specific to an antigen of interest. Each step that is used in the development of the first computationally designed AU-007 mAb involves a machine learning method, showing us the potential power of using computers and machine learning methods in pharmaceutical industry. Biotechnology companies specialized in antibody design are working in collaboration with computational biologists to accelerate their design processes. At this point, new state-of-the-art computational methods in protein design and engineering would help reduce the number of failures at any stage during the development and production of better antibody binders.

As we live longer, the number of people diagnosed with cancer across the globe is increasing. Systemic administration of conventional chemotherapy drugs are not the best treatment options for patient's quality of life. Therefore, immunogenicity risk-reduced new drugs and treatment methods are urgently needed in personalized medicine. As can be seen from the SWOT analysis (figure 11.7), antibody

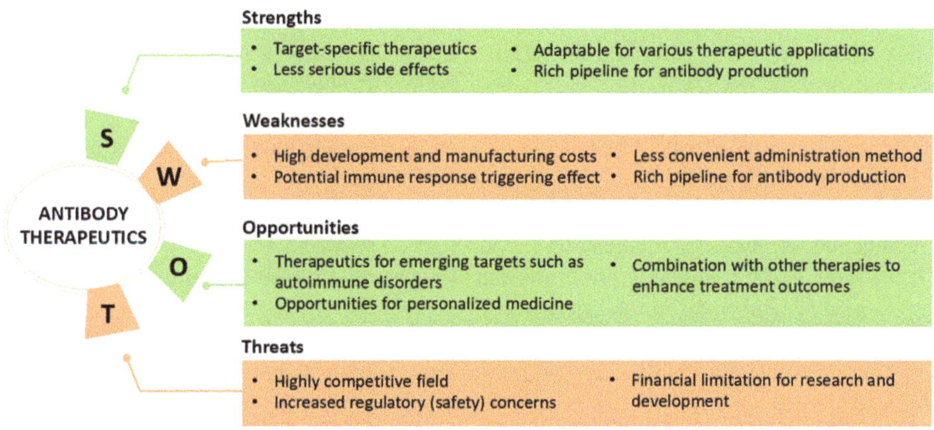

Figure 11.7. SWOT analysis of antibody therapeutics.

therapeutics are target-specific with reduced side effects, and are one of the major components in personalized medicine and targeted therapy.

In the last section, we discussed the market value of biologics and how they are becoming the dominant molecules in the pharmaceutical industry due to their potential in targeted treatment. These molecules offer huge benefits in a patient's quality of life because of reduced side effects during treatment. The big differences between biologics and small molecules can be considered as their molecular weight, complexity, stability, characterizability, production methods, and immunogenicity [192]. In developing and underdeveloped parts of the world, small molecules are more accessible than biologics because of the costs and existing government policies. Most patients have been forced to choose small molecules over more expensive biologics, despite proven superior outcome with biologics treatment simply because these treatments are not accessible or affordable. This leads to a growing biosimilar industry especially in developing countries. As biologics are becoming dominant players in pharmaceutical industry, governments should adopt policies to support biosimilar production and additional assistance programs should be established to make these treatments more accessible to a wider population [193].

Acknowledgments

The authors would like to thank The Scientific and Technological Research Institution of Türkiye with project number: TUBITAK-117C013 (for HTS), Health Institutes of Türkiye with project number: TUSEB-27642 (for SBA, IA, AU and HTS), and Izmir Institute of Technology Scientific Research Projects with project numbers: 2020İYTE0088 (for HTS), 2022-İYTE-3-0005 (for HTS), 2023IYTE-1-0055 (for SG, AU and HTS), and 2022-İYTE-3-0041 (for AU) for financial support. Figures 11.1 through 11.5 are created with BioRender.

References

[1] Lu R M, Hwang Y C, Liu I J, Lee C C, Tsai H Z and Li H J *et al* 2020 Development of therapeutic antibodies for the treatment of diseases *J. Biomed. Sci.* **27** 1

[2] Marovich M, Mascola J R and Cohen M S 2020 Monoclonal antibodies for prevention and treatment of COVID-19 *JAMA* **324** 131–2

[3] World Preview 2022 Outlook to 2028: Patents and Pricing. 2022

[4] Mahase E 2021 COVID-19: Pfizer's paxlovid is 89% effective in patients at risk of serious illness, company reports *Brit. Med. J.* **375** n2697

[5] Cox P B and Gupta R 2022 Contemporary computational applications and tools in drug discovery *ACS Med. Chem. Lett.* **13** 1016–29

[6] Chiu M L, Goulet D R, Teplyakov A and Gilliland G L 2019 Antibody structure and function: the basis for engineering therapeutics *Antibodies* **8** 55

[7] Parham P 2009 Antibody structure and the generation of B-Cell diversity *The Immune System* (Taylor and Francis Group)

[8] Hamers-Casterman C, Atarhouch T, Muyldermans S, Robinson G, Hammers C and Songa E B *et al* 1993 Naturally occurring antibodies devoid of light chains *Nature* **363** 446–8

[9] Muyldermans S 2021 Applications of nanobodies *Annu. Rev. Anim. Biosci.* **9** 401–21

[10] Goulet D R and Atkins W M 2020 Considerations for the design of antibody-based therapeutics *J. Pharm. Sci.* **109** 74–103

[11] Pettersen E F, Goddard T D, Huang C C, Couch G S, Greenblatt D M and Meng E C *et al* 2004 UCSF chimera—a visualization system for exploratory research and analysis *J. Comput. Chem.* **25** 1605–12

[12] Sela-Culang I, Kunik V and Ofran Y 2013 The structural basis of antibody-antigen recognition *Front Immunol* **4** 302

[13] Janeway C, Travers P, Walport M and Shlomchik M 2001 *Immunobiology* (Garland) 5th edn

[14] Vidarsson G, Dekkers G and Rispens T 2014 IgG subclasses and allotypes: from structure to effector functions *Front. Immunol.* **5** 520

[15] Woof J M and Burton D R 2004 Human antibody-Fc receptor interactions illuminated by crystal structures *Nat. Rev. Immunol.* **4** 89–99

[16] Zhou Y and Marks J D 2016 Mechanism of action for therapeutic antibodies *Biosimilars of Monoclonal Antibodies* (Wiley) pp 85–111

[17] Golay J and Introna M 2012 Mechanism of action of therapeutic monoclonal antibodies: promises and pitfalls of *in vitro* and *in vivo* assays *Arch. Biochem. Biophys.* **526** 146–53

[18] Suzuki M, Kato C and Kato A 2015 Therapeutic antibodies: their mechanisms of action and the pathological findings they induce in toxicity studies *J. Toxicol. Pathol.* **28** 133–9

[19] Narayanan H, Dingfelder F, Butté A, Lorenzen N, Sokolov M and Arosio P 2021 Machine learning for biologics: opportunities for protein engineering, developability, and formulation *Trends Pharmacol. Sci.* **42** 151–65

[20] Norman R A, Ambrosetti F, Bonvin A M J J, Colwell L J, Kelm S and Kumar S *et al* 2020 Computational approaches to therapeutic antibody design: established methods and emerging trends *Brief Bioinform.* **21** 1549–67

[21] Kim J, McFee M, Fang Q, Abdin O and Kim P M 2023 Computational and artificial intelligence-based methods for antibody development *Trends Pharmacol. Sci.* **44** P175–89

[22] Kuroda D, Shirai H, Jacobson M P and Nakamura H 2012 Computer-aided antibody design *Protein Eng. Des. Sel.* **25** 507–22

[23] Liang S, Liang Z, Wu Z, Huang B and Wang X 2022 A benchmark study of protein folding algorithms on nanobodies *bioRxiv*

[24] Lefranc M P, Giudicelli V, Duroux P, Jabado-Michaloud J, Folch G and Aouinti S *et al* 2015 IMGT R, the international immunogenetics information system R 25 years on *Nucleic Acids Res.* **43** D413–22

[25] Tsumoto K and Kuroda D 2023 *Computer-aided Antibody Design* ed K Tsumoto and D Kuroda (New York: Springer)

[26] Swindells M B, Porter C T, Couch M, Hurst J, Abhinandan K R and Nielsen J H *et al* 2017 abYsis: integrated antibody sequence and structure-management, analysis and prediction core view metadata, citation and similar papers at core.ac.uk provided by UCL Discovery *J. Mol. Biol.* **429** 356–64

[27] Corrie B D, Marthandan N, Zimonja B, Jaglale J, Zhou Y and Barr E *et al* 2018 iReceptor: a platform for querying and analyzing antibody/B-cell and T-cell receptor repertoire data across federated repositories *Immunol. Rev.* **284** 24–41

[28] Kovaltsuk A, Leem J, Kelm S, Snowden J, Deane C M and Krawczyk K 2018 Observed antibody space: a resource for data mining next-generation sequencing of antibody repertoires *J. Immunol.* **201** 2502–9

[29] Młokosiewicz J, Deszyński P, Wilman W, Jaszczyszyn I, Ganesan R and Kovaltsuk A *et al* 2022 AbDiver: a tool to explore the natural antibody landscape to aid therapeutic design *Bioinformatics* **38** 2628–30

[30] Ruffolo J A, Gray J J and Sulam J 2021 Deciphering antibody affinity maturation with language models and weakly supervised learning *Machine Learning for Structural Biology Workshop, NeurIPS 2021*

[31] Ehrenmann F, Kaas Q and Lefranc M P 2009 IMGT/3dstructure-DB and IMGT/domaingapalign: a database and a tool for immunoglobulins or antibodies, T cell receptors, MHC, IgSF and MHcSF *Nucleic Acids Res.* **38** D301–7

[32] Dunbar J, Krawczyk K, Leem J, Baker T, Fuchs A and Georges G *et al* 2014 SAbDab: the structural antibody database *Nucleic Acids Res.* **42** D1140–6

[33] Ferdous S and Martin A C R 2018 AbDb: antibody structure database—a database of PDB-derived antibody structures *Database* **2018** bay040

[34] Vita R, Zarebski L, Greenbaum J A, Emami H, Hoof I and Salimi N *et al* 2009 The immune epitope database 2.0 *Nucleic Acids Res.* **38** D854–62

[35] Berman H M, Westbrook J, Feng Z, Gilliland G, Bhat T N and Weissig H *et al* 2000 The protein data bank *Nucleic Acids Res.* **28** 235–42

[36] Wang R, Fang X, Lu Y, Yang C Y and Wang S 2005 The PDBbind database: methodologies and updates *J. Med. Chem.* **48** 4111–9

[37] Moal I H and Fernández-Recio J 2012 SKEMPI: a structural kinetic and energetic database of mutant protein interactions and its use in empirical models *Bioinformatics* **28** 2600–7

[38] Sirin S, Apgar J R, Bennett E M and Keating A E 2016 AB-bind: antibody binding mutational database for computational affinity predictions *Protein Sci.* **25** 393–409

[39] Walsh S J, Bargh J D, Dannheim F M, Hanby A R, Seki H and Counsell A J *et al* 2021 Site-selective modification strategies in antibody-drug conjugates *Chem. Soc. Rev.* **50** 1305–53

[40] Briney B *et al* 2019 Commonality despite exceptional diversity in the baseline human antibody repertoire *Nature* **566** 393–7

[41] Weitzner B D, Jeliazkov J R, Lyskov S, Marze N, Kuroda D and Frick R *et al* 2017 Modeling and docking antibody structures with Rosetta *Nat. Protoc.* **12** 401–16

[42] Abanades B, Georges G, Bujotzek A and Deane C M 2022 ABlooper: fast accurate antibody CDR loop structure prediction with accuracy estimation *Bioinformatics* **38** 1877–80

[43] Adolf-Bryfogle J, Kalyuzhniy O, Kubitz M, Weitzner B D, Hu X and Adachi Y *et al* 2018 RosettaAntibodyDesign (RAbD): a general framework for computational antibody design *PLoS Comput. Biol.* **14** 1–38

[44] Liberis E, Velickovic P, Sormanni P, Vendruscolo M and Lio P 2018 Parapred: antibody paratope prediction using convolutional and recurrent neural networks *Bioinformatics* **34** 2944–50

[45] Ambrosetti F, Olsen T H, Olimpieri P P, Jiménez-García B, Milanetti E and Marcatilli P *et al* 2020 proABC-2: prediction of antibody contacts v2 and its application to information-driven docking *Bioinformatics* **36** 5107–8

[46] Honorato R V, Koukos P I, Jiménez-García B, Tsaregorodtsev A, Verlato M and Giachetti A *et al* 2021 Structural biology in the clouds: the weNMR-EOSC ecosystem *Front Mol. Biosci.* **8** 708

[47] Choi Y and Deane C M 2010 FREAD revisited: accurate loop structure prediction using a database search algorithm *Proteins: Struct. Funct. Bioinform.* **78** 1431–40

[48] Khan A, Cowen-rivers A I, Grosnit A, Wang J, Storkey A and Bou-ammar H 2023 Toward real-world automated antibody design with combinatorial bayesian optimization *Cell Rep. Methods* **3** 100374

[49] Robert P A, Akbar R, Frank R, Pavlović M, Widrich M and Snapkov I *et al* 2022 Unconstrained generation of synthetic antibody-antigen structures to guide machine learning methodology for real-world antibody specificity prediction *bioRxiv* 451258
[50] Jumper J, Evans R, Pritzel A, Green T, Figurnov M and Ronneberger O *et al* 2021 Highly accurate protein structure prediction with AlphaFold *Nature* **596** 583–9
[51] Ingraham J, Baranov M, Costello Z, Frappier V, Ismail A and Tie S *et al* 2022 Illuminating protein space with a programmable generative model bioRxiv:518682
[52] Klausen M S, Anderson M V, Jespersen M C, Nielsen M and Marcatili P 2015 LYRA, a webserver for lymphocyte receptor structural modeling *Nucleic Acids Res.* **43** W349–55
[53] Zheng L, Lan H, Shen T, Wu J, Wang S and Liu W *et al* 2021 tFold-TR: combining deep learning enhanced hybrid potential energy for template-based modeling structure refinement ArXiv:2105.04350
[54] Cohen T, Halfon M, Schneidman-Duhovny D, Rachel T and Benin S 2022 NanoNet: rapid end-to-end nanobody modeling by deep learning at sub angstrom resolution *Front. Immunol.* **13** 958584
[55] Rohl C A, Strauss C E M, Misura K M S and Baker D 2004 Protein structure prediction using rosetta *Methods Enzymol.* **383** 66–93
[56] Shapovalov M V and Dunbrack R L 2011 A smoothed backbone-dependent rotamer library for proteins derived from adaptive kernel density estimates and regressions *Structure.* **19** 844–58
[57] Weitzner B D, Jeliazkov J R, Lyskov S, Marze N, Kuroda D and Frick R *et al* 2017 Modeling and docking antibody structures with Rosetta HHS public access author manuscript *Nat. Protoc.* **12** 401–16
[58] Leem J, Dunbar J, Georges G, Shi J and Deane C M 2016 Abodybuilder: automated antibody structure prediction with data–driven accuracy estimation *MAbs* **8** 1259–68
[59] Ruffolo J A, Sulam J and Gray J J 2022 Antibody structure prediction using interpretable deep learning *Patterns* **3** 100406
[60] Ruffolo J A, Chu L-S, Mahajan S P and Gray J J F 2022 accurate antibody structure prediction from deep learning on massive set of natural antibodies *Biophys. J.* **121** 155A–6A
[61] Fernández-Quintero M L, Pomarici N D, Math B A, Kroell K B, Waibl F and Bujotzek A *et al* 2020 Antibodies exhibit multiple paratope states influencing VH–VL domain orientations *Commun. Biol.* **3** 589
[62] Fernández-Quintero M L, Derose E F, Gabel S A, Mueller G A and Liedl K R 2022 Nanobody paratope ensembles in solution characterized by MD simulations and NMR *Int. J. Mol. Sci.* **23** 5419
[63] Fernández-Quintero M L, Kokot J, Waibl F, Fischer A L M, Quoika P K and Deane C M *et al* 2023 Challenges in antibody structure prediction *MAbs* **15** 2175319
[64] Evans R, O'Neill M, Pritzel A, Antropova N, Senior A and Green T *et al* 2022 Protein complex prediction with alphafold-multimer BioRxiv:202110.04.463034
[65] Lee J H, Yadollahpour P, Watkins A, Frey N C, Leaver-Fay A and Ra S *et al* 2022 EquiFold: protein structure prediction with a novel coarse-grained structure representation Biorxiv: 2022.10.07.511322
[66] Daberdaku S and Ferrari C 2019 Antibody interface prediction with 3D Zernike descriptors and SVM *Bioinformatics.* **35** 1870–6
[67] Leem J, Mitchell L S, Farmery J H R, Barton J and Galson J D 2022 Deciphering the language of antibodies using self-supervised learning *Patterns* **3** 100513

[68] Myung Y, Pires D E V and Ascher D B 2021 MmCSM-AB: guiding rational antibody engineering through multiple point mutations *Nucleic Acids Res.* **48** W125–31
[69] Myung Y, Rodrigues C H M, Ascher D B and Pires D E V 2020 MCSM-AB2: guiding rational antibody design using graph-based signatures *Bioinformatics* **36** 1453–9
[70] Kunik V, Ashkenazi S and Ofran Y 2023 Paratome: an online tool for systematic identification of antigen-binding regions in antibodies based on sequence or structure *Nucleic Acids Res.* **40** 521–4
[71] Saha S and Raghava G P S 2006 Prediction of continuous B-cell epitopes in an antigen using recurrent neural network *Proteins: Struct. Funct. Bioinform.* **65** 40–8
[72] Larsen J E P, Lund O and Nielsen M 2006 Improved method for predicting linear B-cell epitopes *Immunome Res.* **2** 2
[73] Manavalan B, Govindaraj R G, Shin T H, Kim M O and Lee G 2018 iBCE-EL: a new ensemble learning framework for improved linear b-cell epitope prediction *Front. Immunol.* **9** 1695
[74] Yao B, Zhang L, Liang S and Zhang C 2012 SVMTriP: a method to predict antigenic epitopes using support vector machine to integrate tri-peptide similarity and propensity *PLoS One* **7** 0045152
[75] Sela-Culang I, Ashkenazi S, Peters B and Ofran Y 2015 PEASE: predicting b-cell epitopes utilizing antibody sequence *Bioinformatics.* **31** 1313–5
[76] Scarabelli G, Morra G and Colombo G 2010 Predicting interaction sites from the energetics of isolated proteins: a new approach to epitope mapping *Biophys.* J. **98** 1966–75
[77] Montefiori M, Pilotto S, Marabelli C, Moroni E, Ferraro M and Serapian S A *et al* 2019 Impact of mutations on NPAC structural dynamics: mechanistic insights from MD simulations *J. Chem. Inf. Model.* **59** 3927–37
[78] Marchetti F, Capelli R, Rizzato F, Laio A and Colombo G 2019 The subtle trade-off between evolutionary and energetic constraints in protein-protein interactions *J. Phys. Chem. Lett.* **10** 1489–97
[79] Pittala S and Bailey-Kellogg C 2020 Learning context-aware structural representations to predict antigen and antibody binding interfaces *Bioinformatics* **36** 3996–4003
[80] Zhou C, Chen Z, Zhang L, Yan D, Mao T and Tang K *et al* 2019 SEPPA 3.0-enhanced spatial epitope prediction enabling glycoprotein antigens *Nucleic Acids Res.* **47** W388–94
[81] Rubinstein N D, Mayrose I, Martz E and Pupko T 2009 Epitopia: a web-server for predicting B-cell epitopes *BMC Bioinformatics* **10** 287
[82] Rubinstein N D, Mayrose I, Halperin D, Yekutieli D, Gershoni J M and Pupko T 2008 Computational characterization of B-cell epitopes *Mol. Immunol* **45** 3477–89
[83] Kringelum J V, Lundegaard C, Lund O and Nielsen M 2012 Reliable B cell epitope predictions: impacts of method development and improved benchmarking *PLoS Comput. Biol.* **8** 1002829
[84] Brenke R, Hall D R, Chuang G-Y, Comeau S R, Bohnuud T and Beglov D *et al* 2023 Application of asymmetric statistical potentials to antibody-protein docking *Bioinformatics* **28** 2608–14
[85] Kozakov D, Hall D R, Xia B, Porter K A, Padhorny D and Yueh C *et al* 2017 The cluspro web server for protein-protein docking *Nat. Protoc.* **12** 255–78
[86] Sircar A and Gray J J 2023 SnugDock: paratope structural optimization during antibody-antigen docking compensates for errors in antibody homology models *PLoS Comput. Biol.* **6** 1000644

[87] Ramírez-Aportela E, López-Blanco J R and Chacón P 2016 FRODOCK 2.0: fast protein–protein docking server *Bioinformatics* **32** 2386–8

[88] De Vries S J, Schindler C E M, Chauvot De Beauchêne I and Zacharias M 2015 A web interface for easy flexible protein-protein docking with ATTRACT *Biophys. J.* **108** 462–5

[89] Dominguez C, Boelens R and Bonvin A M J J 2003 HADDOCK: a protein-protein docking approach based on biochemical or biophysical information *J. Am. Chem. Soc.* **125** 1731–7

[90] De Vries S J, Van Dijk A D J, Krzeminski M, Van Dijk M, Thureau A and Hsu V *et al* 2007 HADDOCK versus HADDOCK: new features and performance of HADDOCK2.0 on the CAPRI targets *Proteins: Struct., Funct. Bioinform.* **69** 726–33

[91] Macindoe G, Mavridis L, Venkatraman V, Devignes M-D and Ritchie D W 2010 HexServer: an FFT-based protein docking server powered by graphics processors *Nucleic Acids Res.* **38** 445–9

[92] Tovchigrechko A and Vakser I A 2006 GRAMM-X public web server for protein–protein docking *Nucleic Acids Res.* **1** 310–4

[93] Duhovny D, Nussinov R and Wolfson H J 2002 Efficient unbound docking of rigid molecules *Algorithms in Bioinformatics. WABI 2002* (Berlin: Springer) Lecture Notes in Computer Science (including subseries Lecture Notes in Artificial Intelligence and Lecture Notes in Bioinformatics) vol 2452 pp 185–200

[94] Schneidman-Duhovny D, Inbar Y, Nussinov R and Wolfson H J 2005 PatchDock and SymmDock: servers for rigid and symmetric docking *Nucleic Acids Res.* **33** W363

[95] Jiménez-García B, Pons C and Fernández-Recio J 2013 pyDockWEB: a web server for rigid-body protein–protein docking using electrostatics and desolvation scoring *Bioinformatics* **29** 1698–9

[96] Torchala M, Moal I H, Chaleil R A G, Fernandez-Recio J and Bates P A 2013 SwarmDock: a server for flexible protein–protein docking *Bioinformatics* **29** 807–9

[97] Kozakov D, Brenke R, Comeau S R and Vajda S 2006 PIPER: an FFT-based protein docking program with pairwise potentials *Proteins: Struct., Funct., Bioinform.* **65** 392–406

[98] Chuang G-Y, Kozakov D, Brenke R, Comeau S R and Vajda S 2008 DARS (decoys As the reference state) potentials for protein-protein docking *Biophys.* J. **95** 4217–27

[99] 2022 Aulos Bioscience Inc. Our pipeline https://aulosbio.com/our-pipeline/ (accessed 23 February 2023)

[100] Lund J, Pound J D, Jones P T, Duncan A R, Bentley T and Goodall M *et al* 1992 Multiple binding sites on the CH2 domain of IgG for mouse FcγR11 *Mol. Immunol* **29** 53–9

[101] 2022 AULOS-preclinical-data-poster-Aulos Biosci.2022 https://f9p5g3w9.rocketcdn.me/wp-content/uploads/2022/03/AULOS-Preclinical-Data-Poster-2022MAR21.pdf (accessed 10 May 2023)

[102] Case D A, Cheatham T E, Darden T, Gohlke H, Luo R and Merz K M *et al* 2005 The Amber biomolecular simulation programs *J. Comput. Chem.* **26** 1668–88

[103] Brooks B R, Brooks Iii C L, Mackerell A D, Nilsson L, Petrella R J and Roux B *et al* 2009 CHARMM: the biomolecular simulation program NIH public access *J. Comput. Chem.* **30** 1545–614

[104] Bowers K J, Chow E, Xu H, Dror R O, Eastwood M P and Gregersen B A *et al* 2006 Scalable algorithms for molecular dynamics simulations on commodity clusters *Proc. of the 2006 ACM/IEEE Conf. on Supercomputing, SC'06* https://dl.acm.org/doi/10.1145/1188455.1188544 (accessed 7 April 2023)

[105] Abraham M J, Murtola T, Schulz R, Páll S, Smith J C and Hess B *et al* 2015 Gromacs: high performance molecular simulations through multi-level parallelism from laptops to supercomputers *SoftwareX* **1–2** 19–25

[106] Phillips J C, Hardy D J, Maia J D C, Stone J E, Ribeiro J V and Bernardi R C *et al* 2020 Scalable molecular dynamics on CPU and GPU architectures with NAMD *J. Chem. Phys.* **153** 044130

[107] Fine R M, Wang H, Shenkin P S, Yarmush D L and Levinthal C 1986 Predicting antibody hypervariable loop conformations II: minimization and molecular dynamics studies of MCPC603 from many randomly generated loop conformations *Proteins: Struct., Funct. Bioinform.* **1** 342–62

[108] Shenkin P S, Yarmush D L, Fine R M, Wang H and Levinthal C 1987 Predicting antibody hypervariable loop conformation. I. Ensembles of random conformations for ringlike structures *Biopolymers* **26** 2053–85

[109] Browne C B, Powley E, Whitehouse D, Lucas S M, Cowling P I and Rohlfshagen P *et al* 2012 A survey of monte carlo tree search methods *IEEE Trans. Comput. Intell. AI Games* **4** 1–43

[110] Shin K, Tran D P, Takemura K, Kitao A, Terayama K and Tsuda K 2019 Enhancing biomolecular sampling with reinforcement learning: a tree search molecular dynamics simulation method *ACS Omega* **4** 13853–62

[111] Bongini L, Fanelli D, Piazza F, De Los Rios P, Sandin S and Skoglund U 2004 Freezing immunoglobulins to see them move *Proc. Natl Acad. Sci. USA* **101** 6466–71

[112] Zhang X, Zhang L, Tong H, Peng B, Rames M J and Zhang S *et al* 2015 3D structural fluctuation of igg1 antibody revealed by individual particle electron tomography *Sci. Rep.* **5** 9803

[113] Nishigami H, Kamiya N and Nakamura H 2016 Revisiting antibody modeling assessment for CDR-H3 loop *Protein Eng. Des. Sel* **29** 477–84

[114] Bekker G J and Kamiya N 2023 Thermal stability estimation of single domain antibodies using molecular dynamics simulations *Methods Mol. Biol.* **2552** 151–63

[115] Shimba N, Kamiya N and Nakamura H 2016 Model building of antibody-antigen complex structures using GBSA scores *J. Chem. Inf. Model.* **56** 2005–12

[116] Best R B, Hummer G and Eaton W A 2013 Native contacts determine protein folding mechanisms in atomistic simulations *Proc. Natl Acad. Sci. USA* **110** 17874–9

[117] Song Y, Dimaio F, Wang R Y R, Kim D, Miles C and Brunette T *et al* 2013 High resolution comparative modeling with RosettaCM *Structure* **21** 1735–42

[118] Park H, Bradley P, Greisen P, Liu Y, Mulligan V K and Kim D E *et al* 2016 Simultaneous optimization of biomolecular energy function on features from small molecules and macromolecules *J. Chem. Theory Comput.* **12** 6201

[119] Qiao X, Qu L, Guo Y and Hoshino T 2021 Secondary structure and conformational stability of the antigen residues making contact with antibodies *J. Phys. Chem.* B **125** 11374–85

[120] Bai G, Ge Y, Su Y, Chen S, Zeng X and Lu H *et al* 2021 Computational construction of a single-chain Bi-paratopic antibody allosterically inhibiting TCR-Staphylococcal enterotoxin B binding *Front. Immunol.* **12** 1–13

[121] Aguilar Rangel M, Bedwell A, Costanzi E, Taylor R J, Russo R and Bernardes G J L *et al* 2022 Fragment-based computational design of antibodies targeting structured epitopes *Sci. Adv.* **8** 1–14

[122] Jones Lellouch E, Hubbard W B, Sicardy B, Vilas F and Bouchet P 1986 Replacing the complementarity-determining regions in a human antibody with those from a mouse *Nature* **324** 227–31

[123] Tan P, Mitchell D A, Buss T N, Holmes M A, Anasetti C and Foote J 2002 'Superhumanized' antibodies: reduction of immunogenic potential by complementarity-determining region grafting with human germline sequences: application to an Anti-CD28 *J. Immunol.* **169** 1119–25

[124] Roguska M A, Pedersen J T, Keddy C A, Henry A H, Searle S J and Lambert J M *et al* 1994 Humanization of murine monoclonal antibodies through variable domain resurfacing *Proc. Natl Acad. Sci. USA* **91** 969–73

[125] Clavero-Álvarez A, Di Mambro T, Perez-Gaviro S, Magnani M and Bruscolini P 2018 Humanization of antibodies using a statistical inference approach *Sci. Rep.* **8** 14820

[126] Tennenhouse A, Khmelnitsky L, Yeshaya N, Noronha A, Lindzen M and Khalaila R *et al* 2022 Reliable energy-based antibody humanization and stabilization bioRxiv 2022.08.14.503891

[127] Sang Z, Xiang Y, Bahar I and Shi Y 2022 Llamanade: an open-source computational pipeline for robust nanobody humanization *Structure* **30** 418–29 e3

[128] Choi Y, Hua C, Sentman C L, Ackerman M E and Bailey-Kellogg C 2015 Antibody humanization by structure-based computational protein design *MAbs* **7** 1045–57

[129] Jayakody R S, Jasin Arachchige L I and Japahuge A 2021 Computational elucidation and validation of the three-dimensional structure of humanized aldolase catalytic antibody 38C2 *J. Biomol. Struct. Dyn.* **39** 2463–77

[130] Sormanni P, Aprile F A and Vendruscolo M 2015 The camsol method of rational design of protein mutants with enhanced solubility *J. Mol. Biol.* **427** 478–90

[131] Wolf Pérez A M, Sormanni P, Andersen J S, Sakhnini L I, Rodriguez-Leon I and Bjelke J R *et al* 2019 In vitro and in silico assessment of the developability of a designed monoclonal antibody library *MAbs* **11** 388

[132] Liang S and Zhang C 2020 Prediction of immunogenicity for humanized and full human therapeutic antibodies *PLoS One* **15** e0238150

[133] Raybould M I J and Deane C M 2022 The therapeutic antibody profiler for computational developability assessment *Methods Mole. Biol.* **2313** 115–25

[134] Sormanni P, Aprile F A and Vendruscolo M 2018 Third generation antibody discovery methods: in silico rational design *Chem. Soc. Rev.* **47** 9137

[135] Raybould M I J, Marks C, Krawczyk K, Taddese B, Nowak J and Lewis A P *et al* 2019 Five computational developability guidelines for therapeutic antibody profiling *Proc. Natl Acad. Sci. USA* **116** 4025–30

[136] Hassanzadeh-Ghassabeh G, Devoogdt N, De Pauw P, Vincke C and Muyldermans S 2013 Nanobodies and their potential applications *Nanomedicine* **8** 1013–26

[137] Salvador J-P, Vilaplana L and Marco M-P 2019 Nanobody: outstanding features for diagnostic and therapeutic applications *Anal. Bioanal. Chem.* **411** 1703–13

[138] Aghebati-Maleki A and Aghebati-Maleki L 2018 Nanobodies: emerging tools for clinical applications *Int. J. Res. Appl. Basic Med. Sci.* **4** 81–90

[139] Verhaar E R, Woodham A W and Ploegh H L 2021 Nanobodies in cancer *Semin. Immunol.* **52** 101425

[140] Siontorou C G 2013 Nanobodies as novel agents for disease diagnosis and therapy *Int. J. Nanomed.* **8** 4215–27

[141] De Meyer T, Muyldermans S and Depicker A 2014 Nanobody-based products as research and diagnostic tools *Trends Biotechnol.* **32** 263–70

[142] Hu Y, Liu C and Muyldermans S 2017 Nanobody-based delivery systems for diagnosis and targeted tumor therapy *Front Immunol* **8** 1442

[143] Wesolowski J, Alzogaray V, Reyelt J, Unger M, Juarez K and Urrutia M *et al* 2009 Single domain antibodies: promising experimental and therapeutic tools in infection and immunity *Med. Microbiol. Immunol* **198** 157–74

[144] Bao G, Tang M, Zhao J and Zhu X 2021 Nanobody: a promising toolkit for molecular imaging and disease therapy *EJNMMI Res.* **11** 1–13

[145] Steeland S, Vandenbroucke R E and Libert C 2016 Nanobodies as therapeutics: big opportunities for small antibodies *Drug Discov. Today* **21** 1076–113

[146] Asaadi Y, Jouneghani F F, Janani S and Rahbarizadeh F 2021 A comprehensive comparison between camelid nanobodies and single chain variable fragments *Biomark. Res.* **9** 1–20

[147] Bannas P, Hambach J and Koch-Nolte F 2017 Nanobodies and nanobody-based human heavy chain antibodies as antitumor therapeutics *Front. Immunol.* **8** 1–13

[148] Boulenouar H, Bouchoutrouch N, Cherrah Y and Sefrioui H 2020 Nanobodies and their medical applications *GMR* **19** 1–12

[149] Hwang T J, Carpenter D, Lauffenburger J C, Wang B, Franklin J M and Kesselheim A S 2016 Failure of investigational drugs in late-stage clinical development and publication of trial results *JAMA Intern. Med.* **176** 1826–33

[150] Pfizer discontinues global development of bococizumab, its investigational PCSK9 inhibitor *Pfizer* 2016 https://pfizer.com/news/press-release/press-release-detail/pfizer_discontinues_global_-development_of_bococizumab_its_investigational_pcsk9_inhibitor (accessed 7 April 2023)

[151] Cheng X, Wang J, Kang G, Hu M, Yuan B and Zhang Y *et al* 2019 Homology modeling-based in silico affinity maturation improves the affinity of a nanobody *Int. J. Mol. Sci.* **20** 4187

[152] Valdés-Tresanco M S, Molina-Zapata A, Pose A G and Moreno E 2022 Structural insights into the design of synthetic nanobody libraries *Molecules* **27** 2198

[153] Pérez-Hernández G and Noé F 2016 Hierarchical time-lagged independent component analysis: computing slow modes and reaction coordinates for large molecular systems *J. Chem. Theory Comput.* **12** 6118–29

[154] Baroroh U, Setiani N A, Mardiah I, Astriany D and Yusuf M 2022 Computational design of nanobody binding to cortisol to improve their binding affinity using molecular docking and molecular dynamics simulations *Indones. J. Chem.* **22** 515–25

[155] Hacisuleyman A and Erman B 2020 ModiBodies: a computational method for modifying nanobodies in nanobody-antigen complexes to improve binding affinity and specificity *J. Biol. Phys.* **46** 189–208

[156] Cheng X, Wang J, Kang G, Hu M, Yuan B and Zhang Y *et al* 2019 Homology modeling-based in silico affinity maturation improves the affinity of a nanobody *Int. J. Mol. Sci.* **20** 4187

[157] Vivcharuk V, Baardsnes J, Deprez C, Sulea T, Jaramillo M and Corbeil C R *et al* 2017 Assisted design of antibody and protein therapeutics (ADAPT) *PLoS One* **12** e0181490

[158] Ponziani S, Di Vittorio G, Pitari G, Cimini A M, Ardini M and Gentile R *et al* 2020 Antibody-drug conjugates: the new frontier of chemotherapy *Int. J. Mol. Sci.* **21** 1–28

[159] Debnath U, Verma S, Patra J and Mandal S K 2022 A review on recent synthetic routes and computational approaches for antibody drug conjugation developments used in anti-cancer therapy *J. Mol. Struct.* **1256** 132524

[160] Melo R, Lemos A, Preto A J, Almeida J G, Correia J D G and Sensoy O *et al* 2018 Computational approaches in antibody-drug conjugate optimization for targeted cancer therapy *Curr. Top. Med. Chem.* **18** 1091–109

[161] Coumans E, Ariaans G J, Spijker H J, Renart Verkerk P, Beusker P H and Kokke A *et al* 2020 A platform for the generation of site-specific antibody–drug conjugates that allows for selective reduction of engineered cysteines *Bioconjug. Chem.* **31** 2136–46

[162] Papageorgiou L, Papakonstantinou E, Salis C, Polychronidou E, Hagidimitriou M and Maroulis D *et al* 2020 Drugena: a fully automated immunoinformatics platform for the design of antibody-drug conjugates against neurodegenerative diseases *GeNeDis 2018* (Springer) Advances in Experimental Medicine and Biology vol 1194 pp 203–15

[163] Kim S, Thiessen P A, Bolton E E, Chen J, Fu G and Gindulyte A *et al* 2016 PubChem substance and compound databases *Nucleic Acids Res.* **44** D1202–13

[164] Brun M P and Gauzy-Lazo L 2013 Protocols for lysine conjugation *Methods Mol. Biol.* **1045** 173–87

[165] Gupta N, Ansari A, Dhoke G V, Chilamari M, Sivaccumar J and Kumari S *et al* 2019 Computationally designed antibody–drug conjugates self-assembled via affinity ligands *Nat. Biomed. Eng.* **3** 917–29

[166] Sakamoto K M, Kim K B, Kumagai A, Mercurio F, Crews C M and Deshaies R J 2001 Protacs: chimeric molecules that target proteins to the Skp1-Cullin-F box complex for ubiquitination and degradation *Proc. Natl Acad. Sci. USA* **98** 8554–9

[167] Kargbo R B 2022 Emerging proteolysis targeting antibodies (PROTABs) for application in cancer therapy *ACS Med. Chem. Lett.* **13** 1833–4

[168] Cotton A D, Nguyen D P, Gramespacher J A, Seiple I B and Wells J A 2021 Development of antibody-based PROTACs for the degradation of the cell-surface immune checkpoint protein PD-L1 *J. Am. Chem. Soc.* **143** 593–8

[169] Maneiro M, Forte N, Shchepinova M M, Kounde C S, Chudasama V and Baker J R *et al* 2020 Antibody-PROTAC conjugates enable HER2-dependent targeted protein degradation of BRD4 *ACS Chem. Biol.* **15** 1306–12

[170] Marei H, Tsai W T K, Kee Y S, Ruiz K, He J and Cox C *et al* 2022 Antibody targeting of E3 ubiquitin ligases for receptor degradation *Nature* **610** 182–9

[171] Dawn M, Ecker T J C and P S 2020 The therapeutic monoclonal antibody product market https://bioprocessintl.com/business/economics/the-market-for-therapeutic-mab-products/

[172] Market Data Forecast 2023 2023 https://marketdataforecast.com/market-reports/antibodies-market (accessed 2 April 2023)

[173] Lu R M, Hwang Y C, Liu I J, Lee C C, Tsai H Z and Li H J *et al* 2020 Development of therapeutic antibodies for the treatment of diseases *J. Biomed. Sci.* **27** 1–30

[174] WORLD PREVIEW 2022 Outlook to 2028: patents and pricing evaluate pharma®. 2022

[175] Grilo A L and Mantalaris A 2019 Science & Society the increasingly human and pro fi table monoclonal antibody market *Trends Biotechnol.* **37** 9–16

[176] Kelley B 2009 Industrialization of mAb production technology: the bioprocessing industry at a crossroads *MAbs.* **1** 443–52

[177] Farid S S, Baron M, Stamatis C, Nie W and Coffman J 2020 Benchmarking biopharmaceutical process development and manufacturing cost contributions to R&D *MAbs* **12** 1754999

[178] Klutz S, Holtmann L, Lobedann M and Schembecker G 2016 Cost evaluation of antibody production processes in different operation modes *Chem. Eng. Sci.* **141** 63–74
[179] Mahal H, Branton H and Farid S S 2021 End-to-end continuous bioprocessing: impact on facility design, cost of goods, and cost of development for monoclonal antibodies *Biotechnol. Bioeng.* **118** 3468–85
[180] FDA approves LEQEMBI^{TM} (lecanemab-irmb) under the accelerated approval pathway for the treatment of Alzheimer's disease *Eisai Inc* 2023 https://media-us.eisai.com/2023-01-06-FDA-Approves-LEQEMBI-TM-lecanemab-irmb-Under-the-Accelerated-Approval-Pathway-for-the-Treatment-of-Alzheimers-Disease (accessed 30 May 2023)
[181] Search of: lecanemab—list results—clinicaltrials.gov national library of medicine (U.S.). https://clinicaltrials.gov/ct2/results?cond=&term=Lecanemab&cntry=&state=&city=&dist= (accessed 30 May 2023)
[182] A Study to evaluate safety, tolerability, and efficacy of lecanemab in subjects with early Alzheimer's disease. Identifier NCT01767311 *National Library of Medicine (U.S.)* 2023 https://clinicaltrials.gov/ct2/show/NCT01767311 (accessed 30 May 2023)
[183] A Study to confirm safety and efficacy of lecanemab in participants with early Alzheimer's disease. Identifier NCT03887455 *National Library of Medicine (U.S.)* 2022 https://clinicaltrials.gov/ct2/show/NCT03887455 (accessed 30 May 2023)
[184] AHEAD 3–45 study: a study to evaluate efficacy and safety of treatment with lecanemab in participants with preclinical Alzheimer's disease and elevated amyloid and also in participants with early preclinical Alzheimer's disease and intermediate amyloid. Identifier NCT04468659 *National Library of Medicine (U.S.)* 2023 https://clinicaltrials.gov/ct2/show/NCT04468659 (accessed 30 May 2023)
[185] Dominantly inherited Alzheimer network trial: an opportunity to prevent dementia. a study of potential disease modifying treatments in individuals with a type of early ons*et Al*zheimer's disease caused by a genetic mutation (DIAN-TU). Identifier NCT05269394 *National Library of Medicine (U.S.)* 2023 https://clinicaltrials.gov/ct2/show/NCT05269394 (accessed 30 May 2023)
[186] Dominantly inherited Alzheimer network trial: an opportunity to prevent dementia. a study of potential disease modifying treatments in individuals at risk for or with a type of early ons*et Al*zheimer's disease caused by a genetic mutation. master protocol DIAN-TU-001. Identifier NCT01760005 *National Library of Medicine (U.S.)* 2023 https://clinicaltrials.gov/ct2/show/NCT01760005 (accessed 30 May 2023)
[187] An extension study of TS-152 in subjects with rheumatoid arthritis. Identifier NCT04077567 *National Library of Medicine (U.S.)* 2023 https://clinicaltrials.gov/ct2/show/NCT04077567 (accessed 30 May 2023)
[188] Study of AU-007 2022 A Monoclonal antibody that binds to IL-2 and inhibits IL-2Rα binding, in patients with unresectable locally advanced or metastatic cancer. Identifier NCT05267626 *National Library of Medicine (U.S.)* https://clinicaltrials.gov/ct2/show/NCT05267626 (accessed 5 March 2023)
[189] Beckman R A, Weiner L M and Davis H M 2007 Antibody constructs in cancer therapy *Cancer* **109** 170–9
[190] Brinkmann U and Kontermann R E 2017 The making of bispecific antibodies *MAbs* **9** 182–212
[191] Wang Q, Chen Y, Park J, Liu X, Hu Y and Wang T *et al* 2019 Design and production of bispecific antibodies *Antibodies* **8** 43

[192] Declerck P J 2012 Biologicals and biosimilars : a review of the science and its implications *Gener. Biosim. Initiative J.* **1** 13–6
[193] Makurvet F D 2021 Biologics vs. small molecules: drug costs and patient access *Med. Drug Discov.* **9** 100075

Chapter 12

Physiologically-based pharmacokinetic modeling for pharmaceuticals—institute, industry and agencies perspective

Ajay S Lale, Maitri S Sanghavi and Anuj K Saini

This chapter offers an overview of physiologically-based pharmacokinetic (PBPK) modeling and its expanding applications across academia, the pharmaceutical industry, and regulatory agencies. PBPK models use physiological and compound-specific parameters to predict *in vivo* performance of drugs. These models aid in determining the suitable study designs, identifying the critical bioavailability attributes, predicting doses, and assessing drug–drug interactions (DDIs), which can ultimately contribute in drug discovery, development, and regulatory submissions. Moreover, the chapter emphasizes the significance of a well-constructed PBPK model in drug development, enhancing our mechanistic understanding of clinical observations, facilitating regulatory communication, and guiding decision making. The authors also highlight the potential for personalized dosing based on PBPK models, emphasizing the need for continued research to enhance their effectiveness. It also offers a promising approach to address specific biopharmaceutical challenges in drug development while overcoming ethical and logistical hurdles. The chapter acknowledges the challenges encountered by PBPK researchers, including the ongoing necessity for optimizing and validating PBPK platforms. Additionally, it calls for further research to enhance the effectiveness of PBPK models in predicting the systemic exposure of novel and generic drug candidates, ultimately benefiting the pharmaceutical industry and regulatory agencies.

12.1 Introduction

Model-informed drug development (MIDD) has revolutionized the pharmaceutical industry by providing a powerful tool for predicting clinical study outcomes and optimizing drug development processes. It is an approach employed to inform drug development and the decision-making process using exposure-based, biological and

doi:10.1088/978-0-7503-5613-8ch12

statistical models derived from preclinical and clinical data sources [1]. One of the key techniques within MIDD is PBPK modeling, which plays a pivotal role in understanding and predicting drug absorption, distribution, metabolism, and excretion [2, 3]. PBPK modeling is a sophisticated approach that integrates physiological, physicochemical, and biochemical processes to simulate the pharmacokinetic behavior of drugs in the body. It considers various factors, including the properties of the active pharmaceutical ingredient (API) and the dosage form, along with the dynamic environment of the gastrointestinal tract. Additionally, PBPK modeling incorporates *in vitro* measurements of properties like solubility, permeability, and dissolution performance. These *in vitro* data are crucial for establishing correlations between the *in vitro* drug release and *in vivo* drug absorption profiles, known as *in vitro–in vivo* correlation (IVIVC), and for predicting *in vivo* drug release from *in vitro* dissolution data, known as *in vitro–in vivo* relationship (IVIVR). By integrating IVIVC and IVIVR concepts into PBPK modeling, it becomes possible to further optimize drug formulations, assess bioequivalence (BE), predict *in vivo* drug performance, and understand biopharmaceutical risk associated with different formulations. A number of different *in silico* PBPK modeling tools are currently available, such as GastroPlus™ by Simulations Plus (simulations-plus.com), SimCYP™ PBPK Simulator by Certara and PK-Sim® by Open Systems Pharmacology (open-systems-pharmacology.org) [4–8].

The historical origin of PBPK modeling can be traced back to Teorell's pioneering proposal in 1937 [9]. Since then, it has evolved into a powerful tool that employs mathematical techniques to depict the organism under investigation as interconnected compartments representing specific organs or tissues. These compartments are interconnected by the circulatory system, and mass-balance equations describe the fate of drug substances within the body [10]. PBPK models combine physiological knowledge with substance-specific factors to solve mass-balance equations and simulate concentration-time curves, providing a temporal depiction of drug concentrations in blood or plasma. These models enable the prediction of drug pharmacokinetics in specific individuals and under various physiological or pathological conditions, offering valuable insights for optimizing dosing regimens and improving therapeutic outcomes [10]. PBPK modeling plays a crucial role in understanding and optimizing drug behavior in different dosage forms and routes of administration. By considering the specific characteristics and mechanisms associated with each route, PBPK models provide valuable insights into drug disposition, aiding in formulation development, dosing regimen optimization, and the assessment of factors affecting drug delivery and systemic exposure.

The concept of 'mechanistic absorption modeling' has been included under the umbrella of 'physiologically-based biopharmaceutics modeling (PBBM)', which is integrated and optimized in current PBPK platforms used by formulation scientists in the pharmaceutical industry. This approach considers the complex interactions a drug undergoes before entering systemic circulation, including luminal precipitation, transporter-dependent absorption, and interactions with colloidal species and endogenous constituents. By accounting for these interactions, PBPK modeling enhances the accuracy of predictions regarding drug absorption and its subsequent behavior in the body [5].

The benefits of PBPK modeling extend beyond drug development. The ability to predict drug concentrations using PBPK models has opened avenues for exploring alternative testing approaches and strategies that align with the principles of the 3Rs (reduce, refine, replace) [11]. Continuous refinement and improvement of PBPK models through parameterization and validation enhance their accuracy and predictive capabilities. Validated PBPK models support decision-making in drug development, regulatory submissions, and facilitate discussions with regulatory agencies. However, it is essential to continually optimize and validate PBPK models to ensure their reliability and applicability across different scenarios. [12, 13]

This process includes assessing the model's ability to reproduce concentration-time profiles, clearance rates, and predicting DDIs. Approaches such as the top-down, bottom-up, and middle-out are used to serve the purpose. The top-down approach fits the model to observable pharmacokinetic data, while the bottom-up approach uses physiological and substance-specific factors to solve mass-balance equations. The middle-out approach combines both approaches to bridge scientific gaps [6].

The scientific community, including academia, health authorities, and industries, are actively involved in sharing their approaches, discussing the difficulties of development and applications, and presenting their modeling work in this field. While some applications have been successful, there are still many limitations and challenges to overcome. Scientists are continuously working to address these limitations of the field and improve them in the future. [4, 6, 7, 14, 15]. In this chapter, we have explained the basic considerations for modeling, its applications, limitations and its future prospects from institute, industry and agencies perspective.

12.2 PBPK model development

Generally, PBPK model development is a process of five stages such as [1] general model structure specifications, [2] tissue/organs model specifications, [3] arrangement of PBPK model equations, [4] parameterization of the model, and [5] parameter estimation and simulation using PBPK modeling softwares [10]. Figure 12.1 describes all the steps and key points in each step which are explained in below content.

12.2.1 General model structure specification

In the initial stages of drug discovery, PBPK models are developed by combining *in silico*, *in vitro*, and animal PK data to guide molecular design towards optimized ADME properties in humans and to predict the PK profile for the FIH dosing regimen. This process is iterative and improves confidence in identifying clinical candidates with a higher likelihood of success in development. Subsequently, during the clinical testing phase, several 'learn and confirm' cycles integrate all accumulated knowledge to create a validated model capable of predicting untested clinical scenarios throughout the early and late stages of drug development [9].

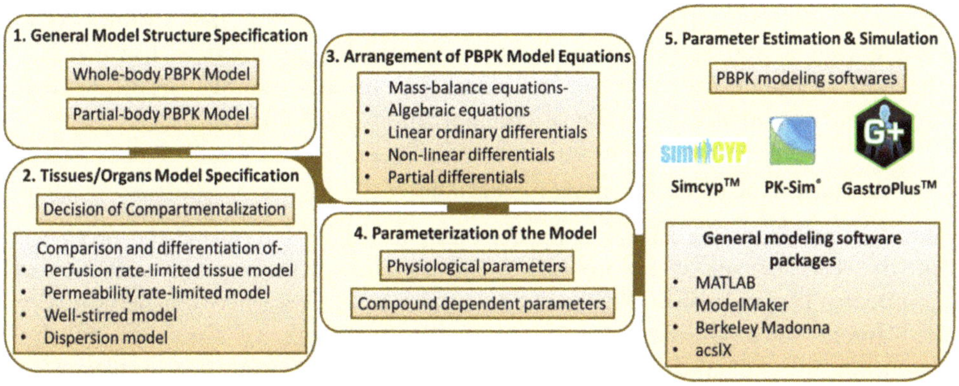

Figure 12.1. Stages in the PBPK model development.

Tissues showing similar physiological, physicochemical, and biochemical characteristics can be considered as lumped together and combined as one compartment, while tissues with different properties, including liver, where metabolism occurs, or target tissues-are separated from lumped compartments [10].

PBPK models are ranging from whole-body PBPK models including nearly all body tissues and are either represented as separated compartments or lumped compartments to partial-body PBPK models containing specific body systems or tissues, to minimal PBPK model coupled with the advanced compartmental absorption transit (ACAT) model [16]. The minimal PBPK model, first proposed by Cao and Jusko,[17] is a commonly used approach to quantitatively assess the drug exposure and target engagement at the tissue site of action [18]. The complexity of the models and the amount of incorporated information increase with the increasing number of represented tissues/organs; however, due to the fact that the main features of drug distribution can be described with few details, a common strategy called 'lumping', can be implemented for building the structure of a PBPK model [16, 19].

12.2.2 Tissues/organs model specification

It is necessary to specify the model of each specific tissue or organ (i.e., selection of the subcompartments that correspond to each organ or tissue). For each tissue or organ, there are typically one to four compartments in PBPK models. The decision of compartmentalization is totally on the basis of tissue kinetics and biochemical processes occurring after the entry of drug into the tissues [16]. Comparison and differentiation between many assumptions made at this level is crucial. Perfusion rate-limited tissue model is based on the assumption that the drug distributes freely and instantaneously across the membranes without diffusion barriers after entry into blood circulation; hence, the rate limiting step is drug distribution by the blood [10].

The permeability rate-limited model is more complicated as it gives at least two compartment tissue structures when diffusion is the rate limiting step in the distribution of a drug within tissues, which was assumed and can be physiologically identified. It can be explained with the example of blood–brain barrier for some hydrophilic molecules, i.e., capillary membranes, or cellular membrane, or both. As per a well-stirred model, there is no concentration gradient within a tissue or organ compartment. In contrast, the dispersion model assumes the absence of a diffusion barrier but the presence of concentration gradients [10].

12.2.3 Arrangement of PBPK model equations

Equations on which the PBPK is model built, are mass-balance equations derived from the law of mass action, since the kinetic processes are mass transfer phenomena. The tissues in PBPK models have been described mathematically in four different ways viz., algebraic equations, linear ordinary differentials, nonlinear differentials and partial differentials [20]. Algebraic equations can be explained with the processes of alveolar and inhaled air concentrations, which are used when processes are assumed to equilibrate instantly and can be presented statistically. The most popular descriptions for describing dynamic PK processes are linear ordinary differentials. Nonlinear differential and partial differential equations are employed with the dispersion tissue model to depict nonlinear processes in a specific tissue, such as concentration-dependent clearance and/or binding [10].

12.2.4 Parameterization of the model

It is necessary to specify and/or estimate the parameters of model equations after they have been set. Two types of parameters can be incorporated into the PBPK models viz., physiological and compound dependent parameters.

12.2.4.1 Physiological parameters

These include organ/tissue volume, heart output and blood flow, tissue composition, surface area, pH values, and/or GI tract transit durations etc, characterizing the anatomical structure and physiological processes of the species being modeled. Values of these parameters are known to change with age, physiological/pathological state, and species [10]. Despite the abundance of literature reporting such physiological data in many species, most notably the annals of the International Committee on Radiological Protection (ICRP) for human values [21] and Brown *et al* [22] for animal values, allometric scaling, or extrapolation from another species or age group is still used when different physiological parameters required for a PBPK model are partially or completely absent. Even if it is mostly assumed that physiological parameters are meant to be compound independent, drugs can alter/affect the physiology of the body, for instance, change in cardiac output and blood flow due to induction of anaesthesia [23]. Hence, in such circumstances, it is necessary to take into account any potential pharmacological effects of particular compounds on the physiological variables.

12.2.4.2 Compound dependent parameters

A PBPK model requires a second set of parameters that are compound dependant and contain details like permeability—surface area products (P × SA) and the partitioning of the substance between body tissues and the blood and plasma (KpT). *In vitro* experiments, extrapolating experimental *in vivo* results from animals to people, or estimation/prediction utilizing particular algorithms can all be used to get these parameters. Algorithms, such as those created by Poulin and Theil, Rodgers and Rowland, or Schmitt to determine tissue: plasma partition coefficients, are present in a large portion of specialized PBPK modeling software. Using this software, simple compound characteristics can be obtained, such as molecular weight (MW), lipophilicity (log P or log D value), ionization constant (pK_a value), and plasma fraction unbound (fu). These algorithms use the information previously mentioned along with tissue composition (lipids, proteins, and water) for the estimation of partition coefficients. Since clearance is a compound or species-specific characteristic that significantly affects a drug's PK behaviour, it is an essential input to the PBPK model. It is up to the researcher to choose how to input this data into the PBPK model [10]. PBPK models often use *in vitro–in vivo* extrapolations (IVIVE) to make predictions. They use data from laboratory studies on microsomes or hepatocytes. In these models, experimental measurements of blood or plasma clearance are commonly used as direct inputs, like half-lives or residual fractions. Additional information such as liver volume, liver blood flow, or microsomal binding is used to calculate the hepatic intrinsic clearance in the body based on the input parameters.[10]

12.2.5 Parameter estimation and simulation using PBPK modeling softwares

The final stage couples the entire system, and equations describing the model are implemented in a specific programming language allowing subsequent simulation and/or parameter estimates. General modeling software packages like MATLAB (The MathWorks, Inc., Natick, Massachusetts, USA), ModelMaker (University of Illinois at Urbana-Champaign) Berkeley Madonna (University of California at Berkeley, California, USA), and acslX (AEgis Technologies Group, Huntsville, Alabama, USA) provide programming languages for the model code, numerical solutions for the ordinary differential equations that define the system being modeled, and a graphical presentation of the simulation results. These software packages provide the PBPK model developer with a great deal of flexibility, but they also demand more experienced and advanced modeling and programming abilities, making them less ideal for beginners. Less flexibility in model construction is offered by the PBPK modeling software packages PK-Sim®, SimCYP™, and Gastroplus™, but they also demand less experience of mathematics and modeling [10].

These computer programmes give users the option of building a model from scratch by clicking and dragging a pre-built model. They can also simulate specific PK-relevant processes such as intestinal absorption or metabolism or create a generic whole-body PBPK model. The simulation of complex absorption, distribution, metabolism, and excretion outcomes involving various drug interactions and parent drug and metabolite profiles is made possible by extra features offered by these softwares. Additionally, they include a clearance prediction model that considers information about the growth, development, and maturation of different organs and tissues involved in drug metabolism and elimination across paediatric age groups to predict clearance in children, and they enable the simulation of virtual patient populations such as obese/morbidly obese individuals and patients with renal impairment or liver cirrhosis [24].

Specialized PBPK modeling software programmes are still difficult to use even though they do not require knowledge of programming language like general-purpose software does. Users need good scientific understanding of clinical pharmacology with the background knowledge of PK and pharmacodynamics (PD) processes of drugs, pharmacogenetics and also the molecular processes involved in these terms—to understand the difference among the models and model equations and assumptions so as to conduct PK analyses [10].

12.3 Platforms for PBPK modeling

Over the last 20 years, a multitude of scientists have focused their efforts on developing pharmaceutical drugs and have utilized specialized PBPK platforms. These platforms differ from standard PBPK modeling tools commonly used in toxicity and environmental science, such as acslX or general-purpose differential equation solvers like Berkeley Madonna and MATLAB. While some exclusive PBPK software, like IDEA™ (LION Bioscience, n.d.), have been phased out. Some new tools have emerged in the drug development field over the past two decades, including the Gastroplus™, SimCYP™ Simulator and remain widely used in the pharmaceutical industry. Some researchers have even transitioned from using commercial platforms to freeware, such as PK-Sim®b [25]. Table 12.1 provides a comparison of user-friendly PBPK modeling software along with their features.

Most general-purpose software uses conventional scripting for their equations and algorithms instead of providing a graphical user interface (GUI) for pre-set PBPK equations and databases. Consequently, PBPK users have typically preferred GUI-based tools that offer a library of pre-defined models (from which the user can select) and a well-defined database containing system parameters [26]. A notable advantage of the aforementioned tools is their ability to efficiently develop models for intricate clinical situations, such as those that involve multiple inhibitors or inducers. These tools are also useful for mechanistically examining the influence of complex factors across different age groups or disease states. As a result, these tools are particularly effective for predicting 'what-if scenarios' and understanding the kinetics of drugs and their effects in situations where several clinical and experimental factors may exist [27].

12.4 Revisiting the journey of PBPK

12.4.1 In the past

The majority of PBPK's applications over the past century were restricted to toxicology and environmental science [12]. This means that scientists who were not directly involved in the advancements of PBPK may have a different understanding of what it is compared to those who have been working with it for the past 20 years. For a number of reasons, the focus of modeling is shifted from applications in toxicology and environmental science to a widespread practice, within the pharmaceutical industry [28].

Table 12.1. Comparison of PBPK software platforms.

Platform (Software)	Company	Key features
GastroPlus® (Latest version: GastroPlus® 9.8.3)	Simulations Plus Inc.	• ACAT model • Consideration of PEAR physiology • Can incorporate *in vitro* data to predict *in vivo* outcomes • Has a user-friendly interface and can perform sensitivity analyses • Can simulate DDIs and food effects
SimCYP™ (Latest version: SimCYP™ 22.0)	Certara USA Inc.	• The advanced dissolution, absorption and metabolism (ADAM) model • Has a database of population-based models for various ethnicities and age groups • Can incorporate *in vitro* data to predict *in vivo* outcomes • Can simulate drug–drug interactions and genetic polymorphisms
PK-Sim® (Latest version: PK-Sim® 10.0)	Bayer TechnologyServices	• Whole-body-PBPK model • Various PBPK calculation methods • Open-source and freely available, useful for beginners to learn modeling • Has a library of pre-defined physiological models for various organs and tissues • Can perform sensitivity analyses and Monte Carlo simulations • Can simulate clinical trial designs and predict outcomes

The integration of *in vitro* systems and quantitative/mechanistic models has enabled the shift from PBPK models to PBPK combined with IVIVE. The IVIVE model is based on physiological, biochemical, and biopharmaceutical factors and various *in vitro* clearance data. These data are incorporated into the model to provide valuable insight into drug properties and evidence to guide decision-making in the drug discovery-development process [29]. This advancement has been made possible by the successful development of various *in vitro* systems and the ability to extrapolate their results to predict *in vivo* outcomes. Previously, when the models were developed as separate sets of equations, it became challenging to maintain consistency and quality as their usage increased. While PBPK is now recognized as a systems biology modeling approach, this was not the case before IVIVE was incorporated into PBPK [28].

12.4.2 Current scenario

Instead of concentrating on a single problem, the advancements in PBPK modeling aim to provide a framework that offers the best rational solutions to a number of issues about the fate of the drug in various populations and under different conditions. The acceptance of results and the interpretation of findings do not have equal status and worth in different areas of application due to these advancements in PBPK modeling. While some fields are relatively well-established, others continue to be the point of scholarly discussion [28].

According to Rowland *et al* PBPK had transitioned from an academic curiosity to an industrial necessity and a level of regulatory acceptance associated with issuing guidance notes for industry [30]. The issue of several regulatory guidances on PBPK was a clear indication that the predictions of PBPK's influence were factual. The US FDA's Office of Clinical Pharmacology regularly publishes its findings on the wide range of areas where PBPK can be applied from a regulatory standpoint [14].

12.4.3 Ongoing debates

There are sceptics and critics of PBPK and mechanistic biological systems modeling. These models are becoming increasingly complex and detailed, which is seen as a positive aspect, but it has also received a lot of criticism. The pharmaco-statistical community often criticizes these models for being too complicated, with too many parameters, and facing difficulties in determining which values to use. They also argue that these models are limited because they rely on assumptions and preconceived ideas, which can prevent the data from speaking for itself [31].

12.4.4 Immediate future

The idea of creating a common toolset is now widely accepted and acknowledged, especially with precompetitive collaboration amongst pharmaceutical companies (albeit not unanimously). The PBPK researchers will soon be challenged by the problem of input parameter quality (whether drug- or system-specific). Beyond the mechanics of the tools and the values themselves, which are tied to the policies and infrastructure for operationalizing the regular usage of PBPK as part of MIDD, there is a lot that needs to be optimized [31].

12.4.5 Long-term prospects

The current generation of PBPK models is based on virtual populations and attributes that define any sub-groups using a combination of system information when it is known that they differ (e.g., abundance of enzymes and transporters, frequency of specific genotypes, demography) and conventional top-down modeling of the available clinical data through reverse translation [32]. Previously, there was no practical technique to determine an individual's protein abundance in different tissues that was important to the drug's fate (enzymes/transporters). We are now closer to utilizing PBPK as the foundation for producing 'virtual twins' and, as a result, personalized dosing due to the invention of liquid biopsy and the potential to correlate measured values in plasma to real protein levels in tissues [33]. Leading pharmaceutical companies are already debating whether or not to use such approaches for individualized dosing. Of course, this may raise the price of the medication, but this might be compensated by possibly diminished side effects or a lack of effectiveness. No matter how far-fetched individualized dosage may seem right now, it will become more appealing as the reimbursement models for the cost of medicines shift towards outcome-based methods [31].

12.5 Institute perspective

From the institutional perspective, it is interesting to assess the influence of certain physiological variables on the systemic outcome of a drug and to what extent a PBPK model should be as basic, complicated, or even more sophisticated as necessary to accurately depict the luminal and systemic behaviour of a drug [5]. It is the responsibility of institutional researchers to determine (a) whether the underlying mathematical equations make any sense and (b) whether they accurately and bio-relevantly describe the physiological variables (physiological range). For instance, all of these programmes assume that a drug will be evenly dispersed throughout the whole stomach following oral delivery and refer to the stomach as a single, well-stirred compartment. It was clearly demonstrated using measured gastric concentrations of the non-absorbable markers phenol red and paromomycin that these markers were not evenly distributed across the various stomach regions (i.e., fundus, body and antrum) [34]. It is worth noting that these topics are relatively new and have only recently started to be included in academic curricula, although their inclusion is not universal. Hence, it is important to consider incorporating it as a subject into graduate pharmacy programs. Moreover, the utilization of PBPK modeling in PhD and postdoctoral research is currently limited, indicating a valuable prospect for further exploration and utilization.

12.6 Industry perspective

Using a stochastic modeling method, PBPK models may simulate individual concentration-time profiles under the assumption that every individual is unique. To get the whole picture, these underlying physiological processes must take variability into account. Moreover, a parameter sensitivity analysis (PSA) can be used to demonstrate how a physiological variable (from a minimal to a maximal value) affects the systemic effect of the drug [35]. Industrial scientists need to be aware of the regulatory requirements for building PBPK workspaces and more importantly, how regulatory authorities will assess their implementation [7]. When adjusting the biopharmaceutical input data (solubility, dissolution, and permeability in the presence and absence of these constituents) and running simulations for the target population, the impact of excipients/manufacturing process/buffers/surfactants can be thoroughly explored for NDA and generic drug products. Figure 12.2 has depicted the applications of PBBM and PBPK modeling in different stages of drug product development. These applications are described in the following section [5, 36].

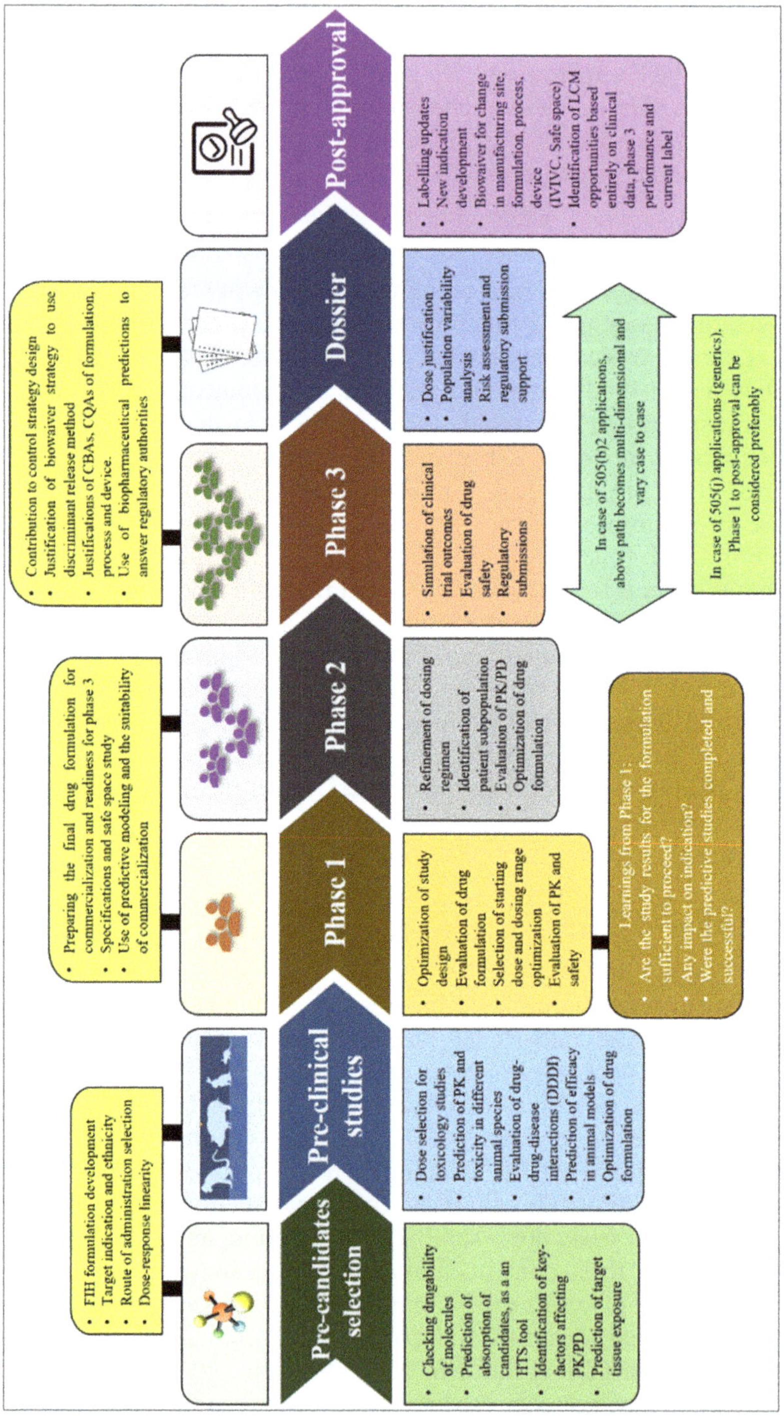

Figure 12.2. Application of PBBM and PBPK modeling in different stages of drug product development.

12.7 Agencies perspective

In addition to the pharmaceutical industry, several regulatory agencies are paying close attention to the use of PBBM/PBPK to ensure the quality of drug products. The use of PBPK modeling was introduced in European Medicines Agency's (EMA) regulatory guidelines less than a decade ago. The 'Investigation of drug interactions' guideline that appeared in 2012 mentioned that 'PBPK models need to be qualified for its purpose. In general, the performance of the model needs to be supported by relevant *in vivo* data.' [7] The increasing recommendations and use of PBPK modeling by regulatory agencies across the world signify the significant advancements in the field of drug development and regulatory science. The proactive efforts of these agencies to promote the use of PBPK modeling through workshops, seminars, and other knowledge-sharing initiatives further contribute to its widespread adoption and the overall improvement of regulatory decision-making processes.

The US Food and Drug Administration (FDA) has provided guidance on PBBM model development and validation. According to it, the incorporation of clinically relevant dissolution data is crucial, as it assists in manufacturing/control changes and establishes a clear correlation between *in vitro* dissolution testing and pharmacokinetics (PK). While biorelevant dissolution data are not obligatory, performing such tests alongside conventional dissolution testing can be beneficial for significant CMC changes and bridge studies. The FDA supports the development of innovative modeling techniques to ensure the quality of medicinal products without facing regulatory hurdles. While traditional or physiologically-based 'mechanistic' IVIVCs are regarded as the 'gold standard' for achieving regulatory flexibility throughout the life cycle of a drug product, US FDA supports their development [14].

When these routes fail, it may be feasible to establish a safe space using the data collected during drug product development and the execution of specific PK studies (where possible). In order to support the quality of drug products, US FDA supports the use of PBBM techniques in regulatory submissions. Establishing trust in this strategy is crucial and a first step towards regulating regulation. In short, creating a safe zone is important for acquiring regulatory flexibility as well as a first step towards developing therapeutic products that are 'patient-centric' and with clinically relevant specifications [14]. In a nutshell, safe space offers a chance to make a significant improvement in hastening and reducing the price of drug product development [7, 14].

Despite the fact that modeling is frequently employed in the pharmaceutical sector, regulatory authorities are rarely getting simulated data. The reasons of this issue are: (i) lack of recognised regulatory framework or guidance; (ii) lack of alignment in vision and strategy across regulatory regions; and (iii) lack of relevant public case studies where PBPK models have been applied in regulatory interactions [37]. To address this, new guidelines aim to outline the expected content in PBPK modeling and simulation (M&S) reports submitted as part of regulatory submissions.

12.8 Applications

PBPK models can be particularly useful in the early stages of drug development where only limited data are available, as well as in the later stages of development where large amounts of data are available [38, 39]. The main functions of PBPK modeling can be grouped into three categories, to enhance the mechanistic understanding of clinical observations, to inform regulatory communications, and to guide decision-making in clinical development [40]. The application of PBPK modeling is highly prevalent in clinical pharmacology for IND/NDA submissions and is now increasingly being adopted in BE/biowaiver assessments for ANDA submissions [41–43]. Specifically, PBPK models have been applied to candidate selection, determination of appropriate first-in-human (FIH) dosing, evaluation of DDI potential, and establishment of suitable study designs, which includes defining inclusion and exclusion criteria for clinical trials involving drugs metabolized by polymorphic enzymes [44, 45] several applications along with their challenges and limitations are presented in table 12.2.

The PBBM/PBPK modeling approach holds great appeal in the scientific community due to its ability to connect *in vitro* drug product attributes, such as dissolution profile and particle size, to *in vivo* performance measures such as PK behavior [46–49]. A well-constructed PBPK model can significantly aid in the design of preclinical and clinical pharmacology studies [44].

Sensitivity analysis can be conducted to provide insights into individual variability and the critical factors that impact PK profiles in human subjects. PBPK modeling is especially advantageous in situations where performing clinical PK studies is difficult, such as in populations with distinct ethnic, age, or disease-related characteristics. By using PK data from a single dose regimen, PBPK modeling can effectively evaluate the PK profile associated with different dosing schedules and/or administration routes [40].

The 'critical bioavailability attributes' (CBAs) refer to the attributes related to formulation or process that are expected to have a significant impact on the bioavailability of a drug product, including its rate and extent of absorption. For poorly soluble drugs and extended-release products, if CBAs cannot be clearly identified and controlled, such as by using a discriminating dissolution specification, then the initial biopharmaceutical risk is considered high to very high. In such cases, the use of the PBBM approach is crucial to understand how CBAs may affect clinical performance, establish IVIVR, and develop biopharmaceutical risk mitigation strategies [50, 51]. In addition, the use of PBPK modeling in biopharmaceutics to identify CBAs and determine the optimal range can assist in establishing a quality target product profile (QTPP) and facilitate drug product development through a quality by design (QbD) approach [14, 46]. In the preclinical stage, PBPK modeling can be used to make predictions related to animal or human PK, as well as efficacious dose projections, oral absorption, and DDI modeling [39].

In drug discovery, the size of a dose has important implications for the safety of the molecule, the costs of production, and the requirements for formulation. At the early stages, predicting the therapeutic dose can inform decisions related to structure–activity relationships, compound design, compound prioritization, and

Table 12.2. Applications of PBPK modeling with level of confidence, limitations and challenges [39].

Applications		Level of confidence	Challenges
Preclinical and clinical PK prediction	CYP cleared substrates	Moderate to high	*In vitro* systems for Biopharmaceutical Classification System (BCS) class I and II drugs do not present significant limitations or challenges for liver metabolism. However, intestinal metabolism poses greater challenges.
	Non-CYP metabolically cleared substrates	Low to moderate	Hepatocytes are reliable predictors of glucuronidation and certain other non-P450 metabolic processes. However, the expression patterns and scaling factors for many non-CYP enzymes are not well-defined, which can pose a challenge.
	Clearance/absorption by active transport	Low	The scaling factors for transporter abundances and activity are not well understood.
	Elimination by combination of metabolism and transport	Low	It is very challenging to understand the interplay between multiple transporters and metabolic enzymes.
	Passive distribution/absorption processes	High	No significant limitations or challenges.
DDI prediction	Involving reversible CYP inhibition alone or CYP induction alone	Moderate to high	Accurate *in vitro* estimation of fraction metabolized by P450, especially when non P450 enzyme involved. Cl and mass-balance data for victim (substrate) not readily available at early stages of drug development. Uncertainty in CYP phenotyping and measured *in vitro* inhibitor constant (Ki) Accurately estimating the fraction metabolized by CYP450 *in vitro* can be challenging, particularly when non-P450 enzymes are involved. At the early stages of drug development, CL and mass-balance data for the victim (substrate) are not readily available, which adds to the uncertainty. There can also be uncertainty in CYP phenotyping and the measured *in vitro* inhibitor constant (Ki).

	Involving time dependent CYP inhibition	Low to moderate	In addition to the aforementioned limitations, there is a tendency for *in vitro* data to over-predict DDI *in vivo*.
	Involving combined reversible, time dependent inhibition and induction of CYPs.	Low	Evaluating mechanisms can be difficult when multiple processes are involved, particularly due to limited clinical data.
	Involving modulation of non-CYP pathways.	Low to moderate	There is a lack of prospective evaluation.
	Involving apical active transport	Moderate	Inappropriate inhibition constants may be provided by some *in vitro* assays.
	Involving basolateral active transport	Low	Similar to the above challenges, predicting intracellular inhibitor concentrations from uptake and efflux transport activity can be challenging.
Absorption, food effect and formulation prediction	For high solubility, high permeability compounds (B(DD)CS I drugs)	High	There are no significant limitations or challenges for predicting absorption in the fasted or fed state.
	For low solubility, high permeability compounds (B(DD)CS II drugs)	Low to moderate	It is necessary to ensure that *in vitro* data and/or *in vivo* models for solubility, dissolution, and precipitation are relevant to humans.
	For high solubility, low permeability compounds (B(DD)CS III drugs)	Low	The effect of food on bile-micelle binding, P-gp, and permeability can be unclear.
	For low solubility, low permeability compounds (B(DD)CS IV drugs)	Low	There is a complex interplay between multiple factors, including solubility, permeability, and transporter interactions, making it difficult to verify the model. The involvement of multiple mechanisms that cannot be independently verified of each other adds to this challenge.

(*Continued*)

Table 12.2. (*Continued*)

Applications		Level of confidence	Challenges
Special population PK prediction	Ethnic variations, smokers, pregnancy, obese, elderly	Low to moderate	The abundance of CYP, non-CYP enzymes, and transporters may not be well-known or understood, and knowledge of changes in gut physiology is also limited. However, as more human data becomes available, confidence in predictions is strengthened.
	Pediatrics	Low to moderate	The metabolism of drugs via non-CYP enzymes and transporters is not well-defined, and the developmental changes in very young individuals for enzymes and transporters are not well understood. Furthermore, there is only limited clinical data available to verify these processes.
	Renal insufficiency	Low	The effect of renal impairment on CYP expression and transporter activities is unknown, and only limited clinical data is available to validate this impact.
	Hepatic insufficiency	Low	The impact of cirrhosis on enzymes and transporters is not fully defined, and there is only limited clinical data available to validate this impact.
	Pharmacogenetics	Moderate to high	The lack of clinical data for infrequent genotypes can limit the accuracy of predictions.
Large-molecule PK prediction	Using reduced PBPK model	Moderate	There are no significant limitations or challenges in predicting plasma or tissue PK for large molecules with linear PK. However, for large molecules with target-mediated drug disposition (TMDD), the predictability of plasma and tissue PK is much more challenging.
	Using full whole-body PBPK model	Low	Some drug disposition mechanisms, such as FcRn recycling, are not fully characterized.
PBPK-PD prediction and target organ distribution	For small passively permeable molecules	High	No significant limitations or challenges.
	For active transporter substrates	Low	The uncertainty of the partition coefficient for target tissue is a challenge when tissue concentrations are limited by permeability, as in the case of biologics, or by transporter-mediated processes, as in the case of the brain, liver, kidney, etc

the identification of ADME-related risks for potential series [38, 52]. While PBPK modeling has been used to address regulatory queries, it is also more commonly used for internal decision-making purposes such as predicting the FIH dose, selecting compounds, assessing food effects, or predicting DDIs. The level of confidence in PBPK modeling and its frequency of use vary from low to high, depending on the complexity of the model. DDI and absorption modeling are used by all companies, but less frequent applications have been reported for specific sub-populations such as pregnant women [39].

Jones *et al* developed and validated a PBPK-based approach for the design of FIH studies. The method involves an initial animal PBPK simulation, which incorporates animal *in vitro* data and compound-specific physicochemical data, followed by a comparison of the simulation with *in vivo* animal data. If the animal simulation is deemed reasonable, a human PBPK simulation is performed using a human PBPK model, human *in vitro* data, and compound-specific physicochemical data. However, if the animal simulation is inaccurate, it may suggest a violation of one or more of the model assumptions, and additional experiments may be necessary to address the discrepancy [38, 53].

In the drug discovery phase, PBPK modeling can be utilized to predict the exposure of a drug candidate in populations that may have varying levels of metabolic enzyme activity, such as poor metabolizers. This can help to determine whether exclusion of certain populations is necessary in FIH trials, and the model can be refined with data from FIH healthy volunteer trials to design DDI studies, including dose adjustments for poor metabolizers [40]. During drug development, DDI risk simulation is a commonly used application of PBPK modeling. Simulations are typically run using the most potent perpetrator or the most sensitive substrate in order to assess the worst-case scenario, and if safety margins are sufficient, clinical trials may be waived for moderately sensitive substrates or perpetrators. PBPK modeling can also be used to predict exposure in patients with organ impairment and to simulate the use of CYP3A4/5 inhibitor to enhance exposure of high clearance compounds and substrates. In cases where DDI liability cannot be avoided, M&S can help to evaluate alternative routes of administration, such as intravenous, to reduce the risk. For drugs targeted for inhalation or non-conventional routes, PBPK modeling is particularly useful to evaluate feasibility [40, 54, 55].

The compressed timelines of clinical development programs have shortened the technical development phase for drug products, which can limit the ability to quickly provide new therapeutics to patients. To accelerate the drug development process, it is essential to have a deep understanding of the biopharmaceutical properties of the active ingredient and the product, and to use advanced biopharmaceutics models that go beyond the BCS-based biowaivers. Combining *in vitro* systems with *in silico* PBBM and dynamic clinical study designs can facilitate rapid development and change management of drug products with optimal performance. These tools can be used to select and optimize drug substance properties, formulations, and manage changes during development, commercialization, and scale-up. Although biopharmaceutics models are already being used to accelerate internal decision-making in the pharmaceutical industry, greater regulatory acceptance and understanding of such approaches can lead to the development of high-quality medicines and provide early access to new medicines for patients [56].

PBPK modeling can be used multi-dimensionally in 505(b)2 applications to aid in drug development. A 505(b)2 application is a type of new drug application (NDA) submitted to the US FDA. These applications also referred as hybrid NDAs. The term 'hybrid' is used to distinguish them from traditional NDAs. These applications involve an approved molecule with a new indication, route of administration, dose, formulation, or new formulation strategy [57].

As depicted in figure 12.2, NDAs progress in a specific direction from pre-candidate selection to post-approval changes. PBPK modeling can be applied at various stages of drug development, with particular objectives and applications depending on the specific drug product and requirements of the situation. Similarly, PBBM or PBPK modeling can be used in 505(b)2 applications according to specific requirements which can vary case to case. The advantage of a 505(b)2 application is that, it may allow a drug product to be approved more quickly and with less expense than a traditional NDA, due to availability of some of the information required for approval. This available information can make impact on the PBPK modeling and can help for better simulations and predictions. However, the applicant must still provide data to support the safety and effectiveness of the new drug product [58–60].

In order to ensure that variant drug batches can be considered bioequivalent to each other or the pivotal clinical batch(es), a 'safe space' or BE space is established based on the ranges of *in vitro* specifications for drug product quality attributes such as dissolution and drug substance particle size. There are multiple ways to construct this safe space, including classical IVIVC or IVIVR (rank-order relationship) and exposure-response analysis. However, the PBBM-based IVIVR/IVIVC approach is currently the most recent method used to build a safe space and obtain regulatory flexibility for both NDA and ANDA applications [7, 46, 61, 62].

The PBBM approach allows for the use of prior knowledge of CBAs and their impact on dissolution, enabling predictions about potential expansion of the CBA ranges. In a study by Pepin *et al* for instance, this approach was applied to a weakly acidic API. PSA was conducted on factors such as permeability, solubility, and particle size distribution. The results showed that the particle size of API, at 100 μm, had the potential to affect C_{max} levels. PBBM approaches have also been employed to facilitate scale-up and post-approval changes (SUPACs), obtain biowaivers, and make bridging formulation changes [6, 46, 58, 63].

The establishment of an *in vivo* and *in vitro* link is crucial for biopredictive methods, but it alone is insufficient to establish quality standards that are patient-centred. To guarantee that commercial batches perform similarly to clinical batches, drug product specifications such as dissolution acceptance criteria are established. Conventionally, these criteria are based on the average dissolution data of pivotal clinical batches (for example, a ±10% variation range for extended-release drug products where $Q = 80\%$ dissolution occurs for immediate-release drug products). However, if the relationship between the critical quality attributes (CQAs), *in vitro* dissolution, and *in vivo* performance is unclear, these acceptance criteria may be too strict, too broad, or irrelevant to clinical performance. Therefore, using PBBM, establishing the *in vitro/in vivo* link, constructing a safe space, and establishing clinically significant dissolution acceptance criteria that are related to clinical performance, are neither too tight nor too broad, and can reject non-bioequivalent batches, is highly significant [46, 64, 65].

PBPK modeling can be used to determine the washout period in a crossover study design. This approach can establish the shortest clinical trial duration required in the DDI prediction area. Moreover, it can substitute DDI studies in certain groups such as paediatrics and organ-impaired patients where DDI trials are not feasible due to logistical or ethical issues. This may result in waiving the requirement for unnecessary clinical DDI trials and thus accelerating drug development while alleviating patient discomfort. Additionally, conducting DDI studies in patients with multiple perpetrators is unethical and impractical, but PBPK modeling can predict the potential effects of co-administering all the drugs in this situation [40].

PBPK modeling has become increasingly popular in the development and application of biotechnological products such as gene therapy, monoclonal antibodies, and antisense oligonucleotides (ASOs) due to their specificity in treating genetic and rare diseases. To develop PBPK models for large-molecule drugs, commercially available software can be used. A user-friendly PBPK module for monoclonal antibodies in humans is available in SimCYP™, which is based on a comprehensive PBPK model developed in mice. The model consists of various compartments such as lymph node and plasma compartments, interstitial spaces, and FcRn recycling, as well as endogenous IgG models [6].

In summary, PBPK models offer several benefits, including the ability to predict drug PK based on food and formulation, which can inform clinical trial design before the FIH trial. They can also predict drug–drug interactions mediated by drug-metabolizing enzymes or drug transporters, which can help with dose selection and inclusion/exclusion criteria, potentially eliminating costly clinical DDI studies. Additionally, PBPK models can propose dosages for paediatric patients, select appropriate sampling times, and estimate dosing regimens. PBPK models can also predict drug exposure in patients with impaired renal and/or hepatic organ function, potentially informing the design of organ impairment studies or the decision to skip them. They can also estimate drug distribution in pregnant women and their foetuses to optimize the therapeutic benefit/risk ratio. Furthermore, PBPK models can predict pH-mediated DDIs in patients using proton pump inhibitors/acid-reducing agents, helping direct formulation development and food interactions. Lastly, PBPK models can help identify CQAs and risks, establish *in vitro–in vivo* links, predict bioequivalent safe space, establish clinically relevant dissolution acceptance criteria, and specify drug product parameters beyond dissolution.

In addition, PBPK models that incorporate mechanistic assumptions can replicate PK and identify the primary causes of atypical PK findings. They can also simulate how modifications in intrinsic and/or extrinsic factors influence the drug's PK profile in plasma or tissues. Due to the availability of PBPK modeling software packages with predetermined system parameters, constructing and improving models has become more straightforward and efficient [6].

12.9 Limitations

The increasing use of PBPK models to address regulatory and therapeutic questions is in line with their ability to circumvent the ethical and logistical difficulties posed by PK and toxicology studies involving various populations. While PBPK models have been evaluated for their regulatory applications in several publications by different regulatory agencies, there have been very few assessments of their general applicability beyond regulatory applications, both in terms of quantity and scope [25].

The current status of PBPK applications may not be accurately reflected in regulatory filings due to the lengthy procedures required for their preparation and evaluation by industries and regulatory authorities. Although there are no standardized criteria for PBPK model validation, predicted values within a two-fold range of observed values are generally deemed acceptable. Model credibility is established through verification, which involves evaluating model components such as computer codes and equations to ensure they accurately represent the model assumptions; and validation, involves assessing the model performance in comparison with observed *in vivo* data [14]. Credibility assessments are used to develop verification and validation plans, as well as criteria for each element of credibility. However, there is no specific range of acceptable prediction errors recommended. Depending on the regulatory purpose, models are classified into three levels of scale: low, medium, and high [6]. In the most general terms, verification refers to an assessment of model components, for example by examining computer codes and equations, to evaluate whether they accurately implement model assumptions; and validation refers to an assessment of the model performance in comparison with observed *in vivo* data.

Further investigation is necessary as we have limited knowledge regarding the impact of the complex gastrointestinal (GI) environment on the behaviour of drugs or formulations. One of the major obstacles in advancing the development of PBPK models is the insufficient and unreliable data. As models become more complex, a deeper understanding of the system is required, and although significant efforts have been made to identify and generate missing information, there is still a long way to go. The scarcity of systems data, including information on non-CYP enzymes and transporters' distribution and activity in different tissues, as well as the effects of age and disease state on absorption, is a common issue. Developing mechanistic PBPK models for biologics and for investigating drug efficacy and safety presents even greater challenges in this regard. The applicability of PBPK models could be further expanded if they could be adequately prepared to interact with other tools and platforms (interoperability), such as quantitative system pharmacology models of various disease progressions [66].

12.10 Opportunities and future scope

Opportunities offered by modeling are:

- Determining and interpreting crucial aspects of *in vivo* performance;
- Better and faster commercial formulation selection;
- More predictable outcomes of BE studies;

- Eliminating the need for critical-path BE studies, which generally take six months or more to complete, in order to facilitate formulation optimization and other project changes that need to be made quickly (e.g., to particle size, manufacturing process, scale-up, etc);
- Development of therapeutically applicable dissolution acceptance criteria without BE studies and without exposing healthy volunteers inadvertently;
- Support and encourage scale-up and supply chain robustness, support the overall control strategy, and provide supply continuity for these essential products while reducing the possibility of a supply deficit;
- Consider the impact of food on drug at an early stage of development [56].

In spite of the progress made by mechanism-based *in silico* models in addressing critical issues in the development of new oral drug products, several poorly understood aspects need to be integrated to enhance their effectiveness in predicting systemic effects of both novel and generic drug candidates. Biopharmaceutics models are frequently used in the pharmaceutical industry to accelerate internal decision-making, and developing a framework to use data from these models in a regulatory setting could accelerate patient access to innovative medications without compromising their safety.

Recent discoveries demonstrate the importance of making predictions in a biorelevant environment, which involves the use of simulated GI media, multi-compartmental *in vitro* models, and an analysis of the interaction between solubility and permeability, to obtain more accurate results. The IMI/EFPIA-funded 'Oral Bioavailability Tools (OrBiTo)' project (http://www.imi.europa.eu/content/orbito) has created a decision tree to aid formulation scientists in selecting the best biopredictive dissolution test based on biopharmaceutical properties of the drug molecule and the type of formulation. These variables are critical in a biopredictive dissolution test, and the decision tree focuses on specific biorelevant aspects of the GI tract that are important and have a significant impact on the luminal behaviour of a drug product. By utilizing these tools, it is possible to move beyond traditional BCS thinking and understand the relationship between *in vitro* and *in vivo* on a product-specific basis, enabling the development of clinically relevant *in vitro* tests and acceptance standards [67, 68].

During the non-clinical stage of drug development, various commercially available software tools, including SimCYP™ simulator, Gastroplus™, and PK-Sim®, are widely used to predict how a therapeutic product will perform in patients. Innovative applications of PBPK models are being documented in the literature, such as incorporating time-varying physiology into paediatric PBPK models, modeling drug disposition in organs like kidney, brain, and lung, conducting virtual BE studies, and modeling antibody drug conjugates. With the integrative nature of PBPK models, it is possible to incorporate patient-specific characteristics for precision dosing, which may become more prevalent in the future. Additionally, if relevant and cost-effective biomarkers for enzyme and transporter activity become available, such data can be incorporated into PBPK models to optimize doses in scenarios like DDIs [66].

The integration of techniques such as AyurGenomics and AyurPharma cometabolomics into drug development pipelines has the potential to revolutionize the field, enabling the development of drugs that are not only faster and more economical but also safer and more effective. By the impact of AyurGenomics and AyurPharmacometabolomics, the clinical translational process could be significantly streamlined, reducing costs, and minimizing the risk of adverse events [69–71].

PBPK modeling can be used to predict the PK of Ayurvedic medicines and their active ingredients, as well as to optimize dosing regimens based on individual patient characteristics. In Ayurgenomics, PBPK modeling can be used to predict the effects of Ayurvedic medicines on gene expression and metabolism, allowing for the identification of personalized treatment options based on an individual's genetic makeup. In Ayurpharmacometabolics, PBPK modeling can be used to predict the PK profile of Ayurvedic medicines in different populations and to identify factors that may influence their metabolism and efficacy. PBPK modeling has great potential in the field of Ayurgenomics and Ayurpharmacometabolics, and its use is likely to increase as these fields continue to develop and mature.

PBPK modeling can be used in personalized medicine to incorporate pharmacogenotypic and pharmacophenotypic data to predict individual drug exposure and response, and optimize drug dosing for maximum efficacy and safety. Both Pharmacogenotyping and pharmacophenotyping can be incorporated into PBPK models to personalize drug dosing. Pharmacogenotyping involves the analysis of genetic variations that affect drug metabolism, while pharmacophenotyping involves the analysis of phenotypic variations that affect drug response. These factors can both influence drug PK and PD, and thus can be used to individualize drug dosing based on the patient's genetic makeup and clinical characteristics [39, 44]. By using patient-specific parameters, such as genetic information, body weight, age, and organ function, PBPK models can generate individualized drug dosing recommendations that maximize drug efficacy while minimizing toxicity.

12.11 SWOT analysis

SWOT analysis is a commonly used tool for evaluating the strengths, weaknesses, opportunities, and threats of a business or organization. However, it can also be applied to scientific research methods such as PBPK modeling. In this section, SWOT analysis has given considering all points mentioned in the chapter to examine the potential strengths, weaknesses, opportunities, and threats associated with PBPK modeling. By doing so, it will be helpful to gain a more comprehensive understanding of the current state of PBPK modeling and identify areas for future improvement (figure 12.3).

12.12 Epilogue

The chapter highlights the expansion of PBPK modeling in MIDD, which has been facilitated by various factors such as the availability of software platforms, current regulatory guidance, new *in silico* ADMET (ADME and toxicity) tools, and

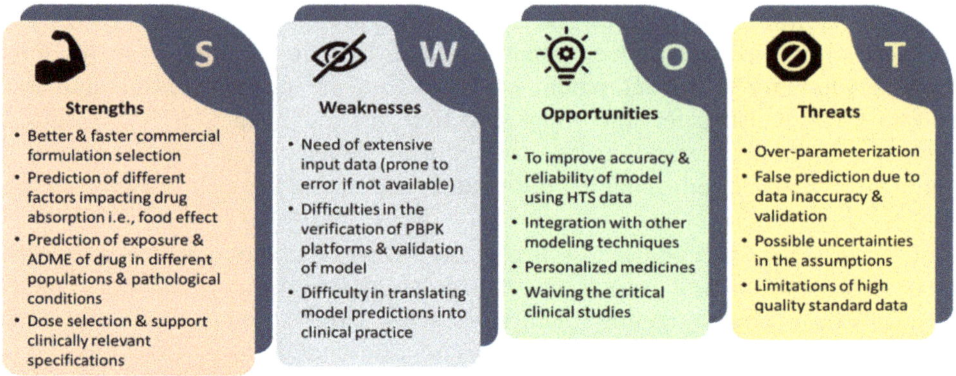

Figure 12.3. Brief overview of SWOT Analysis for PBBM/PBPK Modeling

increasing awareness in academic institutions. PBPK has emerged as a significant tool in the pharmaceutical industry that enables the detection of drug development risks and facilitates regulatory interactions or approvals.

Valid PBPK models provide a mechanistic understanding of ADME processes and their impact on drug efficacy and safety. For instance, PBPK modeling can be used to investigate the impact of dietary factors on drug absorption and to assess the potential for DDI based on the metabolic pathway of the drug. PBPK models can also aid in clinical trial designs and biowaiver studies by predicting drug behaviour in different populations based on physiological differences. Furthermore, this modeling can help in the creation of dosage regimens for specific populations, such as paediatrics or patients with impaired liver or kidney function. Overall, PBPK modeling provides a valuable tool for drug development, helping to optimize drug development and regulatory approval processes, and ultimately improving patient outcomes.

About the author

Maitri is a highly dedicated and passionate individual in the field of biopharmaceutics. With a master's degree from NIPER (Mohali) and over 10 years of professional experience (Dr Reddy's and Zydus), she has made significant contributions to the pharmaceutical industry. Currently, she is working with SimCYP (Certara). Her expertise lies in bioequivalence studies, *in vitro*/*in vivo* correlation, and the application of PBPK modeling for formulation optimization and regulatory submissions. Maitri's knowledge and insights have been shared through her published articles, showcasing her commitment to advancing the field. For those seeking support or collaboration in biopharmaceutics research, Maitri can be contacted at smaitri2010@gmail.com. Her dedication and willingness to contribute make her a valuable asset to the field.

Ajay is a highly motivated research fellow with a passion for scientific research and development in the pharmaceutical field. With two years of experience, he is focused on exploring biopharmaceutics, dissolution science, and *in silico* modeling to enhance drug development processes and improve therapeutic outcomes. Ajay's dedication and commitment make him well-equipped to contribute to the future of pharmaceutical research and make a positive impact on the field. He can be contacted at ajaylale.06@gmail.com.

Anuj Kumar Saini is an esteemed leader in the pharmaceutical industry, currently holding the position of Vice President and Head of Biopharmaceutics and Clinical Development at Zydus Lifesciences in Ahmedabad, India. With a strong academic background (NIPER, Mohali) and over two decades of experience, Anuj has held key leadership roles in reputable organizations such as Lambda Therapeutic Research Ltd, Quintiles India Research Pvt Ltd, Jubilant Organosys Ltd and Cadila Healthcare Ltd. His expertise spans areas such as biopharmaceutics, clinical development, and global regulatory affairs. Anuj has made notable contributions to the field through his research publications, particularly in the field of pharmacokinetics modeling in biopharmaceutics. His knowledge and accomplishments have earned him a respected reputation in the industry. He can be contacted at anuj.saini@zyduslife.com.

Acknowledgments

We would like to acknowledge the insightful suggestions and ideas provided by Swapnil P Borse, PhD while writing this chapter. Additionally, we extend our heartfelt gratitude to Mr M E Kannan—President and Head, Pharmaceutical Technology Center, Zydus Lifesciences Ltd for his valuable support and guidance. His encouragement has been instrumental in writing and submitting this book chapter.

References

[1] Madabushi R and Seo P *et al* 2022 Role of model-informed drug development approaches in the lifecycle of drug development and regulatory decision-making *Pharm. Res.* **39** 1669–80

[2] Zhang X and Yang Y *et al* 2020 Application of PBPK modeling and simulation for regulatory decision making and its impact on us prescribing information: an update on the 2018–2019 submissions to the US FDA's office of clinical pharmacology *J. Clin. Pharm.* **60** S160–78

[3] Wagner C and Zhao P *et al* 2015 Application of physiologically based pharmacokinetic (PBPK) modeling to support dose selection: report of an FDA public workshop on PBPK. CPT: pharmacometrics and systems *Pharmacology.* **4** 226–30

[4] Heimbach T and Chen Y *et al* 2021 Physiologically-based pharmacokinetic modeling in renal and hepatic impairment populations: a pharmaceutical industry perspective *Clin. Pharmacol. Ther.* **110** 297–310

[5] Suarez-Sharp S and Lindahl A *et al* 2020 Translational modeling strategies for orally administered drug products: academic, industrial and regulatory perspectives *Pharm. Res.* **37** 95

[6] Lin W and Chen Y *et al* 2022 Applications, challenges, and outlook for PBPK modeling and simulation: a regulatory, industrial and academic perspective *Pharm. Res.* **39** 1701–31

[7] EMA 2018 Guideline on the reporting of physiologically based pharmacokinetic (PBPK) modelling and simulation. EMA/CHMP/4 (December) 3–15. www.ema.europa.eu/contact

[8] Nguyen M A and Flanagan T *et al* 2017 A survey on IVIVC/IVIVR development in the pharmaceutical industry—past experience and current perspectives *Eur. J. Pharm. Sci.* **102** 1–13

[9] Jones H M and Chen Y *et al* 2015 Physiologically based pharmacokinetic modeling in drug discovery and development: a pharmaceutical industry perspective *Clin. Pharm. Ther.* **97** 247–62
[10] Läer S and Khalil F 2011 Physiologically based pharmacokinetic modeling: methodology, applications, and limitations with a focus on its role in pediatric drug development *J. Biomed. Biotechnol.* **2011** 907461
[11] Bessems J G and Loizou G *et al* 2014 PBTK modelling platforms and parameter estimation tools to enable animal-free risk assessment. Recommendations from a joint EPAA—EURL ECVAM ADME workshop *Regul. Toxicol. Pharm.* **68** 119–39
[12] Rostami-Hodjegan A 2012 Physiologically based pharmacokinetics joined with *in vitro–in vivo* extrapolation of ADME: a marriage under the arch of systems pharmacology *Clinical Pharmacol. Ther.* **92** 50–61
[13] Kostewicz E S and Aarons L *et al* 2014 PBPK models for the prediction of *in vivo* performance of oral dosage forms *Eur. J. Pharm. Sci.* **57** 300–21
[14] U.S. Food and Drug Administration 2020 The use of physiologically based pharmacokinetic analyses—biopharmaceutics applications for oral drug product development, manufacturing changes, and controls. draft 61953–5. (https://fda.gov/drugs/guidance-compliance-regulatory-information/guidances-drugs)
[15] Wang J *et al* 2021 Progress in drug development–pediatric dose selection: workshop summary *J. Clin. Pharmacol* **61** S13–21
[16] Nestorov I 2007 Whole-body physiologically based pharmacokinetic models *Expert Opin. Drug Metab. Toxicol.* **3** 235–49
[17] Cao Y and Jusko W J 2012 Applications of minimal physiologically-based pharmacokinetic models *J. Pharmacokinet. Pharmacodyn.* **39** 711–23
[18] Ayyar V S and Song D *et al* 2021 Minimal physiologically based pharmacokinetic-pharmacodynamic (mPBPK-PD) model of N-acetylgalactosamine–conjugated small interfering rna disposition and gene silencing in preclinical species and humans *J. Pharmacol. Exp. Ther.* **379** 134–46
[19] Brochot C and Tóth J *et al* 2005 Lumping in pharmacokinetics *J. Pharmacokinet. Pharmacodyn.* **32** 719–36
[20] Nestorov I 2003 Whole body pharmacokinetic models *Clin. Pharmacokinet.* **42** 883–908
[21] Valentin J and Streffer C 2002 Basic anatomical and physiological data for use in radiological protection: reference values—ICRP Publication 89 *Ann. ICRP* **32** 1–277
[22] Brown R P and Delp M D *et al* 1997 Physiological parameter values for physiologically based pharmacokinetic models *Toxicol. Ind. Health* **13** 407–84
[23] Sasaki Y and Measurement H N W 1971 of the distribution of cardiac output in anesthesized rats *J. Appl. Physiol.* **30** 879–84
[24] Willmann S and Lippert J *et al* 2005 From physicochemistry to absorption and distribution: predictive mechanistic modelling and computational tools *Expert Opin. Drug Metab. Toxicol.* **1** 159–68
[25] El-Khateeb E and Burkhill S *et al* 2021 Physiological-based pharmacokinetic modeling trends in pharmaceutical drug development over the last 20-years; in-depth analysis of applications, organizations, and platforms. 42 *Biopharm. Drug Dispos.* 107–17
[26] Bouzom F and Ball K *et al* 2014 Physiologically based pharmacokinetic (PBPK) modelling tools: how to fit with our needs? *Biopharm. Drug Dispos.* **33** 55–71

[27] Maher E M and Ali A M A *et al* 2016 *In vitro/in vivo* evaluation of an optimized fast dissolving oral film containing olanzapine co-amorphous dispersion with selected carboxylic acids *Drug Deliv.* **23** 3088–100
[28] Gibson G G and Rostami-Hodjegan A 2007 Modelling and simulation in prediction of human xenobiotic absorption, distribution, metabolism and excretion (ADME): *in vitro–in vivo* extrapolations (IVIVE) *Xenobiotica* **37** 1013–4
[29] Cho H Y and Choi G W *et al* 2019 Interpretation of non-clinical data for prediction of human pharmacokinetic parameters: *in vitro–in vivo* extrapolation and allometric scaling *Pharmaceutics* **11** 168
[30] Rowland M and Lesko L J *et al* 2015 Physiologically based pharmacokinetics is impacting drug development and regulatory decision making *CPT: Pharmacomet. Syst. Pharmacol.* **4** 313–5
[31] Rostami-Hodjegan A and Toon S 2020 Physiologically based pharmacokinetics as a component of model-informed drug development: where we were, where we are, and where we are heading *J. Clin. Pharmacol.* **60** S12–6
[32] Rostami-Hodjegan A 2018 Reverse translation in PBPK and QSP: going backwards in order to go forward with confidence *Clin. Pharmacol. Ther.* **103** 224–32
[33] Polasek T M and Rostami-Hodjegan A 2020 Virtual twins: understanding the data required for model-informed precision dosing *Clin. Pharmacol. Ther.* **107** 742–5
[34] Bermejo M and Hens B *et al* 2020 A mechanistic physiologically-based biopharmaceutics modeling (PBBM) approach to assess the *in vivo* performance of an orally administered drug product: from IVIVC to IVIVP *Pharmaceutics* **12** 74
[35] Hens B, Talattof A and Paixão P *et al* 2018 Measuring the impact of gastrointestinal variables on the systemic outcome of two suspensions of posaconazole by a PBPK model *AAPS* J. **20** 57
[36] Cristofoletti R and Patel N *et al* 2017 Assessment of bioequivalence of weak base formulations under various dosing conditions using physiologically based pharmacokinetic simulations in virtual populations. case examples: ketoconazole and posaconazole *J. Pharm. Sci.* **106** 560–9
[37] Flanagan T and Van Peer A *et al* 2016 Use of physiologically relevant biopharmaceutics tools within the pharmaceutical industry and in regulatory sciences: where are we now and what are the gaps? *Eur. J. Pharm. Sci.* **91** 84–90
[38] Jones H M and Dickins M *et al* 2012 Application of PBPK modelling in drug discovery and development at Pfizer *Xenobiotica* **42** 94–106
[39] Jones H M and Chen Y *et al* 2015 Physiologically based pharmacokinetic modelling in drug discovery and development: a pharmaceutical industry perspective *Clin. Pharmacol. Ther.* **97** 247–62
[40] Zhuang X and Lu C 2016 PBPK modeling and simulation in drug research and development *Acta Pharm. Sinica B.* **6** 430–40
[41] Zhao P and Zhang L *et al* 2011 Applications of physiologically based pharmacokinetic (PBPK) modeling and simulation during regulatory review *Clin. Pharmacol. Ther.* **89** 259–67
[42] Tsakalozou E and Alam K *et al* 2022 Physiologically-based pharmacokinetic modeling to support determination of bioequivalence for dermatological drug products: scientific and regulatory considerations *Clin. Pharmacol. Ther.* **111** 1036–49
[43] Madabushi R and Seo P *et al* 2022 Applications of model informed drug development (MIDD) in drug development lifecycle and regulatory review *Pharm. Res.* **39** 1663–7

[44] Jones H M and Rowland-Yeo K 2013 Basic concepts in physiologically based pharmacokinetic modeling in drug discovery and development *CPT: Pharm. Syst. Pharmacol.* **2** 1–12

[45] Chena Y and Jinb J Y *et al* 2012 Application of IVIVE and PBPK modeling in prospective prediction of clinical pharmacokinetics: strategy and approach during the drug discovery phase with four case studies *Biopharm. Drug Dispos.* **33** 85–98

[46] Anand O and Pepin X J H *et al* 2022 The use of physiologically based pharmacokinetic analyses—in biopharmaceutics applications -regulatory and industry perspectives *Pharm. Res.* **39** 1681–700

[47] Mitra A and Suarez-Sharp S *et al* 2021 Applications of physiologically based biopharmaceutics modeling (PBBM) to support drug product quality: a workshop summary report *J. Pharm. Sci.* **110** 594–609

[48] Kato T and Nakagawa H *et al* 2020 Establishment of a clinically relevant specification for dissolution testing using physiologically based pharmacokinetic (PBPK) modeling approaches *Eur. J. Pharm. Biopharm.* **151** 45–52

[49] Zhao Y and Suarez S 2019 FDA expectations in building a safe space to gain regulatory flexibility based on physiologically based biopharmaceutics modeling (PBBM) Disclaimer this presentation reflects the views of the *REdl & M-CERSI Workshop*

[50] Clinically Relevant Dissolution Specifications 2021 A biopharmaceutics' risk based approach: an FDA perspective

[51] Raines K 2021 PBPK biopharmaceutics guidance and progress on risk assessment *Regulatory Utility of Mechanistic Modeling to Support Alternative Bioequivalence Approaches Workshop*

[52] Smith D A and Obach R S 2009 Metabolites in safety testing (MIST): considerations of mechanisms of toxicity with dose, abundance, and duration of treatment *Chem. Res. Toxicol.* **22** 267–79

[53] Jones H M and Parrott N *et al* 2006 A novel strategy for physiologically based predictions of human pharmacokinetics *Clin. Pharmacokinet.* **45** 511–42

[54] Shardlow C E and Generaux G T *et al* 2013 Impact of physiologically based pharmacokinetic modeling and simulation in drug development *Drug Metab. Dispos.* **41** 1194–2003

[55] Lu C and Suri A *et al* 2014 Assessment of cytochromeP450- mediated drug–drug interaction potentialo for teroneland exposure changes inpatients with renal impairment using physiologically based pharmacokinetic modeling and simulation *Biopharm. Drug Dispos* **35** 543–52

[56] 2020 EFPIA Biopharmaceutics modelling as a fundamental tool to support accelerated access *Executive Summary* European Federation of Pharmaceutical Industries and Associations 1–20

[57] USFDA, CDER, OGDP 2019 Nonbinding recommendations determining whether to submit an ANDA or a 505(b)(2) application guidance for industry **505**(May). http://fda.gov/Drugs/GuidanceComplianceRegulatoryInformation/Guidances/default.htm

[58] USF&DA 2018 Physiologically based pharmacokinetic analyses—format and content. Guidance (August)

[59] Freije I and Lamouche S *et al* 2020 Review of drugs approved via the 505(b)(2) pathway: uncovering drug development trends and regulatory requirements. therapeutic innovation and regulatory *Science* **54** 128–38

[60] Dong Z and Li J *et al* 2020 Application of physiologically-based pharmacokinetic modeling to predict gastric pH-dependent drug–drug interactions for weak base drugs *CPT: Pharm. Systems Pharmacol.* **9** 456–65

[61] Abend A and Heimbach T *et al* 2018 Dissolution and translational modeling strategies enabling patient-centric drug product development: the M-CERSI workshop summary report *AAPS* J. **20** 60

[62] Wu D and Sanghavi M *et al* 2023 Physiologically based pharmacokinetics modeling in biopharmaceutics: case studies for establishing the bioequivalence safe space for innovator and generic drugs *Pharm. Res.* **40** 337–57

[63] Pepin X J H and Flanagan T R *et al* 2016 Justification of drug product dissolution rate and drug substance particle size specifications based on absorption PBPK modeling for lesinurad immediate release tablets *Mol. Pharm.* **13** 3256–69

[64] Suarez-Sharp S and Li M *et al* 2016 Regulatory experience with *in vivo* in vitro correlations (IVIVC) in new drug applications *AAPS* J. **18** 1379–90

[65] Wu F and Shah H *et al* 2021 Biopharmaceutics applications of physiologically based pharmacokinetic absorption modeling and simulation in regulatory submissions to the u.s. food and drug administration for new drugs *AAPS* J. **23** 31

[66] Jamei M 2016 Recent advances in development and application of physiologically-based pharmacokinetic (PBPK) models: a transition from academic curiosity to regulatory acceptance *Curr. Pharmacol. Rep.* **2** 161–9

[67] Butler J and Hens B *et al* 2019 *In vitro* models for the prediction of *in vivo* performance of oral dosage forms: recent progress from partnership through the IMI OrBiTo collaboration *Eur. J. Pharm. Biopharm.* **136** 70–83

[68] Kostewicz E S and Abrahamsson B *et al* 2014 *In vitro* models for the prediction of *in vivo* performance of oral dosage forms *Eur. J. Pharm. Sci.* **57** 342–66

[69] Govindaraj P and Nizamuddin S *et al* 2015 Genome-wide analysis correlates Ayurveda Prakriti *Sci. Rep.* **5** 1–12

[70] Joshi K and Ghodke Y *et al* 2011 Traditional medicine to modern pharmacogenomics: ayurveda Prakriti type and CYP2C19 gene polymorphism associated with the metabolic variability *Evid.-based Complement. Altern. Med.* **2011** 1–5

[71] Mukerji M and Asher B P R 2011 Ayurgenomics : a new approach in personalized and preventive medicine *Sci. Cult.* **77** 10–7

IOP Publishing

Advances in Drug Delivery Systems for Healthcare
From concept to clinic
Piyush Pradeep Mehta and Arpana Parihar

Chapter 13

Computational approaches for antibody-based targeted drug delivery strategies

Jayesh Dharwadkar[1#], Darshana Khandge[1#], Sangeeta Ballav[1] and Soumya Basu[1*]**

Antibodies have become essential diagnostic and therapeutic tools for a variety of disorders. The development of antibodies has progressed from a trial-and-error technique to a logical design approach as technology has advanced. As a result, databases and computational tools that can aid in the characterization and development of therapeutic antibodies, are in high demand. This chapter provides an overview of the numerous antibody sequences and accessible structural databases, also computational approaches utilized in antibody production. It also examines emerging trends in the industry, such as data mining, next-generation sequencing data and the use of alternative antibody forms such as nanobodies. The chapter also discusses the difficulties involved with the pharmacokinetics and formulation of therapeutic antibodies. Overall, this chapter gives insight into the current status of the field and emphasizes the significance of continuous growth in the area of computational-based antibody development.

13.1 Introduction

Antibodies, also known as immunoglobulins, are proteins produced by the immune system in response to the presence of foreign substances called antigens. They play a crucial role in the immune response, specifically in the adaptive immune system [1]. Antibodies are large proteins composed of two identical heavy chains and two identical light chains. These chains are interconnected via disulfide bonds, forming a Y-shaped structure. The variability in the N-terminal ends of the heavy and light chains contributes to the antigen-binding specificity of antibodies. The heavy chains, larger in size, consist of constant and variable regions. The variable region, located

[#] Equal contribution.
[*] Corresponding Author Email ID: soumya.bs@gmail.com
[**] Co-Corresponding Author Email ID: sangeetaballav@gmail.com

at the N-terminal end, includes hypervariable regions or complementarity-determining regions (CDRs) responsible for antigen recognition. Light chains, smaller in size, also possess a variable region. The unique combination of heavy and light chain variable regions determines the antigen specificity of antibodies. They consist of CDRs, which directly interact with antigens. The high diversity of CDRs allows antibodies to recognize a wide range of antigens [2]. The constant regions, located at the C-terminal ends of the heavy and light chains, provide structural stability to antibodies. These regions exhibit less diversity compared to the variable regions and determine the functional properties of antibodies, such as effector functions and interaction with immune cells. The two arms of the 'Y' form the antigen-binding fragments (Fab), while the stem of the 'Y' is called the constant fragment (Fc). Each arm contains a variable region that is responsible for binding to specific antigens. The constant regions, on the other hand, determine the functional properties of antibodies, such as their ability to activate other components of the immune system (figure 13.1) [3].

Antibody-based targeted medication delivery has emerged as a potential technology for the treatment of a wide range of diseases, including cancer, autoimmune disorders, and infectious diseases [4]. The use of antibodies allows for the specific

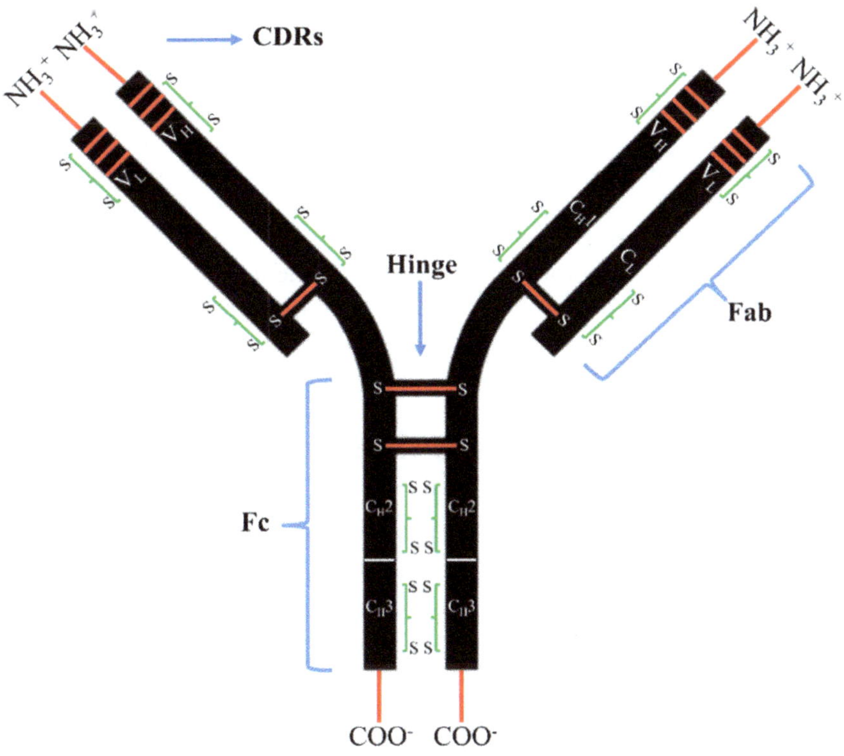

Figure 13.1. Schematic structure of an antibody. COO^-: Carboxy terminal end; NH_3^+: Amino terminal end; CDR: Complementarity-determining region; ScFv: Fab: Antigen-binding fragment; Fc: Constant fragment; C_H: Constant domain of heavy chain; C_L: Constant domain of light chain; S-S: Disulfide bond; V_H: Variable domain of heavy chain; V_L: Variable domain of light chain.

delivery of drugs to target cells or tissues, resulting in increased efficacy and reduced toxicity compared to traditional systemic drug administration. Computational methods have been critical in the development of antibody-based tailored medication delivery techniques. Researchers can use computational tools to create and enhance therapeutic antibody characteristics, predict their pharmacokinetic and pharmacodynamic profiles, and simulate their interactions with target molecules [5]. Besides, developing successful antibody-based drug delivery systems might be a difficult undertaking. Antibodies must be carefully developed to have the necessary qualities for drug administration, such as high affinity and specificity to the target molecule, biological stability, and minimal immunogenicity.

Computational techniques have played a critical role in the development of antibody-based specific drug delivery strategies to solve these issues. Researchers can use computational tools to create and optimize therapeutic antibody characteristics, predict pharmacokinetic and pharmacodynamic profiles, and simulate interactions with target molecules [6]. The utilization of antibody databases, which contain huge repertoires of antibody sequences and structures, is a key part of computational antibody engineering [7]. These databases can be used to find possible lead candidates for further optimization as well as acquire insights into the features of existing therapeutic antibodies. In addition to databases, a huge suite of predictors of various biophysical and other properties of antibodies has been established. These predictors can be used to guide the development of antibodies with desirable features, such as improved affinity or specificity to a target molecule [7]. Advancement of deep learning techniques is also boosting the performance of antibody structure prediction, particularly CDRs. Furthermore, large language models generating functional protein sequences or protein language models are yielding encouraging outcomes in terms of improving antibody activity and characteristics [8]. In this chapter, we will look at the computational tools and techniques that have been employed in the development of antibody-based targeted drug delivery schemes, such as antibody design and optimization, pharmacokinetic modelling, and molecular simulation. We will also explore the obstacles and potential developments in this subject.

13.2 Databases for antibody sequences and structures

13.2.1 Antibody databases

Antibody databases are repositories of information on antibodies, including their sequences, structures, and functions. These databases are essential resources for researchers working in fields such as immunology, cancer biology, and drug development. Some popular antibody databases include Antibody Registry, Protein Data Bank (PDB), ABCD database and Antibodypedia (https://www.antibodypedia.com/) [9, 10]. The Antibody Registry is a comprehensive database of antibodies developed by various manufacturers, while the PDB provides information on the 3D structures of proteins, including antibodies [9]. Antibodypedia is a free resource that provides detailed information on antibody products and their applications [10] (table 13.1).

Table 13.1. List of databases for antibody sequences and structures.

Database name	Description	Website	Reference
IMGT/GENE-DB	A comprehensive database of immunoglobulin (IG) and T-cell receptor (TR) gene sequences from human and other vertebrate species.	https://www.imgt.org/genedb/	[17]
IMGT/LIGM-DB	A database of antibody and T-cell receptor (TCR) three-dimensional structures with associated sequences and other information.	https://www.imgt.org/ligmdb/	[31]
Protein Data Bank (PDB)	PDB is a repository of experimentally determined 3D structures of proteins, including antibody structures.	https://www.rcsb.org/	[25]
Kabat Database	A database containing amino acid sequences and structures of antibodies. It also includes information on antibody numbering schemes and other related data.	https://www.bioinf.org.uk/abs/	[32]
Chothia Database	A database of antibody structures, derived from the analysis of PDB entries. It provides information on antibody domains, framework regions, and complementarity-determining regions (CDRs).	https://opig.stats.ox.ac.uk/webapps/newsabdab/sabdab/	[33]
GenBank	A comprehensive database of nucleotide sequences, including DNA and RNA sequences from various organisms.	https://www.ncbi.nlm.nih.gov/genbank/	[34]
European Nucleotide Archive (ENA)	A database that hosts a wide range of nucleotide sequences, including genomic DNA, cDNA, and RNA sequences.	https://www.ebi.ac.uk/ena/browser/home	[19]
UniProt	A comprehensive resource that provides curated and annotated protein sequences, including information on protein function, structure, and interactions.	https://www.uniprot.org/	[35]
Antibody Database (AbDb)	A database dedicated to antibody structures, providing comprehensive information on antibody sequences, structures, and antigen–antibody complexes.	http://www.abybank.org/abdb/	[13]
Structural Antibody Database (SAbDab)	A resource that provides access to curated antibody structures and related data, including antigen recognition and CDR loop information.	https://opig.stats.ox.ac.uk/webapps/newsabdab/sabdab/	[14]
ClinicalTrials.gov	A registry and database of clinical trials worldwide, including trials involving antibody-based drug delivery systems.	https://www.clinicaltrials.gov/	[36]

Antibodypedia	A database that provides information on antibody therapeutics, including clinical trials and approved antibodies for drug delivery purposes.	https://www.antibodypedia.com/	[10]
DrugBank	A comprehensive database that provides information on drugs, including antibody-based therapeutics, their targets, and drug delivery mechanisms.	https://go.drugbank.com/	[37]
Therapeutic Antibody Database (TAB)	A database that focuses on therapeutic antibodies, providing information on approved and investigational antibodies, including their targets and drug delivery aspects.	https://tabs.craic.com/users/sign_in	[38]
Antibody–drug Conjugate (ADC) Review	A database providing information and reviews on antibody–drug conjugates (ADCs), which are antibody-based drug delivery systems.	https://www.adcreview.com/	[39]
Abysis	A database and analysis system dedicated to antibody structure information	http://www.abysis.org/	[26]
DIGIT	Antibody sequence database	http://circe.med.uniroma1.it/digit/help.php	[40]
Ireceptor	A database and analysis platform specifically designed for immune receptor repertoires	http://ireceptor.irmacs.sfu.ca/	[41]
Observed Antibody Space	NGS sequence data on B-cell receptors/antibodies	http://antibodymap.org/oas	[21]
Immune Epitope Database	Manually curated epitope data for immune epitopes and their interactions with immune receptors.	http://iedb.org	[42]
PDBBind	A database for binding interactions between proteins and small molecules, including drugs and ligands	http://www.pdbbind.org.cn/	[28]
Ab-Bind	Mutational antibody data related to binding affinities	https://github.com/sarahsirin/AB-Bind-Database	[29]
Structural Kinetics and Energetics of Mutant Protein Interactions (SKEMPI)	A database comprising experimentally measured changes in protein–protein interaction kinetics and energetics due to mutations.	https://life.bsc.es/pid/skempi2/	[30]
Single-Domain Antibody Database	Sequence and structural data on nanobodies	http://sdab-db.ca/	[43]

Antibody research heavily relies on the availability of appropriate datasets. Several curated resources are available that provide information on therapeutic antibodies, including TABS-Therapeutic Antibody Database and Therapeutic Structural Antibody Database (Thera-SAbDab) [11]. Antibody databases can be classified based on the type of information they provide, such as sequence, structure, or experimental data, with some databases providing a combination of these types [12]. In contrast, PDB has a large number of antibody structures that have been retrieved and collected into various datasets [11]. For instance, the Antibody Structure Database (AbDb) has updated Fv regions from the antibody using information from the Summary of Antibody Crystal Structures (SACS) dataset [13] (table 13.1). Similarly, the Structural Antibody Database (SAbDab) lists antibody structures from the PDB based on specific criteria, and abYsis offers resources for antibody structure prediction and design [14].

Thera-SAbDab is another valuable resource that provides structural information on therapeutic antibodies and nanobodies [15]. This database tracks 748 unique therapeutics, including monoclonal antibodies (mAbs) and bispecific therapeutics, as of July 2022. Additionally, RAPID is a repertoire sequencing dataset analysis platform that includes a large antibody database, which incorporates 521 therapeutic antibodies and 88 059 antibodies targeting specific antigens or arising in patients with particular diseases [16]. This platform provides information on antibody–antigen (Ab–Ag) interactions, potentially enabling a purely sequence-based solution to the Ab–Ag problem in the future. Access to these curated Ab–Ag information databases and resources is critical for researchers to analyse and predict antibody function, improve therapeutic antibody design, and develop new treatments for diseases. The availability of large-scale datasets has the potential to transform the field of antibody research and accelerate the development of effective therapies.

13.2.2 Sequences database

Antibody sequence databases can be broadly categorized into two types: databases specialized in single sequence depositions and databases that store bulk raw reads produced by next-generation sequencing (NGS) experiments. The most widely used database for germline antibody sequences is the International Immunogenetics Information System (IMGT), which is comprehensive and includes information on nucleotide sequences, genetic polymorphisms, and other features of immunoglobulin and T-cell receptor genes [17]. Other resources that specialize in single sequence depositions include DIGIT, Abysis, and the Kabat database [18] (table 13.1). DIGIT and Abysis source their data from the European Nucleotide Archive (ENA) [19] and the National Center for Biotechnology Information (NCBI) [20]. The Kabat database is a curated database of amino acid sequences of immunoglobulin variable domains. While NGS databases derive their contents from raw sequence reads deposited in multiple repositories, including ENA and NCBI. Typically, these databases only provide the unpaired heavy and light chains. Some examples of NGS databases include iReceptor and Observed Antibody Space [21]. iReceptor is a repository of raw immunological sequencing data, while

Observed Antibody Space offers an annotation of the predicted sequence errors. Other databases curate information based on the content of the dataset, such as structure or experimental information, which may include antibody sequence information as well. For example, Antibodypedia is a comprehensive database of antibody products, including information on suppliers, validation, and characterization data [22]. Another example is the VBASE2 database which is a database of germline sequences of immunoglobulin variable domains [23].

13.2.3 Structure database

A structural antibody database is a collection of information on the three-dimensional structures of antibodies, including their sequences, interactions, and conformational changes [24]. These databases are essential for researchers investigating antibody structure and function, as well as those developing antibody-based therapies. By providing access to this data, these resources have facilitated the discovery of novel binding sites, the rational design of therapeutic antibodies, and the optimization of antibody affinity and specificity. The PDB is the primary global repository for protein structure information [25]. There are several resources available that mine the PDB for antibody fragments, including PyIg-Classify, PCLICK, IMGT/3D-Structure-DB, SabDAb, Abysis, and AbDb [14] (table 13.1). SabDAb allows for a bulk download of its weekly updated database, providing a current resource for applications such as antibody modeling or docking. SabDAb and Abysis enable retrieval of particular structures based on a query antibody sequence (SAbDab) or using advanced features such as canonical classes of the CDRs (Abysis) [26]. Other resources, such as the Immune Epitope Database (IEDB), connect structural data to experimentally derived epitope data [27].

13.2.4 Experimental database

In addition to sequence and structure data, experimental information specific to antibodies can also enrich the understanding of their properties. One such source of experimental data is the Immune Epitope Database (IEDB), which provides information on the epitopes targeted by antibodies and links this information to epitope-specific antibody sequences [28]. Another crucial piece of information for characterizing antibody–epitope interactions is the binding affinity, which can be found in resources such as the SAbDab and PDBBind [28]. Additionally, specialized resources such as Ab-Bind [29] contain data on 1101 mutations across 32 antibody complexes, while Structural Kinetics and Energetics of Mutant Protein Interactions (SKEMPI) (table 13.1) [30] curates binding energy data for available structures, not limited to antibody information alone. The availability of experimental databases for antibody development, such as Antibodypedia, Antibody Registry, PDB-CCD, RCSB Ligand Explorer, and ChEMBL, has enabled the identification of novel binding sites, rational design of therapeutic antibodies, and optimization of antibody affinity and specificity in antibody-based targeted drug delivery applications. These resources provide a wealth of information on antibodies and their potential use in research, allowing researchers to identify promising candidates for further development and optimization.

13.3 Computational-based characterization of antibody development

Computational-based characterization plays a vital role in engineering therapeutic antibodies by utilizing bioinformatics tools such as homology modelling and protein–protein docking when antibody-specific sequence, structure, and experimental data are accessible. The development of antibody-based therapeutics involves two critical phases, lead identification and lead optimization [44]. The lead identification stage produces a large number of 'hit' molecules through animal immunization or surface display technologies, which are further screened and evaluated during the lead optimization phase to select a few high-affinity lead candidates that exhibit favourable characteristics [45]. During both lead identification and optimization phases, computational methods such as homology modeling, docking, or interface prediction are utilized to design and optimize antibodies by creating 3D models of antibodies and identifying crucial residues involved in antigen binding. These methods assist in improving the antibodies' binding affinity, specificity, and stability. Moreover, computational-based characterization of antibody candidates can assist in assessing the 'developability' risk to ensure the development of stable, manufacturable, safe, and effective therapeutics.

13.3.1 Antibody numbering

Antibody numbering is a useful method used by researchers to identify and label individual amino acids in an antibody's variable regions, which include the CDRs and framework regions (FRs). This allows for the comparison and analysis of different antibodies and their respective regions [46]. The IMGT unique numbering system serves as the basis for the antibody numbering system. It provides a standardized nomenclature for the amino acid positions in the variable regions of immunoglobulins (antibodies) and T-cell receptors. The IMGT unique numbering codes (e.g., CDR-IMGT) are used to designate the different regions of the antibody [31]. Meanwhile, a numbering scheme (e.g., Kabat or Chothia) is employed to identify the individual amino acids within those regions. To begin the antibody computational analysis, the first step is to map the antibody sequences onto a standardized reference framework. The raw nucleotide sequences of the variable regions can be translated into amino acids through the alignment with germline sequences. Programs such as IgBLAST and IMGT V-Quest can be used for this purpose [47]. Antibody amino acid sequences are then used to create a standardized reference framework or numbering scheme [46]. This assigns an identifier to each variable region amino acid. The Kabat, Chothia, and IMGT schemes are the most commonly adopted numbering schemes, while others such as Contact, North, WolfGuy, and Aho are less prevalent. The antibody numbering system places each position inside an antibody's structure in context, making it easier to quickly distinguish CDR and FR regions. Finally, three freely available software packages, ANARCI, Abnum, and AbRSA, are available for the numbering of antibodies.

These software packages are used as the first step in computational antibody analysis, such as homology modelling.

13.3.2 Antibody modelling

The process of constructing an antibody structure from its sequence alone is known as structural antibody modelling. This involves using existing knowledge of antibody and protein structures to follow five steps: selecting a suitable framework template, determining the relative orientation of V_H and V_L domains, modelling CDR loops, building and refining side-chains, and optimizing the molecule's energetic packing [48]. To begin, a suitable framework template is selected based on close sequence matches to H and L chains in databases [14]. The relative orientation of V_H and V_H domains is determined using specific algorithms like AbAngle, which is essential to shape the correct paratope [49, 50]. CDR loops are then modelled, with knowledge-based methods currently accurate for predicting the five canonical loops, though CDRH3 remains challenging [51]. Antibody-specific knowledge-based methods are fast and accurate if a template is available, but more computationally expensive *ab initio* approaches can be used to generate a large set of novel loops when no suitable template is available [53].

Hybrid methods like Sphinx combine knowledge-based and *ab initio* approaches to provide better predictions regardless of the availability of prior structural information. The final step involves building and refining side-chains, which can be achieved through either protein-generic approach like SCWRL or antibody-focused approaches like PEARS [52, 53]. The final antibody model can be further refined by optimizing the molecule's energetic packing through packages like Rosetta [54]. Various tools are available for structural antibody modelling, such as PIGS, AbodyBuilder, Biovia, SmrtMolAntibody, MOE, BioLuminate, AbPredict, and Rosetta, which vary in run-times and output quality. Though run-times vary, with some tools producing a model in as little as 60 s and others taking several hours, the tools produce comparable results, as shown by the Antibody Modelling Assessment II benchmarking experiment. Structural antibody modelling is useful for selecting surface-exposed paratope residues for mutations or characterizing binding with respect to the cognate epitope during the Lead Identification stage [55, 56]. Accurate structural information can be used during the lead optimization stage to assess various developability indicators like hydrophobicity, which require accurate models of the molecular surface of the paratope and epitope [57].

13.3.3 Folding stability

The stability of antibody conformation is critical for their usage as therapeutic agents since it keeps their integrity under a variety of manufacturing, formulation, and physiological conditions [58–60]. When antibodies become unfolded, they lose their activity and form protein aggregates, which can be immunogenic or toxic [61, 62]. Despite being inherently stable, antibodies chosen as lead candidates for drug development may require further optimization for other properties such as affinity or immunogenicity, which can result in a decrease in folding stability due to the inherent trade-offs between these biophysical properties. There are known experimental approaches for screening and choosing stable antibody candidates during early-stage evaluation of vast panels or libraries of natural and synthetic antibodies [63, 64].

A recent study demonstrated the utility of mutagenizing sites in the V_H/V_L interface for improving antibody affinity and stability [65]. The study identified a cluster of eight residues at the V_H/V_L interface of an anti-lysozyme single-chain variable fragment (scFv) that were tolerant to mutations via a deep mutational scan. The scFv was re-engineered with mutations introduced at all eight sites, and the resulting variant was found to have greatly improved affinity and folding stability, indicating promise for this method of antibody optimization. Computational approaches such as AbLIFT and Computationally Driven Antibody Humanization (CoDAH) have also been developed to identify favorable mutations at the V_H/V_L interface and predict humanizing mutations that maintain folding stability.

When antibodies are discovered through animal immunization, they can be immunogenic to humans, so a process called humanization is required to reduce this effect [66, 67]. However, humanization can also lead to reduced folding stability, which is a major challenge as stability is crucial for antibody therapeutics. To address this issue, a computational approach called CoDAH was developed. CoDAH uses structural energy information from homology models to identify humanizing mutations that maintain folding stability. It evaluates humanness using a human string content score and Pareto optimization of the humanness score. The structural energies help in identifying stable humanizing mutations. CoDAH was successful in predicting sets of humanizing mutations for antibodies that retained both binding affinity and stability while maintaining humanness. In contrast, conventional humanization methods such as grafting CDRs failed to maintain stability. CoDAH-guided humanization of cetuximab was also successful in maintaining high stability [68].

13.3.4 Interface prediction of antibody–antigen properties

To understand the interactions between an antibody and its target antigen, experimental determination of the 3D structure of the Ab–Ag complex using x-ray crystallography is the gold standard. Computational approaches that predict Ab–-Ag contact surfaces, on the other hand, can give a quick alternative during therapeutic discovery efforts. These methods can predict the paratope, the epitope, or the entire Ab–Ag complex. Predictors of paratopes and epitopes offer useful information on Ab–Ag recognition, which can be exploited for therapeutic design [69].

Antibodies have regions called CDRs that come into direct contact with the antigen and form the paratope. Computational predictors of paratopes can help to guide the mutational choices for affinity engineering of therapeutics during lead optimization. They can also provide valuable information to guide the modeling of Ab–Ag complexes during lead identification. Statistical approaches, such as Antibody i-Patch, assign a score to each residue based on its propensity to be part of the paratope [56]. Paratope residues are not all constrained to the CDRs, so tools such as Paratome can be used to identify other positions that might contribute to antigen recognition [70, 71]. Machine learning approaches such as proABC, AntibodyInterfacePrediction, Parapred, and AG-Fast-Parapred have outperformed these statistical approaches recently [72].

There are two main ways to identify epitopes, which are regions of antigens that interact with antibodies. Experimental methods can be used, or computational protocols can be applied. Computational methods can be further divided into two types: linear epitope predictors and conformational epitope predictors. Conformational epitope predictors are generally more accurate because most epitopes have a specific 3D shape. However, many epitope prediction methods do not take into account the specific antibody being used, and instead focus on identifying generic immunogenic regions. This approach can be problematic because it is difficult to distinguish between immunogenic regions and actual epitopes [73]. Therefore, newer epitope prediction methods include information about the specific antibody, which has led to the development of antibody-specific predictors. Examples of antibody-specific predictors include ASEP, BEPAR, ABEpar, EpiPred, PEASE, MabTope, and Jespersen [74]. Current methods, such as those utilised by MabTope and Jespersen combine protein–protein docking with antibody-specific epitope prediction to identify paratope-epitope pairs.

Predicting paratope and epitope regions can provide valuable information for designing therapeutics. However, such predictions do not offer insights into the actual interactions that occur between an antibody and its antigen. To address this limitation, Ab–Ag docking is utilized. This method is a specialized application of molecular docking, which aims to predict the complex structure of two unbound proteins. Ab–Ag docking involves two main steps: sampling, which generates thousands of potential complex conformations using programs like antibody-specific ClusPro, SnugDock, and general protein HADDOCK and ZDOCK; and scoring, which uses specific scoring functions like DockSorter and general protein ZRANK, FireDock, and SIPPER to rank the generated conformations and identify those that closely resemble the native structure [75].

13.3.5 Pharmacokinetic clearance

Pharmacokinetic clearance is a crucial pharmacological parameter that determines how quickly an antibody drug is eliminated from the body. It helps in estimating the half-life of the antibody, which is the time taken for the drug concentration in the body to decrease by half. Several factors such as isoelectric point, viscosity, immunogenicity, non-specificity, aggregation, and stability are known to affect the clinical pharmacokinetic clearance rate of the antibody. Researchers have developed a number of computational models that evaluate these factors to predict the clearance rate of antibodies [76]. It was reported that the clearance rate of 64 mAbs that had been approved or were in clinical trials could be predicted using a random forest classifier [77]. Among the factors used to distinguish fast clearing antibodies from slow clearing antibodies, the isoelectric point played a crucial role.

In another study, researchers employed structure-based charge calculations to predict the pharmacokinetic clearance rate of antibodies [78].

13.4 Computational chemistry and methods for therapeutic antibody discovery

The process of developing antibodies for therapeutic reasons consists of three major steps: antibody design, immunogenicity assessment, and biophysical property evaluation. The antibody is designed *in silico* utilizing various tools and methodologies in the initial phase using computer-based models. This process entails determining and modifying the structure of the antibody in order to maximize its qualities for therapeutic usage [44]. The immunogenicity of the developed antibody is evaluated in the second stage. Immunogenicity refers to capacity of therapeutic proteins to elicit an immunological response in the body. This phase entails evaluating the antibody to confirm that it can be utilized in a variety of therapies and that it can elicit the required immune response. The last stage is to assess the antibody's biophysical characteristics. This includes looking for concerns like solubility and aggregation-prone areas, which might have an influence on the antibody's usefulness as a therapeutic agent [79]. By following these three processes, scientists may create antibodies that have been designed for therapeutic use, efficient in stimulating an immune response, and have the physicochemical qualities required for successful clinical application.

13.4.1 Antibody design

The use of techniques for interface prediction and analysis and antibody modelling can help in the development of novel compounds during lead identification or as support equipment during lead optimization. For the *ab initio* design of paratopes through CDR generation, modelling, Ab–Ag docking, and binding energy assessment, four techniques can be used: OptCDR, OptMAVEn, AbDesign, and RosettaAntibodyDesign [38]. By optimizing conformational and free energy shift following alteration of particular residues, these techniques can increase antibody stability and affinities. Other strategies that use pre-existing structures to increase antibody affinity include hot-spot grafting and re-epitoping [81]. The development of medicinal lead candidates can be accelerated by using these computational frameworks to guide conventional discovery approaches, although more industry validation is required.

13.4.1.1 OptCDR

The OptCDR approach is a broad computational method for creating new antibodies with high affinity and specificity to bind particular antigens [81]. It creates a number of different and diverse libraries of antibody CDRs, which may then be grafted into an antibody framework utilizing humanization procedures. The approach entails selecting canonical structures for CDRs that are most likely to bind the antigen positively, followed by simultaneous refining of the backbones of the CDR structures and optimum amino acid selection [80]. OptCDR was tested against three different test scenarios and observed to be capable of producing varied antibody libraries of a predetermined size with promising antigen affinity potential, as demonstrated by computationally computed binding metrics. OptCDR is a four-step workflow for designing libraries of antibody CDRs to bind a specified antigen epitope. The first step involves selecting the combination of CDR canonical structures (only backbones) that are most likely to have favourable binding with the antigen. A scoring system based purely on backbone atom-antigen distance information is devised to evaluate the potential of canonical structures for CDRs to display good binding with antigens [81]. In the second step, the amino acid sequences of the selected structures are initialized one at a time using a rotamer library, energy functions, and mixed integer linear programming (MILP) optimization formulation. Using energy functions, a rotamer library, and a previously described MILP rotamer optimization formulation, the amino acid sequences of selected canonical structures are initialized one at a time [81]. The third step of OptCDR entails running several thousand iterations of a modified version of iterative protein redesign and optimization (IPRO), which involves randomly perturbing the phi and psi dihedral angles of each CDR residue, re-determining the amino acid sequence using the rotamer selection MILP, and performing an energy minimization. The fourth step of OptCDR involves generating a library by accumulating the most-promising mutations for the CDRs. This library can then be screened to identify antibodies with high specificity and affinity for the targeted antigen epitope [81].

13.4.1.2 OptMAVEn

OptMAVEn is used in drug development that predicts the binding affinity of small molecule ligands to target proteins using molecular docking and virtual screening. The procedure entails creating a library of molecularly imprinted polymers (MIPs) that have been computationally tuned to identify the target protein. The ligand molecules are then docked into the MIPs, and the docking scores obtained are used to estimate the ligand's binding affinity to the protein [82]. The use of MIPs allows for the prediction of ligand binding with great accuracy and specificity, and has been effectively employed in the development of new therapeutic candidates for diverse diseases. OptMAVEn has been employed in a variety of research, including the discovery of prospective cancer medication candidates and the prediction of small molecule inhibitors for the Zika virus [83]. To begin an experiment using software, OptMAVEn-2.0, the user executes a command/OptMAVEn-2.0 on UNIX terminal, giving the experiment name, antigen structure file, chains, heteroatoms to exclude, and epitope area residues. The application automatically pre-processes the antigen structure file by deleting unnecessary chains and heteroatoms, simplifying the experimentation procedure [84]. OptMAVEn-2.0 enables users to pick antigen chains, heteroatoms, and epitope residues using a simple, single-line syntax that lists the various antigen molecule chains for selection. The application automatically downloads the molecule from the Protein Data Bank (PDB) using a BioPython library and conducts the next stages, making antibody creation studies easier for the user [84].

13.4.1.3 AbDesign

The AbDesign technique is used for creating proteins with highly efficient and specialized functional locations, such as antibodies and enzymes. The method uses several protein families' innate modularity by merging naturally available modular pieces to construct new backbones. This results in a huge combinatorial universe of backbone conformations that can outnumber the variety of the whole PDB (figure 13.2) [85]. The approach enables the construction of huge, atomically precise proteins with hundreds of mutations from any natural protein. The resultant proteins have sub-angstrom level control over the location of active-site groups, which provides the precision required for highly active proteins [85]. The AbDesign pipeline is publicly accessible on GitHub and serves as a guide for implementing it.

a. **Segmenting homologous structures**

   The first step in implementing the AbDesign process for a protein family is to obtain all known structures from freely available resources such as the Pfam database. Manually selected amino acid locations with the highest structural conservation are then used as segmentation points to assemble modular pieces into new backbones [85].

b. **Structure idealization**

   AbDesign performs all design computations in torsion space solely, with no optimization of bond lengths and angles. This is owing to the fact that experimentally derived structures frequently deviate from ideal bond lengths and angles, which may be attributed to uncertainty in structure determination from low-to-medium resolution x-ray crystallographic data [85]. All structures are subjected to the Rosetta idealize technique, which imposes ideal bonds and relaxes dihedral angles with harmonic backbone coordinate restrictions to match the coordinates of the PDB entry, to eliminate noise in energy estimates produced by such aberrations. As a result, model structures with outstanding stereo-chemical characteristics are produced, as measured by MolProbity [85]. In continuing research, idealized protein architectures have been successfully employed to construct functional enzymes.

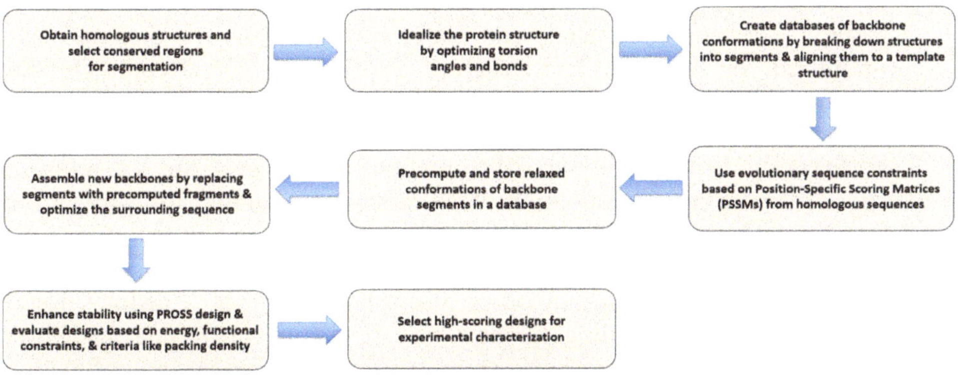

Figure 13.2. Schematic representation of workflow for designing antibody with AbDesign.

c. **Computing backbone-conformation databases**
Backbone-conformation databases are built for each segment of the protein family in this stage of the AbDesign workflow by segmenting the original structure files (PDB format) into pieces at the segmentation points. One of the protein family's structures is assigned as the template, from which all other structures will be segmented [85]. To improve the smooth assembly of fragments into full-length backbones, all structures are aligned to the template, and all fragments belonging to the same segment are aligned. Clustering of fragments can be done for protein families with several members in the PDB to minimize computational cost without reducing backbone diversity.
d. **Evolutionary sequence constraints**
For each backbone segment, AbDesign employs position-specific sequence restrictions based on position-specific scoring matrices (PSSMs), which are constructed by creating a multiple sequence alignment (MSA) based on homologous sequences. BLAST is used to retrieve sequences from the nr sequence database, with cutoffs of 35% sequence identity and $\geqslant$ 75% template protein coverage [85].
e. **Pre-computation of the backbone database.**
To minimize computational time, AbDesign employs modular assembly to pre-compute a relaxed conformation for each backbone segment, keep it in a database, and swiftly combine it during backbone assembly. During pre-computation, each segment of the template protein is removed one at a time, and each structurally aligned fragment from each homolog is relaxed in the context of the template using cyclic-coordinate descent (CCD) backbone relaxation. AbDesign additionally allows for sequence optimization (limited by the PSSMs) in the modelled fragment and its immediate surroundings [85]. Before entering the segment's backbone torsion angles into the database, AbDesign automatically verifies that the backbone main chain is continuous and that the RMSD to the segment as observed in the source structure is low (0.2) [85].
f. **Assembly of new backbones from protein fragments**
In AbDesign, the design process begins with the template structure and proceeds to replace different segments with pre-computed fragments from a database, with PSSM constraints adjusted accordingly. Under these constraints, the new fragments and their surroundings are then sequence-optimized for the backbone structure. PROSS (Protein Repair One-Stop Shop) stability design is used to enhance the fit between fragments and raise the stability of the new backbone to build a seamless structure, often yielding seven designs, with the second-to-highest design in terms of mutations chosen for further investigation. This process is required for good protein stability and expressibility [85].
g. **Selecting designs for experimental characterization**
The backbone design method creates a large number of distinct designs, which are rated according to their system energy. However, the Rosetta energies used to estimate protein stability do not take into account functional constraints, such as the requirement for catalytic residues to adopt the proper

conformation. Thus, designs with incorrect active-site constellations may be eliminated, and other criteria, such as internal packing density or shape complementarity with a binding partner, may be used to select designs. To choose designs based on numerous criteria, utilize a fuzzy-logic expression to characterize the design's fitness relative to each criterion, then integrate them into an optimization objective function to discover a good balance among all characteristics. Designs with close to 1 objective-function scores are chosen [85].

13.4.1.4 Rosetta antibody design (RAbD)

RAbD is a computational approach and platform for developing antibodies to specific targets. It collects antibody sequences and structures using a fully customizable technique that incorporates a database of CDR structures labelled according to CDR cluster nomenclature [86]. RAbD employs a flexible-backbone design approach that integrates cluster-based CDR restrictions and sequence design based on each cluster's amino acid sequence profile. It has been thoroughly benchmarked and experimentally evaluated, with excellent success rates in developing antibodies with increased affinities. The RAbD framework is accessible in RosettaScripts and comprises over 50 new Rosetta classes and over 20 000 lines of code [86].

13.4.2 Immunogenicity prediction

Immunogenicity is a significant factor to consider while developing protein therapeutics since it might cause side effects that impair the therapy's efficacy. Anti-drug antibodies can render protein medicines ineffective, modify their pharmacokinetics, and potentially cause severe side consequences. To avoid such difficulties, it is critical to establish the drivers of immunogenicity. The delivery route, delivery vehicle, dosing regimen, aggregation, innate immune system activation, and the protein's capacity to interface with the humoral and cellular immune systems are all factors that contribute to immunogenicity. To reduce the risk of immunogenicity in clinical trials and after licensure, these parameters must be assessed throughout preclinical development. It is worth emphasizing that the factors of immunogenicity for autologous or human-like proteins are not entirely known, necessitating more research to improve protein therapy design. In this context, regulatory authorities are creating risk-based immunogenicity screening recommendations in order to reduce the risk of adverse events related with protein medication treatment [87].

13.4.2.1 RANKPEP

RANKPEP is an online tool that predicts peptide-MHC binding for the discovery of CD8 T-cell epitopes. It has been expanded to incorporate peptide-MHCII binding prediction for CD4 T-cell epitopes. Currently, the library covers 88 and 50 distinct MHCIs and MHCII molecules, respectively. The server incorporates a proteasomal cleavage site prediction model, which is critical for MHCI-restricted epitopes. A variability masking function was also added in order to focus on conserved protein regions expressed by infectious genomes, pinpointing invariant T-cell epitopes to impede mutation as an immune evasion method [88].

13.4.2.2 NetMHCII

NetMHCII is a method for predicting MHC-peptide binding affinities, whereas NetMHCIIpan is a pan-specific approach for predicting binding affinities for any MHC molecule with a given protein sequence. Both methods were trained using a five-fold cross-validation setup, and for each fold, a network ensemble of individual networks was generated and trained for 500 cycles without early stopping with 10, 15, 40, and 60 hidden neurons using 10 different initial configurations, yielding a total of 40 networks [89]. The BLOSUM50 matrix was used to encode the peptide and the MHC pseudo sequence, and the PFR was encoded using the average BLOSUM scores on a maximum window of three amino acids at each end of the binding core. The peptide core, PFRs, peptide length, and length of the C-terminal and N-terminal PFRs were fed into the neural network for each peptide core. NetMHCII can only estimate binding affinities for MHC molecules discovered in the training data, but NetMHCIIpan can use a pseudo sequence of 34 residues to predict binding affinities for any MHC molecule having a known protein sequence [89].

13.4.3 Biophysical properties

Successful therapeutic antibody development is dependent on desirable biophysical features such as solubility, colloidal stability, and avoidance of aggregation, which can result in loss of function or immunogenicity. Several algorithms and machine learning methods have been developed to predict aggregation-prone regions (APRs) and solubility, as well as to generate a score, such as the developability index (DI), which combines hydrophobicity, SAP score, and molecule net charge [38]. Natural antibody sequences can be exploited to determine advantageous biophysical features in antibody therapies. Computational criteria, such as a hydrophobicity score based on structure, can be utilized to detect developability hazards and guide therapeutic antibody production [38].

Antibody solubility and aggregation can provide substantial obstacles during therapeutic development, since aggregates can elicit immunogenic responses in patients and raise safety concerns. Analytical methods such as size-exclusion chromatography (SEC) and dynamic light scattering can be used to characterize existing aggregates, but high-throughput screening methods are required to evaluate the aggregation potential of large numbers of antibodies during early-stage discovery and development, when they are available in low concentrations, quantities, and purities [90]. APRs are short lengths of protein residues that self-associate and produce organized intermolecular beta-sheet structures known as 'cross-beta' spines. These beta-sheets pack in layers and create stable structures known as 'steric zippers' because the side-chains of nearby layers interlock securely. Backbone hydrogen bonds stabilize APRs, which are generally 5–15 residues long.

13.4.3.1 AggScore

The pharmaceutical business and scientific community are interested in detecting protein aggregation, although doing so experimentally may be expensive. Current aggregation prediction algorithms rely heavily on the main sequence and are trained on beta amyloid peptides, which may be inaccurate when applied to larger protein systems. A novel technique named 'AggScore' has been created to identify aggregation-prone areas in proteins using 3D structural input. AggScore takes into account the distribution of hydrophobic and electrostatic patches on the protein's surface, as well as their intensity and relative orientation. It was trained on a collection of 31 adnectin proteins and can identify aggregation-prone areas as well as changes in aggregation behavior owing to residue mutation. AggScore is relevant to globular proteins as well as tiny proteins. AggScore is applicable to globular proteins, short peptides, and antibodies and is unaffected by the environment of amyloid aggregation [91].

13.4.3.2 SolPredict

Solpredict is a machine learning-based tool that predicts the solubility of antibody molecules. SolPredict is a system that predicts the apparent solubility of mAbs in histidine (pH 6.0) buffer conditions using protein language modeling and machine learning [92]. To predict solubility, it leverages embeddings taken from a pretrained protein language model from single sequences and feeds them into a shallow neutral network. SolPredict was trained on a dataset of 220 different in-house mAbs and tested on an independent test set of 40 mAbs using extrapolated protein solubility data collected from a PEG-induced precipitation technique. SolPredict has a strong correlation with experimental data, enabling quick, large-scale, and high-throughput screening of mAbs during the early stages of antibody development.[92].

13.5 Antibody formulation

In order to meet the unique requirements of storage, freeze–thaw cycles, and administration method, it is necessary to optimize a variety of pharmaceutical additives while creating antibody therapies. In order to decrease injection volume while keeping the appropriate dose, antibody-based therapies are increasingly being made with higher concentrations. The goal of this is to facilitate more flexible administration routes and better therapeutic outcomes [93]. Antibody formulations are commonly administered systemically via intravenous (IV) infusion, but intramuscular (IM) and subcutaneous (SC) injections are potentially preferable due to their simpler accessibility, possibility for prolonged release kinetics and half-life [94]. Smaller injection quantities can nevertheless achieve therapeutically relevant delivery when antibodies are concentrated to high levels. Although exceptionally high viscosities may make it difficult to administer a substance using small-bore needles, viscosity physical factors must also be taken into account throughout the formulation process. As each delivery route, molecular entity, and target requires distinct formulation conditions to ensure stability and shelf life, antibody therapeutic formulation should be considered early in the development phase [95]. It is essential to comprehend how the antibody reacts to stresses such as freeze–thaw, agitation, heat stability, and pH/buffer changes. Excipients, or inactive chemicals, are added to products to reduce protein instability. However, due to the regulatory difficulties involved in introducing novel excipients, there are only a finite number of excipients that the FDA has allowed for use in antibody formulation. Due to their tendency to aggregate, mAbs can make it difficult to achieve high concentrations with long shelf lives. When working with polyclonal antibodies, ADCs, or combinations of mAbs, the formulation process becomes more difficult. To create the most stable formulation, optimization steps, buffer selection and excipient addition in sequence are used [96]. The stability and activity of compounds are evaluated under stressful conditions using a variety of characterization techniques, such as chromatography, mass spectrometry, and potency assays. Dynamic light scattering, molecular modelling, and other methods aid in assessing formulation properties [97]. A typical antibody formulation includes an antibody, an excipient to regulate tonicity or osmolality, a lyoprotectant (lyophilized powders), a buffer(s), and a surfactant.

13.5.1 Antibody concentration

Antibody concentrations in formulations range from 0.012 to 200 mg ml^{-1}. In order to fit into small dosing amounts, subcutaneous formulations frequently have greater concentrations (100–200 mg ml^{-1}), whereas intravenous formulations normally range from 80 mg ml^{-1} [98]. Benlysta®, Cimzia®, and Kevzara® are a few examples of subcutaneous preparations with a high concentration. Actemra®, Benlysta®, Stelara™, Herceptin®, and Rituxan® are some medicines that provide both intravenous and subcutaneous formulations with dramatically differing antibody concentrations [97].

13.5.2 Tonicity and osmolality excipients

Sodium chloride is the main excipient used to regulate tonicity in antibody formulations, whereas sucrose, trehalose, sorbitol, mannitol, and maltose are used to adjust osmolality. The most widely used ingredients are sugar and sodium chloride. There are also other excipients used, including maltose, sorbitol, mannitol, and trehalose. In addition to adjusting tonicity, sodium chloride can also lessen the viscosity of solutions. In some formulations, a positive charge arginine helps modify the tonicity and is utilised to reduce viscosity [97].

13.5.3 Viscosity-lowering excipients

In antibody products, arginine is found in quantities of 5–26 mg ml^{-1}. Subcutaneous solutions are the main sources of it. Arginine is present in a number of high-concentration subcutaneous solutions (150–200 mg ml^{-1}) [99]. Glycine is present in many formulations, both as lyophilized powders and intravenous solutions, with values ranging from 0.1 to 22.5 mg ml^{-1}. Three subcutaneous solutions with proline concentrations between 15 and 25 mg ml^{-1} are available. Sodium chloride is frequently combined with other excipients like sucrose and mannitol to adjust tonicity and reduce viscosity [97].

13.5.4 Lyoprotectants

The two lyoprotectants that are most frequently utilized in lyophilized powders are sucrose and trehalose. The amount of sucrose in a solution after reconstitution ranges from 19 to 160 mg ml^{-1}. Examples are Besponsa™ and Ebanga™, which have sucrose concentrations of 45 mg ml^{-1} and 82 mg ml^{-1}, respectively, and Nucala®, has the greatest sugar content at 160 mg ml^{-1} [100]. After reconstitution, trehalose concentrations range from 7.8 to 95 mg ml^{-1}. OgivriTM lyophilized powder contains sorbitol, together with other excipients, in a concentration of 16 mg ml^{-1} following reconstitution [97]. Simulect® is a lyophilized powder that contains mannitol and sucrose with a mannitol concentration of 16 mg ml^{-1} following reconstitution. Lumoxiti™ is a lyophilized powder made up of 33% sucrose and 66% glycine [97].

13.5.5 pH range and buffers

Antibody compositions typically have a pH range of 4.8 to 8.0. Histidine, phosphate, citrate, acetate, succinate, lactic acid, tromethamine, aspartic acid, glutamate and adipic acid are just a few of the buffers utilized to reach the required pH [101]. The pH range with the highest frequency among the formulas evaluated is 6.0–6.9, with 53 products falling within this range. The pH ranges of 5.0–5.9 and 7.0–7.9 are then followed by 44 and 14 items, respectively. A few formulations are also available at pH 4.8 and pH 8.0. The most widely used buffer is histidine, which is used in 49 formulations [102]. Phosphate (22), citrate (20), acetate (14), succinate (4), tromethamine (2), and adipic acid, lactic acid is only used once each [97].

13.5.6 Surfactants

The most widely utilized choices for surfactants in antibody formulations are polysorbate 20 and polysorbate 80. Poloxamer 188 and PEG 3350 are additional surfactants. However, the latter is a polymer rather than a conventional surfactant [97].

13.6 Drug delivery vehicles in targeted antibody therapy

13.6.1 Albumin nanoparticles

Albumin, the most abundant protein in plasma, is widely used as a carrier for drug delivery. Recent research has shown that albumin can effectively bind to various molecules and substances, such as drugs, genes, peptides, vaccines, and antibodies, making it a versatile carrier [103]. mAbs are designed to target overexpressed tumor markers and have been modified by attaching them to albumin nanoparticles. These modified nanoparticles loaded with drugs have been successfully taken up by breast cancer cells and released the drug payload [104]. In the normal human serum, IgG-albumin complexes naturally form through disulfide linking. These complexes have been found to accumulate in solid tumors due to the enhanced permeability and retention (EPR) effect, potentially enhancing the process of cellular uptake [105]. Human serum albumin possesses a free cysteine residue, enabling the formation of heterodimers between PEGylated antibodies and albumin [106]. Oxidative stress in tumors facilitates the formation of disulfide bonds, which can be safely cleaved in endosomes [106]. Researchers have fused an albumin-binding domain to an anti-HER2 nanobody, resulting in its internalization into cells and improved efficacy against tumors *in vivo*. The relevance of albumin to the EPR effect suggests its significance in drug delivery [105].

13.6.2 Liposomes

Based on developments in antibody/protein engineering and targeted liposome design, targeted liposomes are prospective therapeutic agents for the treatment of cancer. The targeting moiety, which is commonly an antibody, should be attached to the free termini of PEGylated lipids in the ideal arrangement [107]. Successful *in vivo* targeting is influenced by density, PEG chain length, and surface charge. Although cationic liposomes may be useful for gene therapy due to their ability to connect with endosomal membranes, they could also result in unfavourable immunological reactions [108]. Target cell populations are favoured by zwitterionic liposomes' decreased interactions in circulation. The ideal PEG chain length and density are found empirically. PEGylation impacts how liposomes interact with proteins and cells.

At tumor sites, targeted liposomes interact more frequently with target cells and promote fusion or internalization. There is no comprehensive comparison of the possible non-uniform spatial distribution inside solid tumors. Recombinant proteins are used for mass synthesis, and advances in antibody and, protein engineering help to target moieties. Targeted liposomes have been utilized to deliver gene expression modifiers for both gene therapy and diagnostic imaging [109]. While radionuclide, chemo-, and radio-sensitizer delivery applications are emerging, the majority of investigations focus on chemotherapy delivery. In the future, multifunctional liposomes with stacked functionalities might be used. Preclinical studies show the adaptability and potential of tailored liposomes in cancer detection and therapy, however clinical research is still in the early phases of development [110].

13.6.3 Nanocarriers

Nanocarrier-driven targeted intracellular delivery offers several advantages, including systemic delivery of a large cargo amount with reduced side effects, lower off-target organ toxicity, sustained release, and protection against premature degradation. Nanocarriers can be easily decorated with functional moieties for cell targeting without compromising reactivity. They can be designed to respond to stimuli such as temperature, enzymes, pH, light, or combinations thereof, enabling controlled payload release. Examples of nanocarriers include inorganic nanoparticles, polymersomes, liposome-based nanocarriers, modified viral particles, and virus-like particles. These nanocarriers have shown promising results for intracellular antibody delivery [111].

13.7. Clinical trials of antibody-targeted drugs

Clinical trials are essential for the advancement of medical research and the development of new treatments in many different fields. In recent years, the focus on antibody-targeted drugs, or monoclonal antibodies, has been particularly important in clinical trials, including cancer, mental illness, respiratory disease and influenza. By delaying the onset of disease, enhancing immune responses and targeting therapeutic molecules, these drugs have revolutionized medicine. These drugs bind selectively to certain disease-related proteins or receptors. Clinical trials investigating tumors in the breast, lung, colon and other organs have shown promise for antibody-targeted drugs. These trials test whether the treatment is effective in reducing side effects, improving patient outcomes and reducing cancer progression. The trials will highlight specific receptors or proteins associated with mental disorders such as schizophrenia and explore the use of antibody-targeted drugs to regulate psychopathology. People with mental health problems can see a positive change in their lives as a result of this method. The effectiveness and safety of the treatment of influenza and respiratory infections have also been evaluated in clinical trials. These studies are necessary to determine the effectiveness of treatment, the safety of vaccinations and their general characteristics. They also provide important information on better disease control and prevention methods. Complete information about these clinical trials can be found at ClinicalTrials.gov (https://www.clinicaltrials.gov), a comprehensive resource for obtaining trial data and researching ongoing research projects. Some of the antibody-targeted drugs which have passed the clinical trials are listed in (table 13.2).

13.8. Commercial aspects of antibody-based drug delivery

The development of antibody-based drug delivery systems has revolutionized the field of medicine by providing targeted and effective therapies for various diseases, including cancer. Monoclonal antibodies (mAbs) and antibody–drug conjugates (ADCs) have emerged as powerful tools in the realm of commercial antibody-based drug delivery. These innovative approaches combine the specificity of mAbs with the cytotoxic potential of drugs, allowing for precise targeting and delivery of therapeutic payloads to disease-associated cells or tissues [4].

13.8.1 Gemtuzumab ozogamicin

The first FDA-approved ADC, Gemtuzumab ozogamicin Mylotarg® (https://mylotarg.pfizerpro.com/), faced initial challenges but was later reapproved with improved dosing regimens and safety profiles [112]. It utilizes a calicheamicin-derived payload, known for its potent anti-tumor activity through the generation of DNA double-strand breaks [113]. The conjugation chemistry of Mylotarg® involves an amide bond between the antibody and a linker-payload, forming an acyl hydrazone linkage with the payload [114]. The ADC's acid-cleavable hydrazone

Table 13.2. Clinical trials of antibody-targeted drugs.

Product name OR Active Ingredient	Condition or disease	Intervention/ treatment	Phase	Identifier	Sponsor
Sym004 in SCCHN patients failing Anti-EGFR based therapy	Carcinoma, squamous cell of head and neck	Sym004 will be administered at the dose of 12 milligram per kilogram (mg kg^{-1}) as an intravenous infusion every week up to disease progression or withdrawal from treatment.	Phase 2	NCT01417936	Symphogen A/S
Chemotherapy and Lapatinib or Trastuzumab	HER2/Neu-positive metastatic breast cancer	Drug: docetaxel 75 mg m^{-2} IV q 3 weekly, day 1 of a 3-week cycle for 8 cycles plus G-CSF (when given together with lapatinib). Drug: lapatinib ditosylate 1250 mg po daily (while given with taxane). 1500 mg PO daily (when given alone after taxane completion). Drug: paclitaxel 80 mg m^{-2} IV q weekly days 1, 8 and 15 of a 4-week cycle for 6 cycles. Biological: trastuzumab IV q weekly (loading dose 4 mg kg^{-1}; subsequent doses 2 mg kg^{-1}) or IV q 3 weekly (loading dose 8 mg kg^{-1}, subsequent doses 6 mg kg^{-1})	Phase 3	NCT00667251	Novartis Pharmaceuticals
Abraxane with or without Tigatuzumab	Breast cancer Triple-negative breast cancer	Drug: Abraxane + Tigatuzumab Tigatuzumab will be administered as a loading dose of 10 mg kg^{-1} on Day 1, then 5 mg kg^{-1} on Day 15 and then every other week on Days 1 and 15 of subsequent cycles. It will be given as an IV	Phase 2	NCT01307891	University of Alabama at Birmingham

(*Continued*)

Table 13.2. (*Continued*)

Product name OR Active Ingredient	Condition or disease	Intervention/ treatment	Phase	Identifier	Sponsor
	Stage IV BREAST CANCER Metastatic breast cancer	infusion over 60 min or less. No dose reductions will be allowed. Tigatuzumab will be administered in combination with the Abraxane according to the intervention described for it. Drug: Abraxane alone 100 mg m^{-2} weekly X 3 doses (days 1, 8, 15) at 28-day intervals until disease progression or unacceptable toxicity. Abraxane will be administered on an outpatient basis by an IV infusion over 30 min. Patients will be evaluated for response every 2 cycles (every 8 weeks).			
Mediplex	a) Colorectal cancer b) Pancreatic cancer c) Metastatic cancer d) Advanced cancer	DURVALUMAB (MEDI4736): therapeutic Class anti-PD-L1 mAb, given IV every 4 weeks at a fixed dose of 1500 mg, AstraZeneca PEXIDARTINIB (PLX3397): therapeutic Class Kinase inhibitor targeting CSF1-R, Flt3 and Kit. Administered daily as split dose regimen, orally. Five dose levels possible in dose escalation part: 400 mg 5 days on 2 days off (intermittent schedule), 400 mg, 600 mg, 800 mg or 1000 mg. In this combination trial, Pexidartinib should be taken first and the Durvalumab IV infusion should be scheduled 1 h after the Pexidartinib morning dose	Phase 1	NCT02777710	Centre Leon Berard

Rovalpituzumab tesirine	Recurrent small cell lung cancer	Rovalpituzumab tesirine will be administered as a single agent, at increasing dose levels as permitted based on real-time assessment of safety and tolerability, intravenously over 30 min. Doses will be repeated on day 1 of each 21-day or 42-day cycle until either unacceptable toxicity or evidence of disease progression occurs.	Phase 1 Phase 2	NCT01901653	Stemcentrx
RO6958688	Solid tumors	Drug: RO6958688 RO6958688 is given as an intravenous (IV) infusion as a single administration in Part I, and QW, Q3W, or as a combined QW/Q3W step up dosing regimen (cycle = 7 days in the QW regimen and cycle = 21 days in the Q3W regimen) in Part II of the study. Drug: Tocilizumab Tocilizumab will be administered as an IV infusion as necessary to treat adverse events. Drug: Obinutuzumab Obinutuzumab is given as an IV infusion at a dose level of 2000 mg on Day −13 or 1000 mg on Days −13 and −12 prior to the treatment start with RO6958688 on Cycle 1 Day 1	Phase 1	NCT02324257	Hoffmann-La Roche
Olaratumab	Prostate cancer	Biological: Olaratumab 15 milligrams per kilogram (mg kg^{-1}) intravenous (IV) Days 1 and 8 Drug: Mitoxantrone	Phase 2	NCT01204710	Eli Lilly and Company

(Continued)

Table 13.2. (*Continued*)

Product name OR Active Ingredient	Condition or disease	Intervention/ treatment	Phase	Identifier	Sponsor
		Mitoxantrone 12 milligrams per square meter (mg m^{-2}) IV Day 1. Mitoxantrone is to be administered for up to 12 cycles (total cumulative dose of mitoxantrone is restricted to $\leqslant$144 mg $m^{-1\ 2}$) Drug: Prednisone 5 mg orally (PO) twice daily (BID) on each day			
DS-8201a	HER2-expressing breast cancer	DS-8201a is supplied as a lyophilized powder which is reconstituted for infusion	Phase 1	Daiichi Sankyo Co., Ltd	NCT03366428
Atezolizumab	Non-small cell lung cancer	Drug: Atezolizumab (MPDL3280A) [TECENTRIQ], an engineered anti-PDL1 antibody Atezolizumab 1200 mg IV on Day 1 of each 21-day cycle until disease progression.	Phase 2	Genentech, Inc.	NCT01846416
Tocilizumab	Schizophrenia	Therapeutic/Pharmacologic Class of Drug: Tocilizumab is a recombinant humanized anti-human interleukin-6 (IL-6) receptor monoclonal antibody of the immunoglobulin (Ig) gamma-1 subclass. Type of Dosage Form: Concentrate for solution for infusion. Route of Administration: Intravenous (i.v.) infusion.	Phase 1	Brian Miller	NCT01696929

Pembrolizumab	Neuroendocrine tumors	Drug: Pembrolizumab Pembrolizumab given intravenously at a fixed dose of 200 mg every 3 weeks	Phase 2	Fox Chase Cancer Center	NCT02939651
Anti-EGFR immunoliposomes	Solid tumors	Drug: anti-EGFR immunoliposomes loaded with doxorubicin All patients were treated with anti-EGFR immunoliposomes Different dose levels (5, 10, 20, 30, 40, 50 and 60 mg doxorubicin m^{-2}), at least 3 patients per dose level, treatment was given every 4 weeks	Phase 1	University Hospital, Basel, Switzerland	NCT01702129
2017 A/H7N9 IIV revaccination	Avian influenza Influenza immunisation	Biological: A/H7N9 Monovalent split 2017 A/H7N9 Inactivated Influenza Virus Vaccine containing the Hemagglutinin (HA) and Neuraminidase (NA) from low pathogenic avian influenza A/Hong Kong/125/2017 (H7N9) and the PB2, PB1, PA, NP, M and NS from A/Puerto Rico/8/1934 (H1N1). The HA content of the 2017 A/H7N9 vaccine formulations were determined by Single Radial Immunodiffusion (SRID) assay to be approximately two times higher (14.45 mcg of HA per 0.5 ml dose) than the targeted HA content on the label (7.5 mcg of HA per 0.5 ml dose). Drug: AS03 AS03 oil-in-water emulsion-based adjuvant system containing DL-alpha-tocopherol, squalene, polysorbate 80, and a buffer.	Phase 2	National Institute of Allergy and Infectious Diseases (NIAID)	NCT03738241

(*Continued*)

Table 13.2. (*Continued*)

Product name OR Active Ingredient	Condition or disease	Intervention/ treatment	Phase	Identifier	Sponsor
AVE0005 (VEGF trap)	a) Pulmonary diseases b) Neoplasms, lung	Drug: Aflibercept (ziv-aflibercept, AVE0005, VEGF trap, ZALTRAP®) Aflibercept 4.0 mg kg^{-1} administered intravenously (IV) over a period of at least 1 h once every 2 weeks. Aflibercept could be reduced by 1 dose level (to 3.0 mg kg^{-1}) or 2 dose levels (to 2.0 mg kg^{-1}) in case of uncontrolled hypertension or urinary protein >3.5 g 24 h^{-1}. Intrapatient dose escalation was not to be permitted. Participants requiring more than 2 dose level reductions would be withdrawn from study treatment.	Phase 2	Sanofi	NCT00284141
IMMU-132	Epithelial cancer	Drug: Sacituzumab Govitecan-hziy (SG) Administered via intravenous (IV) infusion	Phase 1 Phase 2	Gilead Sciences	NCT01631552

linker allows for selective release of the payload within target cells. Mylotarg® in the realm of acute myeloid leukemia, Mylotarg has emerged as a significant milestone in antibody-based drug delivery. Through its specific targeting of CD33, a protein expressed on leukemic cells, Mylotarg delivers a potent cytotoxic agent directly to the cancer cells, augmenting the therapeutic outcome while minimizing off-target toxicity [114].

13.8.2 Inotuzumab ozogamicin

Inotuzumab ozogamicin, marketed as Besponsa®, has obtained FDA approval ADC (https://besponsa.pfizerpro.com/). Inotuzumab ozogamicin (CMC-544) targets CD22, a cell surface antigen found in the majority of B-cell acute lymphoblastic leukemia (B-ALL). It consists of a humanized monoclonal antibody linked to a cytotoxic N-acetyl-γ-calicheamicin with an average drug-to-antibody ratio (DAR) of 5–7 [115, 116]. Clinical studies have shown that inotuzumab ozogamicin leads to a higher rate of complete remission (CR) in relapsed or refractory B-ALL patients compared to alternative chemotherapy regimens. The most common adverse events include neutropenia, thrombocytopenia, leukopenia, and febrile neutropenia. In August 2017, Besponsa® (inotuzumab ozogamicin) became the first and only CD22-directed ADC approved by the FDA for the treatment of adults with relapsed or refractory B-cell precursor ALL [117]. Besponsa exemplifies the transformative potential of antibody-based drug delivery in hematological malignancies. This ADC has gained approval for the treatment of relapsed or refractory B-cell acute lymphoblastic leukemia. By selectively binding to CD22, a protein expressed on B-cells, Besponsa facilitates the targeted delivery of a cytotoxic payload, offering a lifeline to patients with limited treatment options [115].

13.8.3 Brentuximab vedotin

Brentuximab vedotin, commercially known as Adcetris®, has received FDA approval as a remarkable drug (https://www.adcetris.com) developed by Seagen. Brentuximab vedotin (SGN-35) is an antibody–drug conjugate (ADC) approved by the FDA in 2011 for the treatment of relapsed or refractory CD30-positive Hodgkin lymphoma (HL) and systemic anaplastic large cell lymphoma (sALCL). It consists of a chimeric monoclonal antibody that targets CD30, a dipeptide-based linker, and the cytotoxic agent MMAE. The ADC is internalized into cancer cells via CD30 binding and undergoes linker hydrolysis to release MMAE, which inhibits tubulin polymerization, leading to cell cycle arrest and apoptosis [118]. Brentuximab vedotin has demonstrated high response rates in clinical trials, leading to its accelerated approval for HL and sALCL. It has also received additional approvals for primary cutaneous anaplastic large cell lymphoma (pcALCL), mycosis fungoides (MF), certain types of peripheral T-cell lymphoma (PTCL), and previously untreated stage III or IV classical Hodgkin lymphoma (cHL). The common adverse events include neutropenia, peripheral sensory neuropathy, thrombocytopenia, and anemia [119].

13.8.4 Ado-trastuzumab emtansine

Kadcyla® (Ado-trastuzumab emtansine) stands as an FDA-approved medication (https://www.kadcyla.com/) innovatively developed by Roche, a renowned pharmaceutical company. Ado-trastuzumab emtansine (T-DM1) is an antibody–drug conjugate used to target HER2-positive breast cancer. It consists of an antibody linked to a potent cytotoxic agent. T-DM1 releases the drug inside cancer cells, inhibiting HER2 signalling and inducing cell death. It received FDA approval in 2013 for metastatic breast cancer patients who had previously received trastuzumab and taxane chemotherapy. It showed improved survival compared to other treatments. In 2019, it received approval for adjuvant treatment of early breast cancer patients with residual disease after neoadjuvant treatment [120, 121].

13.8.5 Polatuzumab vedotin

Polatuzumab vedotin, commercially known as Polivy®, has attained FDA approval as a notable ADC, developed by Roche (https://www.polivy.com/newly-diagnosed/rchp.html). Polatuzumab vedotin is used for the treatment of relapsed or refractory diffuse large B-cell lymphoma (DLBCL). It consists of a humanized antibody targeting CD79b, a protein expressed on B-cell non-Hodgkin lymphomas, linked to a microtubule-disrupting agent called MMAE. The linker used in Polivy is protease-cleavable, allowing for the release of MMAE inside the cancer cells. In combination with bendamustine and rituximab, Polivy has shown positive results in a phase Ib/II study [122]. Patients treated with Polivy combination therapy had higher complete response rates and longer response durations compared to those treated with bendamustine and rituximab alone. Common grade 3–4 adverse events observed with Polivy combination therapy include neutropenia, thrombocytopenia, anemia, lymphopenia, and febrile neutropenia. The FDA approved Polivy in July 2019 as the first antibody–drug conjugate for the treatment of DLBCL.

13.8.6 Moxetumomab pasudotox

Moxetumomab pasudotox, marketed as Lumoxiti®, is a drug developed by AstraZeneca (https://www.lumoxiti.com/). It is specifically used in the treatment of hairy cell leukemia (HCL), a rare type of blood cancer characterized by the accumulation of abnormal B lymphocytes. CD22, a protein expressed on B-cells, is targeted for the treatment of HCL. Moxetumomab pasudotox is an antibody–drug conjugate used in HCL treatment. It consists of moxetumomab, which targets CD22, linked to a fragment of Pseudomonas exotoxin A [123]. When moxetumomab pasudotox binds to CD22, it enters the cancer cells and releases a toxin that inhibits protein translation, leading to apoptosis. A phase 3 clinical study enrolled HCL patients who had received prior treatment with at least two systemic therapies. The study evaluated moxetumomab pasudotox monotherapy. The overall response rate (ORR) was 75%, with a complete response (CR) rate of 41%. The durable complete response rate was 30%. Common grade 3–4 adverse events included decreased lymphocyte count, anemia, and asymptomatic hypophosphatemia.

In September 2018, the FDA approved Lumoxiti® (moxetumomab pasudotox) for the treatment of relapsed or refractory HCL in patients who had previously received at least two systemic therapies [124]. This approval marked a significant milestone in HCL treatment, as it was the first new drug approved for HCL in the past 20 years.

13.8.7 Loncastuximab tesirine-lpyl

Zynlonta® (loncastuximab tesirine-lpyl), developed by ADC Therapeutics (https://www.zynlonta.com/) it is specifically designed for the treatment of relapsed or refractory large B-cell lymphoma. It targets CD19 and received accelerated approval from the FDA in April 2021.Zynlonta® consists of a humanized monoclonal antibody (IgG1κ) linked to a cytotoxic pyrrolobenzodiazepine (PBD) dimer alkylating agent called SG3199 through a protease-cleavable valine-alanine linker. SG3199 is highly potent and selectively alkylates the minor groove of DNA, inhibiting nucleic acid synthesis. The connection between the linker and SG3199 occurs at the N10 position of the PBD, forming a carbamate moiety. When Zynlonta® binds to CD19 on cancer cells, the linker-payload connection undergoes a spontaneous 1,6-elimination, releasing the active drug. Each antibody has an average of 2.3 linker-payload molecules attached, and a pegylated spacer is used to enhance stability. Zynlonta® represents a significant advancement in ADC therapy, as it utilizes the highly cytotoxic SG3199, making it the most potent payload used in a marketed ADC to date [125].

13.8.8 Sacituzumab govitecan-hziy

Sacituzumab govitecan-hziy, marketed as Trodelvy®, is an FDA-approved ADC developed by Immunomedics (https://www.trodelvy.com/). It received accelerated FDA approval in 2020 for the treatment of metastatic triple-negative breast cancer (mTNBC) and later gained additional approvals for locally advanced or metastatic urothelial cancer [126]. Trodelvy® combines a humanized antibody targeting TROP2 with SN-38, an active cancer-fighting drug [127, 128]. It has a high drug-to-antibody ratio and delivers SN-38 more effectively than the standard drug irinotecan [129]. Trodelvy® has demonstrated commercial success and an improved toxicity profile compared to irinotecan, making it a promising ADC in the field.

13.8.9 Belantamab mafodotin-blmf

Belantamab mafodotin-blmf, marketed as Blenrep®, is an ADC developed by GlaxoSmithKline (GSK) (https://www.gsk.com/en-gb/media/press-releases/gsk-provides-update-on-blenrep-us-marketing-authorisation/). It stands as the first FDA-approved anti-BCMA (B-cell maturation antigen) therapy, receiving accelerated approval in 2020 for the treatment of relapsed or refractory multiple myeloma. Blenrep® combines a humanized antibody targeting BCMA with the tubulin inhibitor MMAF. It uses a non-cleavable linker and an afucosylated Fc-engineered antibody to enhance ADCC activity. Blenrep® has high specificity for target cells and requires high levels of BCMA expression for effectiveness [130].

13.8.10 Cetuximab sarotalocan

Cetuximab sarotalocan, marketed as Akalux® and also referred to as RM-1929, is a highly innovative ADC developed by Rakuten Medical (https://www.adcreview.com/tag/akalux-iv-infusion-250mg/). This cutting-edge ADC integrates the anti-EGFR antibody cetuximab with the potent photosensitizing dye IRDye®700DX [131]. It targets EGFR, which is highly expressed in various solid tumors. Cetuximab sarotalocan utilizes a red laser to activate the photosensitizing dye and induce cell death in cancer cells while sparing normal tissues. It received approval in Japan for the treatment of unresectable locally advanced or recurrent head and neck squamous cell carcinoma (HNSCC) based on positive results from a phase 2a trial. The treatment showed an overall response rate (ORR) of 28%, including a complete response (CR) rate of 14%. The most common grade ⩾3 adverse events included skin reactions, paronychial cracking, and allergic reactions. Cetuximab sarotalocan is currently undergoing a global Phase 3 trial and has not been approved outside of Japan [132].

13.9. Potential developing trends

13.9.1 Data mining—NGS

NGS is a DNA sequencing method that has transformed the science of genomics. NGS enables the simultaneous sequencing of millions of tiny pieces of DNA, resulting in tremendous data depth and accuracy [133]. It can sequence complete genomes as well as specific areas of interest, such as all 22 000 coding genes or a small number of individual genes. By mapping individual reads to the human reference genome, bioinformatics methods are employed to put together these fragments (figure 13.3). NGS has significantly boosted the speed and efficiency of DNA sequencing, allowing a full human genome to be sequenced in a single day, compared to nearly a decade with older methods such as Sanger sequencing [136].

NGS technique has transformed genomic research by allowing the sequencing of a full human genome in a single day. NGS platforms employ various sequencing methods to simultaneously sequence millions of tiny DNA fragments, which are subsequently stitched together by bioinformatics analysis. NGS may be used to sequence complete genomes or specific regions of interest, including all 22 000 coding genes or a subset of a few genes. The great depth of sequencing gives reliable data and insights on unexpected DNA variation. Despite its success in genome research, next-generation sequencing (NGS) has yet to be translated into routine clinical practice [137].

13.9.1.1 Applications of NGS

a. NGS-based antibody discovery using illumina's cluster mapping capabilities

Due to the short read length of NGS, reconstructing entire antibody sequences is difficult, especially if the CDRs are randomized. The scientists employed Illumina's cluster mapping capabilities to couple non-overlapping reads to rebuild entire Fab sequences with precise V_L:V_H pairings to overcome this problem (figure 13.4). Their technique is based on *in silico* cluster coordinate information, making it simple to

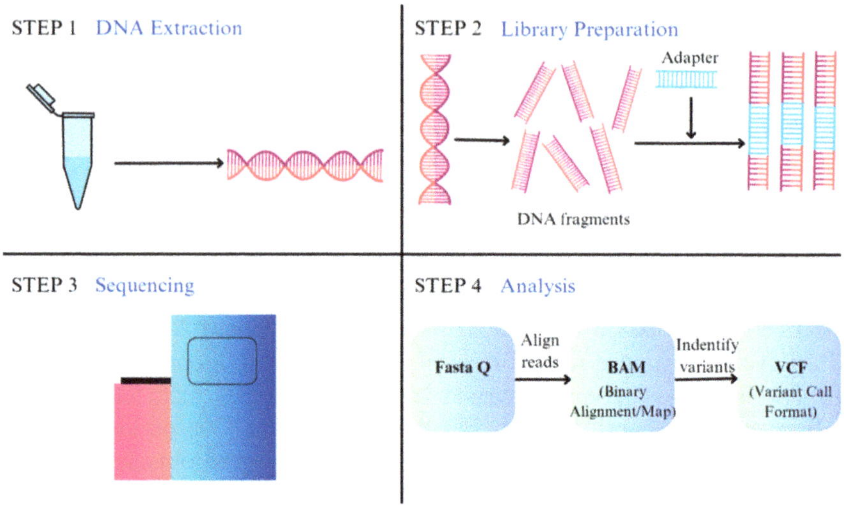

Figure 13.3. A schematic representation of the NGS workflow: extraction, library preparation, sequencing, and analysis. Step 1: Extraction isolates DNA/RNA from the sample. Step 2: Library preparation fragments and ligates the DNA/RNA, adding adapters for sequencing. Step 3: Sequencing employs NGS technologies to sequence the library. Step 4: FASTA files contain DNA or protein sequences, Q files store base quality scores, BAM files store aligned reads, and VCF files capture genetic variant information.

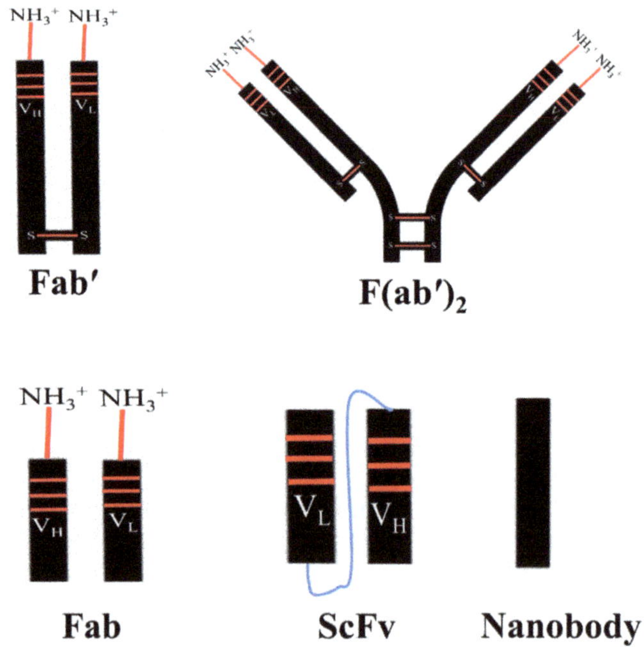

Figure 13.4. Examples of antibody derived fragment technologies and next-generation antibodies.

implement and less susceptible to PCR-derived mistakes. This strategy preserves the throughput required for antibody discovery campaigns while also enhancing NGS-driven analysis of naive and immune libraries [134].

b. NGS for screening clones from phage display libraries

NGS might be used to screen clones from a library for a higher number of clones than traditional approaches during bio-panning, a procedure utilized in phage display technology to find binding molecules. The researchers looked at three chicken immunological scFv libraries that had been bio-panned on prostate-specific antigen (PSA). The heavy chain complementarity-determining region 3 (HCDR3) sequences of the scFv clones were analyzed using NGS. The scFv clones returned by NGS analysis included all of the clones identified by the traditional colony screening approach, as well as many more. The enrichment of the HCDR3 sequence throughout the bio-panning process was a favorable predictor of PSA-reactive scFv clone selection (figure 13.4) [135].

13.9.2 Alternative antibody formats—nanobodies

Nanobodies, also known as variable domains of heavy chain-only antibodies (VHHs), are tiny antibody fragments obtained from camelid (camels, llamas, and alpacas) heavy-chain-only antibodies. They are approximately one-tenth the size of a standard antibody and are made up of a single monomeric variable domain that can identify and bind to a specific antigen [136]. Nanobodies have various benefits over traditional antibodies due to their tiny size and unique binding capabilities, including better tissue penetration, stability, and manufacturability. They are being researched as possible treatments for a variety of ailments, including cancer, viral infections, and inflammatory disorders (figure 13.4).

13.9.2.1 Nanobody databases

a. Integrated nanobody database for immunoinformatics (INDI)

INDI is a comprehensive nanobodies database that incorporates sequence and structure data from a variety of public sources, including patents, GenBank, next-generation sequencing repositories, structures, and scientific publications. It now has access to over 11 million nanobody sequences and excellent nanobody-specific sequence and text search capabilities [137]. The goal of INDI is to speed the discovery and development of nanobody-based treatments by facilitating the creation of innovative nanobody-specific computational techniques. This database improves on prior efforts in nanobody data gathering, which featured a small quantity of publicly available nanobody data and were focused on manual antibody identification. INDI's automated technique enables it to keep up with the ever-increasing volume of publicly available biological sequencing data [138].

b. The single-domain antibody database (sdAb-DB)

sdAb-DB is a free, open-source database that contains curated data on single-domain antibodies (sdAbs) from diverse sources such as protein databases, research articles, and user contributions. It is intended to serve as a community platform for sdAb researchers and synthetic biologists to exchange data, access performance data, and create new sdAbs and proteins using basic bioinformatic techniques. The sdAb-DB is the first of its type, with the goal of becoming a reference resource for the scientific community. Other high-affinity, single-domain binders can be added to the framework. Feedback and recommendations for the database's future growth are welcome using the website's 'Contact us' form [43].

c. Institute collection and analysis of nanobodies (iCAN)

iCAN is the world's first comprehensive database of nanobodies, with the goal of providing searchable, consistent annotation, and integrated analysis tools to academic and industry researchers alike. It comprises 2391 entries, including 74 nanobodies from the RCSB PDB, 156 nanobodies from EMBL, and 2131 nanobodies from patents, as well as information about the parent organism's nanobody sequence, structure, target antigens, function, and taxonomy. For sequence analysis and distinctive feature extraction, iCAN additionally includes online bioinformatic tools such as Blast, Clustal Omega, Motif extraction, and CDR prediction tool. It will help the scientific and industrial communities analyze nanobody properties and discover new uses for them [139].

13.9.2.2 Applications of nanobodies

Nanobodies are tiny, stable, and simple to make, making them a possible future treatment approach for COVID-19 and maybe other developing coronaviruses. The possible application of nanobodies in COVID-19 diagnostics also warrants further investigation [140]. Nanobodies can be coupled with diagnostic agents for targeted tumor imaging as well as anti-tumor medications to improve treatment efficacy and decrease side effects. To increase therapeutic targeting to particular malignancies, nanobodies can also be painted on nanodrug delivery devices [141]. Chromobodies are fluorescent, antigen-binding nanobodies created by fusing the epitope-recognizing portion of heavy-chain antibodies from Camelidae sp. with fluorescent proteins. Throughout S phase and mitosis, chromobodies can recognize and trace antigens in various subcellular compartments, potentially enabling new functional studies. According to the scientists, chromobodies have the ability to target and track any antigenic structure in live cells, making them valuable for a variety of applications [142]. They can target previously inaccessible antigens in cancer immunotherapy due to their small size, improved solubility, and stability.

Nanobodies outperform traditional antibodies and are expected to have a large influence on the antibody reagent industry. Nanobodies offer enormous promise for application in next-generation diagnostics and therapeutic tools, according to preliminary studies on functional heavy chain antibodies in alpaca. Further investigation of their potential may lead to their use as medications in regular clinical practice [143]. Anti-tumor effectiveness of nanobodies and nanobody-based heavy chain antibodies has been demonstrated in multiple preclinical investigations. They have good biodistribution and tissue penetration and may be combined with human immunoglobulin to generate highly soluble and versatile antibodies. They can also be coupled to other chemical moieties for optimal tumor cell targeting.

Before nanobody-based anticancer treatments may be used, further preclinical and clinical research is required. Nanobodies might possibly be employed to designate tumor cells for assault by T and NK cells [144].

13.10 Pharmacokinetic limitations and formulation challenges

Therapeutic proteins such as mAbs often have short *in vivo* half-lives, limiting their efficacy and resulting in frequent dosing and higher costs. Additionally, their large size limits their ability to penetrate and accumulate in tissues, making delivery to target tissues challenging. Most biotherapeutics are transported via the lymphatic system rather than through blood capillaries. Subcutaneous administration is a desired route of administration, but macromolecules are likely to be restricted to the interstitial space after injection. The subcutaneous administration of some therapeutic proteins is enabled by the use of permeation enhancers such as recombinant human hyaluronidase. Protein-based drugs, such as mAbs, are susceptible to enzymatic degradation and are often provided parenterally due to the difficulties of oral administration [145]. Even when given parenterally, pre-systemic breakdown by enzymes and immunogenicity might hasten clearance, reducing effectiveness. High dosages of protein-based medicines can also cause quicker elimination, and receptor saturation can affect bioavailability [146]. Furthermore, frequent dosing regimens may be necessary to maintain therapeutic levels, and infusion reactions are a common side effect of parenteral therapy. Because immune responses differ between species, animal models are unreliable predictors of human immunogenicity.

The complicated tertiary structures of biological macromolecules, including mAbs, are maintained through a balance of intra- and intermolecular interactions. Any stimuli that disrupt this equilibrium might cause the structure to alter, resulting in an unstable state and eventual aggregation. Structural change can happen at any point in the manufacturing process, from protein expression through processing and storage. Non-native proteins must be avoided since aggregation can result in non-uniform dosing and undesirable consequences such as the production of neutralizing anti-drug antibodies (NAbs). Producing mAbs in eukaryotic cells is time-consuming and expensive, resulting in high medication costs that limit patient access [147]. Overall, therapeutic protein delivery, such as mAbs, has problems such as short half-life, limited tissue penetration, enzymatic degradation, and immunogenicity. Subcutaneous delivery using permeability enhancers is a possibility, although structural alterations and aggregation must be closely monitored throughout production and storage. Patient access is limited due to the high cost of manufacturing in eukaryotic cells. Future research should concentrate on novel techniques to improving medication delivery and stability.

13.11 Concluding remarks

Computational approaches have emerged as valuable tools in developing antibody-based targeted drug delivery strategies. These methods, including antibody characterization, modeling, folding stability assessment, interface prediction, and

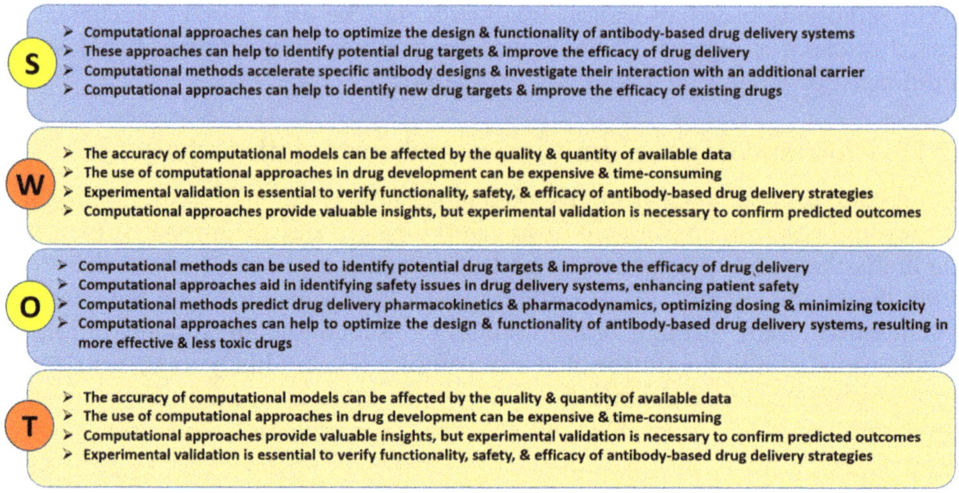

Figure 13.5. Strengths, weaknesses, opportunities and threats (SWOT) analysis of antibody-based targeted drug delivery.

pharmacokinetic clearance prediction, contribute to the design and optimization of therapeutic antibodies as shown in (figure 13.5). By utilizing bioinformatics tools and techniques, researchers can analyze antibody sequences and structures, predict binding interactions with target antigens, optimize folding stability, and assess pharmacokinetic properties. Computational approaches provide valuable insights into the molecular mechanisms underlying antibody–drug interactions and enable the rational design of effective and safe targeted drug delivery systems. OptCDR and OptMAVEn are two computational methods that have shown promise in antibody design and drug discovery. OptCDR utilizes diverse antibody libraries and optimization procedures to generate antibodies with high specificity and affinity for target antigens. While, OptMAVEn, predicts the binding affinity of small molecule ligands to target proteins through molecular docking and virtual screening. These approaches offer a streamlined and efficient way to design antibodies and predict their binding potential, ultimately accelerating the development of therapeutic candidates. Additionally, the AbDesign technique allows for constructing specialized proteins by combining modular pieces from different protein families. This method enables the creation of antibodies and enzymes with high precision and activity, offering further opportunities for targeted drug delivery strategies. Immunogenicity assessment is a critical aspect of therapeutic protein development, as it impacts efficacy and safety. Computational tools such as RANKPEP and NetMHCII aid in predicting T-cell epitopes and MHC-peptide binding affinities, facilitating the assessment of immunogenicity and informing protein therapeutic design. Furthermore, NGS has revolutionized genomics research and holds the potential for advancing antibody discovery and transforming clinical practice. Nanobodies, derived from camelids, offer advantages in various applications and can be explored as part of targeted drug delivery strategies.

Despite the progress made in computational approaches for antibody-based targeted drug delivery challenges remain, including limited half-lives, tissue penetration, and immunogenicity of therapeutic proteins. Future research should focus on improving protein stability, delivery methods, and production techniques to overcome these challenges and enhance the efficacy and safety of targeted drug delivery strategies. In summary, computational approaches serve as valuable tools in the development of antibody-based targeted drug delivery strategies. They enable the design of antibodies with optimized properties, prediction of binding affinity, assessment of immunogenicity, and exploration of novel protein structures. These computational methods, combined with experimental validation, have the potential to revolutionize the field of targeted drug delivery and enhance the development of effective therapeutic interventions. As computational techniques continue to advance, they hold great potential in accelerating the development of novel antibody-based therapeutics for various diseases and improving the efficacy and safety of targeted drug delivery strategies.

Acknowledgments

The authors are thankful to Dr D Y Patil Biotechnology and Bioinformatics Institute, Dr D Y Patil Vidyapeeth, Pune for the physical infrastructure. Sangeeta Ballav is thankful to Dr D Y Patil Vidyapeeth, Pune for Junior Research Fellowship (DPU/291/2021).

Conflict of interest

There are no conflicts of interest.

References

[1] Dowd K A, Mukherjee S, Kuhn R J and Pierson T C 2014 Combined effects of the structural heterogeneity and dynamics of flaviviruses on antibody recognition *J. Virol.* **88** 11726–37

[2] Chailyan A, Marcatili P and Tramontano A 2011 The association of heavy and light chain variable domains in antibodies: implications for antigen specificity *FEBS J.* **278** 2858–66

[3] Kaur H 2021 Characterization of glycosylation in monoclonal antibodies and its importance in therapeutic antibody development *Crit. Rev. Biotechnol.* **41** 300–15

[4] Chen Z, Kankala R K, Yang Z, Li W, Xie S, Li H, Chen A Z and Zou L 2022 Antibody-based drug delivery systems for cancer therapy: mechanisms, challenges, and prospects *Theranostics* **12** 3719–46

[5] Tang Y and Cao Y 2021 Modeling pharmacokinetics and pharmacodynamics of therapeutic antibodies: progress, challenges, and future directions *Pharmaceutics* **13** 422

[6] Wang B, Gallolu Kankanamalage S, Dong J and Liu Y 2021 Optimization of therapeutic antibodies *Antibody Therap.* **4** 45–54

[7] Kim J, McFee M, Fang Q, Abdin O and Kim P M 2023 Computational and artificial intelligence-based methods for antibody development *Trends Pharmacol. Sci.* **44** 175–89

[8] Hie B L, Shanker V R, Xu D, Bruun T U J, Weidenbacher P A, Tang S, Wu W, Pak J E and Kim P S 2023 Efficient evolution of human antibodies from general protein language

models *Nat. Biotechnol.* (Advance online publication) https://doi.org/10.1038/s41587-023-01763-2

[9] Lima W C, Gasteiger E, Marcatili P, Duek P, Bairoch A and Cosson P 2020 The ABCD database: a repository for chemically defined antibodies *Nucleic Acids Res.* **48** D261–4

[10] Björling E and Uhlén M 2008 Antibodypedia, a portal for sharing antibody and antigen validation data *Mol. Cell. Proteomics: MCP* **7** 2028–37

[11] Raybould M I J, Marks C, Lewis A P, Shi J, Bujotzek A, Taddese B and Deane C M 2020 Thera-SAbDab: the therapeutic structural antibody database *Nucleic Acids Res.* **48** D383–8

[12] Gao S H, Huang K, Tu H and Adler A S 2013 Monoclonal antibody humanness score and its applications *BMC Biotech.* **13** 55

[13] Ferdous S and Martin A C R 2018 AbDb: antibody structure database-a database of PDB-derived antibody structures *Database: J. Biol. Databases Curation* **2018** bay040

[14] Dunbar J, Krawczyk K, Leem J, Baker T, Fuchs A, Georges G, Shi J and Deane C M 2014 SAbDab: the structural antibody database *Nucleic Acids Res.* **42** D1140–6

[15] Obrezanova O, Arnell A, de la Cuesta R G, Berthelot M E, Gallagher T R, Zurdo J and Stallwood Y 2015 Aggregation risk prediction for antibodies and its application to biotherapeutic development *mAbs* **7** 352–63

[16] Zhang Y *et al* 2021 RAPID: a Rep-Seq dataset analysis platform with an integrated antibody database *Front. Immunol.* **12** 717496

[17] Lefranc M P 2001 IMGT, the international ImMunoGeneTics database *Nucleic Acids Res.* **29** 207–9

[18] Cuenca A G, Delano M J, Kelly-Scumpia K M, Moreno C, Scumpia P O, Laface D M, Heyworth P G, Efron P A and Moldawer L L 2011 A paradoxical role for myeloid-derived suppressor cells in sepsis and trauma *Mol. Med.* **17** 281–92

[19] Cummins C *et al* 2022 The European nucleotide archive in 2021 *Nucleic Acids Res.* **50** D106–10

[20] NCBI Resource Coordinators 2016 Database resources of the national center for biotechnology information *Nucleic Acids Res.* **44** D7–D19

[21] Kovaltsuk A, Leem J, Kelm S, Snowden J, Deane C M and Krawczyk K 2018 Observed antibody space: a resource for data mining next-generation sequencing of antibody repertoires *J. Immunol.* **201** 2502–9

[22] Peng H P, Lee K H, Jian J W and Yang A S 2014 Origins of specificity and affinity in antibody–protein interactions *PNAS* **111** E2656–65

[23] Retter I, Althaus H H, Münch R and Müller W 2005 VBASE2, an integrative V gene database *Nucleic Acids Res.* **33** D671–4

[24] Marcatili P, Rosi A and Tramontano A 2008 PIGS: automatic prediction of antibody structures *Bioinformatics* **24** 1953–4

[25] Berman H M *et al* 2002 The protein data bank *Acta Crystallogr. Section D, Biol. Crystallogr.* **581** 899–907

[26] Swindells M B, Porter C T, Couch M, Hurst J, Abhinandan K R, Nielsen J H, Macindoe G, Hetherington J and Martin A C 2017 abYsis: integrated antibody sequence and structure-management, analysis, and prediction *J. Mol. Biol.* **429** 356–64

[27] Vita R, Zarebski L, Greenbaum J A, Emami H, Hoof I, Salimi N, Damle R, Sette A and Peters B 2010 The immune epitope database 2.0 *Nucleic Acids Res.* **38** D854–62

[28] Wang R, Fang X, Lu Y, Yang C Y and Wang S 2005 The PDBbind database: methodologies and updates *J. Med. Chem.* **48** 4111–9

[29] Sirin S, Apgar J R, Bennett E M and Keating A E 2016 AB-Bind: antibody binding mutational database for computational affinity predictions *Protein Sci.* **25** 393–409
[30] Moal I H and Fernández-Recio J 2012 SKEMPI: a structural kinetic and energetic database of mutant protein interactions and its use in empirical models *Bioinformatics* **28** 2600–7
[31] Lefranc M P, Pommié C, Ruiz M, Giudicelli V, Foulquier E, Truong L, Thouvenin-Contet V and Lefranc G 2003 IMGT unique numbering for immunoglobulin and T cell receptor variable domains and Ig superfamily V-like domains *Dev. Comp. Immunol.* **27** 55–77
[32] Johnson G and Wu T T 2001 Kabat Database and its applications: future directions *Nucleic Acids Res.* **29** 205–6
[33] Murzin A G, Brenner S E, Hubbard T and Chothia C 1995 SCOP: a structural classification of proteins database for the investigation of sequences and structures *J. Mol. Biol.* **247** 536–40
[34] Benson D A, Cavanaugh M, Clark K, Karsch-Mizrachi I, Ostell J, Pruitt K D and Sayers E W 2018 GenBank *Nucleic Acids Res.* **46** D41–7
[35] UniProt Consortium 2015 UniProt: a hub for protein information *Nucleic Acids Res.* **43** D204–12
[36] Zarin D A, Tse T, Williams R J, Califf R M and Ide N C 2011 The clinicaltrials.gov results database—update and key issues *New Engl. J. Med.* **364** 852–60
[37] Wishart D S *et al* 2018 DrugBank 5.0: a major update to the drugbank database for 2018 *Nucleic Acids Res.* **46** D1074–82
[38] Norman R A, Ambrosetti F, Bonvin A M J J, Colwell L J, Kelm S, Kumar S and Krawczyk K 2020 Computational approaches to therapeutic antibody design: established methods and emerging trends *Briefings. Bioinform.* **21** 1549–67
[39] Bargh J D, Isidro-Llobet A, Parker J S and Spring D R 2019 Cleavable linkers in antibody-drug conjugates *Chem. Soc. Rev.* **48** 4361–74
[40] Chailyan A, Tramontano A and Marcatili P 2012 A database of immunoglobulins with integrated tools: DIGIT *Nucleic Acids Res.* **40** D1230–4
[41] Corrie B D *et al* 2018 iReceptor: a platform for querying and analyzing antibody/B-cell and T-cell receptor repertoire data across federated repositories *Immunolo Rev.* **284** 24–41
[42] Vita R *et al* 2015 The immune epitope database (IEDB) 3.0 *Nucleic Acids Res.* **43** D405–12
[43] Wilton E E, Opyr M P, Kailasam S, Kothe R F and Wieden H J 2018 sdAb-DB: the single domain antibody database *ACS Synth. Biol.* **7** 2480–4
[44] Lu R M, Hwang Y C, Liu I J, Lee C C, Tsai H Z, Li H J and Wu H C 2020 Development of therapeutic antibodies for the treatment of diseases *J. Biomed. Sci.* **27** 1
[45] Sliwoski G, Kothiwale S, Meiler J and Lowe E W 2013 Computational methods in drug discovery *Pharmacol. Rev.* **66** 334–95
[46] Dondelinger M, Filée P, Sauvage E, Quinting B, Muyldermans S, Galleni M and Vandevenne M S 2018 Understanding the significance and implications of antibody numbering and antigen-binding surface/residue definition *Front. Immunol.* **9** 2278
[47] Ye J, Ma N, Madden T L and Ostell J M 2013 IgBLAST: an immunoglobulin variable domain sequence analysis tool *Nucleic Acids Res.* **41** W34–40
[48] Chiu M L, Goulet D R, Teplyakov A and Gilliland G L 2019 Antibody structure and function: the basis for engineering therapeutics *Antibodies (Basel, Switzerland)* **8** 55

[49] Bujotzek A, Dunbar J, Lipsmeier F, Schäfer W, Antes I, Deane C M and Georges G 2015 Prediction of VH-VL domain orientation for antibody variable domain modeling *Proteins* **83** 681–95

[50] Dunbar J, Fuchs A, Shi J and Deane C M 2013 ABangle: characterising the VH-VL orientation in antibodies *Protein Eng. Sel: PEDS* **26** 611–20

[51] Marks C and Deane C M 2017 Antibody H3 structure prediction *Comput. Struct. Biotechnol. J.* **15** 222–31

[52] Marks C, Nowak J, Klostermann S, Georges G, Dunbar J, Shi J, Kelm S and Deane C M 2017 Sphinx: merging knowledge-based and *ab initio* approaches to improve protein loop prediction *Bioinformatics* **33** 1346–53

[53] Leem J, Georges G, Shi J and Deane C M 2018 Antibody side chain conformations are position-dependent *Proteins* **86** 383–92

[54] Weitzner B D, Jeliazkov J R, Lyskov S, Marze N, Kuroda D, Frick R, Adolf-Bryfogle J, Biswas N, Dunbrack R L and Gray J J 2017 Modeling and docking of antibody structures with Rosetta *Nat. Protoc.* **12** 401–16

[55] Krawczyk K, Liu X, Baker T, Shi J and Deane C M 2014 Improving B-cell epitope prediction and its application to global antibody–antigen docking *Bioinformatics* **30** 2288–94

[56] Krawczyk K, Baker T, Shi J and Deane C M 2013 Antibody i-Patch prediction of the antibody binding site improves rigid local antibody–antigen docking *Protein Eng. Des. Sel.: PEDS* **26** 621–9

[57] Raybould M I J, Marks C, Krawczyk K, Taddese B, Nowak J, Lewis A P, Bujotzek A, Shi J and Deane C M 2019 Five computational developability guidelines for therapeutic antibody profiling *PNAS* **116** 4025–30

[58] Le Basle Y, Chennell P, Tokhadze N, Astier A and Sautou V 2020 Physicochemical stability of monoclonal antibodies: a review *J. Pharm. Sci.* **109** 169–90

[59] Perchiacca J M and Tessier P M 2012 Engineering aggregation-resistant antibodies *Ann. Rev. Chem. Biomol. Eng.* **3** 263–86

[60] Lowe D, Dudgeon K, Rouet R, Schofield P, Jermutus L and Christ D 2011 Aggregation, stability, and formulation of human antibody therapeutics *Adv. Protein Chem. Struct. Biol.* **84** 41–61

[61] Rosenberg A S 2006 Effects of protein aggregates: an immunologic perspective *AAPS J.* **8** E501–7

[62] Frokjaer S and Otzen D E 2005 Protein drug stability: a formulation challenge *Nat. Rev. Drug Discov.* **4** 298–306

[63] Stimple S D, Smith M D and Tessier P M 2020 Directed evolution methods for overcoming trade-offs between protein activity and stability *AIChE* J **66** e16814

[64] Rabia L A, Desai A A, Jhajj H S and Tessier P M 2018 Understanding and overcoming trade-offs between antibody affinity, specificity, stability and solubility *Biochem. Eng. J.* **137** 365–74

[65] Warszawski S *et al* 2019 Optimizing antibody affinity and stability by the automated design of the variable light-heavy chain interfaces *PLoS Comput. Biol.* **15** e1007207

[66] Clark M 2000 Antibody humanization: a case of the 'Emperor's new clothes'? *Immunol. Today* **21** 397–402

[67] Choi Y, Hua C, Sentman C L, Ackerman M E and Bailey-Kellogg C 2015 Antibody humanization by structure-based computational protein design *mAbs* **7** 1045–57

[68] Choi Y, Ndong C, Griswold K E and Bailey-Kellogg C 2016 Computationally driven antibody engineering enables simultaneous humanization and thermostabilization *Protein Eng. Des. Sel. : PEDS* **29** 419–26

[69] Kazi A, Chuah C, Majeed A B A, Leow C H, Lim B H and Leow C Y 2018 Current progress of immunoinformatics approach harnessed for cellular- and antibody-dependent vaccine design *Pathog. Glob. Health* **112** 123–31

[70] Kunik V, Peters B and Ofran Y 2012 Structural consensus among antibodies defines the antigen binding site *PLoS Comput. Biol.* **8** e1002388

[71] Kunik V, Ashkenazi S and Ofran Y 2012 Paratome: an online tool for systematic identification of antigen-binding regions in antibodies based on sequence or structure *Nucleic Acids Res.* **40** W521–4

[72] Daberdaku S and Ferrari C 2019 Antibody interface prediction with 3D Zernike descriptors and SVM *Bioinformatics* **35** 1870–6

[73] Zhang W, Xiong Y, Zhao M, Zou H, Ye X and Liu J 2011 Prediction of conformational B-cell epitopes from 3D structures by random forests with a distance-based feature *BMC Bioinf.* **12** 341

[74] Sela-Culang I, Ofran Y and Peters B 2015 Antibody specific epitope prediction-emergence of a new paradigm *Curr. Opin. Virol.* **11** 98–102

[75] Pedotti M, Simonelli L, Livoti E and Varani L 2011 Computational docking of antibody–antigen complexes, opportunities and pitfalls illustrated by influenza hemagglutinin *Int. J. Mol. Sci.* **12** 226–51

[76] Ovacik M and Lin K 2018 Tutorial on monoclonal antibody pharmacokinetics and its considerations in early development *Clin. Trans. Sci.* **11** 540–52

[77] Grinshpun B, Thorsteinson N, Pereira J N, Rippmann F, Nannemann D, Sood V D and Fomekong Nanfack Y 2021 Identifying biophysical assays and in silico properties that enrich for slow clearance in clinical-stage therapeutic antibodies *mAbs* **13** 1932230

[78] Thorsteinson N, Gunn J R, Kelly K, Long W and Labute P 2021 Structure-based charge calculations for predicting isoelectric point, viscosity, clearance, and profiling antibody therapeutics *mAbs* **13** 1981805

[79] Harding F A, Stickler M M, Razo J and DuBridge R B 2010 The immunogenicity of humanized and fully human antibodies: residual immunogenicity resides in the CDR regions *mAbs* **2** 256–65

[80] Entzminger K C *et al* 2017 De novo design of antibody complementarity determining regions binding a FLAG tetra-peptide *Sci. Rep.* **7** 10295

[81] Pantazes R J and Maranas C D 2010 OptCDR: a general computational method for the design of antibody complementarity determining regions for targeted epitope binding *Protein Eng. Des. Sel. : PEDS* **23** 849–58

[82] Torres P H M, Sodero A C R, Jofily P and Silva-Jr F P 2019 Key topics in molecular docking for drug design *Int. J. Mol. Sci.* **20** 4574

[83] Wang L, Liang R, Gao Y, Li Y, Deng X, Xiang R, Zhang Y, Ying T, Jiang S and Yu F 2019 Development of small-molecule inhibitors against Zika virus infection *Front. Microbiol.* **10** 2725

[84] Chowdhury R, Allan M F and Maranas C D 2018 OptMAVEn-2.0: De novo design of variable antibody regions against targeted antigen epitopes *Antibodies* **7** 23

[85] Lipsh-Sokolik R, Listov D and Fleishman S J 2021 The AbDesign computational pipeline for modular backbone assembly and design of binders and enzymes *Protein Sci.* **30** 151–9

[86] Adolf-Bryfogle J, Kalyuzhniy O, Kubitz M, Weitzner B D, Hu X, Adachi Y, Schief W R and Dunbrack R L 2018 RosettaAntibodyDesign (RAbD): a general framework for computational antibody design *PLoS Comput. Biol.* **14** e1006112
[87] De Groot A S, McMurry J and Moise L 2008 Prediction of immunogenicity: in silico paradigms, *ex vivo* and *in vivo* correlates *Curr. Opin. Pharmacol.* **8** 620–6
[88] Reche P A, Glutting J P, Zhang H and Reinherz E L 2004 Enhancement to the RANKPEP resource for the prediction of peptide binding to MHC molecules using profiles *Immunogenetics* **56** 405–19
[89] Jensen K K, Andreatta M, Marcatili P, Buus S, Greenbaum J A, Yan Z, Sette A, Peters B and Nielsen M 2018 Improved methods for predicting peptide binding affinity to MHC class II molecules *Immunology* **154** 394–406
[90] Makowski E K, Wu L, Gupta P and Tessier P M 2021 Discovery-stage identification of drug-like antibodies using emerging experimental and computational methods *mAbs* **13** 1895540
[91] Sankar K, Krystek S R, Carl S M, Day T and Maier J K X 2018 AggScore: prediction of aggregation-prone regions in proteins based on the distribution of surface patches *Proteins* **86** 1147–56
[92] Feng J, Jiang M, Shih J and Chai Q 2022 Antibody apparent solubility prediction from sequence by transfer learning *iScience* **25** 105173
[93] Laptoš T and Omersel J 2018 The importance of handling high-value biologicals: physico-chemical instability and immunogenicity of monoclonal antibodies *Exp. Ther. Med.* **15** 3161–8
[94] Ryman J T and Meibohm B 2017 Pharmacokinetics of monoclonal antibodies *CPT: Pharmacometr. Syst. Pharmacol.* **6** 576–88
[95] Zhang W, Wang H, Feng N, Li Y, Gu J and Wang Z 2022 Developability assessment at early-stage discovery to enable development of antibody-derived therapeutics *Antibody Therap.* **6** 13–29
[96] Alves N J 2019 Antibody conjugation and formulation *Antibody Therap.* **2** 33–9
[97] Strickley R G and Lambert W J 2021 A review of formulations of commercially Available Antibodies *J. Pharm. Sci.* **110** 2590–608
[98] Dani B, Platz R and Tzannis S T 2007 High concentration formulation feasibility of human immunoglubulin G for subcutaneous administration *J. Pharm. Sci.* **96** 1504–17
[99] Oki S, Nishinami S, Nakauchi Y, Ogura T and Shiraki K 2022 Arginine and its derivatives suppress the opalescence of an antibody solution *J. Pharm. Sci.* **111** 1126–32
[100] Snell J R, Kumar N S K, Suryanarayanan R and Randolph T W 2020 Nanobubbles in reconstituted lyophilized formulations: interaction with proteins and mechanism of formation *J. Pharm. Sci.* **109** 284–92
[101] Ghosh I, Gutka H, Krause M E, Clemens R and Kashi R S 2023 A systematic review of commercial high concentration antibody drug products approved in the US: formulation composition, dosage form design and primary packaging considerations *mAbs* **15** 2205540
[102] Martin K P, Grimaldi C, Grempler R, Hansel S and Kumar S 2023 Trends in industrialization of biotherapeutics: a survey of product characteristics of 89 antibody-based biotherapeutics *mAbs* **15** 2191301

[103] Karimi M, Bahrami S, Ravari S B, Zangabad P S, Mirshekari H, Bozorgomid M, Shahreza S, Sori M and Hamblin M R 2016 Albumin nanostructures as advanced drug delivery systems *Expert Opin. Drug Deliv.* **13** 1609–23

[104] Anhorn M G, Wagner S, Kreuter J, Langer K and von Briesen H 2008 Specific targeting of HER2 overexpressing breast cancer cells with doxorubicin-loaded trastuzumab-modified human serum albumin nanoparticles *Bioconjug. Chem.* **19** 2321–31

[105] Tashima T 2022 Delivery of drugs into cancer cells using antibody-drug conjugates based on receptor-mediated endocytosis and the enhanced permeability and retention effect *Antibodies* **11** 78

[106] Kawakami A, Kubota K, Yamada N, Tagami U, Takehana K, Sonaka I, Suzuki E and Hirayama K 2006 Identification and characterization of oxidized human serum albumin. A slight structural change impairs its ligand-binding and antioxidant functions *FEBS J.* **273** 3346–57

[107] Sawant R R and Torchilin V P 2012 Challenges in development of targeted liposomal therapeutics *AAPS J.* **14** 303–15

[108] Liu C, Zhang L, Zhu W, Guo R, Sun H, Chen X and Deng N 2020 Barriers and strategies of cationic liposomes for cancer gene therapy *Mol. Ther. Methods Clin. Dev.* **18** 751–64

[109] Wang S, Chen Y, Guo J and Huang Q 2023 Liposomes for tumor targeted therapy: a review *Int. J. Mol. Sci.* **24** 2643

[110] Sofou S and Sgouros G 2008 Antibody-targeted liposomes in cancer therapy and imaging *Expert Opin. Drug Deliv.* **5** 189–204

[111] Cook N, Hansen A R, Siu L L and Abdul Razak A R 2015 Early phase clinical trials to identify optimal dosing and safety *Mol. Oncol.* **9** 997–1007

[112] Jen E Y *et al* 2018 FDA approval: gemtuzumab ozogamicin for the treatment of adults with newly diagnosed CD33-positive acute myeloid leukemia *Clin. Cancer Res.* **24** 3242–6

[113] Bhattacharya P, Basak A, Campbell A and Alabugin I V 2018 Photochemical activation of enediyne warheads: a potential tool for targeted antitumor therapy *Mol. Pharmaceutics* **15** 768–97

[114] Vollmar B S *et al* 2021 Calicheamicin antibody-drug conjugates with improved properties *Mol. Cancer Ther.* **20** 1112–20

[115] Shah N N, Stevenson M S, Yuan C M, Richards K, Delbrook C, Kreitman R J, Pastan I and Wayne A S 2015 Characterization of CD22 expression in acute lymphoblastic leukemia *Pediatr. Blood Cancer* **62** 964–9

[116] Lanza F, Maffini E, Rondoni M, Massari E, Faini A C and Malavasi F 2020 CD22 Expression in B-Cell acute lymphoblastic leukemia: biological significance and implications for inotuzumab therapy in adults *Cancers* **12** 303

[117] Kantarjian H M *et al* 2016 Inotuzumab ozogamicin versus standard therapy for acute lymphoblastic leukemia *New Engl. J. Med.* **375** 740–53

[118] Katz J, Janik J E and Younes A 2011 Brentuximab vedotin (SGN-35) *Clin. Cancer Res.* **17** 6428–36

[119] Younes A *et al* 2012 Results of a pivotal phase II study of brentuximab vedotin for patients with relapsed or refractory Hodgkin's lymphoma *J. Clin. Oncol.* **30** 2183–9

[120] Wedam S *et al* 2020 FDA approval summary: ado-trastuzumab emtansine for the adjuvant treatment of HER2-positive early breast cancer *Clin. Cancer Res.* **26** 4180–5

[121] Mamounas E P *et al* 2021 Adjuvant T-DM1 versus trastuzumab in patients with residual invasive disease after neoadjuvant therapy for HER2-positive breast cancer: subgroup analyses from Katherine *Annals Oncol.* **32** 1005–14

[122] Sehn L H *et al* 2022 Polatuzumab vedotin plus bendamustine and rituximab in relapsed/refractory DLBCL: survival update and new extension cohort data *Blood Adv.* **6** 533–43

[123] Kreitman R J and Pastan I 2011 Antibody fusion proteins: anti-CD22 recombinant immunotoxin moxetumomab pasudotox *Clin. Cancer Res.* **17** 6398–405

[124] Mullard A 2019 2018 FDA drug approvals *Nat. Rev. Drug Discov.* **18** 85–9

[125] Lee A 2021 Loncastuximab tesirine: first approval *Drugs* **81** 1229–33

[126] Bardia A *et al* 2019 Sacituzumab govitecan-hziy in refractory metastatic triple-negative breast cancer *New Engl. J. Med.* **380** 741–51

[127] Syed Y Y 2020 Sacituzumab govitecan: first approval *Drugs* **80** 1019–25

[128] Cardillo T M, Govindan S V, Sharkey R M, Trisal P and Goldenberg D M 2011 Humanized anti-Trop-2 IgG-SN-38 conjugate for effective treatment of diverse epithelial cancers: preclinical studies in human cancer xenograft models and monkeys *Clin. Cancer Res.* **17** 3157–69

[129] Goldenberg D M, Cardillo T M, Govindan S V, Rossi E A and Sharkey R M 2015 Trop-2 is a novel target for solid cancer therapy with sacituzumab govitecan (IMMU-132), an antibody-drug conjugate (ADC) *Oncotarget* **6** 22496–512

[130] Tong J T W, Harris P W R, Brimble M A and Kavianinia I 2021 An insight into FDA approved antibody-drug conjugates for cancer therapy *Molecules (Basel, Switzerland)* **26** 5847

[131] Li J, Wang R and Gao J 2021 Novel anticancer drugs approved in 2020 *Drug Dis. Ther.* **15** 44–7

[132] Kitamura N, Sento S, Yoshizawa Y, Sasabe E, Kudo Y and Yamamoto T 2020 Current trends and future prospects of molecular targeted therapy in head and neck squamous cell carcinoma *Int. J. Mol. Sci.* **22** 240

[133] Davis T A, Grillo-López A J, White C A, McLaughlin P, Czuczman M S, Link B K, Maloney D G, Weaver R L, Rosenberg J and Levy R 2000 Rituximab anti-CD20 monoclonal antibody therapy in non-Hodgkin's lymphoma: safety and efficacy of re-treatment *J. Clin. Oncol.* **18** 3135–43

[134] Yang Y, Xie B and Yan J 2014 Application of next-generation sequencing technology in forensic science *Genom. Proteom. Bioinf.* **12** 190–7

[135] Gupta N and Verma V K 2019 Next-generation sequencing and its application: empowering in public health beyond reality *Microbial Technology for the Welfare of Society* (Singapore: Springer) Microorganisms for Sustainability vol 17 pp 313–41

[136] Moura-Sampaio J, Faustino A F, Boeuf R, Antunes M A, Ewert S and Batista A P 2022 Reconstruction of full antibody sequences in NGS datasets and accurate VL:VH coupling by cluster coordinate matching of non-overlapping reads *Comput. Struct. Biotechnol. J.* **20** 2723–7

[137] Yang W, Yoon A, Lee S, Kim S, Han J and Chung J 2017 Next-generation sequencing enables the discovery of more diverse positive clones from a phage-displayed antibody library *Exp. Mol. Med.* **49** e308

[138] Bannas P, Hambach J and Koch-Nolte F 2017 Nanobodies and nanobody-based human heavy chain antibodies as antitumor therapeutics *Front. Immunol.* **8** 1603

[139] Deszyński P, Młokosiewicz J, Volanakis A, Jaszczyszyn I, Castellana N, Bonissone S, Ganesan R and Krawczyk K 2022 INDI-integrated nanobody database for immunoinformatics *Nucleic Acids Res.* **50** D1273–81

[140] Zuo J, Li J, Zhang R, Xu L, Chen H, Jia X, Su Z, Zhao L, Huang X and Xie W 2017 Institute collection and analysis of Nanobodies (iCAN): a comprehensive database and analysis platform for nanobodies *BMC Genomics* **18** 797

[141] Ezzikouri S, Nourlil J, Tsukiyama-Kohara K, Kohara M, El Ossmani H, Windisch M P and Benjelloun S 2022 Nanobodies: an unexplored opportunity to combat COVID-19 *J. Biomol. Struct. Dyn.* **40** 3129–31

[142] Liu M, Li L, Jin D and Liu Y 2021 Nanobody—a versatile tool for cancer diagnosis and therapeutics *Wiley Interdiscip. Rev. Nanomed. Nanobiotechnol.* **13** e1697

[143] Rothbauer U *et al* 2006 Targeting and tracing antigens in live cells with fluorescent nanobodies *Nat. Methods* **3** 887–9

[144] Sun S *et al* 2021 Nanobody: a small antibody with big implications for tumor therapeutic strategy *Int. J. Nanomed.* **16** 2337–56

[145] Bruno B J, Miller G D and Lim C S 2013 Basics and recent advances in peptide and protein drug delivery *Ther. Deliv.* **4** 1443–67

[146] Liu L 2018 Pharmacokinetics of monoclonal antibodies and Fc-fusion proteins *Protein Cell* **9** 15–32

[147] Awwad S and Angkawinitwong U 2018 Overview of antibody drug delivery *Pharmaceutics* **10** 83

IOP Publishing

Advances in Drug Delivery Systems for Healthcare
From concept to clinic
Piyush Pradeep Mehta and Arpana Parihar

Chapter 14

Medical electronics—future trends and market potential

Kalpesh V Bhavsar, Maargavi Singh, Manav Shirodkar and Mikhail Vora

This chapter looks at the evolving discipline of medical electronics and how it might affect healthcare. It offers a thorough review of the current and most recent developments in medical technology and its business potential. It addresses the possible uses of cutting-edge technologies in healthcare, including wearable technology, telemedicine options, artificial intelligence, and robotics, providing improved patient outcomes through personalized therapies and increased diagnostics efficiency and accuracy. It examines market trends, growth factors, industry player problems, and business potential. The chapter also clarifies the standards and regulatory environment that govern medical electronics, assuring the protection of patients and product efficacy. To fully realize the potential of medical electronics in altering healthcare delivery, it emphasizes the need for ongoing innovation, a partnership between innovators in technology and medical professionals, and funding for research and development. The chapter comes to a close with a glance toward the future of medical electronics.

14.1 Introduction

The modern strategies and methods of study that use electronics are capturing the interest of research scientists working in the vast field of the biological sciences. Conversely, the electronics expert is discovering that live things have a variety of engineering systems that, if comprehended, could be helpful in the advancement of man-made electrical components. Diagnoses have been made using x-rays ever since Röntgen first discovered them in 1895. De Forest created a triode vacuum tube in 1907 to enhance heartbeat and central nervous system impulses [1]. In the 1940s, electroconvulsive treatment (ECT) was attempted to lessen the impact of several psychiatric illnesses. During the 1960s, electrical stimulation of the heart was being used, first in defibrillators to revive or resynchronize a dysfunctional heart and then

doi:10.1088/978-0-7503-5613-8ch14

in miniature pacemakers which could be worn over time to avoid actual injury to the heart's structural components [2]. One of the key developments in the field of medical imaging has been the use of computerized tomography in 1972, which has made it feasible to see inside components in a way that was previously inconceivable. Ultrasound is another method that has changed the medical industry. The development of those devices served as a basis for the incorporation of electronics into medical applications.

A rising understanding of the need for medical structures that are more effective and patient-centered has emerged in recent years. The weight of chronic diseases, limited access to medical services, and rising expenses have all been problems for the conventional medical model. By utilizing innovations in technology, medical electronics have the potential to improve healthcare delivery and address these issues significantly. Medical electronics, a discipline that includes a wide range of technologies to enhance patient care and revolutionize the healthcare sector, emerged due to the fusion of electronics and healthcare. With its multidisciplinary nature, medical electronics is emerging as a crucial enabler in tackling these issues and providing cutting-edge healthcare solutions. Medical electronics offers unheard-of prospects for tracking, detecting, telemedicine, and curing various diseases using pioneering technology, bioengineering, and data methodologies.

The development of medical electronics is heavily influenced by sectors other than medicine. Medical electronic devices underwent a movement towards mobility and miniaturization in the 1980s and 1990s. Handheld ECG monitors and ultrasound tools are examples of lighter, more compact gadgets that have been made possible through microelectronics and battery management innovations. The introduction of digital equipment in the 2000s revolutionized medical electronics. With greater reliability, precision, and computational capability, digital equipment gradually supplanted analogue ones. Additionally, the combination of wireless and communication technologies' inclusion allowed medical devices to be connected, enabling remote monitoring and the transfer of immediate information. The use of wearable technology and remote surveillance technologies increased dramatically in the 2010s. Wearable activity monitors and biological sensors have all been developed as a result of developments in sensor tech and data analytics. Individuals can gauge their exercise activities, keep track of their health markers, and communicate data to medical professionals for distant observation and assistance. Furthermore, implanted sensors have made tremendous strides. Biological characteristics that can be monitored by implantable sensors in real time include blood pressure, brain activity, and glucose levels.

Medical electronics promptly use machine learning (ML) and artificial intelligence (AI) technologies. By allowing the analysis of massive quantities of healthcare data, these technologies support precise diagnosis, predictive modeling, and the creation of individualized therapies. In order to optimize resource allocation algorithms based on machine learning and AI can help healthcare professionals recognize trends, predict consequences, and suggest the best course of treatment. Progress in privacy and data protection are essential nowadays as medical electronics depend more and more on gathering and processing private information from patients. To preserve the integrity and security of medical information, it is now a top priority to build strong encryption methods, secure cloud platforms, and adhere to privacy regulations. The development of robotics in surgical treatment and minimally-invasive techniques will be aided by medical electronics. Robotic surgery will improve accuracy and efficiency, allowing for smaller incisions, less scarring, and quicker postoperative recovery. Robotics will also help with orthopedic rehabilitation and therapy. The fusion of cutting-edge technologies like AI, IoT, and robotics will define the next phase of medical electronics. These developments will spur innovation, enhance healthcare results, and change how healthcare is provided.

The chapter focuses on essential topics such as organ-on-a-chip technology, MRI advancements, and wearable technology to give a thorough picture of the upcoming trends in medical electronics. The chapter addresses the new developments influencing the direction of medical electronics. The chapter examines technological developments as well as the business prospects for medical electronics. It evaluates the state of the market and pinpoints the chances for growth and acceptance. The chapter culminates with a glimpse of medical electronics, imagining an era in which personalized, effective, and easily accessible healthcare services will be provided through integrated technology, information analysis, and computational intelligence in the future healthcare environment. To promote growth and realize the full potential of medical electronics, it emphasizes the necessity of coordinated efforts of all parties involved, including researchers, healthcare professionals, legislators, and technology innovators.

14.2 Microelectromechanical systems

Microelectromechanical systems (MEMS) emerged at the start of the 1980s when mechanical and electronic elements were merged into a single chip with a number of small components. This was made possible by important developments in microelectronic systems, as well as the utilization of parallel production and miniaturization [3]. Decreased reagent and cell requirements and high-throughput screening are a few benefits of such miniaturized devices. Additionally, it has a decreased need for quick responses, is portable, has a flexible design, and may work independently or in tandem with other miniature instruments [4]. A subgroup of MEMS called BioMEMS is used for biological or biomedical purposes. Applications for BioMEMS devices are poised to expand thanks to current developments in biotechnology. The practical implications of the advancements in micro-technologies include BioMEMS for detection, surveillance, drug delivery, and cell culture similar to organ-on-a-chip (OOC) platforms [5].

14.2.1 Organ-on-a-chip

With the ever-advancing pharmaceutical industry, research and testing on models are necessary. Testing provides a better knowledge of the medication's effectiveness and negative effects. For a long time, traditional two-dimensional (2D) cultured cell methods were the cornerstone of research. By cultivating individual cells or their by-products, 2D models are used to investigate the roles of diverse cell types. The physiological state of biological tissues and organs, as well as microenvironmental elements, cannot be sufficiently simulated by 2D models, which is why they typically need to be verified using *in vivo* animal models [6]. Animal models typically do not replicate precisely how human biology reacts to illnesses and medications. The main cause of this is that the disease patterns, pathophysiology, symptoms, concurrent illnesses, and genetic effects vary greatly between species [7]. The practice of using animals in drug testing has come under criticism since it is expensive and unethical [8]. One of the major factors impacting the rise of OOC tech is the absence of adequate clinical applications of animals used to assess the effectiveness or harmful effects of pharmacological drugs [9, 10]. OCC can be utilized for *in vivo* pharmacokinetic and pharmacodynamic research as well as studies on toxicity, drug absorption, circulation, metabolism, and elimination [11]. The era of OOCs officially began in 2010. In 2010, L Griffith and D Huh made the first liver-on-chip and lung-on-chip, respectively [12, 13]. In 2012, the first gut-on-a-chip was by H J Lim [14], in 2013 first kidney-on-chip was by J Himmelfarb [15] and the first heart-on-chip was by M Radisic [16]. Over the year many organizations funded the research for OOC like Defence Advanced Research Projects Agency (DARPA) in 2011, NCATS in 2012 and 2016, and the National Institute of Health in 2014 [17].

OOC technologies imitate the *in vitro* system of living organs in order to produce more precise *in vitro* replicas of important human organs. OOC has the ability to accurately replicate physiological indicators and modify the environment when paired with microfluidics and cell biology [18]. The kinetic, physiological, biochemical, and microstructural aspects of the milieu of biological organs are better modeled by OOC systems. Microchannel cell culture-based systems enable the production of metabolic gradients of enzymes, biomolecules, mediators, and other substances in the physiological milieu [18]. The goal is to simulate the tiniest functional unit of an organ, these microfluidic cell culture systems replicate the cell environment, interactions, and biomechanical features of a fully functioning organ [19]. Working at the microscopic level offers a singular chance to gain more influence on the milieu that assures tissue survival as well as a way to study cell/tissue activity directly. With its capability to deal with complicated cell cultures and better-tailored microenvironments to maximize the model, OOC might be viewed as an interlinking technology [19].

The purpose of the chips is to mimic and duplicate the organ characteristics that can react to biochemical and physiological inputs to preserve organ function. OOC systems are crucial because they enable multi-parametric functional status indicators, giving insight into the integrated biochemistry of humans and animals. One or more cell types are typically cultivated on the chip inside a 3D framework that allows for extracellular matrix or porous membrane attachment. To sustain their life and capacity to function, cells are constantly perfused with fluid containing nutrients and oxygen. Physical cues like shear stress can also be applied. More recent developments have enabled tracking cellular and physiological adaptations with structures with greater aspect ratios and detectors [20].

14.2.1.1 Construction of organ-on-a-chip

The intended application and expected output are specified in the scope of use, which acts as a guide for OOC building [21]. When building and conceptualizing the OOC system, it is important to take into account the number of organ models, the ways in which they communicate, and the cultural settings of each organ model. A design and prototyping program would be used to create the necessary design after taking into account numerous aspects to mimic the requirements of a particular organ. The biological functioning and the actual operability of the device must be balanced when choosing the cell sources. The cell sources can be primary, immortalized, or stem cell-derived. The device will then be constructed using a microfabrication technology that is suited to the device's goals [17].

The chip will be used for cell or tissue cultivation to replicate an organ's functions, carry out pharmacological or biophysical tests, and conduct drugs assessment. There are two options available: single-organ system and multi-organ system. Single-organ devices normally attain an elevated degree of physiological realism, allowing investigation of a specific organ's response to a substance or combination of substances. The prospective involvement of one organ with at minimum one other can be examined in multi-organ systems, primarily through the transfer of substrates or soluble communication substances [22]. Microfabrication techniques like photolithography, stereolithography, and soft lithography are employed for the fabrication of OOC. Lithographic techniques are used to produce nano- and micrometer-scale structures [23]. Numerous variables, such as the ultimate device's functioning, the microfabrication method, and biocompatibility, influence substrate selection. Due to its superior micro- and nanostructure reproducibility, biocompatibility, optical transmittance, and gas permeability, poly(dimethyl siloxane) (PDMS) has become the most popular substrate for the manufacture of OOC devices. PDMS's flexibility has also been used to apply a physical stimulus to cells [13]. OOCs are designed to provide cells with the ideal *in vivo* environment so that they can amass to form 3D tissues that can mimic several or more functions at the organ level or grow organoid tissue while keeping function. The cell/tissue that will be used in OOCs will depend on the purpose for which they are being produced. Sometimes OOCs simulate physiological alterations in individuals or a particular person to evaluate their health or test potential disease treatments. In these circumstances, the same person's primary cells or stem cells may be utilized.

Another key element is the flow of nutrients and biomolecules on the chip. At the microscopic level, the liquid typically exhibits a unidirectional regime, resulting in a continuous gradient of controlled biomolecules [24]. Biological activities such as angiogenesis, incursion, and motility employ various physiological signals that are regulated by concentration gradients [25]. Every organ experiences various pressure throughout including bone pressure, air pressure, and blood pressure [26]. To mimic such pressure conditions, periodic physical pressures are created using elastic porous membranes. This mechanical stimulus is regarded as a crucial factor in physiological functions [27]. As with any other biological system, it is essential to keep the system sterile. It is essential to ensure the sterility of the OOC to prevent microbiological contamination, especially in the numerous microfluidic parts and cell cultures that will be utilized to assemble the overall OOC system.

The planned use and the cell growth method can greatly influence the structural design of the chip. Currently, there are four such structural configurations of OOC, namely microchannel-based, chamber-based, membrane structure-based, and multi-structure-based [28]. Microchannel-based systems are OOCs that have a relatively simpler structure. To control fluid movement, diverse mechanical characteristics can be applied to various channels, and microchannels of various diameters can be constructed as desired. Also, it is possible to create 3D-structured OOC by raising the number of parallel microchannels. As is the fact with many physiological systems, chamber-based organ chips provide fluid flows with specific durations in each chamber. Additionally, each chamber might correspond to a distinct organ or tissue. Certain membranes can simulate the contraction and expansion of cells and help to maintain homeostasis and provide mechanical strength. Membrane structure-based OOCs are created by utilizing this characteristic of membranes, such as those found in PDMS [29]. Many organ chips contain multiple structures that are combined to create a highly integrated chip structure based on functional parameters. OOC includes both culture chambers and microchannels [28].

The OOC technology's present applications centre on assessing drug effectiveness and safety, cell/tissue/organ function, response, and sensitivity to stimuli. Liver-on-a-chip, heart/cardiac-on-a-chip, lungs-on-a-chip, and several other organs and tissues are examples of current OOCs.

14.2.1.2 Liver on-a-chip

The liver is an important organ for the body. Among the many processes it performs are bile secretion, detoxification, protein—and carbohydrate metabolism, and drug metabolism [30]. Hence liver is an important organ associated with drug testing. Chitosan [31], collagen [32], alginate [33], and fibrin [34] are a few examples of biomaterials employed in liver-on-chip. Appropriate evaluation of the cell types and origins is crucial due to the complicated anatomy of the liver and the necessity for a correct representation of it in mechanical components [35]. Multiple cell sources include primary hepatocytes [36], hepatocytes derived from animals [37], hepatic cell lines of humans [38], Kupffer cells [39], stellate cells [40], and induced and embryonic pluripotent cells [41, 42]. Hurel creates revolutionary micro-liver tissue and is an expert in cell-based examination techniques that use microfluidics. Professionals can reproduce the pharmacokinetic responses across different parts of the body using the micro-liver tissue since it has biochemical competence and cell culture durability [43].

14.2.1.3 Heart-on-a-chip

The circulatory system's most crucial element is the heart. The circulatory system is in charge of moving nutrients and gases throughout the body. The heart is the organ in charge of maintaining blood flow. The heart is made of cardiac tissues which undergo rhythmic beating. The selection of the source of cells, culture setup, and environmental stimuli all significantly affect the ability to recreate functional heart tissue [20]. Blood flow, muscle tissue, endothelial cells, and other intricate components of blood vessels cause fluid stress and vessel deformations. Microfluidic substrates can be used to apply uniquely designed shear patterns to the cells being grown in the system [19]. Materials employed for the construction of heart-on-a-chip are polystyrene [44], polydopamine and polycaprolactone nanofibers [45], and polydimethylsiloxane [46]. Several heart-on-a-chip prototypes have been developed for a variety of purposes, such as drug testing, heartbeat simulation, mimicking myocardial lesions, and replicating the intricate physiological anatomy of blood vessels. TARA Biosystems has created a biotechnology platform that transforms the development of heart medication by utilizing anticipatory cardiac tissue models, human physiology, and analytics. The technology generates heart cells from stem cells, eliminating the requirement for human testing and enabling the assessment of changes in human cardiac function. This makes it possible to develop new medications [47].

14.2.1.4 Lung-on-a-chip

To put it in simple words, the lungs are responsible for the exchange of gases. The alveoli are the site of the exchange of gases. Various diseases are associated with malfunctioning or damage to the lungs like asthma, influenza, occupational disorder, and acute respiratory disorder. By simulating organ-level functions, OOCs have become a ground-breaking platform that can shed light on the pathophysiology and capabilities of the human lung [10]. Materials like polydimethylsiloxane [48], Matrigel membrane [49], Poly (lactic-co-glycolic) acid (PLGA), collagen, elastin [50], etc have been used. Using lung-on-a-chip models, researchers can examine various ailments and test for nanotoxicity in addition to researching lung cancer [51]. In more recent research, a lung-on-a-chip model with alveolar cell layers was used to assess the harm caused by SARS-CoV-2 [52].

The OrganDOT platform from BioIVT replicates tissue structure and activities by combining superior primary cultures with a reliable air–liquid connection. Using this approach, established replicas of the lung airway epithelium and pancreatic islets have been created [53]. For drug screening, AlveoliX has created *in vitro* pulmonary products. With the help of the goods manufactured by them, it is possible to simulate the biophysical properties of lungs, foresee the consequences of potential respiratory pharmaceutical candidates in people, and decrease the sum of candidates that need to be evaluated in clinical studies [54].

14.2.2 Future prospects of organ-on-a-chip

A thorough understanding of human anatomy and the more thorough advancement of associated technologies have made OOC recognized as a high-end strategy in the healthcare industry. OOCs are going to prove to be a really useful tool. OOC seems to have the potential to revolutionize a number of industries and medical fields, particularly in both preclinical and clinical pharmaceutical applications. Recent exhibits of several key works for linked multiple-organ devices for drug testing showed that the 'human-on-a-chip' concept was rapidly moving toward commercialization [55]. OOC is driven by a variety of established systems engineering, such as microfluidic devices, microfabrication, microscopy, sensing, etc. Recent developments in the combination of 3D (bio) printing with microfluidic systems, OOCs, and other technologies have helped the technology and its commercialization [56].

Due to its intriguing applications, there has been a noticeable rise in OOC research. Machine learning and AI-powered innovations may be used in the coming years to resolve the significant challenges posed by huge amounts of data, realize automatic and smart analysis of data, aid researchers in comprehending disease mechanisms more quickly, monitor patients, and recognize more suited medications for specific individuals, and ultimately achieve precise personalized medicine [55]. Personalized medicine is based on such goals, and has been developed to improve healthcare through earlier detection, risk evaluation, superior therapy, and reduced costs [57].

In order to help stakeholders implement MPS technology more widely, NA3RsC established a special project with the purpose of facilitating regulatory acceptability [58]. The European Organ-on-Chip Society (EUROOCS), which features special advisory committees for both the government and industry, has been instrumental in bringing together academic innovators on the educational front [59]. A network in the United Kingdom called Organ-On-a-Chip Technologies Network seeks to foster and advance OOC research by encouraging cooperation between academic institutions and businesses [60].

Utilizing human tissues, TissUse has created a novel 'Multi-Organ-Chip' technology that delivers outstanding preliminary information on a systemic level. This multi-organ-on-chip contains four organs on one chip. An updated human-on-a-chip with ten organs is being researched and developed [61]. MesoBioTech concentrates on cutting-edge stem cell innovations that make use of monolayers of active proteins and gelatin nanofibers to create synthetic bottom membranes. In order to create OOC, which is essential for ailment modeling, toxicology studies, drug assessment, and regenerative medicine experiments, the patches may then be reversibly combined with microfluidic devices [62].

14.2.3 Market potential of organ-on-a-chip

The pharmacon manufacturers and the scientific community have responded swiftly against the COVID-19 pandemic. These industries saw a need for cutting-edge techniques to do research work more effectively and quickly. Hence OOC is a suitable alternative. OOC will be a booming industry in the coming years, replacing animal testing and enhancing drug testing, disease diagnosis, and disease treatment. To aid in the acceptance and execution of OOCs in the drug manufacturing procedure, it is essential to maintain contact and interaction with OOC authors, end users, and regulatory bodies. Yole Développemen estimated in 2017 that the global OOC marketplace may increase by 38% annually to create US$117 million in revenue by 2022, with the chance of becoming a multibillion-dollar industry [63].

The market for organs-on-chip was sized at $150.29 million in 2021, and it is anticipated to increase to $1,427.41 million by 2029, increasing at a CAGR of 28.58% over the forthcoming years, i.e., from 2022 to 2029 [64]. Because of the growing number of OOC manufacturing businesses and the expanding demand for organ-on-chip devices, North America currently controls the majority of the sector for OOC globally [64].

14.3 Magnetic resonance imaging

Since the turn of the 20th century, scientists have contributed to our understanding of nuclear magnetic resonance (NMR) and the physics behind magnetic resonance imaging (MRI). The contributions of these people are documented in the literature on MRI. Paul C Lauterbur devised MRI in September 1971 when he created a method to employ magnetic field gradients, spatial data may be gathered from an NMR signal [65]. *For NMR images, Lauterbur invented the word 'zeugmatogram,' which, in Greek, is translated as 'that which is employed for joining.'*

Erik Odeblad and Gunnar Lindström, two scientists and doctors, described the factors causing picture contrast roughly 20 years ago [66]. The procedures utilized to take and analyze MR pictures were improved by Peter Mansfield. Both Mansfield and Lauterbur were jointly presented with the 2003 Nobel Prize in Physiology or Medicine in recognition of the efforts put together for the advancement of MRI. Beginning in the 1980s, MRI machines for medical applications were introduced. Subsequently, the technology underwent tremendous progress, and now it is widely used in medicine. MRI has undergone evolution through the years. In 1937, Columbia University physics professor Isidor Rabi developed a method for calculating the movements of the nucleus of an atom. The technique was given the label nuclear magnetic resonance (NMR). Initially, the main application of Rabi's methodology was to examine chemical compound structures [67].

Dr Raymond Damadian started to question if similar techniques could be used for biological things due to the fact that malignant tissue contains more water than healthy tissue. He came to the conclusion that it might be discovered using devices that exposed a piece of an individual's body to radio frequency and looked at the signals from adjacent atoms of hydrogen. The only task remaining was to build a scanner big enough to fit a human body [68]. Using NMR, scientist Paul Lauterbur was diligently at work generating images of water vials, clams, and green peppers. Reading Damadian's findings from 1971 made him understand that his study might have biomedical relevance [65]. He was the first to understand that viewers may capture two-dimensional photographs of an object using a gradient magnetic field. When two-dimensional photographs are piled together, a three-dimensional image is created [65]. The time constraint was being addressed by physicist Peter Mansfield, who tried to complete scans in a matter of minutes rather than hours. He did this by eschewing the standard 'sensitive point scan' approach in favor of a brand-new technology he named 'line scan imaging.' The first human body component to be triumphantly imaged with NMR was Andrew Maudsley's finger, which only required 15 to 23 min per segment [69].

The full-body scanner was Mansfield's next objective, and Damadian was hard at work building one. On May 11, 1977, while his helpers turned on the imaging equipment, Damadian put on the cardboard-backed antenna coils onto the moving base of Indomitable and laid there without producing an image. After hours of gadget manipulation, someone eventually indicated that Damadian's body-fat content might be too high. Then a slimmer volunteer was called in to assist. After several weeks, there were no noticeable negative effects. For ordinary clinical use, Lauterbur and Mansfield's procedures were chosen after Damadian's were rejected as being too sluggish. Since Lauterbur's sketches and Damadian's cardboard antenna, modern MRI technology has experienced significant advancements [70].

14.3.1 Future prospects in MRI technology

To achieve the best operating potential, MRI has undergone certain advancements in hardware, namely field strength, gradient capabilities, and peripheral nerve stimulation.

14.3.1.1 Field strength

Over 80 MRI systems are currently functioning at magnetic field strengths of seven teslas (T) or higher, making UHF MRI an extensively used technique in research and therapeutic settings. The signal-to-noise ratio (SNR) has significantly improved in UHF MRI [71]. It is very desirable to have mid- to low-field MRI that uses magnetic forces that are 1 Tor weaker than UHF MRI systems. Due to contemporary system engineering, it would be anticipated that they will have lower manufacturing and running expenses while maintaining high-quality imaging [72]. Additionally, the static B_o and transmit B_1 fields' increased homogeneity and lowered specific absorption rates, respectively, show tremendous promise for clinical applications and might be utilized, for instance, to image metallic objects with less artifice.

14.3.1.2 Higher-level gradient capabilities

Only the creation of excellent performance gradient systems allowed for the recent MRI scanner generations' improvements in resolution and speed, are employed to encode the incoming signal spatially, and offer significant advantages for diffusion encoding in diffusion-weighted imaging. The primary attributes and performance of gradient systems are their peak gradient intensity (measured in mT m^{-1}) and rising time (usually expressed as 'slew rate' in T m^{-1} s^{-1}). Owing to improvements in gradient technology, clinically viable whole-body systems may now attain magnitudes of up to 80 mT m^{-1} and simultaneous slew rates of up to 200 T m^{-1} s^{-1}. However, in addition to the amplifier employed, geometric boundary conditions, such as patient bore, significantly affect the possible gradient strength. As a result, utilizing specialized coils like head gradient coils, even greater amplitudes and slew rates (up to 200 mT m^{-1} and up to 1000 T m^{-1} s^{-1}) are feasible [73]. These head gradient coils' ability to generate high amplitudes is one of their main advantages. Due to peripheral nerve stimulation (PNS), switches can typically be made in short-rise periods without limits.

Only with a thorough understanding of all interacting elements of the MR can high gradient performance scanners be developed. One illustration is the interaction of the gradient coil's quickly shifting magnetic fields with the magnet's conducting layers. Simulations and tests result in a system that is optimized for reducing eddy current-related image artifacts. Another factor to take into account is the energy deposition inside the magnet as a result of the gradient coil's stray field.

Another area where high-performance gradients are crucial is functional MRI [74]. However, in this instance, the outcome is decided by the slew rate rather than the peak amplitude. The readout used in MRIs, known as echo-planar imaging (EPI), is based on the signals being recorded in functional blood oxygen level-dependent ways. The slew rate, in turn, is limited by the echo spacing, which controls the achievable sharpness. It may be feasible to elucidate the operation of cortical constructions, such as its foundational units and sections, using slew rates higher than those of clinical scanners (>200 T m^{-1} s^{-1}) [75].

14.3.1.3 Peripheral nerve stimulation

When employing skeletal muscle simulation (SMS) excitation methods like PINS [76] or image-capturing methods like echo-planar [77] and spiral imaging [78], the gradient coils need to be swapped quickly. Recent developments in gradient engineering have made PNS a significant barrier to fully utilizing the capability of the available gradient coil for quick imaging [79]. PNS parameters are only indirectly taken into account during the coil design phase, despite their influence on operating limits. Using coil prototypes to conduct stimulation tests on healthy human volunteers, for instance, or by lowering the linear volume [80]. To impose PNS-optimized gradient winding patterns, this PNS model can be added as an additional constraint to the conventional method for numeric gradient winding optimization. Additionally, such a tool can help evaluate additional PNS mitigation measures. A framework was developed to model the system based on coupled electromagnetic-neurodynamic simulations and provide in-depth information on the PNS capabilities of the coil avoiding having to manufacture expensive coil prototypes. This PNS model might be used as an additional constraint to the traditional method for numeric gradient winding optimization in order to impose PNS-optimized gradient winding patterns. Such a PNS tool can also help evaluate other PNS mitigating measures [79].

14.3.2 Market potential of MRI

The global market for MRI systems was valued at USD 8924 million in 2022, and CAGR growth is predicted at 6.60% from 2022 to 2030, reaching USD 14 880 million. This is brought on by advances in MRI technology, more public awareness of the value of early disease detection, increased government assistance for MRI, a rise in the incidence of long-term illnesses, and an increase in the number of elderly people.

Early detection of chronic conditions enables patients and their families to obtain prompt guidance and assistance for treating the disease. Early disease detection reduces the likelihood of later acquiring a serious condition. This is especially beneficial in the case of cancer, where efforts are being undertaken on a global scale to raise awareness of the value of early diagnosis. If the patient is immediately diagnosed and adequately treated, the early detection of breast cancer can assist to increase survival rates, lessen mortality, and lower healthcare costs [81].

The market for MRI systems is divided into low-field, high-field, and medium-field systems based on field strength. Due to the rising incidence of chronic illnesses in both developed and developing countries, the rising demand for medical imaging, the expansion of government initiatives, and the rapid uptake of medium-field MRI systems in hospitals and healthcare facilities, the medium-field systems segment held the lion's share of the market in 2020 [82]. By controlling more than 37% of the worldwide MRI market in 2021, North America led the market. Imaging analysis is in demand due to the region's rising prevalence of chronic diseases like breast cancer, cardiovascular problems, and neurological conditions.

Fast-developing European nations like the UK, France, and Germany, which have large per-capita incomes and clear healthcare norms, are seeing an increase in demand for advanced diagnostic imaging modalities. Because of the escalating demand for improved imaging modalities and the region's expanding senior population, Asia Pacific is anticipated to develop at the quickest rate during the projection period. Countries like India, China, and Japan are fostering development potential because they have a booming medical care sector, a knowledgeable wellness workforce, along with cutting-edge health clinics and services that are more affordable than industrialized nations in North America and Europe [83].

14.4 Artificial cardiac pacemaker

When a person's heartbeat is erratic (tachycardia) or slow (bradycardia), a pacemaker is used to supervise and regulate the electrical activity of the heart. It is made up of a pulse generator and leads that send electrical impulses to the heart, assisting in keeping it in a regular beat and avoiding arrhythmia. Wired pacemakers can be of different types: single chamber pacemakers that transmit impulses to the right atrium, double chamber pacemakers that send impulses to the right atrium and ventricle, a biventricular pacemaker includes three leads that provide electrical signals to the right atrium, right ventricle, and left ventricle to help both sides of the heartbeat in synchrony. A device the size of a tablet serves as both the pulse generator and electrodes in a wireless pacemaker. Usually, the wireless pacemaker is placed in the right ventricle. A transvenous method is used for implanting the majority of wired pacemakers. This indicates that the electrodes and leads are inserted into your heart through your veins. Usually, veins in the neck, chest, or thigh are used.

14.4.1 Future potential of artificial cardiac pacemaker

The advancement in pacemakers in the near future revolves around the developments in improving cardiac resynchronization, eliminating energy storage devices from the pacemaker, eliminating leads, making the pacemaker MRI compatible, remote monitoring, and reducing hardware [84].

14.4.1.1 Cardiac resynchronization

Pacing as a method of treating a delayed portion of the ventricle was first presented by cardiac resynchronization therapy (CRT). Left bundle branch block [LBBB] most frequently causes the free wall of the left ventricle (LV) to contract with a noticeable delay, failing to make a significant contribution to stroke volume and cardiac output. This condition is called dyssynchrony. CRT has been demonstrated to prevent unfavourable cellular remodelling, enhance cardiac function, decrease heart failure hospitalization, and minimize death. The current focus of CRT research is on expanding the number of pacing sites to enable the simultaneous pacing of many sites.

14.4.1.2 Remote monitoring

In order to treat bradycardias, tachyarrhythmias, or heart failure, seven million people worldwide have a cardiovascular implantable electronic device that they depend on for successful long-term monitoring. Receiving individual patient information from cardiac-implanted electronics and relaying it to a clinic far from the patient to improve care is referred to as remote monitoring (RM) or remote interrogation (RI). Multiple techniques like trans-telephonic monitoring, inductive transmission, and radio-frequency RM are being explored.

14.4.1.3 Pacemaker with no leads

The lead almost always results in issues, despite being dependable and efficient. It is technically difficult to remove leads because they are intrinsically thrombogenic and cause fibrotic reactions that increase the danger of venous rupture, hemothorax, and even mortality. Two different approaches have been used to create leadless pacemakers: single and multiple-component systems. Single-component pacemakers consist of the entire pacemaker, including the battery, circuitry, stimulating electrodes, and sensors. This compact unit is inserted into the heart via a deflectable sheath. A small receiver electrode placed endocardially in the left ventricle is part of the multi-component system. The endocardial seed receives ultrasonic pulses from a subcutaneous pulse generator implanted in the left lateral thorax and converts them to electrical pacing stimuli.

14.4.2 Market potential of artificial cardiac pacemaker

One of the main causes of cardiovascular fatalities worldwide is coronary heart disease. By 2030, it is estimated that these diseases will cost more than USD 1044 billion, underscoring the critical need for cardiac pacemakers. The market for pacemakers was valued at USD 4.51 billion in 2022, and from 2023 to 2030, it is anticipated to expand at a CAGR of 3.6%. In 2022, North America held a commanding 42.0% part of the revenue in the pacemaker market [85]. Over the anticipated period, the market in Asia Pacific is anticipated to display a profitable CAGR of about 4.0%. Due to the leading companies' expanding market share and the vast untapped market potential, the industry is growing. The market for pacemakers that are compatible with MRIs is anticipated to expand at a rate of roughly 4%.

14.5 Wearable medical devices

A wearable medical device is autonomous, non-invasive, and performs a specific medical role over a prolonged period, such as support as well as monitoring. The vast majority of modern devices in use today often depend on user input to track data that is later offline evaluated. Instead of only recording data, the next generation of wearable monitoring devices aims to deliver smart care coordination with real-time feedback through notifications and medical decision support. Since wearable medical devices are one of the most recent alternatives for healthcare monitoring, early identification, and tailored treatment, they will contribute to the development of a more economical and durable healthcare system [86]. In this portion, we will look into the series of events that led to these advancements, the current state of wearable medical devices, and future prospects.

The continued improvement and expansion of wearable medical technology are in line with the general health trend toward personal healthcare as opposed to hospital treatment. Because of this, developers are changing. They have shifted their attention from stationary medical devices to portable and, more lately, wearable ones. Although they are portable and flexible, wearable medical devices rely on established technology for their primary medical purposes [86].

The Holter monitor was the first wearable medical application that was used for the gathering of data that would subsequently be assessed after being saved in a wearable device. Telemedicine was a novel idea in the 1990s, and healthcare professionals primarily used it to consult with patients and get a second opinion, regardless of the time or place. In response to the demand for immediate access to the patient being monitored, real-time wireless telemetry is a type of wearable device that integrates health data gathering and processing capabilities with telemedicine. The earliest such gadgets were created for high-profile uses like the American space program when NASA regularly observed the physiological reactions of men in space. The American army then created wearable battlefield computers as part of the Land Warrior program. Such features are now becoming commercially available in wearable medical devices. Most commonly, they are used to monitor patients' vital signs in high-risk circumstances, to monitor patients remotely when urgent care assistance is unavailable, to monitor athletic events, and for research [86].

Fitbits, smartwatches, and other wearable monitors have been developed by the medical business, which includes insurers, providers, and technology companies, as a result of the advancement of wearable technology and the increased need from consumers to take control of their health [86]. Components that are compact, lightweight, strong, pleasant, and perform the required duties dependably and securely at a reasonable price are needed to create wearable medical devices. It is now possible to address these needs because of recent advancements in wearable tech, particularly the scaling down of detector, computing, and wireless telecommunication technology as well as the novel concept of computational apparel.

14.5.1 Types of modern wearable medical devices

Wearable fitness trackers are bracelets with sensors that monitor a user's heart rate and physical activity. Even though they are among the most basic and innovative types of wearable technology, they are enduring because they easily connect with smartphone applications to offer customers priceless health and fitness tips. Wearable ECG monitors, as opposed to some smartwatches, are at the forefront of consumer technology because they can record electrocardiograms. The Move ECG can measure an electrocardiogram and transmit the results to the user's physician. It can also identify atrial fibrillation. Together with automatic monitoring for biking, walking, running, and swimming, it can measure pace, distance, and elevation. 2019 saw the introduction of HeartGuide, the first wearable blood pressure monitor, by Omron Healthcare. HeartGuide is an oscillometric blood pressure tracker that can track regular activities, including steps taken, kilometers traveled, and calories burned, in addition to blood pressure. It may appear like a conventional wristwatch. Unlike wrist trackers and smartwatches, biosensors are a new generation of wearable medical gadgets. The Philips wearable biosensor is a self-adhesive patch that enables individuals to move around while tracking their activity, temperature, pulse, and breathing rate. According to a study from the Augusta University Medical Center, the number of individuals who encountered needless cardiopulmonary arrest decreased by 89% as a result of the use of this monitoring device. The potential for wearable technology to improve patient outcomes and possibly reduce staff burdens is highlighted by this. Smartwatches, which formerly served merely as timepieces and step counters, have evolved into clinically useful healthcare instruments. Currently, fitness trackers, glucose monitors, blood pressure monitors, pulse oximeters, and sleep trackers are the most popular types of wearable medical devices available. Here are a few startups that are working to develop the greatest wearable medical technology.

1. Proteus: Leading the way in digital medicine is Proteus Digital Health. Proteus Discover, one of its products, is digital medicine that consists of consumable sensors, a tiny wearable sensor patch, a smartphone app, and a provider site. Proteus Discover enables patients to recover quickly by removing uncertainty from diagnosis and therapy.
2. Augmedix: By altering the way operational and record-keeping chores are carried out, Augmedix enables doctors to have more meaningful interactions with their patients. With Augmedix, doctors just put on smart glasses during sessions and communicate with transcriptionists live via a feed. These transcriptionists access each video and audio channel of the doctor–patient conversation, capture records, and edit patient files, sparing medical professionals up to 15 h weekly on client documentation. Augmedix offers AI-enabled products namely Augmedix-Live, Augmedix-Notes, and Augmedix-Prep to manage documentation [87].
3. Neurotech: The cutting-edge in-home visual electroencephalogram (EEG) systems from Neurotech is clinically complete, constantly tracked, and committed to improvement. It offers EEG testing in patients' residences, healthcare facilities, and community centers, enhancing access to care for those who are unable to travel or live in remote places, as well as comfort for children and individuals with special needs who frequently respond well to EEG administered in their own environment [88].

4. Hinge Health: A musculoskeletal (MSK) clinic designed by Hinge Health combines skilled clinical care, state-of-the-art equipment, and computer vision to assist patients in overcoming pain, avoiding unneeded procedures, and using fewer opioids. Hinge Health provides TrueMotion technology, which uses computer vision and sensors to give personalized care, Enso for alleviating pain, HingeConnect, which seamlessly combines online and face-to-face MSK care, physiotherapy for pelvic floor issues, and support for musculoskeletal health [89].
5. Grapheal: The integrated and portable biosensors made by Grapheal are computerized by design, have few parts, and can administer biomarkers and recognize microbes practically with a basic smartphone. Grapheal provides TestNPass a battery-free computerized antigen examination that monitors for Covid-19 infection in mere seconds with a mobile device, GraphLab provides the perfect R&D tool to develop new integration for graphene-based sensors, and WoundLab is an electrical wound patch that persistently gathers and stores wound factors to transmit them to a clinical cloud via a mobile application. By converting any gauze into a personalized assessment tool for precise healthcare, it empowers carers [90].
6. ReTiSense: ReTiSense began working in 2014, emphasizing remedies for sports-related injury anticipating, safeguarding, and athletic performance enhancement using cutting-edge wearable technology. Stridalyzer, ReTiSense's initial product for runners, has won various accolades, including being one of the best running gadgets in *Runner's World*. Specifically designed for runners, Stridalyzer is a tracking and counseling system that may be used to understand better how they run, prevent injuries, and function better [91]. Some medical devices in the current market are summarized in table 14.1.

Table 14.1. Medical electronics in the current market.

Medical device	Type	Function
Computed tomography	Diagnostic system	Imaging
Pulse oximeter	Diagnostic system	Blood oxygen measurement
X-ray machine	Diagnostic system	Imaging
Glucose monitors	Monitoring system	Diabetes management
Continuous positive airway pressure (CPAP)	Monitoring system	Aid individuals to keep their airways open
Insulin pumps	Therapeutic system	Delivery of insulin
Dialysis machine	Therapeutic system	Assist individuals with kidney issues to eliminate waste
Prosthetics & orthotics	Assistive system	Mobility and functionality
Hearing aid	Assistive system	Aid individuals with hearing issues
Orthopaedic braces	Assistive system	Stabilizes joints and aids in recovery

14.5.2 Future prospects in wearable medical devices

The COVID-19 outbreak increased the necessity of advanced wearable gadgets that track the body's oxygen saturation, such as smartwatches. Moreover, remote patient monitoring systems made it easier for patients and medical practitioners to continuously track their health thanks to wearable medical devices. Practitioners remotely assessed patient health data without the individual being in a medical environment. In addition, users learned useful information without visiting hospitals or doctors' offices. Monitors that record daily activities such as consuming water, napping, and exercising made up around 22% of the industry's overall worth in 2022. The healthcare industry will focus on, among other things, identifying emergencies beforehand, assessing individuals' health concerns, determining respiratory system capacity, and even keeping an eye on circulatory hemodynamics [92]. Due to patent changes, the medical instruments business in the US and Europe currently confronts considerable challenges. Firms known as 'patent trolls' buy patents specifically to demand remuneration from businesses they believe are violating their rights through the use of their products or processes. Medical equipment makers were the target of many patent infringement lawsuits brought by patent trolls in 2013 [92].

If companies take the required safeguards to protect the innovations of mobile medical technology through patents, they may ensure the monetary and legal benefits of correctly filed patents and minimize possible losses brought on by patent trolls. Patents must be protected if the clinical-grade wearables industry is to expand and prosper. Securing the innovations of medical technology, including the devices currently under clinical trial (table 14.2), through proper patent safeguards is essential.

Table 14.2. Medical devices in clinical trials [95].

Product name/ active ingredient	Condition/disease	Intervention/ treatment	Identifier	Sponsor
Aerin Medical Device	Nasal obstruction	Vivaer stylus	NCT02914236	Aerin Medical
Caloprothese Connected Kit, CCK	Neuropathic pain, phantom limb pain	KCC active or inactive	NCT04748484	Greg and Innovations
Dermapol	Skin lesion	Dermapol	NCT03796871	University Hospital, Strasbourg, France
Boomerang closure device	Angiography	Boomerang closure device	NCT00732628	University of Michigan
AeviceMD		AeviceMD	NCT05194436	AEvice Health Pte Ltd

(*Continued*)

Table 14.2. (*Continued*)

Product name/ active ingredient	Condition/disease	Intervention/ treatment	Identifier	Sponsor
	Subject presenting wheeze, COPD, asthma			
CBRA	Breast cancer	BRA	CONNECT device	NCT05294016
Hopital Nord Franche-Comte				
SIVA-MVP	Chronic cough	SIVA-MVP	NCT05689307	Siva Health AG
OMNI FIT DTx-MDD	Depressive disorder	OMNI FIT	DTx-MDD	NCT05701345
Omni C&S				
Prototype 0.3	Diabetes mellitus	Prototype 0.3	NCT03781232	RSP Systems A/S
POLARIS	Bacterial vaginosis	Polybactum®	NCT02863536	Effik Italia S.p.A

14.5.3 Market potential of wearable medical devices

Wearable medical gadget sales are expected to reach US$73.48 billion by 2032, expanding at a 28.1% CAGR. The market for wearable medical devices is expected to rise as a result of the rising incidence of chronic illnesses and the expanding world population. Regulations, the growth of the medical industry, and an increase in patients have all resulted in a swift expansion of the health sector's businesses and product approvals [93]. As more people who enjoy sports and exercise seek alternative methods to check their fitness, the global wellness and healthcare system is predicted to expand dramatically. Early adopters, who account for a sizeable fraction of the public, are represented in both the American and Canadian demographics.

14.6 European Union medical device regulations

The highest possible standards of durability and security are ensured when medical devices are manufactured in or exported to Europe by European Union Medical Device Regulations (EU MDR). The EU MDR laws are designed to increase the functionality and security of medical devices, and hence will also increase patient safety in Europe. The EU MDR uses a risk-based framework to categorize medical electronics in use, taking into consideration both the fragility of the human system and any possible hazards posed by the devices in question. This method classifies devices based on a set of variables that can be coupled in different ways, such as the period of their interaction with the patient's body, the level of invasion, the difference between regional and widespread effects, the possibility of toxic

Table 14.3. Classification of medical devices by EU MDR.

Sr. No.	Classification	Risk factor	Description	Examples
1	Class I	Low risk	Pose almost no threat	Stomach tubes, wheelchairs
2	Class IIa	Medium risk	Require regular assessment	Surgical clamps, lancets
3	Class IIb	Medium/ high risk	Mandatory conformity regular assessment	Urethral stents, brachytherapy devices
4	Class III	High risk	Require monitoring	Cardiovascular catheters

consequences, the area of the body impacted by the usage, and whether it is powered by an external source. Medical equipment is classified according to MDR into classes [94] as described in table 14.3.

According to how long they have been used continuously, the device is classified by EU MDR as either transient (constant use for less than an hour), short-term (constant use for between an hour and 30 days), or long-term (constant use for more than 30 days). The type of device provides the basis for yet another classification; invasive, non-invasive, active, and special devices. Devices that do not penetrate the body by an entrance or via the exterior of the body itself are considered non-invasive. Instruments that enter the body entirely or partially, either through a bodily entrance or through the exterior of the body, are referred to as invasive devices. All gadgets that require a means of energy to function are considered active devices. Special medical devices that can be active and invasive, or that integrate medical equipment with an *in vitro* diagnostic tool or a medicament. Any medical equipment must be classified in the following order, beginning with determining the sort of device it is (invasive, non-invasive, active, or special), the appropriate EU MDR rule is examined, the greatest risk rule is addressed when multiple rules are applied, and in case of a special device, one must identify the primary goal.

14.7 Conclusion

Industry 4.0's emerging solutions are on the path of advanced automation allowing for the delivery of improved, value-added, and cheaper production and service operations. The medical electronics sector is expanding along with general technological progress. Healthcare professionals and researchers are investigating options in machine learning, a subset of artificial intelligence that translates to computations that can instantly improve through experience, and data science to supervise and respond to situations more effectively. IoT has quickly and substantially altered the healthcare industry. For instance, connected gadgets significantly improve older people's safety in regular surroundings. Additionally, networked gadgets enable real-time consultations among medical professionals and scientists across the globe on complex situations, the monitoring of patients' chronic illnesses during pauses from other activities, etc. It is clear that future healthcare applications will be made possible by how quickly technology like adaptive hardware and effective algorithms is emerging [96]. It will be achievable to take advantage of enormous quantities of information and use them for all facets of medical care, including residential care, rehabilitative services, personalized healthcare, e-health systems, pharmaceuticals, and disease surveillance, thanks to upcoming advancements in the areas of data management and machine learning.

Due to a number of important variables, the market potential for medical electronics is quickly growing. The aging population is one of the most important factors since it is raising the need for healthcare services and necessitating the development of novel, cutting-edge medical technologies. The future of medical electronics is being significantly shaped by technological advancements as well as demographic and disease-related variables. Medical electronics have huge market potential and present chances for cutting-edge goods and services in a variety of fields, including diagnosis, treatment, and condition monitoring and management. Emerging technologies like wearables, AI, and the Internet of Things, as well as evolving customer preferences and healthcare regulations, will all have an impact on the direction of medical electronics in the future. In order to stay up with the fast-changing environment of medical technology, regulatory policies will need to strike a balance between the requirement for patient safety and the need for innovation. To enhance the understanding and evaluation of the current state of medical electronics and recent technologies, a comprehensive strengths, weaknesses, opportunities, and threats (SWOT) analysis is presented in figure 14.1. This analysis provides valuable insights into each aspect of the SWOT framework. By examining the SWOT analysis, a better understanding of the overall landscape can be achieved.

In conclusion, the foreseeable future of healthcare is quite promising for the discipline of medical electronics. Medical electronics technologies are poised to revolutionize patient care, advance detection, and offer personalized treatment by utilizing technology, statistical analysis, and AI. To promote innovation, address problems, and realize the maximum potential, cooperation between researchers, healthcare professionals, administrators, and entrepreneurs in technology is crucial. Medical experts, engineers, and other stakeholders will increasingly need to work together as the area develops to ensure that novel goods and services are created and commercialized safely, efficiently, and ethically. Medical electronics have the potential to completely change the way healthcare is delivered and significantly enhance patient outcomes with the correct research, development, and funding.

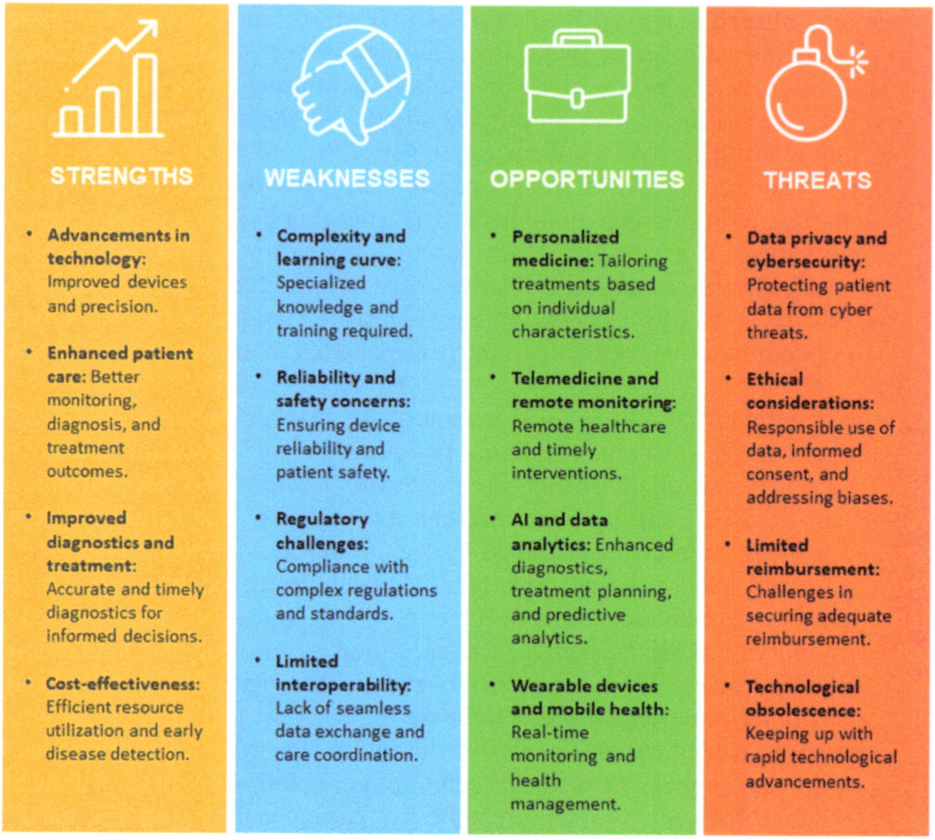
STRENGTHS
• Advancements in technology: Improved devices and precision.
• Enhanced patient care: Better monitoring, diagnosis, and treatment outcomes.
• Improved diagnostics and treatment: Accurate and timely diagnostics for informed decisions.
• Cost-effectiveness: Efficient resource utilization and early disease detection.
WEAKNESSES
• Complexity and learning curve: Specialized knowledge and training required.
• Reliability and safety concerns: Ensuring device reliability and patient safety.
• Regulatory challenges: Compliance with complex regulations and standards.
• Limited interoperability: Lack of seamless data exchange and care coordination.
OPPORTUNITIES
• Personalized medicine: Tailoring treatments based on individual characteristics.
• Telemedicine and remote monitoring: Remote healthcare and timely interventions.
• AI and data analytics: Enhanced diagnostics, treatment planning, and predictive analytics.
• Wearable devices and mobile health: Real-time monitoring and health management.
THREATS
• Data privacy and cybersecurity: Protecting patient data from cyber threats.
• Ethical considerations: Responsible use of data, informed consent, and addressing biases.
• Limited reimbursement: Challenges in securing adequate reimbursement.
• Technological obsolescence: Keeping up with rapid technological advancements.

Figure 14.1. SWOT analysis of medical electronics and recent technologies.

References

[1] Herrick J F 1962 History of bio-medical electronics art *Proc. IRE* **50** 1173–7

[2] Nokes L, Jennings D, Flint T and Turton B 1995 *Introduction to Medical Electronics Applications* (Elsevier)

[3] Verpoorte E and De Rooij N F 2003 Microfluidics meets MEMS *Proc. IEEE* **91** 930–53

[4] Osaki T, Shin Y, Sivathanu V, Campisi M and Kamm R D 2018 *In vitro* microfluidic models for neurodegenerative disorders *Adv. Healthc. Mater.* **7** 1700489

[5] Bashir R 2004Sep22 BioMEMS: state-of-the-art in detection, opportunities, and prospects *Adv. Drug Deliv. Rev.* **56** 1565–86

[6] Sung J H, Esch M B, Prot J M, Long C J, Smith A and Hickman J J *et al* 2013 Microfabricated mammalian organ systems and their integration into models of whole animals and humans *Lab Chip* **13** 1201

[7] Shrestha J, Razavi Bazaz S, Aboulkheyr Es H, Yaghobian Azari D, Thierry B and Ebrahimi Warkiani M *et al* 2020 Lung-on-a-chip: the future of respiratory disease models and pharmacological studies *Crit. Rev. Biotechnol.* **40** 213–30

[8] Al-Lamki R S, Bradley J R and Pober J S 2017 Human organ culture: updating the approach to bridge the gap from *in vitro* to *in vivo* in inflammation, cancer, and stem cell biology *Front. Med. (Lausanne)* **4** 00148

[9] Seyhan A A 2019 Lost in translation: the valley of death across preclinical and clinical divide —identification of problems and overcoming obstacles *Transl. Med. Commun.* **4** 18

[10] Alépée N 2014 State-of-the-art of 3D cultures (organs-on-a-chip) in safety testing and pathophysiology *ALTEX* **31** 441–77

[11] Ishida S 2018 Organs-on-a-chip: current applications and consideration points for *in vitro* ADME-Tox studies *Drug Metab. Pharmacokinet* **33** 49–54

[12] Domansky K, Inman W, Serdy J, Dash A, Lim M H M and Griffith L G 2010 Perfused multiwell plate for 3D liver tissue engineering *Lab Chip* **10** 51–8

[13] Huh D, Matthews B D, Mammoto A, Montoya-Zavala M, Hsin H Y and Ingber D E 2010 Reconstituting organ-level lung functions on a chip *Science (1979)* **328** 1662–8

[14] Kim H J, Huh D, Hamilton G and Ingber D E 2012 Human gut-on-a-chip inhabited by microbial flora that experiences intestinal peristalsis-like motions and flow *Lab Chip* **12** 2165

[15] Kelly E J, Wang Z, Voellinger J L, Yeung C K, Shen D D and Thummel K E *et al* 2013 Innovations in preclinical biology: *ex vivo* engineering of a human kidney tissue micro-perfusion system *Stem. Cell Res. Ther.* **4** S17

[16] Nunes S S, Miklas J W, Liu J, Aschar-Sobbi R, Xiao Y and Zhang B *et al* 2013 Biowire: a platform for maturation of human pluripotent stem cell–derived cardiomyocytes *Nat. Methods* **10** 781–7

[17] Clapp N, Amour A, Rowan W C and Candarlioglu P L 2021 Organ-on-chip applications in drug discovery: an end user perspective *Biochem. Soc. Trans.* **49** 1881–90

[18] Bhatia S N and Ingber D E 2014 Microfluidic organs-on-chips *Nat. Biotechnol.* **32** 760–72

[19] Azizipour N, Avazpour R, Rosenzweig D H, Sawan M and Ajji A 2020 Evolution of biochip technology: a review from lab-on-a-chip to organ-on-a-chip *Micromachines (Basel)* **11** 599

[20] Leung C M, de Haan P, Ronaldson-Bouchard K, Kim G A, Ko J and Rho H S *et al* 2022 A guide to the organ-on-a-chip *Nat. Rev. Methods Primers* **2** 33

[21] Hargrove-Grimes P, Low L A and Tagle D A 2022 Microphysiological systems: stakeholder challenges to adoption in drug development *Cells Tissues Organs* **211** 269–81

[22] Advancing Alternative Methods at FDA. https://fda.gov/science-research/about-science-research-fda/advancing-alternative-methods-fda (accessed 20 January 2023)

[23] Xia Y and Whitesides G M 1998 Soft lithography *Annu. Rev. Mater. Sci.* **28** 153–84

[24] Yang K S, Cheng Y C, Jeng M S, Chien K H and Shyu J C 2014 An experimental investigation of micro pulsating heat pipes *Micromachines (Basel)* **5** 385–95

[25] Song J W, Daubriac J, Tse J M, Bazou D and Munn L L 2012 RhoA mediates flow-induced endothelial sprouting in a 3-D tissue analogue of angiogenesis *Lab Chip* **12** 5000

[26] Sellgren K L, Hawkins B T and Grego S 2015 An optically transparent membrane supports shear stress studies in a three-dimensional microfluidic neurovascular unit model *Biomicrofluidics.* **9** 061102

[27] Kshitiz , Park J S, Kim P, Helen W, Engler A J and Levchenko A *et al* 2012 Control of stem cell fate and function by engineering physical microenvironments *Integr. Biol.* **4** 1008–18

[28] Yan J, Li Z, Guo J, Liu S and Guo J 2022 Organ-on-a-chip: a new tool for *in vitro* research *Biosens. Bioelectron.* **216** 114626

[29] Van Engeland N C A, Pollet A M A O, Den Toonder J M J, Bouten C V C, Stassen O M J A and Sahlgren C M 2018 A biomimetic microfluidic model to study signalling between

endothelial and vascular smooth muscle cells under hemodynamic conditions *Lab Chip* **18** 1607–20
[30] Kuntz E 2008 Biochemistry and functions of the liver *Hepatology Textbook and Atlas* (Berlin, Heidelberg: Springer) pp 35–76
[31] Lee K H, Shin S J, Kim C B, Kim J K, Cho Y W and Chung B G *et al* 2010 Microfluidic synthesis of pure chitosan microfibers for bio-artificial liver chip *Lab Chip* **10** 1328–34
[32] Mi S, Yi X, Du Z, Xu Y and Sun W 2018 Construction of a liver sinusoid based on the laminar flow on chip and self-assembly of endothelial cells *Biofabrication* **10** 025010
[33] Lan S F, Safiejko-Mroczka B and Starly B 2010 Long-term cultivation of HepG2 liver cells encapsulated in alginate hydrogels: a study of cell viability, morphology, and drug metabolism *Toxicol. In Vitro* **24** 1314–23
[34] Miller J S, Stevens K R, Yang M T, Baker B M, Nguyen D H T and Cohen D M *et al* 2012 Rapid casting of patterned vascular networks for perfusable engineered three-dimensional tissues *Nat. Mater.* **11** 768–74
[35] Beckwitt C H, Clark A M, Wheeler S, Taylor D L, Stolz D B and Griffith L *et al* 2018 Liver 'organ on a chip *Exp. Cell. Res.* **363** 15–25
[36] McGinnity D F, Soars M G, Urbanowicz R A and Riley R J 2004 Evaluation of fresh and cryopreserved hepatocytes as *in vitro* drug metabolism tools for the prediction of metabolic clearance *Drug Metab. Dispos.* **32** 1247–53
[37] Lu C and Li A P 2001 Species comparison in P450 induction: effects of dexamethasone, omeprazole, and rifampin on P450 isoforms 1A and 3A in primary cultured hepatocytes from man, Sprague–Dawley rat, minipig, and beagle dog *Chem. Biol. Interact.* **134** 271–81
[38] Gerets H H J, Tilmant K, Gerin B, Chanteux H, Depelchin B O and Dhalluin S *et al* 2012 Characterization of primary human hepatocytes, HepG2 cells, and HepaRG cells at the mRNA level and CYP activity in response to inducers and their predictivity for the detection of human hepatotoxins *Cell Biol. Toxicol.* **28** 69–87
[39] Kitani H, Sakuma C, Takenouchi T, Sato M, Yoshioka M and Yamanaka N 2014 Establishment of c-myc-immortalized Kupffer cell line from a C57BL/6 mouse strain *Res. Immunol.* **4** 68–74
[40] Friedman S L 2008 Hepatic stellate cells: protean, multifunctional, and enigmatic cells of the liver *Physiol. Rev.* **88** 125–72
[41] Takayama K, Inamura M, Kawabata K, Katayama K, Higuchi M and Tashiro K *et al* 2012 Efficient generation of functional hepatocytes from human embryonic stem cells and induced pluripotent stem cells by HNF4α transduction *Mol. Ther.* **20** 127–37
[42] Duan Y, Catana A, Meng Y, Yamamoto N, He S and Gupta S *et al* 2007 Differentiation and enrichment of hepatocyte-like cells from human embryonic stem cells *in vitro* and *in vivo* *Stem Cells* **25** 3058–68
[43] HUREL® micro livers https://hurel.visikol.com/ (accessed 24 June 2023)
[44] Heidi A H T, Cui B, Chu Z E, Veres T and Radisic M 2009 Cell culture chips for simultaneous application of topographical and electrical cues enhance phenotype of cardiomyocytes *Lab Chip* **9** 564–75
[45] Ahn S, Ardoña H A M, Lind J U, Eweje F, Kim S L and Gonzalez G M *et al* 2018 Mussel-inspired 3D fiber scaffolds for heart-on-a-chip toxicity studies of engineered nanomaterials *Anal Bioanal. Chem.* **410** 6141–54

[46] Lind J U, Busbee T A, Valentine A D, Pasqualini F S, Yuan H and Yadid M *et al* 2017 Instrumented cardiac microphysiological devices via multimaterial three-dimensional printing *Nat. Mater.* **16** 303–8

[47] Valo | This is Intelligent Health https://valohealth.com/ (accessed 24 June 2023)

[48] Ren K, Zhou J and Wu H 2013 Materials for microfluidic chip fabrication *Acc. Chem. Res.* **46** 2396–406

[49] Zhang M, Xu C, Jiang L and Qin J 2018 A 3D human lung-on-a-chip model for nanotoxicity testing *Toxicol Res.* **7** 1048–60

[50] Zamprogno P, Wüthrich S, Achenbach S, Thoma G, Stucki J D and Hobi N *et al* 2021 Second-generation lung-on-a-chip with an array of stretchable alveoli made with a biological membrane *Commun. Biol.* **4** 1–10

[51] Francis I, Shrestha J, Paudel K R, Hansbro P M, Warkiani M E and Saha S C 2022 Recent advances in lung-on-a-chip models *Drug Discov Today* **27** 2593–602

[52] Zhang M, Wang P, Luo R, Wang Y, Li Z and Guo Y *et al* 2021 Biomimetic human disease model of SARS-CoV-2-induced lung injury and immune responses on organ chip system *Adv. Sci.* **8** 2002928

[53] Biospecimens and Research Services | BioIVT https://bioivt.com/ (accessed 24 June 2023)

[54] AlveoliX — *in vitro* models inspired by nature https://alveolix.com/ (accessed 24 June 2023)

[55] Ramadan Q and Zourob M 2020 Organ-on-a-chip engineering: toward bridging the gap between lab and industry *Biomicrofluidics.* **14** 041501

[56] Cho S and Yoon J Y 2017 Organ-on-a-chip for assessing environmental toxicants *Curr. Opin. Biotechnol.* **45** 34

[57] Zarrintaj P, Saeb M R, Stadler F J, Yazdi M K, Nezhad M N and Mohebbi S *et al* 2022 Human organs-on-chips: a review of the state-of-the-Art, current prospects, and future challenges. Adv. *Biol.* **6** 2000526

[58] NA3RsC | Advancing Science, Innovation & Research Animal Welfare—NA3RsC https://na3rsc.org/ (accessed 25 January 2023)

[59] Home—EUROoCS https://euroocs.eu/ (accessed 25 January 2023)

[60] The Organ-on-a-Chip Technologies Network https://organonachip.org.uk/ (accessed 25 January 2023)

[61] Emulating Human Biology—TissUse GmbH https://tissuse.com/en/ (accessed 24 June 2023)

[62] MesoBioTech—Inspiration, Invention, and Innovation https://mesobiotech.com/ (accessed 24 June 2023)

[63] Low L A, Mummery C, Berridge B R, Austin C P and Tagle D A 2020 Organs-on-chips: into the next decade *Nat. Rev. Drug Dis.* **20** 345–61

[64] Organ-On-Chip Market Value | Size | Share | 2030 https://datamintelligence.com/research-report/organ-on-chip-market (accessed 25 January 2023)

[65] Lauterbur P C 1973 Image formation by induced local interactions: examples employing nuclear magnetic resonance *Nature* **242** 190–1

[66] Rinck P A 2018 *Magnetic Resonance in Medicine : A Critical Introduction: The Basic Textbook of the European Magnetic Resonance Forum* (The Round Table Foundation) pp 375–90

[67] Rabi I I, Zacharias J R, Millman S and Kusch P 1938 A new method of measuring nuclear magnetic moment *Phys. Rev.* **53** 318

[68] NMR in cancer: XVI. FONAR image of the live human body—PubMed https://pubmed.ncbi.nlm.nih.gov/909957/ (accessed 25 January 2023)Damadian R, Goldsmith M and

Minkoff L 1977 NMR in cancer: XVI. FONAR image of the live human body *Physiol. Chem. Phys.* **9** 97–100
[69] Mansfield P and Grannell P K 1975 'Diffraction' and microscopy in solids and liquids by NMR *Phys. Rev.* B **12** 3618–34
[70] Featured history: magnetic resonance imaging—UW radiology https://rad.washington.edu/blog/featured-history-magnetic-resonance-imaging/ (accessed 25 January 2023)
[71] Ladd M E, Bachert P, Meyerspeer M, Moser E, Nagel A M and Norris D G *et al* 2018 Pros and cons of ultra-high-field MRI/MRS for human application *Prog. Nucl. Magn. Reson. Spectrosc.* **109** 1–50
[72] Zhuang Y, Potchen M J, Kampondeni S D, Tivarus M, Birbeck G L and Zhong J 2018Jan1 Validation of diffusion measurements obtained on a 0.35 T MR in Malawi: Important insights for radiologists in low income settings with low field MRI *Magn. Reson. Imaging* **45** 120–8
[73] Lee S K, Mathieu J B, Graziani D, Piel J, Budesheim E and Fiveland E *et al* 2016 Peripheral nerve stimulation characteristics of an asymmetric head-only gradient coil compatible with a high-channel-count receiver array *Magn. Reson. Med.* **76** 1939–50
[74] Glover G H 2011 Overview of functional magnetic resonance imaging *Neurosurg. Clin. N. Am.* **22** 133–9
[75] MRI corticography: developing next generation microscale human cortex MRI scanner | Brain Initiative https://braininitiative.nih.gov/funded-awards/mri-corticography-developing-next-generation-microscale-human-cortex-mri-scanner (accessed 25 January 2023)
[76] Norris D G, Koopmans P J, Boyacioğlu R and Barth M 2011 Power independent of number of slices (PINS) radiofrequency pulses for low-power simultaneous multislice excitation *Magn. Reson. Med.* **66** 1234–40
[77] Mansfield P, Morris P G, Ordidge R J, Pykett I L, Bangert V and Coupland R E 1980 Human whole body imaging and detection of breast tumours by NMR *Philos. Trans. R. Soc. Lond. B. Biol. Sci.* **289** 503–10
[78] Stark H and Yudilevich E 1988 Spiral sampling: theory and an application to magnetic resonance imaging *J. Opt. Soc. Am.* A **5** 542–53
[79] Davids M, Guérin B, vom Endt A, Schad L R and Wald L L 2019 Prediction of peripheral nerve stimulation thresholds of MRI gradient coils using coupled electromagnetic and neurodynamic simulations *Magn. Reson. Med.* **81** 686–701
[80] Zhang B, Yen Y F, Chronik B A, McKinnon G C, Schaefer D J and Rutt B K 2003 Peripheral nerve stimulation properties of head and body gradient coils of various sizes *Magn. Reson. Med.* **50** 50–8
[81] MRI systems market share, growth and demand forecast to 2030 https://psmarketresearch.com/market-analysis/mri-market (accessed 25 January 2023)
[82] Magnetic resonance imaging (MRI) systems market forecast 2030 https://alliedmarketresearch.com/magnetic-resonance-imaging-mri-systems-market (accessed 25 January 2023)
[83] Magnetic resonance imaging market size, share report, 2030 https://grandviewresearch.com/industry-analysis/magnetic-resonance-imaging-market (accessed 25 January 2023)
[84] Madhavan M, Mulpuru S K, McLeod C J, Cha Y M and Friedman P A 2017 Advances and future directions in cardiac pacemakers: part 2 of a 2-part series *J. Am. Coll. Cardiol.* **69** 211–35
[85] Pacemaker market size, share & growth analysis report, 2030 https://grandviewresearch.com/industry-analysis/pacemaker-market (accessed 28 June 2023)

[86] Fotiadis D I, Glaros C and Likas A 2006 Wearable medical devices *Wiley Encyclopedia of Biomedical Engineering* (Wiley)
[87] AI medical documentation for physicians & hospitals | augmedix. https://augmedix.com/ (accessed 24 June 2023)
[88] Neurotech EEG | EEG Monitoring Company. https://neurotecheeg.com/ (accessed 24 June 2023)
[89] About us | Hinge Health https://hingehealth.com/about/ (accessed 24 June 2023)
[90] GraphLAB | GFET | Grapheal | France https://grapheal.com/graphlab (accessed 24 June 2023)
[91] ReTiSense | stridalyzer sensor insoles—sensor insoles for gait research, physiotherapy, runners and rehab https://retisense.com/ (accessed 24 June 2023)
[92] Wearable tech in healthcare: smart medical devices & trends in 2023 https://insiderintelligence.com/insights/wearable-technology-healthcare-medical-devices/ (accessed 25 January 2023)
[93] Wearable medical devices market size, demand & trend | FMI https://futuremarketinsights.com/reports/wearable-medical-devices-market (accessed 25 January 2023)
[94] Medical devices medical device coordination group document
[95] Home | beta https://clinicaltrials.gov/ (accessed 28 June 2023)
[96] Karatas M, Eriskin L, Deveci M, Pamucar D and Garg H 2022 Big data for healthcare industry 4.0: applications, challenges and future perspectives *Expert Syst. Appl.* **200** 116912

IOP Publishing

Advances in Drug Delivery Systems for Healthcare
From concept to clinic
Piyush Pradeep Mehta and Arpana Parihar

Chapter 15

Human ergonomics in healthcare system: applications and challenges

Kalpesh V Bhavsar, Priya Singh, Angela Shony and M Sureshchandra

In this chapter, human ergonomics is introduced as an influential discipline that addresses the intricate interactions within a healthcare system. It investigates the incorporation of ergonomics into the healthcare system by highlighting elements that constitute the work system model and further categorizing the diverse domains of application within the ergonomic field, including physical, cognitive, and organizational aspects. It delves into the physical domain, focusing on designing workspaces and equipment to optimize human performance and minimize physical strain and injury risks. Evolving design principles and innovative ergonomic interventions such as robotic surgery, 3D printing, and artificial intelligence (AI) have been reported to be revolutionizing the healthcare industry by improving automation, personalization, and precision. When designing clinical decision support systems and enhancing user experiences, cognitive ergonomics places a strong emphasis on understanding human perception, natural motor responses, memory, and decision-making processes. By applying cognitive ergonomics principles, the chapter highlights how healthcare professionals' cognitive workload and potential errors can be reduced, ultimately improving patient care outcomes. Within the organizational domain, the chapter addresses the design of work systems, policies, and procedures to optimize healthcare delivery. It describes strategies to enhance workflow efficiency, staffing levels, and task allocation and further underscores the importance of creating supportive work environments that foster teamwork, communication, and employee wellbeing. Together, these domains provide a comprehensive overview of the multidimensional aspects of ergonomics in healthcare contexts. Ultimately, the chapter reports some of the most significant challenges associated with the widespread adoption of human ergonomics within the healthcare system. It covers impediments such as resistance to change, lack of standardized processes, intricate and slowly changing health legislation, and technical and environmental variables. By recognizing these challenges, the chapter seeks to offer insights and recommendations for overcoming major obstacles, thus advancing the integration of ergonomics principles in healthcare settings.

15.1 Introduction

Ergonomics is a highly interdisciplinary field which is steadily being recognized and adopted within the healthcare industry. The term ergonomics, comes from the Greek word *ergon* meaning work and *nomos* meaning laws, which translates to 'the science of work' [1]. The IEA (International Ergonomics Association) provides the ergonomics definition such as: 'Ergonomics is the field of science which deals with the humans interactions with different elements of a system, and the profession that relates data, principles, designing methods and theory to optimize human welfare and in general system performance' [2].

When the subject of ergonomics was evolving, academics from different fields around the world titled this area of study from a number of facets; as a result, many related subject titles appeared. As ergonomics draws from diverse fields of study, including anthropometry, biomechanics, engineering, industrial design, psychology, physiology, and occupational health and safety, its definition was fluid and subject to frequent revision [3]. 'Ergonomics' was originally known as 'human factor science' or 'human factor engineering,' 'engineering psychology,' or 'man-machine-environment system engineering' [4]. In essence, ergonomics refers to the art and science of designing and structuring systems in a way that humans can safely and effectively optimize their health and general wellbeing.

The tenets of ergonomics are based on sociotechnical principles. The foundational concepts are rooted in regarding humans as assets, promoting sustainability and quality of life, considering accountability to all stakeholders, respecting individual diversity, and using technology as a tool to aid humans [5]. Ergonomics encourages the development of safe and dependable work systems through a unique convergence of fundamental drivers. Design is the driving force behind ergonomics, which takes a systems-based approach and ultimately focuses on maximizing the two interconnected goals of performance and wellbeing [6].

One of the major industries in the world is healthcare, employing around 59 million individuals globally across a range of professions and occupations [7]. The large and diverse sector of healthcare encompasses a diverse array of services and products focused on promoting health, preventing and treating illness and injury, and improving quality of life. It includes hospitals, independent clinics, pharmaceutical firms, nursing homes, rehabilitation facilities, manufacturers of medical devices and equipment, and more. The industry is also heavily regulated and influenced by government policies and market forces such as competition and consumer demand. Between 2021 and 2031, a 13% increase in employment in the healthcare industry is anticipated, generating more than 2 million job opportunities [8].

Although the healthcare sector is vital to safeguarding the health of individuals and communities and contributes significantly to the global economy, millions of fatalities in countries with low and moderate incomes are attributable to subpar medical care and misapplication of the healthcare system [9]. Research has indicated a significantly high-mortality rate caused by low-quality healthcare, about 8.6 million deaths are amenable to healthcare of which 5.0 million are caused by subpar quality of care and 3.6 million fatalities resulting from lack of usage of healthcare services [10]. Many patients are susceptible to medical-related mishaps, and even high-income countries confront a considerable death rate from poor management and misdiagnosis. The same report published by WHO emphasizes that the integration of high-quality healthcare systems could possibly prevent millions of fatalities annually. These figures represent the significance of rebuilding and engineering high-quality healthcare systems which can be rendered feasible by incorporating ergonomics research in the healthcare systems [10].

Healthcare, as an industry, is uniquely positioned to gain from the field of ergonomics since it is a human-centred and human-driven industry [11]. Ergonomics serves a critical role in the healthcare system since it centres on optimizing the interactions between people, the tasks they perform, and the dynamics of their working environment [12].

The healthcare sector began to place more emphasis on ergonomics concepts midway through the 20th century [13]. As the implications of working environments on the productivity and health of healthcare personnel became more generally recognized, ergonomics in healthcare began to take shape. In 1991, Paris played host to the first inaugural conferences on ergonomics in healthcare. Francois Daniellou founded the Technical Committee on Healthcare Ergonomics and Patient Safety under the International Ergonomics Association [14]. Thereafter, since 2005, conferences conducted on clinical patient safety issues have briefly addressed and included sessions and papers on patient safety ergonomics in healthcare. Ergonomics gained relevance in the healthcare sector as a way to enhance patient care and outcomes while also promoting healthcare professionals' wellbeing.

Pandemics and epidemics change healthcare dynamics and highlight the crucial role of ergonomics as they pressurize the building of more dependable and high-quality health services to safeguard the general populace and prevent further outbreaks [15]. A strong health system can quickly detect and respond to outbreaks, provide adequate medical care and resources, and effectively communicate with the public to reduce panic and misinformation. In contrast, underdeveloped health systems struggle to handle the burden of epidemics and may exacerbate the situation, leading to higher mortality rates and further spread of the disease. Such circumstances illustrate the need for creating ergonomic solutions that can adapt to accommodate the changing requirements of patient care [16].

Healthcare facilities, for instance, had to adjust to new problems during the Covid-19 pandemic and put in place infection control procedures that lower the high risk of transmission [17]. Ergonomic design principles were used for the creation and implementation of safety measures like touchless technology, redesigning workstations to achieve physical distancing, and designing practical, accessible, and easy-to-wear personal protection equipment kits [18]. The pandemic further uncovered the need for ergonomic solutions to address the crisis of limited healthcare resources like ventilators. The design of ergonomic devices, such as ventilators with ergonomic interfaces, allowed healthcare professionals to provide life-saving care to critically ill patients. Significant issues were addressed by adopting strategies to minimize the demand for mechanical ventilators, boost supply and generate new supply, and staff supply adequately [19].

This chapter briefly explores the integration of ergonomics in the healthcare system by outlining factors that contribute to the work system and detailing the several domains of ergonomic applications. Special emphasis is placed on the function of ergonomics for the enhancement of healthcare work systems and procedures. The chapter concludes by examining some of the most important impediments to the widespread use of human factor ergonomics within the healthcare system.

15.2 Application

Healthcare, as a service industry, is a highly complex system because there are so many different layers of variation in every aspect of healthcare. Each facet of healthcare has its own complexity [20]. Many more layers become discernible as different components of the greater healthcare system interact with each other. A wide variety of concerns are addressed by the application of ergonomics in healthcare, with an emphasis on patient safety, health technology including clinical decision support, medical devices, and electronic health records (EHRs), as well as process enhancements for caregiving.

In order to effectively incorporate human ergonomics into healthcare, it is crucial to first identify the multiple external, interface, and internal stakeholders [21]. A stakeholder of human factor ergonomics in a healthcare system can be defined as any individual or group that can either have a direct or indirect influence on, is affected by, or believes they are affected by decisions or actions of healthcare system engineering [22, 23]. In the context of healthcare, interconnected stakeholders include *system decision makers*, such as directors, healthcare managers, and administrators, who determines the requirements for the development, implementation, acquisition, and usage of the system; *system influencers*, such as competent authorities like autonomous or government bodies such as Ministry of Health and Family Welfare, other regulatory agencies, and standardization organizations at national and regional levels; and, lastly, *system niche experts*, responsible for managing microsystems in line with their area of competence such as physicians, psychologists, industrial design engineers, and certified human factor engineering specialists, etc.

15.2.1 Work system models in healthcare system

Professionals in the healthcare industry, executives, and regulatory bodies acknowledge the significance of human factor engineering as an area of study in the sciences that can provide information to rethink healthcare operations and procedures to enhance patient safety and treatment quality [24–26]. The term 'work system' describes the intricate network of interrelated components of a system that function together to execute a task or achieve a goal. The work system in healthcare systems involves not only the healthcare workers but also the equipment, technology, rules, and setting in which they operate [26, 27]. For instance, the patient-centred medical home (PCMH) model encompasses the following [28, 29]:

- People: Medical professionals, nurses, and all staff members from the primary clinics constitute the entire healthcare team. Hiring supervisors, whose main duty is caring coordination, is frequently essential for implementing patient-focused medical facilities. The medical home personnel include patients and their family members looking after them.
- Tasks: The actions and duties that healthcare professionals take while providing primary care services are referred to as tasks. These duties involve carrying out patient evaluations, creating care plans, organizing the provision of treatment, educating patients, and keeping track of patients' progress.
- Tools and technologies: Tools, frameworks, and procedures employed by healthcare experts to facilitate the provision of primary care services are covered under this element. The resources include clinical decision support tools, patient portals, telehealth technologies, EHRs, and medical devices.
- Physical environment: This refers to the physical space infrastructure where primary care services are provided by healthcare professionals. It concerns the clinic's layout and design, including its temperature, air quality, lighting, noise levels, equipment, and supplies, as well as its safety and security.
- Organization: The organization and administration of the healthcare system that offers people primary care services are included. It involves management and leadership, rules and regulations, manpower and workload, instruction and training, and coordination and cooperation.

The SEIPS (Systems Engineering Initiative for Patient Safety) model is a framework used to investigate and remediate the work system in healthcare [30]. The concept of the SEIPS system model was developed by Carayon and Smith's macroergonomic work [31–33]. The SPO (Structure-Process-Outcome) model, devised by Donabedian in 1978, is yet another commonly recognized model of healthcare [34]. However, the SEIPS model, which combines the work system model and the SPO model of healthcare, is more widely and universally acknowledged in the industry. The salient features of this model include the following: elucidating the design of a work system along with its interrelated components, embodying the Donabedian-standard model, singling out processes impacting the work system, factoring organizational or personnel variables into account while assessing patient outcomes, and establishing feedback channels between operations and results [35]. People, activities, equipment, technologies, and environment were the four key focuses of the original SEIPS model, which was created in 2006 [36]. The evolution of both healthcare and technology, however, necessitated a change in the SEIPS paradigm. The SEIPS 3.0 model, which improved upon the previous model by adding a number of new features like organization, outcomes, and policies, was introduced in 2019. These newly added features take into account both the policies and procedures that govern healthcare delivery and the culture of healthcare organizations. It focuses on the rules, regulations, and policies that regulate

Table 15.1. An evaluation of performance obstacles through the application of work system model in healthcare system.

Work system, model factors	Performance obstacles	
	Example 1.1	Example 1.2
People	Lack of training in health IT, Knowledge gaps	Unprofessional behaviour
Tasks	Managing and processing patient-related information such as the requirement for repeated data entry in several health IT programmes	Heavy workload
Tools and technologies	Issues with technological design, such as poor reaction times	Inadequate usability
Physical environment	Restricted physical accessibility to computers	Unorganized work space
Organization	Ineffective application of health IT, and ineffective access to patient data	Lack of adherence to rules, system of hierarchy

healthcare delivery, including ethical and professional standards that healthcare workers are supposed to uphold. It also emphasizes reducing healthcare costs and increasing patient satisfaction [37].

To illustrate the application of the work system model in a healthcare system, consider following example 1.1 in table 15.1. In a study [38, 39], an analysis of the performance barriers faced by supervisors who oversee patients with chronic illnesses as they transitioned from hospital was investigated. The study focused on the use of many health-related IT apps by care coordinators which revealed the performance barriers listed below in table 15.1. Consider yet another instance (example 1.2). In order to identify possible risks to patient safety during the perioperative period following cardiac surgery, a multidisciplinary team of investigators—including ergonomic specialists and systems design engineers—conducted a descriptive study. Based on information from 20 cardiac operations, 58 kinds of challenges were found across all work system components [40–42], summarized in table 15.1.

As stated by the International Ergonomics Association, three types of work factors that the ergonomics field addresses are physical, cognitive, and organizational [43]. These aspects will be briefly discussed in this section from the perspective of the healthcare system.

15.2.2 Physical ergonomics

Designing workplaces and technologies that are compatible with individuals' physical abilities and constraints is referred to as physical ergonomics. Ergonomic design plays an essential role in healthcare systems to ensure that healthcare employees are capable of carrying out their tasks safely and effectively without experiencing physical stress or harm [44]. It also entails instructing healthcare personnel in suitable lifting and movement practices, as well as creating workstations and equipment that promote good posture and minimize repetitive motions [45]. Healthcare organizations are likely to prevent several workplace injuries and enhance the general overall wellbeing of their workforce by implementing physical ergonomics concepts [46].

For primary care, consultation, and diagnosis of all types of discomfort and illnesses, patients approach hospitals. Hospitals and clinics frequently prioritize practicality and efficiency over human comfort, which results in ergonomic problems such as insufficient lighting, claustrophobic workplaces, and inadequate room for equipment installation. Medical equipment and tools are made with a generic approach, disregarding the diversity of human anatomy and size. Subsequently, the equipment may not fit well or be used correctly, increasing the risk of harm and decreasing patient comfort [47]. Nonetheless, the capacity to receive the required treatment promptly with minimal time and effort has been improved by advancements in healthcare facilities and medical technology, such as 3D printing, robotic surgery, information technology, etc. In the not-too-distant future, remote patient monitoring will be possible through using AI in healthcare. The breakthroughs in technology and medicine that support the implementation of this endeavour are discussed in this section.

15.2.2.1 Robotic surgery

Robotic surgery is a revolutionary technology that exemplifies the transformation of healthcare systems with the application of physical ergonomics [48]. Robotics is employed to aid or assist the surgeon during the surgical procedure and eventually shorten the patient's hospitalization and recuperation time [49]. This technique combines robotic arms and devices to execute surgical procedures with more control and precision than existing conventional practices like video-assisted surgeries [50]. Robotic surgery lessens the physical effort and exhaustion related to lengthy surgical procedures by enabling physicians to work from a comfortable, sitting position at a console. In addition, it operates with less intrusion than human-assisted surgery and the robotic arms mimic the natural human hand movements, lowering the possibility of human errors and hand tremors. Another benefit of robotic surgery is that it provides the physician with complete access and a wider panoramic view during the process [51].

Microsurgery using microrobots is currently used in a variety of medical procedures, including ophthalmology, neurology, urology, cardiology, and plastic surgery [52]. Recently, researchers developed a snake-like teleoperated robot to extract gastrointestinal tumour cells using least invasive approach of radiosurgery [53]. Many nations are implementing robotic surgery to improve their healthcare systems and the technology is gaining prominence around the world. The market for robotic surgery treatments was valued at USD 5.32 billion in 2019 and is anticipated to reach USD 19.03 billion in 2027, growing at a CAGR of 21.8% between 2020 and 2027 [54]. For instance, with approximately one million robotic operations conducted yearly in the United States [55], it is already a standard component of many surgical procedures. Other nations have also made large expenditures in robotic surgical technology, notably Japan and South Korea [56]. This technology is anticipated to enhance patient outcomes, boost efficiency, and decrease healthcare costs by minimizing hospital stays and the need for follow-up surgeries. Robotic surgery could potentially be improved further and become more readily available to medical professionals with the development of new technologies like haptic feedback systems and augmented reality [57]. Overall, there are a great deal of interesting developments in robotic surgery that point to a promising future.

15.2.2.2 3D printing

A number of industries, including healthcare, have been transformed by 3D printing, which is a form of additive manufacturing. This technology allows healthcare providers to design and manufacture customized products, improving the patient's comfort and overall functionality of medical equipment. Its application in healthcare is extensive, including the printing of casts for amputated limbs, the creation of human body parts, and the manufacturing of medical equipment, etc [58]. Medical equipment such as personalized implants, surgical instruments, implants and prostheses for cardiac, dental, and spinal disorders, among others, are created and tailored to the patient's unique anatomy utilizing 3D printers [59]. It also aids surgeons or medical students in practising before performing an actual operation, investigating potential issues by printing or duplicating various human parts, etc [60]. The *in vivo* behaviour of anti-malignant drugs can be assessed using 3D-printed models of the human heart, ear, limbs, and cancerous tumours [61, 62]. The tumour model aids physicians in their understanding of cancerous cells, their comprehension of current health status of the patient, and their application of appropriate patient care [63]. These printers also make it feasible to synthesize biomaterials for tissue engineering and organ regeneration, for instance, a 3D-printed heart valve can be generated by combining appropriate cardiac cells and polymeric scaffolds as biomaterials [64]. Customized models of patient-specific anatomical features can be made via 3D printing, which can help in the development and execution of personalized medical programmes [65]. For instance, to help in the visualization and comprehension of genetic mutations and variations, 3D printing can be utilized in personalized genomics to build physical representations of DNA sequences [66]. These simulations may be employed to educate patients and their families about hereditary disorders. In general, 3D printing is proving to be an invaluable tool for enhancing physical ergonomic in healthcare systems by enabling the development of customized solutions that are adapted to the patient's unique individual needs.

15.2.2.3 Information technology

Information technology (IT) may improve physical ergonomics by offering tools and systems that increase productivity and lessen physical stress on employees. For instance, EHRs can eliminate the need for manual paperwork and documentation, which can be physically and mentally demanding [67]. This enables healthcare professionals to devote more of their time and attention to providing patient care and less of it on administrative duties. It is crucial to manage and organize the vast amounts of data that are received and maintained at hospitals, laboratories, and various medical departments. Effective data management enables the emergency department of healthcare organizations and physicians to access prior medical records quickly, study the patient's medical history, and proceed with the necessary treatment or post-operative treatment [68].

A further proposal is that of employing sensors to transmit care so that patients receive the same treatment they would conventionally receive from hospitals in the convenience of their homes [69]. It is also a cost-effective alternative. Nanotechnology enables the creation of small, smart gadgets with sensors that can continuously monitor the wellbeing of an individual. Through the use of the appropriate sensors and biotelemetry, data on blood pressure, heart rate, oxygen saturation, and other parameters may be gathered [70]. Constant patient health monitoring is beneficial. For example, it can be applied for early detection of cardiovascular issues. These sensors may be easily found in wearable technology, such as smartwatches [71]. Increased accessibility of telecommunication has been rendered by the collaboration of several niche experts from different disciplines. Through telecommunication, e-healthcare enables doctors to obtain patient information from anywhere around the globe [72]. Mobile technology is used for m-healthcare. The need for healthcare workers to walk about the hospital or clinic to obtain information is reduced by the portability and usability of gadgets such as smartphones and tablets, which can be utilized at the point of service. Medical professionals are better equipped to quickly and accurately diagnose patients by using mobile devices to access medical imaging and diagnostic tools. This can lessen the need to physically move patients for testing and treatments within the hospital or clinic [73].

IT in healthcare has also made it feasible to develop treatments that have been reused and medications based on an individual's distinct gene structure. The development of repurposed drugs and medicines based on the individual gene structure is only possible because of IT in healthcare [74]. In summary, the use of IT in healthcare systems can provide significant physical ergonomic advancements for healthcare workers, by reducing the need for physical movement and offering features improving communication among healthcare workers.

15.2.2.4 Artificial intelligence

AI progress has been remarkably rapid in a short period of time. Heavy jobs like objection detection, voice recognition, translation, fraud prevention, self-driving vehicles, and many more may be handled by AI. After numerous years of research, AI is currently applied in healthcare systems in medical diagnosis, therapy, and medical care. Medical research and a patient's large volume data may be investigated by AI to generate scientific results that can be used to improve diagnosis and treatment [75].

AI is able to diagnose a disease by running a complex algorithm by using millions of patient imaging and other reports data that is extracted from EHRs. In radiology,

AI can identify tumours and categorize, characterize, and analyze images [76]. AI may be applied to medical imaging to help in the analysis of MRIs, x-rays, and CT scans, hence reducing the duration of time that healthcare professionals must devote to analyzing images. Healthcare professionals may identify patients who are at risk for specific illnesses and take early action to avoid problems by using AI in predictive analytics [77]. It also aids in toxicity assessment. By offering real-time monitoring and early warning systems that can identify possible problems before they become serious, AI can also assist to increase patient safety. This may lower the possibility of unfavourable consequences while also improving patient outcomes. After feeding the network a variety of clinical pictures of various skin conditions, machine learning is capable of detecting skin cancer like a dermatologist [78].

Another illustration demonstrates how AI was used to diagnose pneumonia on chest x-rays. AI was employed in a hybrid detection system that found both breast and colon cancer with satisfactory results [79]. Oxford University claims to have the most precise echocardiography software that uses machine learning to assist in the diagnosis of coronary heart disease [80]. A 3D echocardiography (3DE) system with real-time 3DE software was created by a medical university hospital in Italy to evaluate the left ventricular volume and ejection fraction. Results were improved and more precise as a consequence [81]. To identify blood infections, a microscope and AI were combined to create a gadget. Large portions of the samples were effectively categorized without any human intervention [82]. By eliminating the need for manual labour and routine activities, offering real-time monitoring and early warning systems, and aiding with the interpretation of patient data and medical pictures, AI can, overall, make major physical ergonomic gains in healthcare systems.

Several design principles are placed into practice under physical ergonomics: limiting screen time, reducing operation time, optimizing the scope of mobility, and minimizing the need for manual force [83]. Additionally, participatory ergonomics is an effective technique for including system users in the design process [84]. An ergonomics approach known as participatory ergonomics involves including participants of the system, such as physicians, other caregivers, and patients, during the spotting and evaluation of occupational risk factors along with assisting in the planning and execution of ergonomic solutions [85]. Participatory ergonomics in healthcare has taken on a number of physical ergonomic concerns, such as locating and putting into practice strategies to curtail musculoskeletal damage for nursing assistants in city hospitals [86], lowering the physical demands placed on community nurses [87], identifying variables that increase the likelihood of lower back discomfort in caretakers [88], altering the architectural style of hospital rooms and outpatient departments [89], and using assistive technologies to improve patient handling [90].

15.2.3 Cognitive ergonomics

Cognitive ergonomics is an investigation of the methods used to design and arrange work environments to maximize human cognitive skills and to advance employee wellbeing. It refers to the investigation of the elements influencing the stability of mental health like perception, motor response, and memory of the healthcare workers. It also includes human–computer interaction, decision-making, problem-solving and work stress [91]. The goal of cognitive ergonomics is to improve interactions among professionals, patients and other components of the healthcare system.

In the medical industry, mistakes and disputed choices are made often, leading to frequent contentious rulings. An individual in such a position of responsibility is expected to be in optimum form, which calls for them to have the tools necessary to fulfil their duties effectively [92]. An optimum level of cognitive processing, decision-making, and attention to detail are necessary for the demanding nature of the healthcare industry. The interruptions, information overload, and other cognitively taxing circumstances are related to weak job performance and low wellbeing at work [93]. Therefore, it is critical to reduce the negative effects they have on both organizations and employees. Principles of cognitive ergonomics can serve to enhance the working environment, lessen the cognitive load, and encourage better decision-making, which will lead to better patient outcomes and worker satisfaction [94]. This section will give an overview of cognitive ergonomics in healthcare systems, along with a summary of common issues and their proposed remedies.

Healthcare workers make several decisions during work that include judgements about anything from patient care in the medical environment to resource allocation in the administrative setting that can have significant consequences. They must be able to quickly and accurately process enormous amounts of information, recognize crucial facts, and take decisions under pressure [95]. Due to the nature of their work, healthcare workers are frequently exposed to emotionally taxing events, such as dealing with patient suffering or end-of-life care, and might experience emotional overload [96]. This may result in overwhelming sensations of stress and emotional tiredness. Workers experience stress constantly, and ongoing stress can result in problems with their mental and physical wellbeing, causing hypertension, insomnia, anxiety, and depression. The symptoms of burnout, a kind of persistent stress, include emotional depletion, depersonalization, and a diminished feeling of personal accomplishment. Burnout can cause cynicism, alienation, and a lack of empathy for patients, which can eventually result in inadequate care [97]. According to research published by the National Institute of Health in 2020, one in three physicians is experiencing burnout at any given time [98]. Healthcare organizations must therefore place a high priority on the health of their workforce by putting in place policies that encourage work–life balance, offer help and tools for coping with stress and emotional difficulties, and cultivate a culture of compassion and empathy [99].

Making effective sound decisions under a high-pressure environment is an essential skill for healthcare professionals, and processing a lot of information while providing high-quality care is a continual source of stress [100]. This might lead to high cognitive effort and increase the probability of errors. Cognitive ergonomics ideas are utilized to lessen the cognitive load on healthcare professionals by developing efficient and easy-to-use systems, reducing visual clutter, and streamlining information processing. Systems for communication are essential to decision-making in healthcare organizations. To encourage precise decision-making and reduce errors, effective communication is crucial. Systems for communication can be created to encourage productive dialogue and alleviate cognitive strain [101]. Communication systems might, for instance, utilize visual or aural signals to notify healthcare personnel of important information or standardized communication standards to encourage clear and succinct communication.

Designing clinical decision support systems (CDSSs) is one important way cognitive ergonomics is used in decision-making. Real-time data from CDSS can help decision-making and enhance healthcare outcomes. For instance, depending on patient data, CDSS might assist healthcare professionals in identifying potential medication interactions or recommending suitable therapies. Additionally, CDSS can offer decision support in the form of alerts, reminders, and suggestions, lowering cognitive load and improving the precision and effectiveness of decision-making [102, 103]. EHRs are a further variable that can aid in decision-making. EHRs can be made to assist with cognitive functions including prioritizing tasks, recalling information, and making decisions [104]. For instance, EHRs can warn healthcare professionals of possible medication oversights or remind them to do certain duties. EHRs can also make patient data easily accessible, lowering the cognitive strain involved in information retention. Additionally, training programmes may be created to enhance cognitive abilities including concentration, perception, and judgement. For instance, simulation-based training programmes can provide healthcare professionals with an opportunity to practise decision-making under pressure, enhancing their capacity to perform in practical settings [105, 106].

Human error is a major concern for healthcare systems since, it may happen at any point in the process, from diagnosis through treatment and follow-up care [107]. Errors encompass managerial errors, administrative errors, planning errors, and knowledge-based errors. Misdiagnosis, prescription mistakes, inaccurate charting, and poor intersystem communication are a few examples of human errors in the healthcare industry [108]. They may result from several reasons such as insufficient sleep, exhaustion, distractions, performance pressure, memory problems, knowledge gaps, inadequate training, poor communication, system flaws, etc Cognitive biases, which can result in mistakes in judgement and diagnostic reasoning, is also an issue among healthcare practitioners [109].

To prevent the occurrence of these human errors, numerous councils have implemented restrictions on the number of working hours per week, limitations on unnecessary conversations like the prohibition on answering phones in operating rooms, and many other such measures. The use of technology to support precise and timely decision-making, the creation of standard operating procedures to ensure consistency and reliability in healthcare processes, and continuous education and training for healthcare workers are all important measures to take in order to reduce human error in the industry. Service design, behavioural design, and interface design are the labels given to different precautionary approaches [110]. To find areas for improvement and stop recurring errors, healthcare organizations should also promote reporting of errors and near-misses. For instance, the ability of junior doctors to express their opinions and warn their superiors about any possible harm should not be curtailed.

To better understand the causes of accidents and injuries, a variety of models and methods for dealing with human error have been created. Rasmussen and Reason developed one of the most used human error models [111, 112]. In this concept, human error is divided into two categories: errors and slip-ups. Mistakes can then be divided into two categories: knowledge-based behaviour and rule-based behaviour [113]. Three phases are generally used for error recovery. The initial action is to identify the inaccuracies or immediate lapses. The second step is to explain the problem and its causes, and the third step is to take corrective action to return the situation to normal or at least minimize its effects, including recurrences, or even completely omit one or both of these final two steps [114].

Another prominent area in which cognitive ergonomics is used in the healthcare industry is the design of medical devices and equipment [115]. Healthcare workers employ different medical equipment, each having a unique interface and range of settings. Cognitive ergonomics concepts are used to create simple, intuitive, and user-friendly digital programmes that reduce the number of potential errors. This entails speeding the data-entering process and improving the structure and arrangement of the content. This design includes elements such as creating simple labelling and visual displays, streamlining control interfaces and providing users with consistent and comprehensible feedback [116].

In summary, by decreasing cognitive load, enhancing information processing, and fostering effective communication, cognitive ergonomic principles can aid in decision-making, process optimization, problem-solving ability, and the general wellbeing of healthcare professionals.

15.2.4 Organizational ergonomics

Organizational ergonomics relates to the application of ergonomic principles and practices inside organizations to enhance work practices, procedures, and services to provide improved performance, comfort, and safety [117]. Human ergonomics seeks to enhance performance by reducing errors and establishing a comfortable, secure environment for physicians, nurses, patients, and other workers. To ensure high-quality care, patient safety, and staff wellbeing, organizational ergonomics is crucial in healthcare systems. The key goals of human ergonomics in this context are process, product, training, and research to enhance patient safety, workflow efficiency, and the sociotechnical health system [118].

The definition of a work team is 'a small, interconnected group of individuals who are jointly responsible for the outcomes of their corporations.' [119] The healthcare team is viewed as a system made up of many people who collaborate to offer patients healthcare services. Individuals work together in groups in a range of contexts, such interdisciplinary teams that care for patients with certain clinical conditions and operating room crews. A variety of specialities and educational backgrounds are frequently represented in healthcare teams [120]. The workload, resources, leadership, and organizational culture are a few examples of the many variables that can affect the complex and dynamic healthcare system. To ensure that the system operates at its most efficient level and serves the needs of patients, it has to be managed, planned, and monitored effectively by adopting teamwork models.

Our understanding of teamwork in the healthcare sector has benefitted enormously from the ergonomic discipline, as well as from the scientific study of collaborative thinking and performance as a team. A three-dimension model of collaboration in healthcare has been presented by Salas and colleagues [121]. It consists of three components: cooperation, coordination, and communication. They further proposed several approaches for improving collaboration based on data for each aspect. A systematic methodology called Team Strategies and Tools to Enhance Performance and Patient Safety (TeamSTEPPSTM), developed by major agencies, has been embraced by several organizations as a useful strategy for improving teamwork and cooperative reasoning in the healthcare systems [122]. Consequently, TeamSTEPPS^{TM} is used as educational material to enhance patient outcomes by promoting cooperation among healthcare personnel [123]. It has been extensively used throughout the healthcare industry, especially in hospital units like critical care units [124].

To facilitate communication between healthcare practitioners, the Situation-Background-Assessment-Recommendation (SBAR) model is used in organizational ergonomics [125]. The SBAR approach offers a standardized framework for communicating vital details regarding a patient's health and strives to ensure that crucial information is not overlooked, particularly during handoffs and transition of care. It enables important data to be communicated during care transitions in a clear and succinct way, reducing the likelihood of errors and increasing patient outcomes. The SBAR approach is especially helpful when speaking with patients and their families or in interdisciplinary team meetings. Another model used to enable successful communication and information exchange during patient handoffs is I-PASS [126]. The acronym stands for 'Identify, Prioritize, Analyze, Select, and Solve.'

A data-driven strategy utilized in healthcare organizational ergonomics to raise care quality and productivity is the Lean Six Sigma model [127]. The Plan-Do-Study-Act (PDSA) cycle of continuous improvement is used in the model to find and eliminate waste in healthcare procedures [128]. By analyzing data and finding areas for improvement using statistical techniques, the model seeks to improve system outcomes [129]. Healthcare operations are streamlined and variability is decreased using Lean Six Sigma methods like process mapping and value stream mapping [130]. Healthcare providers may provide high-quality treatment while keeping expenses to a minimum by increasing efficiency and minimizing waste.

Patient safety is the first priority of the healthcare industry. To emphasize the necessity of describing, measuring, and analyzing many system levels in patient safety, Karsh and Brown suggested a macroergonomic model [131]. This model was further improved to include descriptions of the three levels of systemic assessment: microergonomics, mesoergonomics, and macroergonomics [132]. Additionally, Rasmussen lists the following as sociotechnical elements that affect patient safety: the government, regulators and associations, the firm, management, personnel, and work [133]. Inefficiency and accidents are a result of interactions and influences between these many sociotechnical elements across time.

Organizational ergonomics may help achieve the objective of patient safety by lowering the likelihood of medical mistakes, unfavourable outcomes, and occupational accidents. Take the case of a healthcare institution that introduces a new kind of infusion pump but does not provide adequate training and guidance to operators, thus jeopardizing patient safety [134]. The implementation of organizational ergonomics requires ongoing education and training for managers, leaders, and healthcare experts. Redesigning a work system is a dynamic process that necessitates extensive learning and continuous adaptation. This includes using ergonomic tools and goods, learning about ergonomic concepts, and following safe and effective work procedures [135]. In order to educate various sections, including medical residents, nurses, and other leaders in healthcare, several healthcare organizations and medical colleges have made attempts to combine problem-based learning (PBL) and scenario simulations. Additionally, each of them receives customized content training based on their individual interests, knowledge, and skills. Examples of residency requirements include methods for illness recognition, diagnosis, and treatment, patient safety, etc. Manikins, patients, trainers, and even cadaveric material are used in these training exercises and simulations [136]. Furthermore, modifying the system to build ergonomic workstations, tools, and equipment can reduce the physical stress placed on healthcare professionals, lowering the likelihood of musculoskeletal problems and repetitive stress injuries [137]. Consequently, there would be a lower chance of medical mistakes and unfavourable outcomes brought on by exhaustion or discomfort.

It is also essential to assess the patient's journey through time and across various treatment settings to comprehend the patient's point of view. The patient journey was described by Carayon and Wooldridge as the spatial and temporal distribution of a patient's encounters with various treatment settings throughout time [138]. Patient journey mapping is a technique used for comprehending and analyzing a patient's journey with the goal of improving patient experience while also enhancing the quality of treatment and increasing the efficacy of the healthcare system [139].

Resilience engineering is one ergonomic safety technique that has been developed and examined in light of unprecedented disease outbreaks and pandemics [140, 141]. The ability of an organization to function despite changes or disruptions, regardless of time constraints and limited resources, has been termed resilience. Workplace variables can either increase or decrease resilience. To increase patient safety in emergency circumstances, the Crisis Resource Management (CRM) model is a collaboration and communication training methodology used in healthcare organizational ergonomics [142]. The approach places a strong emphasis on fostering abilities including situational awareness, communication, leadership, and decision-making. The CRM concept entails teaching healthcare professionals skills to successfully collaborate in high-stress circumstances and make optimum use of the resources at hand. The methodology places a strong emphasis on the value of debriefing and continual development to identify problem areas and draw lessons from past mistakes [143].

A fundamental principle of organizational transformation is user or employee participation. The advantages of job involvement are theoretically and empirically supported. Benefits include improved performance and worker health, higher employee motivation and job satisfaction, quicker organizational and technical change implementation, and more complete ergonomic issue identification and solution development [144]. Feedback is a crucial component of behaviour modification and has been highlighted as a key organizational design component in the healthcare industry [145]. Any implementation process needs good communication between team members, decision makers, and technical support. Successful implementations depend on the principles and techniques of project management [146–148]. A few of the essentials for a successful implementation project include identifying a capable and experienced clinician leader to spearhead the initiative, recruiting a full-time project manager to run the project, and putting together a team of specialists, executive, and technical staff members to serve as the leading committee members.

The commitment of senior management is a requirement for adoption of aforementioned principles covered in this section. The existence of a structured implementation plan is a key sign of senior management commitment [149, 150]. An ideal management committee makes resources available to support new implementation design techniques and ensure that the deployment is successful. Eventually, organizational characteristics that define a successful implementation of a redesigned work system are quantifiable metrics like decreased or limited negative effects on healthcare workers, such as stress and dissatisfaction, and on the organization, such as delays, costs, and decreased performance, as well as more advantageous consequences on individuals, such better work control, willingness to embrace change, and enhanced personal performance.

15.3 Challenges

Regardless of its many merits, applying human ergonomics to healthcare can be challenging. Numerous constraints must be overcome to implement and enforce a shift in healthcare systems. In addition to complicated and slowly evolving health policies, technical and environmental factors also affect advancements in the healthcare industry. Healthcare requirements inevitably evolve as society does. Changes in our healthcare system as a whole are challenged by surges of pandemics, advancing diagnosis techniques, technological advancements and demographics, lack of standardized procedures, and changing healthcare regulations and policies. In this section, some of the contributing factors to this ongoing divergence between the culture of healthcare and ergonomics are reported.

To begin with, nomenclature and definitions, particularly with respect to the word 'system,' is an inconsistent point where ergonomics and healthcare systems contradict. The term 'system' is frequently used and ambiguous in the healthcare sector to describe a broad spectrum of concepts are only loosely related to ergonomic standards [151, 152]. The systems theory viewpoint on the healthcare sector reveals the inherent limited understanding of interrelated connections between engineering, organizational, and behavioural elements [153].

The operations of the healthcare sector are complicated to define because they encompass several different tasks, resources, and amenities that can be provided in several locations, including homes, clinics, operating rooms, and retail pharmacies. Many different occupations fall under the various categories of the health services sector, including management, business, and financial occupations; professional practitioners, research and development scientists; service occupations, and office and administrative support roles. To restructure healthcare systems, structures, and processes, there is a need for more collaboration and partnerships across these domains [154]. The peculiarities of the healthcare system as a workplace, industry, and institution add to this ongoing estrangement. There are many issues that make the integration of ergonomic professionals challenging and lack of explicit understanding of each domain's relationship to the other is one significant factor.

Applying human factors concepts to the healthcare industry will be different from applying them to other sectors because of the social and organizational settings, particularly the deeply engrained discounting of external knowledge. Human beings are the foundation of healthcare; they are exceedingly diverse and need a variety of transformation processes, which may be very challenging to specify in advance or rigorously design. Recognizing the distinctive degree of unpredictability, inconsistency, and dynamism that is a part of the healthcare work system is incredibly challenging. Clinical work in healthcare is very adaptable, seeking the optimal result based on the unique circumstances of the patient. For instance, consider two individuals with the same illness being examined in the same healthcare setting. Their medical histories and other subjective traits could possibly be different. These factors might further complicate clinical practice and dictate various therapy paths. In many areas of healthcare operations, due to unexpected consequences that may arise from a one-size-fits-all approach, standardization becomes implausible [155].

Ergonomic programme design and execution are not standardized, which results in inconsistent procedures among healthcare institutions [156]. Even from the most fundamental system engineering-based perspectives, where known inputs and outputs are acquired through an engineered transformation process, the healthcare industry differs from all other industries. It is also uncertain that understanding the workings of one healthcare environment will be easily transferrable to other equivalent settings, even within the same healthcare institutions. Most physicians only scale their expertise to the breadth of their microsystem, thus making it challenging to acquire accurate information about any system's operation. The lack of sustainability is more frequently linked to employee non-compliance than to the widespread ignorance of ergonomic basic concepts in the healthcare sector [157].

An indicator of healthcare organizations is the frequency of medical malpractice lawsuits and claims. In 2022, the World Health Organization issued a warning that medical misconduct injured more than 138 million people annually. Inaccuracies in diagnosis, discrepancies in pharmaceutical prescriptions and treatments, and improper use of medication are the three primary causes of harm [158]. Due to the healthcare systems' inadequate readiness to handle and address these incidents, these tragedies happen more frequently. One of the reasons for these accidents is that certain institutions lack a clearly defined hierarchy or have inadequate worker communication. A Geneva-based organization estimates that errors, including improper prescriptions for medications, account for $42 billion in healthcare expenses globally [159].

As the population ages and becomes more dependent on programmes like Medicare and Medicaid, the healthcare industry and patient care requirements will change [160]. The ageing population and the rising prevalence of chronic conditions like obesity and arthritis pose a significant challenge for the healthcare industry. It is crucial to take into account potential increases in the demand for workers, medical costs, the older population's increased need for assisted living facilities, and a disparity caused by shifting reliance ratios between the working class and elderly professionals who require medical care [161–163].

The evolving needs and requirements of patients are one of many factors that cause changes in the demands placed on the healthcare system. New solutions and treatments are developed for treatment of prevalent ailments. Each of these developments has an effect on patients as well as the overall healthcare system. The healthcare system has to change in order to address diseases as they grow more prevalent. The Covid-19 outbreak serves as a case in point of how a disease can fundamentally alter the healthcare system by swiftly allocating all resources to tackle a pandemic [164]. Nevertheless, a new upcoming threat is always conceivable. Following the lessons drawn from the previous pandemic, the healthcare sector must identify these adverse parameters and should set supplies and resources in place to meet any anticipated surges.

In the healthcare system, health regulations and rules can pose an ergonomic difficulty in a number of areas, such as resource allocation, regulatory compliance, equipment design, and workforce considerations. Most healthcare reform projects, it has been noted, are bureaucratic dead ends despite being anchored on a consensus of principles [165].

The emergence of value-based quality metrics, evidence-based medicine, considering patient outcomes as the primary indicators of clinical performance illustrate the healthcare environment currently takes a reductionist stance rather than adopting a systemic approach [166–168]. This supports the idea that highly stringent control of the work system will prevent ingrained disharmony in order to deal with continually conflicting goals at the political and administrative levels. These healthcare industry-developed conceptions of labour, or *work as envisioned* do not accurately reflect the reality of healthcare work, or *work as done* [169].

Most healthcare organizations do not prioritize ergonomics in their workplace safety programs, and workers may not be trained on proper body mechanics and safe equipment use. An upcoming practice should be undertaken within the healthcare industry to hire ergonomic specialists in full-time roles inside hospitals and other clinical care-providing organizations as awareness of the crucial role that human factor engineering can play in safety and improvement initiatives among healthcare professionals [170]. Through embedded practice, these practitioners would provide a more complex awareness of the nuances of the language, methods, culture, roles and duties, illnesses, physiology, procedures, organization, and structure of the clinical environments. Interdisciplinary specialists should seek for events to signify the overall organizational gains from an embedded-human factor engineering engagement, and develop productive and efficient change management skills. Addressing these challenges can be complicated because one of the responsibilities is frequently to find proactive solutions to issues, which calls for innovation. On the whole, examining the intrinsic function of ergonomic discipline will furnish awareness for an advanced perspective on resolving these system-specific challenges and inadequacies discussed in this section.

15.4 Conclusion

Human ergonomics has the potential to positively impact and revolutionize the healthcare sector. Adopting ergonomic practices in healthcare concurrently improves worker sustainability, capability, and wellbeing while increasing performance and lowering both direct and indirect expenses resulting from lost productivity and subpar quality. Given that the challenges it tackles are fundamentally structural or systemic in origin, ergonomics takes a multidisciplinary approach to apply concepts and theories gathered from related areas of study to the development and assessment of tasks, products, and processes. Despite several challenges, human ergonomics in healthcare has substantial advantages that cannot be overlooked. The application of ergonomic principles can enhance patient safety, healthcare professionals' wellness, and the overall efficiency of an organization. Healthcare systems that are built using ergonomic principles would have greater performance and yield better return on investments. As a result, it is crucial that healthcare organizations give ergonomics special emphasis and strive to integrate this into their procedures and operations. Human factor engineering in the healthcare system is simply and without a doubt, solid industrial and sustainable business practice.

References

[1] Jastrzębowski W B 2000 An outline of ergonomics, or the science of work based upon the truths drawn from the Science of Nature *International Encyclopedia of Ergonomics and Human Factors* (Taylor & Francis)

[2] What Is Ergonomics (HFE)? | The international ergonomics association is a global federation of human factors/ergonomics societies, registered as a nonprofit organization in Geneva, Switzerland. https://iea.c.c./about/what-is-ergonomics/ (accessed 1 February 2023)

[3] Ghosh S, Bagchi A, Sen D and Bandyopadhyay P 2011 Ergonomics: a bridge between fundamentals and applied research *Indian J. Occup. Environ. Med.* **15** 14

[4] Licht D, Polzella D J, Boff K and Armstrong H G 1989 Human factors, ergonomics, and human factors engineering: an analysis of definitionsHuman factors, ergonomics, and human factors engineering: an analysis of definitions CSERIAC 89-01

[5] Kleiner B M, Hettinger L J, DeJoy D M, Huang Y H and Love P E D 2015 Sociotechnical attributes of safe and unsafe work systems *Ergonomics* **58** 635

[6] Singleton W T 2007 Ergonomics in systems design *Ergonomics* **10** 541–8

[7] Joseph B and Joseph M 2016 The health of the healthcare workers *Indian J. Occup. Environ. Med.* **20** 71

[8] *Healthcare Occupations: Occupational Outlook Handbook* U.S. Bureau of Labor Statistics https://bls.gov/ooh/healthcare/home.htm (accessed 2 April 2023)
[9] Kruk M E, Gage A D, Joseph N T, Danaei G, García-Saisó S and Salomon J A 2018 Mortality due to low-quality health systems in the universal health coverage era: a systematic analysis of amenable deaths in 137 countries *Lancet* **392** 2203
[10] Fact sheet: quality health services https://who.int/news-room/fact-sheets/detail/quality-health-services (accessed 2 April 2023)
[11] Bazzano A N, Martin J, Hicks E, Faughnan M and Murphy L 2017 Human-centred design in global health: a scoping review of applications and contexts *PLoS One* **12** 0186744
[12] Carayon P, Wetterneck T B, Rivera-Rodriguez A J, Hundt A S, Hoonakker P and Holden R *et al* 2014 Human factors systems approach to healthcare quality and patient safety *Appl. Ergon* **45** 14
[13] Fayomi O S I, Akande I G, Essien V, Asaolu A and Esse U C 2021 Advances in concepts of ergonomics with recent industrial revolution *IOP Conf. Ser.: Mater. Sci. Eng.* **1107** 012010
[14] Edworthy J, Hignett S, Hellier E and Stubbs D 2006 Patient safety *Ergonomics* **49** 439–43
[15] Wooldridge A R, Carman E M and Xie A 2022 Human factors and ergonomics (HFE) applications in responses to the COVID-19 pandemic: lessons learned and considerations for methods *Appl. Ergon.* **102** 103733
[16] Kazemi R and Smith A 2022 Overcoming COVID-19 pandemic: emerging challenges of human factors and the role of cognitive ergonomics *Theor. Issues Ergonom. Sci.* **24** 401–12
[17] Plant K L and Fendley M E 2021 Human factors and ergonomics and the response to COVID-19 *Hum.Factors Ergon. Manuf. Serv. Indust.* **31** 329–32
[18] Gurses A P, Tschudy M M, McGrath-Morrow S, Husain A, Solomon B S and Gerohristodoulos K A *et al* 2020 Overcoming COVID-19: what can human factors and ergonomics offer? *J. Patient Saf. Risk Manag.* **25** 49–54
[19] Dar M, Swamy L, Gavin D and Theodore A 2021 Mechanical-ventilation supply and options for the COVID-19 pandemic leveraging all available resources for a limited resource in a crisis *Ann. Am. Thorac. Soc.* **18** 408–16
[20] Lipsitz L A 2012 Understanding health care as a complex system: the foundation for unintended consequences *JAMA* **308** 243
[21] Kaur A and Victoria E L 2017 Major stakeholders in health care system government, non-government and other professionals *Glob. J. Bus. Manag.* **2** 1–7
[22] Berlin C, Bligård L O, Babapour Chafi M and Eriksson S 2022 Development of a stakeholder identification and analysis method for human factors integration in work system design interventions—Change agent infrastructure *Hum. Factors Ergon. Manuf. Serv. Indust.* **32** 151–70
[23] Dul J, Willemse H and Kleef D 2003 Ergonomics standards: identifying stakeholders and encouraging participation *ISO Bulletin* **34** 19–22
[24] Pronovost P J and Weisfeldt M L 2012 Science-based training in patient safety and quality *Ann. Intern. Med.* **157** 1–4
[25] Gurses A P, Ozok A A and Pronovost P J 2012 Time to accelerate integration of human factors and ergonomics in patient safety *BMJ Qual. Saf* **21** 347–51
[26] Carayon P 2012 Emerging role of human factors and ergonomics in healthcare delivery—A new field of application and influence for the IEA *Work.* **41** 5037–40

[27] Karsh B T and Alper S J 2005 Work System analysis: the key to understanding health care systems *Advances in Patient Safety: From Research to Implementation* (Agency for Healthcare Research and Quality) vol 2
[28] Wetterneck T B, Lapin J A, Karsh B T and Beasley J W 2016 Human factors and ergonomics in primary care *Handbook of Human Factors and Ergonomics in Health Care and Patient Safety* (Taylor & Francis)
[29] Stange K C, Nutting P A, Miller W L, Jaén C R, Crabtree B F and Flocke S A *et al* 2010 Defining and measuring the patient-centered medical home *J. Gen. Intern. Med.* **25** 601–12
[30] Carayon P, Schoofs Hundt A, Karsh B T, Gurses A P, Alvarado C J and Smith M *et al* 2006 Work system design for patient safety: the SEIPS model *BMJ Qual. Saf.* **15** i50–8
[31] Carayon P and Smith M J 2000 Work organization and ergonomics *Appl. Ergon.* **31** 649–62
[32] Smith M J and Sainfort P C 1989 A balance theory of job design for stress reduction *Int. J. Ind. Ergon.* **4** 67–79
[33] Carayon P 2009 The Balance theory and the work system model … twenty years later *Int. J. Hum.-Comput. Interact.* **25** 313–27
[34] Donabedian A 1978 The quality of medical care *Science (1979)* **200** 856–64
[35] Carayon P, Wetterneck T B, Rivera-Rodriguez A J, Hundt A S, Hoonakker P and Holden R *et al* 2013 Human factors systems approach to healthcare quality and patient safety *Appl. Ergon* **45** 14–25
[36] Components and elements of the SEIPS model | Download table https://researchgate.net/figure/Components-and-elements-of-the-SEIPS-model_tbl1_6655634 (accessed 29 April 2023)
[37] Carayon P, Wooldridge A, Hoonakker P, Hundt A S and Kelly M M 2020Apr1 SEIPS 3.0: human-centered design of the patient journey for patient safety *Appl. Ergon.* 84
[38] Alyousef B, Carayon P, Hoonakker P, Hundt A S, Cartmill R and Tomcavage J *et al* 2012 Care managers' challenges in using multiple health IT applications *Proc. of the Human Factors and Ergonomics Society Annual Meeting* **56** 1748–52
[39] Carayon P, Alyousef B, Hoonakker P, Hundt A S, Cartmill R and Tomcavage J *et al* 2012 Challenges to care coordination posed by the use of multiple health IT applications *Work* **41** 4468–73
[40] Catchpole K and Wiegmann D 2012 Understanding safety and performance in the cardiac operating room: from 'sharp end' to 'blunt end.' *BMJ Qual. Saf.* **21** 807–9
[41] Pennathur P R, Thompson D, Abernathy J H, Martinez E A, Pronovost P J and Kim G R *et al* 2013 Technologies in the wild (TiW): human factors implications for patient safety in the cardiovascular operating room *Ergonomics* **56** 205–19
[42] Gurses A P, Kim G, Martinez E A, Marsteller J, Bauer L and Lubomski L H *et al* 2012 Identifying and categorising patient safety hazards in cardiovascular operating rooms using an interdisciplinary approach: a multisite study *BMJ Qual. Saf.* **21** 810–8
[43] 22. Ergonomics 101: the definition, domains, and applications of ergonomics https://ergo-plus.com/ergonomics-definition-domains-applications/ (accessed 26 April 2023)
[44] Physical ergonomics | usability body of knowledge https://usabilitybok.org/physical-ergonomics (accessed 26 April 2023)
[45] Salonen H, Lahtinen M, Lappalainen S, Nevala N, Knibbs L D and Morawska L *et al* 2013 Physical characteristics of the indoor environment that affect health and wellbeing in healthcare facilities: a review *Intell. Build. Int.* **5** 3–25
[46] Waters T R 2010 Introduction to ergonomics for healthcare workers *Rehabil. Nurs.* **35** 185–91

[47] Ergonomics and handheld medical devices: five vital elements for design success – medical design briefs (accessed 2023 May 2) https://medicaldesignbriefs.com/component/content/article/mdb/pub/features/articles/29108

[48] The rise of robotic surgery in the healthcare industry https://blog.marketresearch.com/the-rise-of-robotic-surgery-in-the-healthcare-industry (accessed 26 April 2023)

[49] How can robotic surgery revolutionize healthcare? https://healthtechmagazine.net/article/2021/02/what-does-future-hold-robotic-surgery-perfcon (accessed 26 April 2023)

[50] Novellis P, Bottoni E, Voulaz E, Cariboni U, Testori A and Bertolaccini L *et al* 2018 Robotic surgery, video-assisted thoracic surgery, and open surgery for early stage lung cancer: comparison of costs and outcomes at a single institute *J. Thorac. Dis.* **10** 790

[51] Vatandsoost M and Litkouhi S 2019 The future of healthcare facilities: how technology and medical advances may shape hospitals of the future *Hosp. Pract. Res.* **4** 1–11

[52] van Mulken T J M, Schols R M, Qiu S S, Brouwers K, Hoekstra L T and Booi D I *et al* 2018 Robotic (super) microsurgery: feasibility of a new master-slave platform in an *in vivo* animal model and future directions *J. Surg. Oncol.* **118** 826–31

[53] Omisore O M, Han S, Ren L, Zhang N, Ivanov K and Elazab A *et al* 2017 Non-iterative geometric approach for inverse kinematics of redundant lead-module in a radiosurgical snake-like robot *Biomed. Eng. Online* **16** 1–25

[54] Robotic surgical procedures market size, share and growth | report, 2030 https://fortunebusinessinsights.com/industry-reports/robotic-surgical-procedures-market-100124 (accessed 26 April 2023)

[55] Sheetz K H, Claflin J and Dimick J B 2020 Trends in the adoption of robotic surgery for common surgical procedures *JAMA Netw. Open* **3** e1918911

[56] Asian surgical robotics market doubles by 2025—Asian robotics review https://asianroboticsreview.com/home316-html (accessed 26 April 2023)

[57] Yamamoto T, Abolhassani N, Jung S, Okamura A M and Judkins T N 2012 Augmented reality and haptic interfaces for robot-assisted surgery *The Int. J. Med. Robot. Comput. Assist. Surg.* **8** 45–56

[58] Kirkpatrick K 2017 3D-printing human body parts *Commun. ACM* **60** 15–7

[59] Urooj S *et al* 2021 Healthcare applications of 3D printing in human implants: a review *2020 IEEE 17th India Council Int. Conf. (INDICON)*

[60] Lee Ventola C 2014 Medical applications for 3D printing: current and projected uses *Pharm. Ther.* **39** 704

[61] Mathew E, Pitzanti G, Larrañeta E and Lamprou D A 2020 3D printing of pharmaceuticals and drug delivery devices *Pharmaceutics* **12** 266

[62] Schubert C, Van Langeveld M C and Donoso L A 2014 Innovations in 3D printing: a 3D overview from optics to organs *Br. J. Ophthalmol.* **98** 159–61

[63] Kim M P, Ta A H, Ellsworth W A, Marco R A, Gaur P and Miller J S 2015Jan1 Three dimensional model for surgical planning in resection of thoracic tumors *Int. J. Surg. Case Rep.* **16** 127–9

[64] Saidy N T, Fernández-Colino A, Heidari B S, Kent R, Vernon M and Bas O *et al* 2022 Spatially heterogeneous tubular scaffolds for *in situ* heart valve tissue engineering using melt electrowriting *Adv. Funct. Mater.* **32** 2110716

[65] Vaz V M and Kumar L 2021 3D printing as a promising tool in personalized medicine *AAPS Pharm. Sci. Tech.* **22** 1–20

[66] Dobres S, Mula G, Sauer J and Zhu D 2022 Applications of 3D printed chimeric DNA biomaterials *Eng. Regen* **3** 13–23
[67] What is an electronic health record (EHR)? | HealthIT.gov https://healthit.gov/faq/what-electronic-health-record-ehr (accessed 26 April 2023)
[68] Batko K and Ślęzak A 2022 The use of big data analytics in healthcare *J. Big Data* **9** 3
[69] Koch S 2006 Home telehealth—Current state and future trends *Int. J. Med. Inform.* **75** 565–76
[70] Demiris G and Kneale L 2015 Informatics Systems and tools to facilitate patient-centered care coordination *Yearb Med. Inform.* **10** 15–21
[71] Mehrotra A, Jena A B, Busch A B, Souza J, Uscher-Pines L and Landon B E 2016 Utilization of telemedicine among rural medicare beneficiaries *JAMA* **315** 2015–6
[72] Karuppiah M, Li X, Das A K, Kumari S and Liu Q 2018 Introduction to the special section on Big data and IoT in e-healthcare *Comput. Electr. Eng.* **65** 261–4
[73] Dicianno B E, Parmanto B, Fairman A D, Crytzer T M, Yu D X and Pramana G *et al* 2015 Perspectives on the evolution of mobile (mHealth) Technologies and application to rehabilitation *Phys. Ther.* **95** 397–405
[74] Wang Z, Xiong H, Zhang J, Yang S, Boukhechba M and Zhang D *et al* 2022 From personalized medicine to population health: a survey of mHealth sensing techniques *IEEE Internet Things J.* **9** 15413–34
[75] Shaheen M Y 2021 *ScienceOpen Preprints* Applications of artificial intelligence (AI) in healthcare: a review https://www.scienceopen.com/hosted-document?doi=10.14293/S2199-1006.1.SOR-.PPVRY8K.v1
[76] Shortliffe E H 2019 Artificial Intelligence in medicine: weighing the accomplishments, hype, and promise *Yearb Med. Inform.* **28** 257–62
[77] What are the benefits of predictive analytics in healthcare? https://healthitanalytics.com/news/what-are-the-benefits-of-predictive-analytics-in-healthcare (accessed 27 April 2023)
[78] Suzuki K 2012 Pixel-based machine learning in medical imaging *Int. J. Biomed. Imaging* **2012** 792079
[79] Majid A, Ali S, Iqbal M and Kausar N 2014 Prediction of human breast and colon cancers from imbalanced data using nearest neighbor and support vector machines *Comput. Methods Programs Biomed.* **113** 792–808
[80] The Oxford spinout company using AI to diagnose heart disease | Research | University of Oxford https://research.ox.ac.uk/article/2018-10-15-the-oxford-spinout-company-using-ai-to-diagnose-heart-disease (accessed 27 April 2023)
[81] Muraru D, Badano L P, Piccoli G, Gianfagna P, Del Mestre L and Ermacora D *et al* 2010 Validation of a novel automated border-detection algorithm for rapid and accurate quantitation of left ventricular volumes based on three-dimensional echocardiography *Eur. J. Echocardiogr.* **11** 359–68
[82] An AI-equipped microscope can diagnose deadly blood infections https://futurism.com/neo-scope/ai-equipped-microscope-diagnose-deadly-blood-infections (accessed 27 April 2023)
[83] Carayon P, Alvarado C J and Schoofs Hundt A 2009 Work design and patient safety *Theor. Issues Ergonom.* **8** 395–428
[84] 2004 Participatory ergonomics (PE) *Handbook of Human Factors and Ergonomics Methods* (Taylor & Francis) pp 777–84

[85] Effectiveness of participatory ergonomics: summary of a systematic review https://iwh.on.ca/summaries/sharing-best-evidence/effectiveness-of-participatory-ergonomics (accessed 29 April 2023)
[86] Evanoff B A, Bohr P C and Wolf L D 1999 Effects of a participatory ergonomics team among hospital orderlies *Am. J. Ind. Med.* **35** 358–65
[87] Lee E W C, Fok J P C, Lam A T, Law R K Y, Szeto G P Y and Li P P K 2014 The application of participatory ergonomics in a healthcare setting in Hong Kong *Work* **48** 511–9
[88] Rasmussen C D N, Lindberg N K, Ravn M H, Jørgensen M B, Søgaard K and Holtermann A 2017 Processes, barriers and facilitators to implementation of a participatory ergonomics program among eldercare workers *Appl. Ergon.* **58** 491–9
[89] Andersen S N and Broberg O 2015 Participatory ergonomics simulation of hospital work systems: the influence of simulation media on simulation outcome *Appl. Ergon.* **51** 331–42
[90] Jakobsen M D, Aust B, Dyreborg J, Kines P, Illum M B and Andersen L L 2016 Participatory organizational intervention for improved use of assistive devices for patient transfer: study protocol for a single-blinded cluster randomized controlled trial *BMC Musculoskelet. Disord.* **17** 1–11
[91] Colovic G 2011 Ergonomic workplace *Management of Technology Systems in Garment Industry* (Woodhead) pp 80–105
[92] Veselinovic S P n.d. Cognitive ergonomics, socio-technical systems, and the impact of healthcare information technologies https://academia.edu/709131/Cognitive_ergonomics_socio_technical_systems_and_the_Impact_of_healthcare_information_technologies (accessed 29 April 2023)
[93] Jennings B M 2008 Work stress and burnout among nurses: role of the work environment and working conditions *Patient Safety and Quality: An Evidence-Based Handbook for Nurses* (Agency for Healthcare Research and Quality (US))
[94] What is cognitive ergonomics? | IxDF https://interaction-design.org/literature/topics/cognitive-ergonomics (accessed 29 April 2023)
[95] Sbaffi L, Walton J, Blenkinsopp J and Walton G 2020 Information overload in emergency medicine physicians: a multisite case study exploring the causes, impact, and solutions in four North England national health service trusts *J. Med. Internet Res.* **22** e19126
[96] Panari C, Caricati L, Pelosi A and Rossi C 2019 Emotional exhaustion among healthcare professionals: the effects of role ambiguity, work engagement and professional commitment *Acta Bio. Medica: Atenei Parmensis* **90** 60–7
[97] Occupational stress, burnout and fatigue https://who.int/tools/occupational-hazards-in-health-sector/occup-stress-burnout-fatigue (accessed 30 April 2023)
[98] De Hert S 2020 Burnout in healthcare workers: prevalence, impact and preventative strategies *Local Reg. Anesth* **13** 171–83
[99] Søvold L E, Naslund J A, Kousoulis A A, Saxena S, Qoronfleh M W and Grobler C *et al* 2021 Prioritizing the mental health and well-being of healthcare workers: an urgent global public health priority *Front. Public Health* **9** 514
[100] Zolotova M 2020 'ChECk' the Hospital cognitive ergonomics components for the analysis of a human-system interaction in a hospital environment *Int. J. Design. Objects* **15** 1–14
[101] Coiera E 2006 Communication systems in healthcare *Clin. Biochem. Rev.* **27** 89
[102] Sutton R T, Pincock D, Baumgart D C, Sadowski D C, Fedorak R N and Kroeker K I 2020 An overview of clinical decision support systems: benefits, risks, and strategies for success *npj Digital Med.* **3** 1–10

[103] Wasylewicz A T M and Scheepers-Hoeks A M J W 2018 Clinical decision support systems *Fundamentals of Clinical Data Science* (Cham: Springer) pp 153–69

[104] Ohno-Machado L 2011 Use of electronic health record systems for decision support *J. Am. Med. Inform Assoc.* **18** 729

[105] Simulation training: the future of healthcare professional development. https://hurix.com/simulation-training-the-future-of-healthcare-professional-development/ (accessed 30 April 2023)

[106] Holmboe E, Rizzolo M A, Sachdeva A K, Rosenberg M and Ziv A 2011 Simulation-based assessment and the regulation of healthcare professionals *Simul. Healthc.* **6** S58–62

[107] Sameera V, Bindra A and Rath G 2021 Human errors and their prevention in healthcare *J. Anaesthesiol Clin. Pharmacol.* **37** 328

[108] Gluyas H and Morrison P 2014 Human factors and medication errors: a case study *Nurs. Stand.* **29** 37–42

[109] Webster C S, Taylor S and Weller J M 2021 Cognitive biases in diagnosis and decision making during anaesthesia and intensive care *BJA Educ.* **21** 420

[110] Khadilkar P R and Cash P 2020 Understanding behavioural design: barriers and enablers *J. Eng. Des.* **31** 508–29

[111] Skills R J 1983 Rules, and knowledge; signals, signs, and symbols, and other distinctions in human performance models *IEEE Trans. Syst. Man Cybern.* **13** 257–66

[112] Reason J 1990 *Human Error* (Cambridge: Cambridge University Press)

[113] Reason J 2000 Human error: models and management *West. J. Med.* **172** 393

[114] Kanse L, Van Der Schaaf T W, Vrijland N D and Van Mierlo H 2006 Error recovery in a hospital pharmacy *Ergonomics* **49** 503–16

[115] Ranzani F and Parlangeli O 2021 Digital technology and usability and ergonomics of medical devices *Textbook of Patient Safety and Clinical Risk Management* (Springer) pp 455–64

[116] Kalra J, Lightner N J and Taiar R 2021 *Advances in Human Factors and Ergonomics in Healthcare and Medical Devices* (Cham: Springer) p 263

[117] Privitera M R and Privitera M 2020 Human factors/ergonomics (HFE) in leadership and management: organizational interventions to reduce stress in healthcare delivery *Health N. Hav* **12** 1262–78

[118] Santos R 2021 Reengineer healthcare: a human factors and ergonomics framework to improve the socio-technical system *Int. J. Qual. Health Care* **33** 19–24

[119] de Meuse K 1990 *Work teams: applications and effectiveness. American Psychologist* https://academia.edu/28285577/Work_teams_Applications_and_effectiveness (accessed 1 May 2023)

[120] Mitchell P H, Wynia M K, Golden R, McNellis B, Okun S and Webb C E *et al* 2012 Core principles and values of effective team-based health care *NAM Perspectives* https://nam.edu/perspectives-2012-core-principles-values-of-effective-team-based-health-care/

[121] Salas E, Cooke N J and Rosen M A 2008 On teams, teamwork, and team performance: discoveries and developments *Hum. Factors* **50** 540–7

[122] King H B, Battles J, Baker D P *et al* 2008 TeamSTEPPS™: Team strategies and tools to enhance performance and patient safety *Advances in Patient Safety: New Directions and Alternative Approaches (vol 3: Performance and Tools)* ed K Henriksen, J B Battles, M A Keyes et al (Rockville, MD: Agency for Healthcare Research and Quality (US))

[123] Guimond M E, Sole M L and Salas E 2009 TeamSTEPPS *Am. J. Nurs.* **109** 66–8

[124] Mayer C M, Cluff L, Lin W T, Willis T S, Stafford R E and Williams C *et al* 2011 Evaluating efforts to optimize TeamSTEPPS implementation in surgical and pediatric intensive care units *Jt. Comm. J. Qual. Patient Saf.* **37** 365–74
[125] SBAR tool: situation-background-assessment-recommendation | IHI – Institute for healthcare improvement. https://ihi.org/resources/Pages/Tools/sbartoolkit.aspx (accessed 1 May 2023)
[126] Blazin L J, Sitthi-Amorn J, Hoffman J M and Burlison J D 2020 Improving patient handoffs and transitions through adaptation and implementation of I-PASS Across multiple handoff settings *Pediatr. Qual. Saf.* **5** e323
[127] Rathi R, Vakharia A and Shadab M 2022 Lean six sigma in the healthcare sector: a systematic literature review *Mater. Today Proc.* **50** 773–81
[128] Christoff P 2018 Running PDSA cycles *Curr. Probl. Pediatr. Adolesc. Health Care* **48** 198–201
[129] Ahmed S, Manaf N H A and Islam R 2013 Effects of lean six sigma application in healthcare services: a literature review *Rev. Environ. Health* **28** 189–94
[130] Schweikhart S A and Dembe A E 2009 The applicability of lean and six sigma techniques to clinical and translational research *J. Investig. Med.* **57** 748
[131] Karsh B T and Brown R 2010 Macroergonomics and patient safety: the impact of levels on theory, measurement, analysis and intervention in patient safety research *Appl. Ergon.* **41** 674–81
[132] Karsh B T, Waterson P and Holden R J 2014 Crossing levels in systems ergonomics: a framework to support 'mesoergonomic' inquiry *Appl. Ergon* **45** 45–54
[133] Rasmussen J 1997Nov1 Risk management in a dynamic society: a modelling problem *Saf. Sci.* **27** 183–213
[134] Hignett S, Carayon P, Buckle P and Catchpole K 2013 State of science: human factors and ergonomics in healthcare *Ergonomics* **56** 1491–503
[135] Khan R and Hinshaw K 2022 We are only human – effective training in human factors *Best Pract. Res. Clin. Obstet. Gynaecol.* **80** 67–74
[136] Keebler J R and Mancini M E 2021 *The Future of Simulation in Healthcare Safety and System Improvement* (Springer) pp 231–6
[137] Dutta A, Breloff S P, Dai F, Sinsel E W, Warren C M and Carey R E *et al* 2020Sep1 Effects of working posture and roof slope on activation of lower limb muscles during shingle installation *Ergonomics.* **63** 1182–93
[138] Gosbee J 2002 Human factors engineering and patient safety *Qual. Saf. Health Care* **1** 352–4
[139] Bharatan T, Devi R, Huang P H, Javed A, Jeffers B and Lansberg P *et al* 2021 A Methodology for mapping the patient journey for noncommunicable diseases in low- and middle-income countries *J. Healthc. Leadersh.* **13** 35–46
[140] Haldane V, De Foo C, Abdalla S M, Jung A S, Tan M and Wu S *et al* 2021 Health systems resilience in managing the COVID-19 pandemic: lessons from 28 countries *Nat. Med.* **27** 964–80
[141] Armenakis A A, Harris S G and Mossholder K W 1993 Creating readiness for organizational change *Hum. Relat.* **46** 681–703
[142] Lei C and Palm K 2022 *Crisis Resource Management Training in Medical Simulation* (StatPearls)

[143] Bishop R, Porges C, Carlisle M and Strickland R 2020 Crisis resource management in medicine: a clarion call for change *Curr. Treat Options Pediatr* **6** 299–316
[144] Korunka C, Weiss A and Karetta B 1993 Effects of new technologies with special regard for the implementation process per se *J. Organ Behav.* **14** 331–48
[145] Smith K U and Smith M F 1966 *Cybernetic Principles of Learning and Educational Design* (New York: Holt, Rinehart and Winston, Inc)
[146] Boddy D 2000 MacBeth D. Prescriptions for managing change: a survey of their effects in projects to implement collaborative working between organisations *Int. J. Project Manage.* **18** 297–306
[147] Barki H and Pinsonneault A 2005 A model of organizational integration, implementation effort, and performance *Organ. Sci.* **16** 165–79
[148] Gordon A and Pollack J 2018 Managing healthcare integration *Project Manage. J.* **49** 5–21
[149] Smith M J and Carayon P 1995 New technology, automation, and work organization: stress problems and improved technology implementation strategies *Int. J. Hum. Factors in Manuf.* **5** 99–116
[150] Karsh B T 2004 Beyond usability: designing effective technology implementation systems to promote patient safety *Qual. Saf. Health Care* **13** 388–94
[151] Xiao Y and Fairbanks R J 2011 Speaking systems engineering: bilingualism in health care delivery organizations *Mayo Clin. Proc* **86** 719–20
[152] Alper B S and Fox G N 2004 Integrative healthcare: arriving at a definition *Altern. Ther. Health Med.* **10** 14
[153] National Academy of Engineering (US) and Institute of Medicine (US) Committee on Engineering and the Health Care System 2005 A framework for a systems approach to health care delivery *Building a Better Delivery System: A New Engineering/Health Care Partnership* (Washington DC: National Academies Press)
[154] Institute of Medicine, Board on the Health of Select Populations, Committee on Evaluation of the Lovell Federal Health Care Center Merger 2012 Collaboration among health care organizations: a review of outcomes and best practices for effective performance *Evaluation of the Lovell Federal Health Care Center Merger: Findings, Conclusions, and Recommendations* (Washington DC: National Academies Press) Appendix D
[155] Standardized care: does one size fit all in medicine? https://carecloud.com/continuum/standardized-care-does-one-size-fit-all-in-medicine/ (accessed 2 May 2023)
[156] Leider J P, Resnick B, McCullough J, Alfonso Y N and Bishai D 2020 Inaccuracy of official estimates of public health spending in the United States, 2000–2018 *Am. J. Public Health* **110** S194–6
[157] Perry S J, Catchpole K, Rivera A J, Henrickson Parker S and Gosbee J 2021 'Strangers in a strange land': understanding professional challenges for human factors/ergonomics and healthcare *Appl. Ergon* **94** 103040
[158] World Patient Safety Day 2022 https://who.int/campaigns/world-patient-safety-day/2022 (accessed 1 May 2023)
[159] Wrong diagnosis, medication errors, care-related infections adding USD 1 Trillion To spiraling health costs Globally, Warn OECD, WHO, World Bank—Health Policy Watch https://healthpolicy-watch.news/wrong-diagnosis-medication-errors-care-related-infections-adding-usd-1-trillion-to-spiraling-health-costs-globally-warn-oecd-who-world-bank/ (accessed 2 May 2023)

[160] Breyer F, Costa-Font J and Felder S 2010Dec Ageing, health, and health care *Oxf. Rev. Econ. Policy* **26** 674–90

[161] Griffiths A 1997 Ageing, health and productivity: a challenge for the new millennium *Work Stress* **11** 197–214

[162] Cristea M, Noja G G, Stefea P and Sala A L 2020 The impact of population aging and public health support on EU labor markets *Int. J. Environ. Res. Public Health* **17** 1439

[163] Borsch-Supan A 1991 Aging population: problems and policy options in the US and Germany *Econ. Policy* **12** 103–39

[164] Sobral M, Santa-Rosa B and Silvestre M 2021 Resource allocation during the COVID-19 pandemic: contributions to an ethical approach *Acta Med. Port* **34** 7–8

[165] Health care reform: a consensus on values, but an administrative road to nowhere. https://brookings.edu/blog/fixgov/2019/07/16/healthcare-reform-a-consensus-on-values-but-an-administrative-road-to-nowhere/ (accessed 2 May 2023)

[166] Perry S J and Wears R L 2016 Notes from underground: latent resilience in healthcare *Resilience Engineering Perspectives* (Taylor & Francis) vol 2 pp 189–200

[167] Plsek P 1999 Innovative thinking for the improvement of medical systems *Ann. Intern. Med.* **131** 438–44

[168] Porter M E 2009 A strategy for health care reform—toward a value-based system *N. Eng. J. Med.* **361** 109–12

[169] Wears R L and Hollnagel E 2017 Why is work-as-imagined different from work-as-done? Resilient health care *Resilient Health Care* (Taylor & Francis) vol 2 pp 279–94

[170] Israelski E 2010 Using human factors engineering to improve patient safety: problem solving on the front line, second edition, 2010 *Biomed. Instrum. Technol.* **44** 474

www.ingramcontent.com/pod-product-compliance
Ingram Content Group UK Ltd.
Pitfield, Milton Keynes, MK11 3LW, UK
UKHW051910100926
8556IPUK00005B/831